# Type 2 Diabetes - From Pathophysiology to Cyber Systems

*Edited by Anca Pantea Stoian*

Published in London, United Kingdom

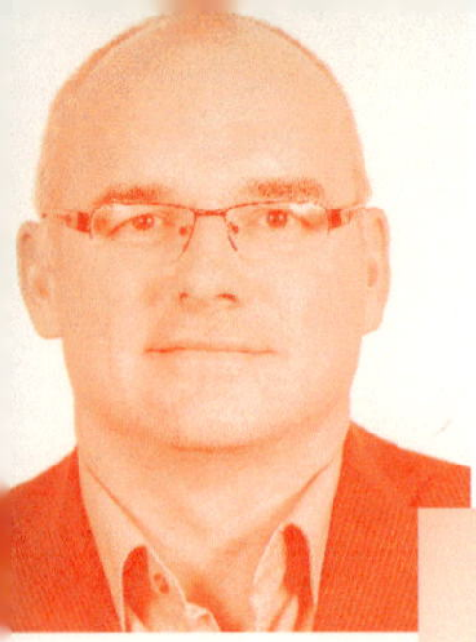
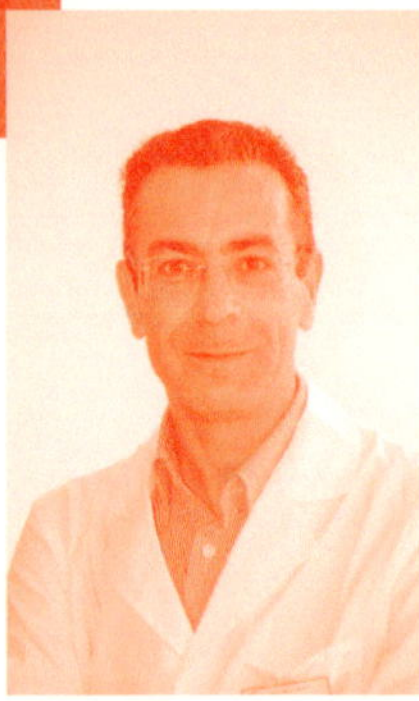
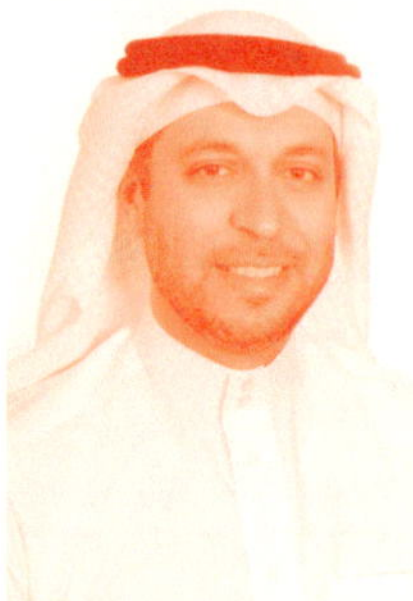
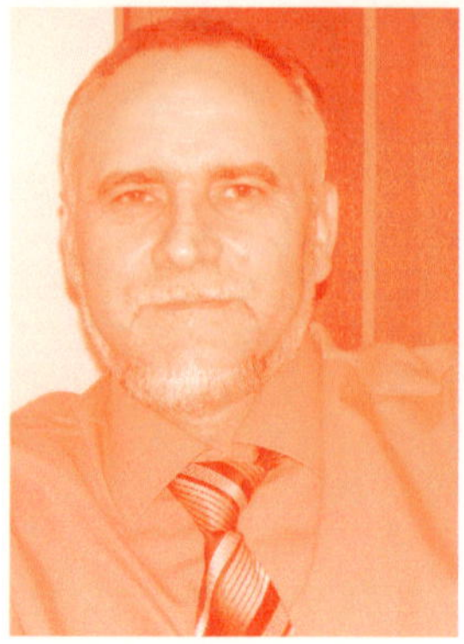
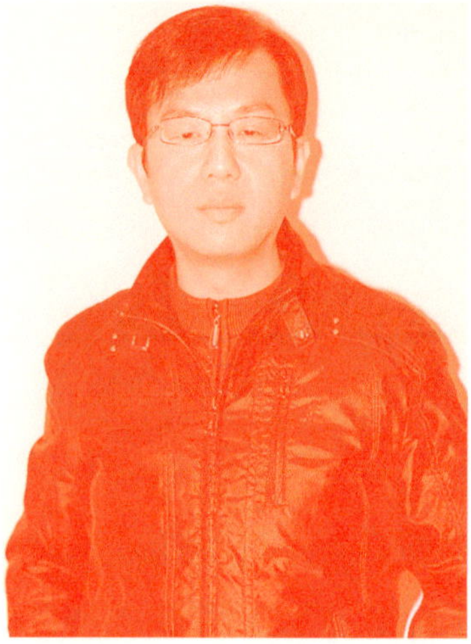
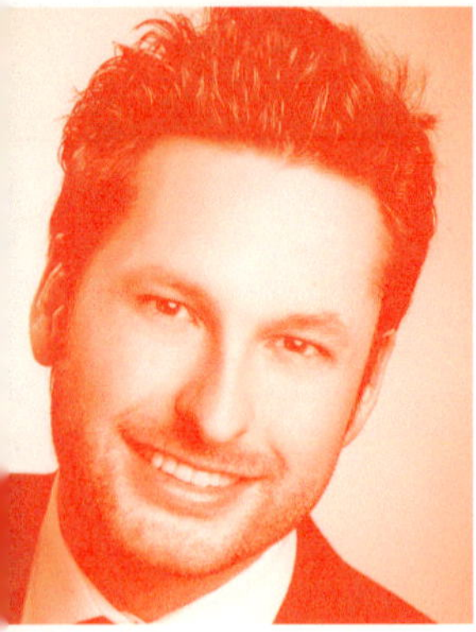
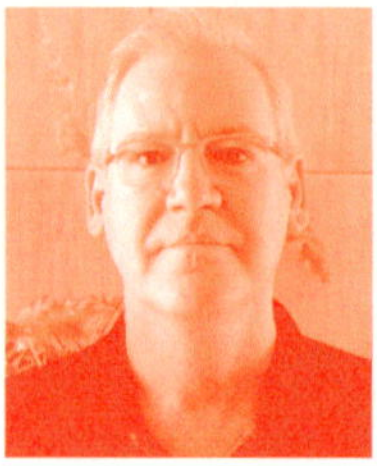

IntechOpen

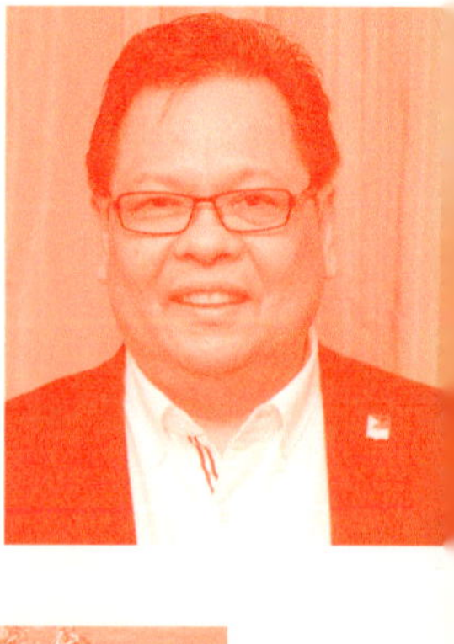
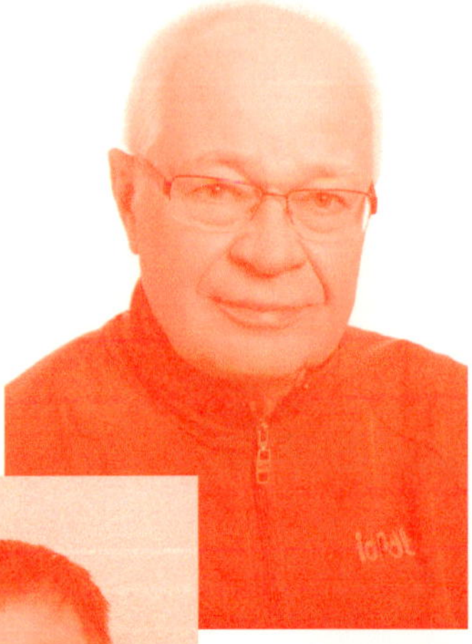
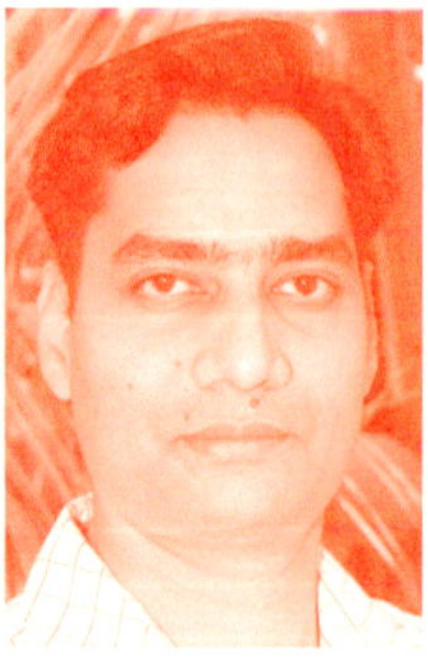
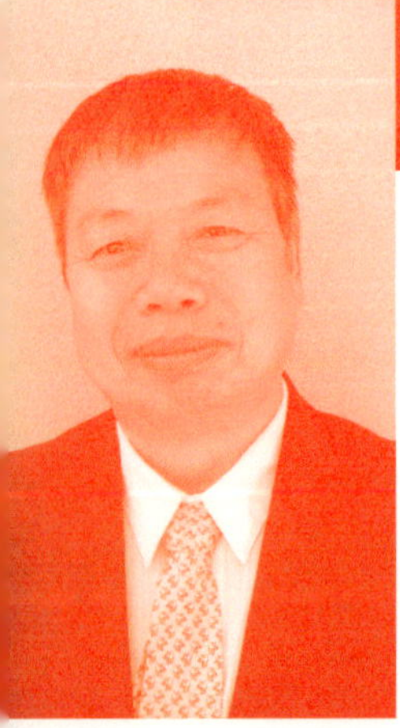
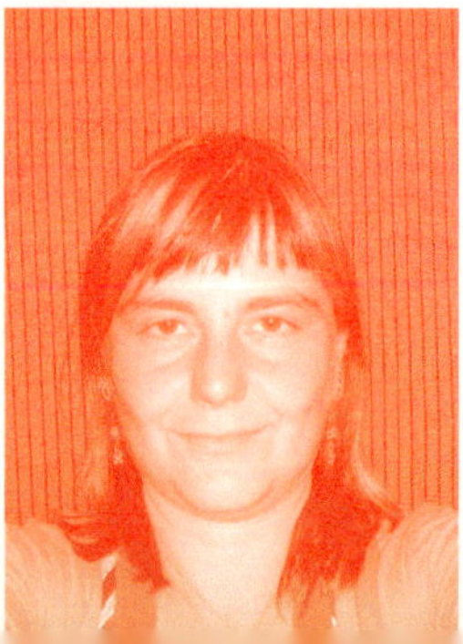
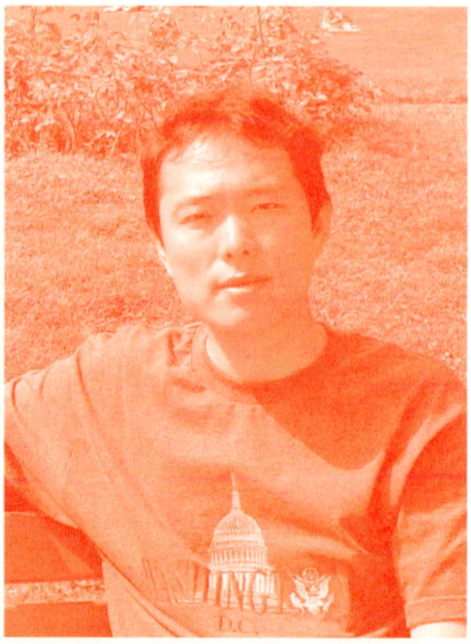

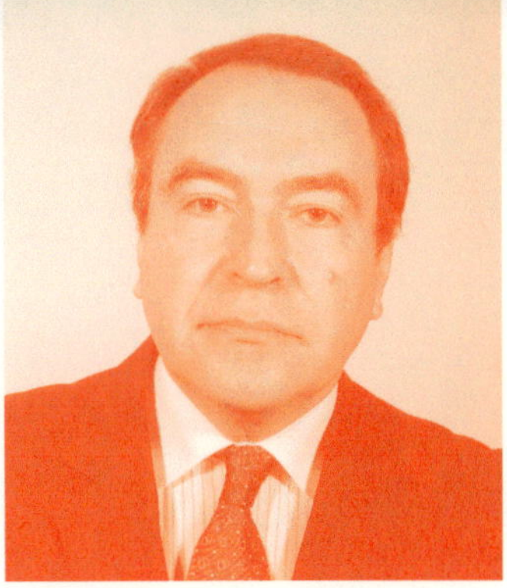

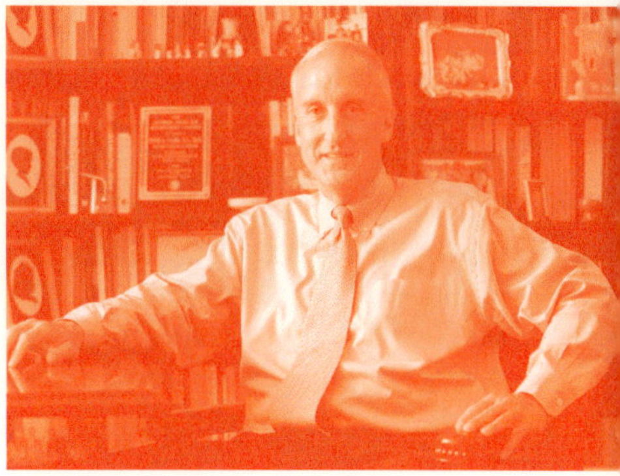

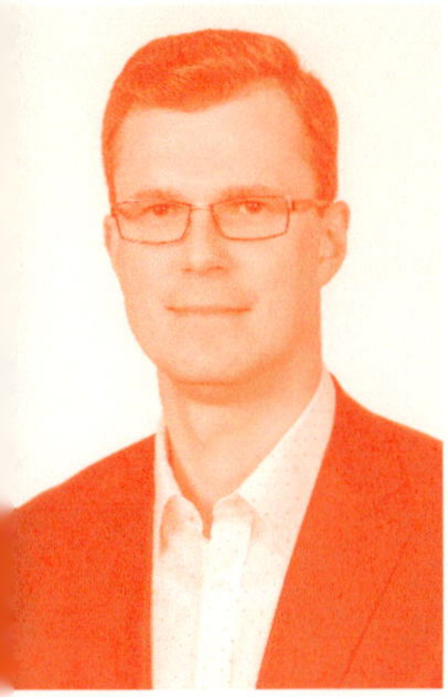

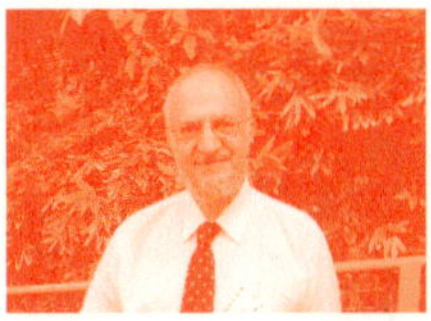

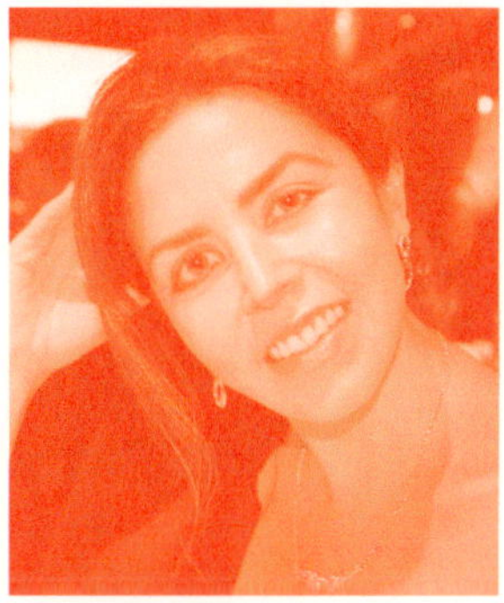

*Supporting open minds since 2005*

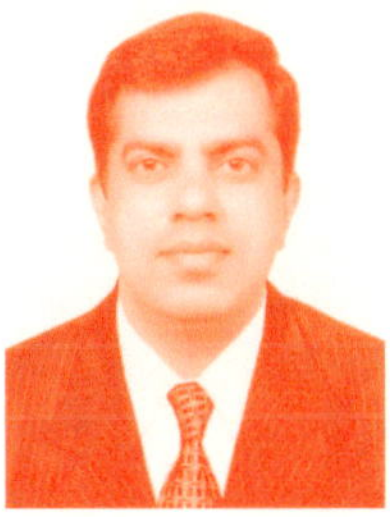

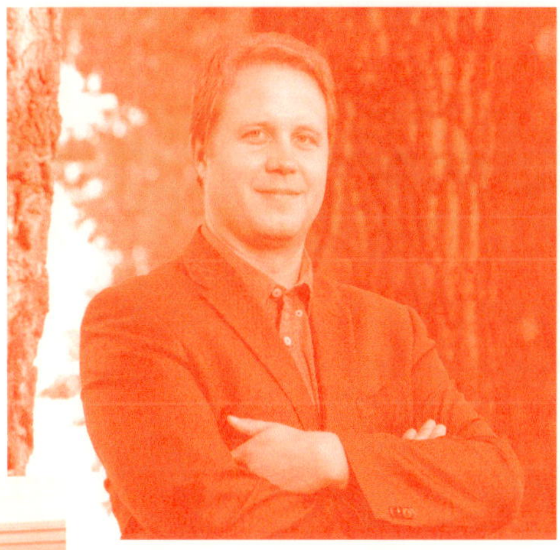

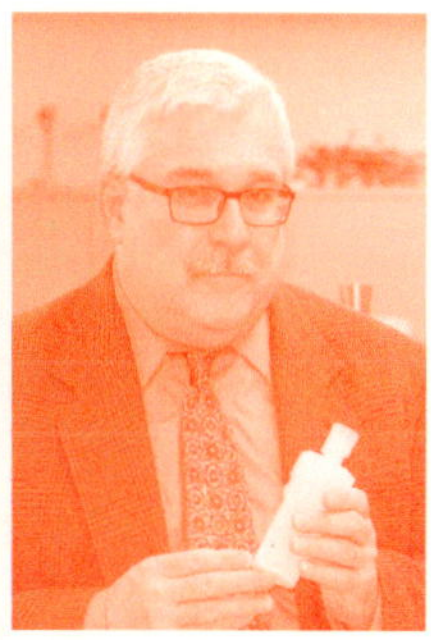

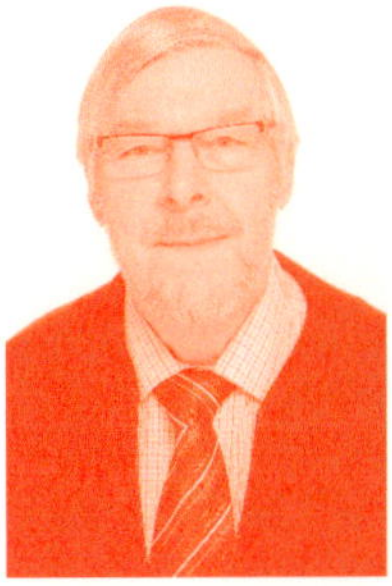

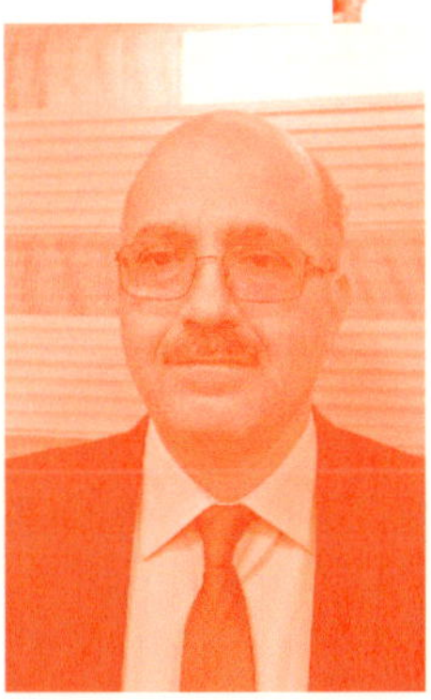

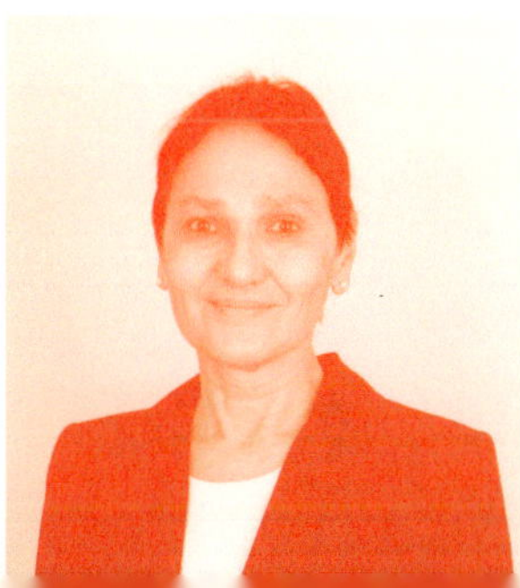

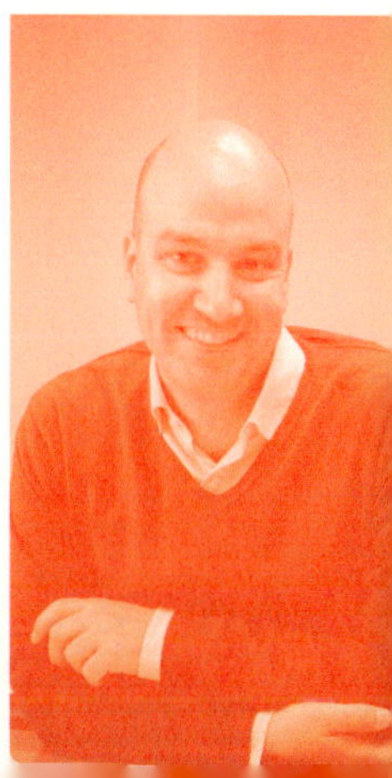

Type 2 Diabetes - From Pathophysiology to Cyber Systems
http://dx.doi.org/10.5772/intechopen.87312
Edited by Anca Pantea Stoian

Contributors
Mimie Noratiqah Jumli, Muhammad Ilyas Nadeem, Shula Shazman, Leila Yousefi, Allan Tucker, Dahiru Saleh Saleh Mshelia, Sani Adamu, Rebecca Mtaku Gali, Jameela Banu, Alena Soboleva, Andrej Frolov, Natalia Vashurina, Carmen Sanz, Elvira Álvarez, Verónica Hurtado-Carneiro, Ana Pérez-García, Zsolt P. Ori, Gabriela Roman, Anca Pantea Stoian, Mioara Petrus, Cristina Popa, Ana-Maria Bratu, Petr Ježek, Lydie Plecitá - Hlavatá, Blanka Holendová, Martin Jabůrek, Jan Tauber, Andrea Dlasková, Féaron C. Cassidy, Cynthia M. M Coleman, Sinead Lafferty, Rudolf Chlup, Richard Kaňa, Lada Hanáčková, Hana Zálešáková, Blanka Doubravová, Farah Qudsia, Samreen Riaz, Dabota Yvonne Yvonne Buowari, Pawan Kumar Kare, Neerja Aggarwal, Sultana Ferdousi, Phurpa Gyeltshen, Ana Maria Dascalu, Dragos Serban, Nikolaos Papanas, Manfredi Rizzo, Daniela Stana, Peter Kempler



First published in London, United Kingdom, 2021 by IntechOpen
IntechOpen is the global imprint of INTECHOPEN LIMITED, registered in England and Wales, registration number: 11086078, 5 Princes Gate Court, London, SW7 2QJ, United Kingdom
Printed in Croatia

British Library Cataloguing-in-Publication Data
A catalogue record for this book is available from the British Library

Additional hard and PDF copies can be obtained from orders@intechopen.com

Type 2 Diabetes - From Pathophysiology to Cyber Systems
Edited by Anca Pantea Stoian
p. cm.
Print ISBN 978-1-83881-903-3
Online ISBN 978-1-83881-904-0
eBook (PDF) ISBN 978-1-83881-905-7

For EU product safety concerns:
IN TECH d.o.o., Prolaz Marije Krucifikse Kozulić 3, 51000 Rijeka, Croatia, info@intechopen.com or visit our website at intechopen.com.

# Meet the editor

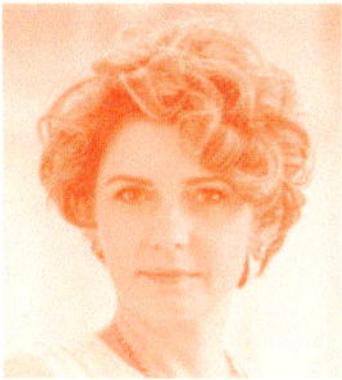

Anca Pantea Stoian is a specialist in diabetes, nutrition, and metabolic diseases as well as health food hygiene. She also has competency in general ultrasonography. She is an associate professor in the Diabetes, Nutrition and Metabolic Diseases Department, Carol Davila University of Medicine and Pharmacy, Bucharest, Romania. She has been chief of the Hygiene Department, Faculty of Dentistry, at the same university since 2019. Her interests include micro and macrovascular complications in diabetes and new therapies. Her research activities focus on nutritional intervention in chronic pathology, as well as cardio-renal-metabolic risk assessment, and diabetes in cancer. She is currently engaged in developing new therapies and technological tools for screening, prevention, and patient education in diabetes. She is a member of the European Association for the Study of Diabetes, Cardiometabolic Academy, CEDA, Romanian Society of Diabetes, Nutrition and Metabolic Diseases, Romanian Diabetes Federation, and Association for Renal Metabolic and Nutrition studies. She has authored or co-authored 160 papers in national and international peer-reviewed journals.

# Contents

# Preface

Diabetes mellitus is one of the most known non-communicable diseases. It is a metabolic disease characterized by chronic high blood glucose levels. There are many types of diabetes, such as prediabetes, type 1 diabetes, type 2 diabetes, and gestational diabetes, with type 2 being the most common.

Nowadays, the prevalence of type 2 diabetes is increasing annually, driven by obesity, aging, sedentarism, and many other factors.

The central symptom of diabetes is chronic hyperglycemia, which can cause serious complications. Therefore, understanding the pathophysiology of diabetes as well as related diagnostic, prevention, and treatment methods is essential for diabetes management.

This book presents a novel approach to preventing and treating type 2 diabetes. Chapters cover such topics as diagnosis, pathogenesis, management, lifestyle and nutritional intervention, and systems to support early diagnosis and prevention of prediabetes.

**Anca Pantea Stoian**
Diabetes, Nutrition and Metabolic Diseases Department,
"Carol Davila" University,
Bucharest, Romania

Section 1

# Pathophysiology of Diabetes

Chapter 1

# Pathophysiologic Approach to Type 2 Diabetes Management: One Centre Experience 1980–2020

*Rudolf Chlup, Richard Kaňa, Lada Hanáčková, Hana Zálešáková and Blanka Doubravová*

## Abstract

This overview summarizes the evolution of pathophysiologic treatment of diabetes type 2 (T2D) in the period of the last 40 years. Randomized Controlled Trials (RCT) and Real World Evidence (RWE) studies resulted in recent Statements of the American Diabetes Association (ADA) and the European Association for the Study of Diabetes (EASD) in the year 2020. Case reports and studies of a single-centre in Czech Republic are reported. The authors demonstrate the impact of (1) multiple doses of rapid insulin, (2) multiple doses of rapid or ultrarapid insulin analogs (3) continuous subcutaneous insulin infusion (CSII) (4) incretin receptor agonists, (5) fixed combination of insulin degludec with liraglutide (IDegLira) and (6) SGLT2 inhibitor dapagliflozin, on plasma glucose concentration, HbA1c, body mass and patient satisfaction. The importance of therapeutic patients' education and technology (personal glucometers, continuous/flash glucose monitors, insulin pens/pumps) is emphasized. Most of the observations were already published. Hence, individually adopted education, lifstyle, technical equipment, incretin receptor agonists and/or metformin and/or gliflozins and/or insulin analogs appear to be the core of an effective pathophysiologic approach. Scientific conclusions from RCTs, RWE trials and own clinical case reports may prevail over clinical inertia and induce early implementation of effective methods into routine T2D treatment.

**Keywords:** insulin analogs, incretins, gliflozins, insulin pen, CSII, glucose monitoring, education, case report, randomized control trial, real world evidence

## 1. Introduction

Type 2 diabetes mellitus (T2D) is a syndrome of disturbed metabolic pathways of sacharides (carbohydrates), proteins and fat due to various influence of eight pathophysiologic mechanisms described as ominous octet: disturbed dynamics of insulin secretion, reduced production of incretins in gut, hyperglucagonaemia, increased production of glucose from liver, disturbed endocrine function of adipose tissue, insulin resistance, increased activity of sodium glucose transporter 2 (SGLT2) resulting in increased reabsorption of glucose from renal tubules and malfunction of hypothalamic centers for satiety and hunger. [1] These mechanisms are induced by different genetic and environmental factors. [2, 3]

In previous centuries, clinical symptoms of T2D lead to therapeutic attempts based on lifestyle, diet and on oral antidiabetic drugs, mostly sulfonylureas.

The discovery of insulin by Paulesco in 1921 [4] and its final introduction to human medicine by Banting, Collip, Best and Macleod in 1922 [5] saved many lives of people with T1D. However, in T2D insulin was mostly used as an ultimate therapeutic alternative.

In 1957, the discovery of metformin resulted in reduction of hyperglycaemia without hypoglycaemias. In the course of several decades, metformin proved to be a relatively effective mean to reduce body mass and cardiovascular complications. In addition, in persons on metformin the frequency of neoplasms appears to be lower. Today, metformin undoubtedly remains the drug worthy of choice for the majority persons with T2D. [6]

At the end of the 20th century, a new concept of pathophysiologic approach to T2D was suggested by Bruns [7] under the descriptive term „complementary therapy", and, independently by Berger [8, 9] as „supplementary therapy".

Important role in the intensification of insulin regimens played insulin pens which were produced since the year 1983. [10] At the beginning of the 21st century, insulin pumps (first implemented by John Pickup in 1978 [11]) and intensive self-monitoring were also applied in people with T2D. [12–14] Despite of pumps many persons with T2D were unable to reach the expected metabolic improvement until incretin receptor agonists and gliflozins have been made available. [15, 16]

In 1974, the first glucometer (Ames) was introduced into clinical practice, followed by tenths of other glucometers [17–19], Continuous Glucose Monitors (CGM) [20] and/or Flash Glucose Monitors (FGM) [21]. Today, these devices have become mandatory means (together with HbA1c analysers [22]) to assess the metabolic control. Scientific inventions from the last 100 years were applied in official statements and guidelines. [23–25]

This overview introduces promoting insights and better understanding of pathophysiologic approach to various treatments of T2D. Purpose of the presented case reports and single-centre „real world trials "is to motivate to education and to implementation of incretins and/or gliflozins and/or insulin analogs and/or insulin pumps in daily routine of diabetes care.

## 2. Prerequisites for a pathophysiologic approach to T2D management

### 2.1 Therapeutic education

Lifestyle and education of people with chronic disorders have been recognised as an essential part of treatment. Many anonymous dedicated enthusiasts have created a solid platform for effective therapy. Some of them became famous educators, however, most of them remained unnoticed in everyday practice.

The Diabetes Education Study Group (DESG) of the European Association for the Study of Diabetes (EASD), was founded in 1977 [26] and the Therapeutic Patient Education (TPE) became a goal of many respected bodies in the world.

The DESG aimed to improve the quality of life through educational programmes designed to foster independence for the patient, to improve the quality of metabolic control, to emphasise the prevention and to encourage research. The DESG organised activities all over the Europe, published more than 30 Teaching letters and Series of the 5-min education basics. In eastern countries, the DESG workshops (Bucharest, 1982, Balatonfuered, 1985, Warsaw, 1987, Weimar, 1989, Olomouc, 1991) supported the cooperation between health care providers (physicians, teachers, psychologists, nurses, dietitians, social workers) and patients. (**Figure 1**) Therefore, the adopted 5- day scheduled teaching programs created by Assal, Berger and Jörgens in Genf and Düsseldorf [27] could be spread throughout Europe. Workshops at Grimentz,

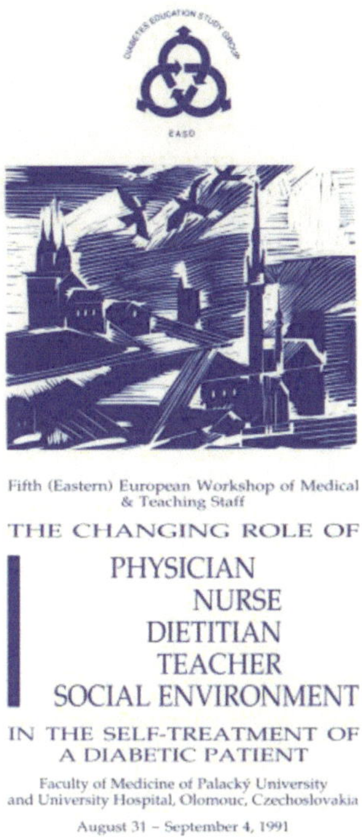


**Figure 1.**
*Abstract Book from the last workshop of the Eastern DESG in Olomouc (1991).*

Capri, Celano, Assisi, Chillworth, Cambridge, Winchester, Windsor, Sesimbra, etc., motivated to look at issues from various angels.

Process of TPE consists of three parts: teaching knowledge, training skills and formating attitudes. These principles have also been considered in our pathophysiologic approach to treatment of T2D in daily routine. [28, 29]

### 2.2 Technical support

#### *2.2.1 Development and clinical implementation of insulin pens*

Insulin pens opened the door to comfortable insulin administration thereby making the intensive regimens acceptable at work, at school, at leisure, during travels, etc.

In 1983, the first models of a MAnual Device for Insulin (MADI) proved to be a useful aid to injection of U-40 insulin either as a needle pen or as a catheter pen. [10] Within a few years other injectors appeared. [30, 31] Six models of a new type of MADI for insulin U-40, U-80 and U-100 were developed. [32] (**Figure 2**) In the needle pen (**Figure 3**) a sliding cover prevents the contamination of the needle which remains invisible in the course of injection and might be reused without sterilization. [33] In the catheter pen (**Figure 4**) the catheter remained inserted in subcutaneous tissue for 3 days. A syringe-like interchangeable plastic reservoir (3 ml) was refilled from insulin vials with any kind of soluble insulin. Actual insulin administration occurred by twisting the cap after subcutaneous insertion of needle or catheter.

To date, about one hundred of various types of insulin or incretin needle-pens have been distributed all over the world. (**Figure 5**) Most of them are disposable pens [34] (prefilled with insulin, to be discarded after emptying), some of them are constructed for cartridged insulin produced by the respective company.

Despite initial enthusiasm, the preference of catheter pens [35] (**Figure 6**) was low over time.

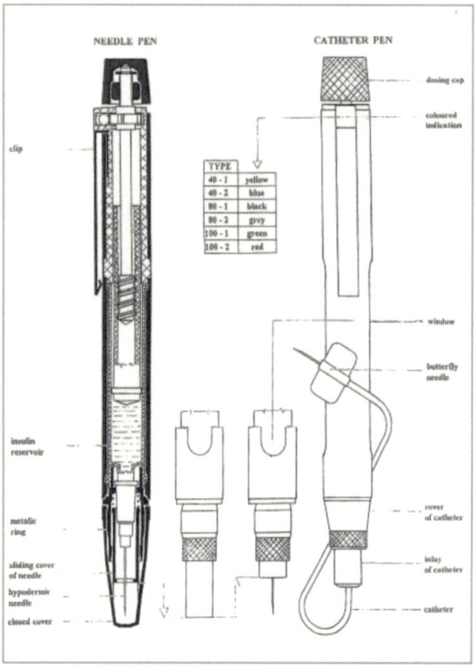


**Figure 2.**
*Scheme of MADI: needle pen with telescopic sliding cover (left) and catheter pen [32] (1991).*

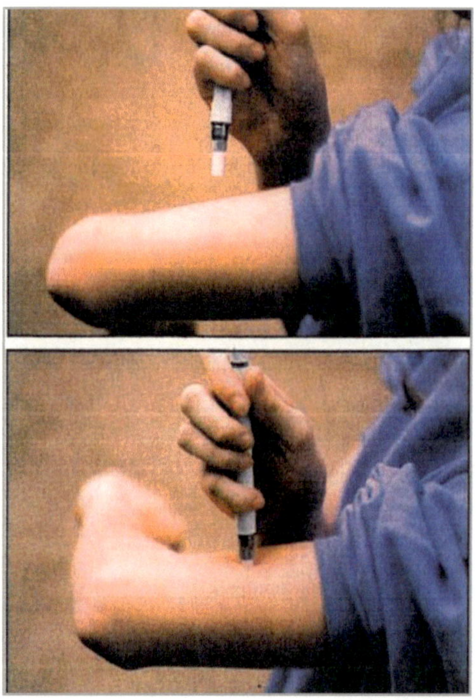

**Figure 3.**
*MADI – needle pen in the course of injection (1994).*

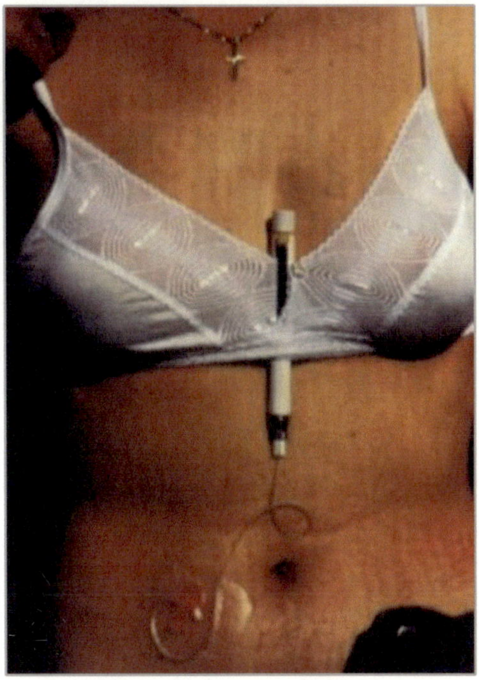

**Figure 4.**
*MADI – catheter pen [35] (1994).*

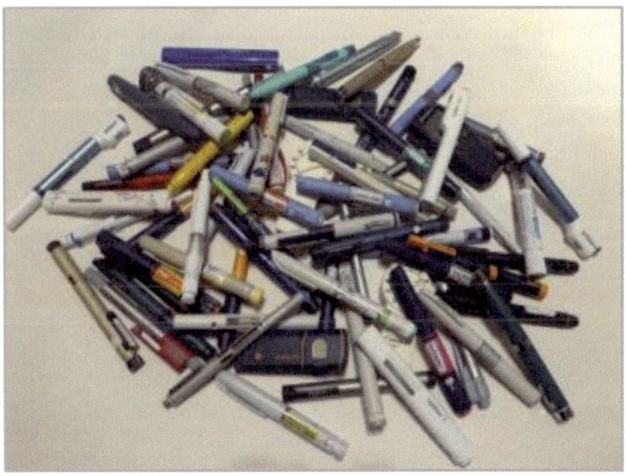

**Figure 5.**
*Heaps of insulin or incretin pens produced by different companies all over the world since 1983. Photo V. Kupčik, Diabetes Museum, Háj ve Slezsku, CR. (2019).*

### 2.2.2 Trials for testing accuracy and precision of glucometer-strips systems

Within the course of 25 years, we have tested the accuracy and precision of glucometer-strips systems Card (Medisense), OPTIUM (Abbott), ADVANCE (Hypoguard, GB) [17] and LINUS (Agamatrix, USA). [18] to support the reliability of our therapeutic recommendations.

The purpose of our last experimental and clinical trial (2010–2013) [19] was (1) to assess the electrochemistry-based glucometers CONTOURLINK (Bayer, Germany) using glucose dehydrogenase strips, CALLA, (Wellion, Austria) and

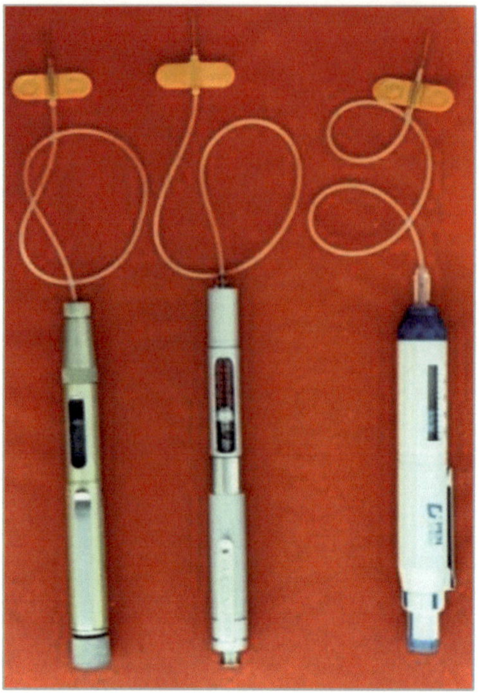

**Figure 6.**
*Various catheter pens: MADI (CR), MD2 (GDR), D pen (CH) (1989).*

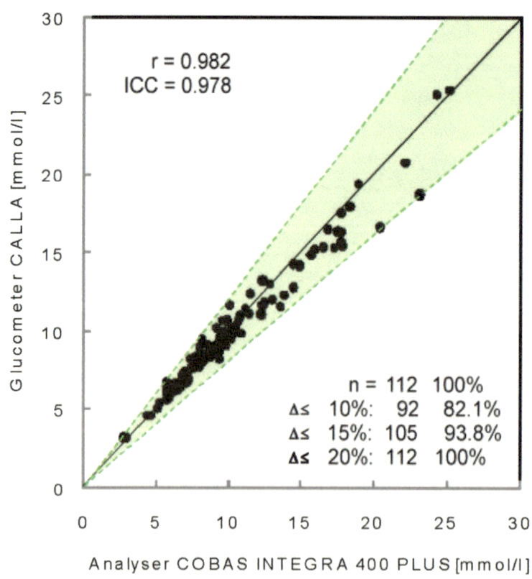


**Figure 7.**
*Correlations (Spearman) between PG estimations on INTEGRA vs. CALLA [19] (2013).*

LINUS (Agamatrix, USA) both using glucose oxidase strips; (2) to evaluate diabetes control using Ambulatory Glycaemic Profiles (AGP) and comparing the results with those of the COBAS INTEGRA 400 Plus analyser. There were 112 sets (each from one person) analysed. Means of 3 PG estimations on glucometers and on INTEGRA analyser were calculated.

Strong correlations between PG values estimated on COBAS INTEGRA analyser vs. individual glucometers (CONTOURLINK, CALLA, LINUS) were shown (**Figure 7**).

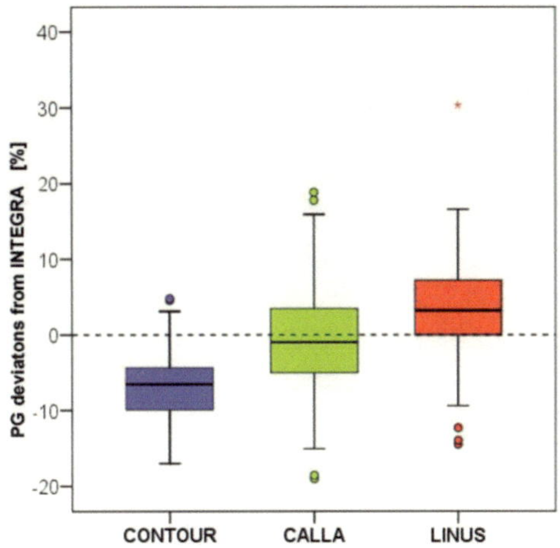


**Figure 8.**
*Relative deviations of glucometer estimations from estimations on analyser Cobas Integra. PG deviations of respective glucometers from INTEGRA PG were within the range ± 15% (i.e. in 94.6%, 93.8%, 97.3% of 112 pairs, resp.) [19] (2013).*

Deviations from INTEGRA were within the range ± 15%. (**Figure 8**) PG variability was measured by SD: SD INTEGRA = 0.061 mmol/l, SD CONTOURLINK = 0.256 mmol/l, SD CALLA = 0.290 mmol/l, SD LINUS = 0.286 mmol/l. The mean INTEGRA PG values ranged from 2.7 to 25.3 mmol/l.

All persons with T2D performed 10-point PG profiles to optimise balance between meals, physical exercise, and insulin boluses. PG differences between the respective glucometer-strips system and COBAS INTEGRA laboratory values were in borderline of ISO 15197. [25]. So, the practical acceptability of all tested glucometer-strips systems was demonstrated. Nevertheless, due to different (even though acceptable) accuracy of individual systems, it is advisable to use one type of glucometer-strips system in each diabetes centre. Since 2013 all our patients are trained in SMPG on glucometer CALLA. If insulin pump MINIMED 640 G is used, glucometer CONTOUR PLUS is sometimes preferred due to wireless signal transmission.

#### *2.2.3 Trials for the efficiency of continuous glucose monitoring (CGM)*

In 2005–2013 we tested benefits of CGM in three independent studies. Two of them were performed in people with T2D and T1D treated by insulin pumps PARADIGM (Medtronic MiniMed, Nordthridge, CA, USA). One study aimed to patients without insulin pump in perioperative care.

The pump PARADIGM 722 communicates with CGM and enables daily reading of 288 PG values determined by a SENsor inserted into subcutaneous tissue (PARASEN study). Real-time PG values are helpful to adapt further treatment.

##### *2.2.3.1 Single center trial for benefits of CGM vs SMPG (2005–2009)*

Aim of this clinical study [36] was to compare the evolution of HbA1c over the 3- month period with CGM vs. a period with conventional SMPG by glucometers.

Two cohorts of T1D + T2D on insulin pumps PARADIGM were investigated.

Cohort 1 comprised 17 persons using CGM sensors for continuous glucose monitoring (CGM group). Cohort 2 comprised 25 people performing self-monitoring as before (3 to 6 times/d) on glucometer LINUS, Wellion, Agamatrix (SMPG group).

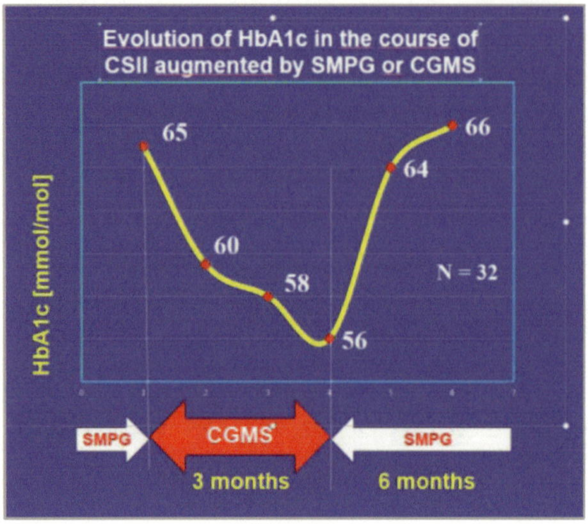


**Figure 9.**
*Benefits of CGM in individuals on insulin pump [36] (2013).*

In the CGM group (but not in the SMPG group) HbA1c significantly dropped within one month and remained reduced as long as the CGM was applied, i.e., until the switch back to SMPG. (**Figure 9**).

Hence, continuous glucose monitoring with transcutaneous sensors appeared to be an important measure for improving metabolic compensation in people with diabetes. With CGM, the evolution of HbA1c showed metabolic improvement. The PARASEN study demonstrated that continuous self-monitoring should become a regular part of treatment in educated persons on insulin pumps.

Several years later, the COMISAIR study [37] demonstrated that also a conventional intensive multiple dose insulin regimen (MDI), if supported by CGM, can be a suitable alternative to CGM augmented insulin pump therapy.

### *2.2.3.2 Multicenter trial on CGM-augmented insulin pump therapy in T1D (2005–2009)*

The multicenter CGM study (2005–2009) [38] aimed to the assessment of benefits of CGM-augmented insulin pump therapy for persons with T1D.

Community or academic practices in six Central and Eastern European/ Mediterranean countries established a registry of people with T1D starting CGM-augmented insulin pump therapy with the pump PARADIGM® X22 under everyday conditions. We compared HbA1c values before and after 3 months of CGM and assessed relationships between insulin therapy and glycaemia-related variables.

Sensor data and HbA1c data were evaluated in 85 of 102 enrolled persons with longstanding T1D, mean age 33.2 ± 16.9 years. Mean HbA1c declined after 3 months of CGM from 59.0 ± 8.9 mmol/mol at baseline to 50.9 ± 11.7 mmol/mol ($P < 0.001$).

Hence, CGM-augmented insulin pump therapy appeared to improve glycaemic control in T1D in everyday practice settings.

### *2.2.3.3 The trial for CGM benefits in perioperative care (2009–2013)*

Our third CGM study (2009–2013) [39] payed attention to the assessment of implementation of CGM in perioperative care of T2D.

PG monitoring was performed by means of GUARDIAN REAL-Time CGMS (Medtronic, Northridge, USA) in perioperative periods of 20 persons with T2D. Sensor was inserted on the day before surgery and continued for 3 days.

This approach was successful in the intensive care unit setting only. Neither electromagnetic interference nor other side effects appeared. No significant difference between sensor and laboratory analyser values was found. Pearson's correlation coefficients between PG by sensor and by Wellion Linus glucometer during the whole perioperative period were significantly strong (0.9). Hypoglycaemia was registered in 4 of 20 persons.

So, transcutaneous CGM appears to be a safe approach offering a detailed insight into perioperative PG homeostasis. However, confirmation of sensor data by an approved method remains necessary.

## 3. Clinical trials on effectiveness of preprandial complementary (= supplementary) insulin boluses in T2D

Disturbed dynamics of insulin secretion in T2D (**Figure 10**) makes the need of small complementary preprandial boluses of rapid insulin understandable.

In the years 1991–2019 we carried out three single centre trials to this topic.

### 3.1 Trial on effectiveness of rapid insulin

In 1991–1994, a nonrandomized uncontrolled study with 251 T2D assessed the effectiveness of supplementary insulin regimen [40, 41] The complementary insulin therapy using insulin pen MADI started in hospital following the baseline PG profile on day 2. The final ten-point PG profile was performed on day 4. (**Figures 11** and **12**) At a check-up 8–10 weeks later a decrease of HbA1c, BMI and improved lipoprotein-spectrum was found (**Figures 13** and **14**).

We concluded that in T2D better metabolic control can be achieved with complementary insulin therapy than with oral antidiabetic drugs or long-acting insulin 1–2 times daily. Our "surprising" results were based on pathophysiologic concept of Bruns, Berger and Kalfhaus. [7–9] To date, intensive insulin therapy in people with T2D appears to be more accepted in daily routine. [6, 23]

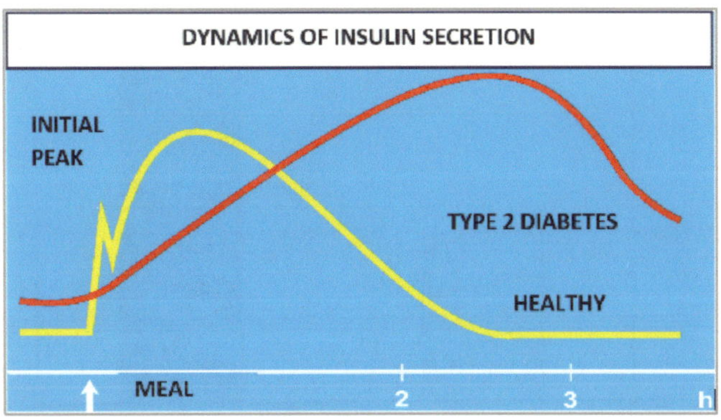


**Figure 10.**
*Dynamics of insulin secretion in blood in healthy people (initial postprandial peak is present, insulin concentration returns to baseline within 3 h); in T2D (missing Initial peak, maximum is delayed and hyperinsulinaemia remains over 3 h) [7] (1995).*

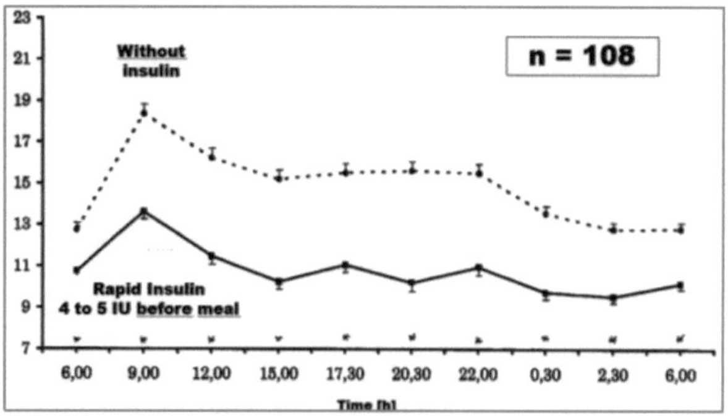


**Figure 11.**
*Ten- point BG profiles (mean ± SE) in insulin-naïve-T2D treated on baseline with oral antidiabetic drugs and/ or diet (upper curve) and then with complementary boluses (4 to 6 U each = 26 U/d) of rapid insulin (lower curve) *P < 0,05. [40] (1997).*

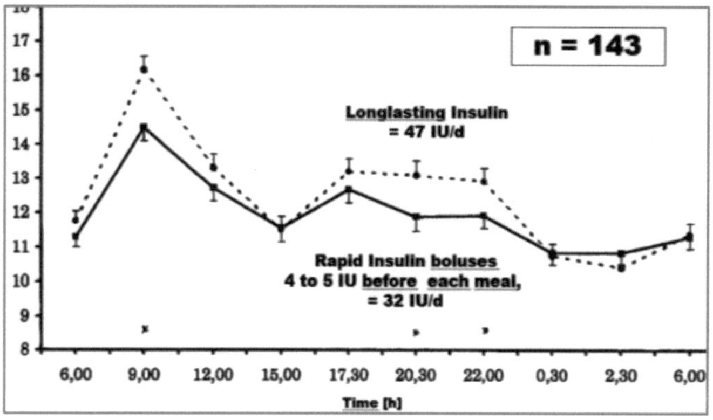


**Figure 12.**
*Ten- point BG profiles (mmol/l, mean ± SE) in T2D treated on baseline with long-acting insulin (1 to 2 boluses/d = 47 U/d) and/or diet and then with complementary boluses (4 to 6 U each = 32 U/d) of rapid insulin (lower curve) *P < 0,05. [40] (1997).*

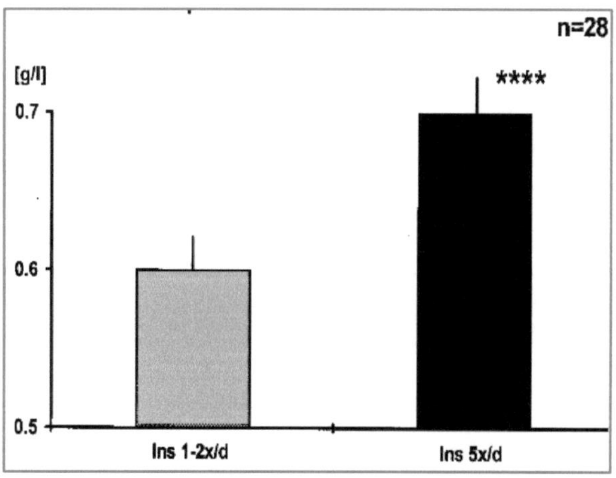


**Figure 13.**
*Lipoprotein apoLpA1 at baseline and after 8–10 weeks of complementary insulin therapy [41] (1997).*

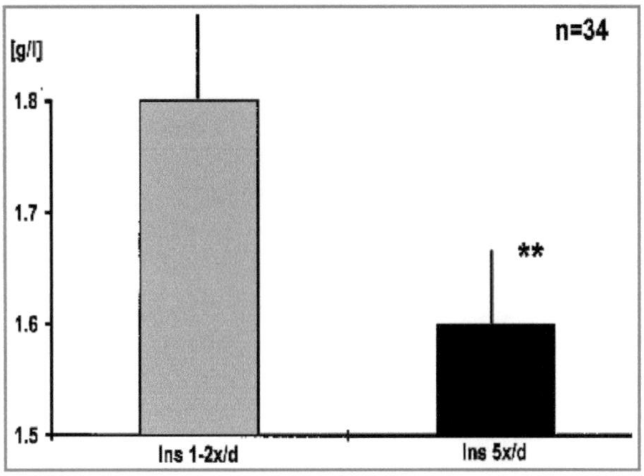


**Figure 14.**
*Lipoprotein apo LpB at baseline and after 8–10 weeks of complementary insulin therapy [41] (1997).*

### 3.2 Trial on effectiveness of complementary boluses of rapid insulin analog

The rapid acting insulin anologs (aspart, lispro and glulisin) are available since the end of the 20th century. Their absorption rates prevail over that of regular human insulin. [42, 43]

The aim of our prospective observational open-label controlled study (2004–2007) [44] was to compare the effects of insulin analog aspart and human regular insulin resulting from their routine administration in small preprandial boluses according to identical algorithms.

Fifty-seven persons with T2D aged 64.0 ± 1.29 (mean ± SE) years, diabetes duration of 12.4 ± 1.06 years, C-peptide positive, were enrolled into the study. Their treatment with human regular insulin lasted 5.2 ± 0.44 years. Human regular insulin was replaced with insulin analog aspart. Two check-ups in the course of 330 ± 11.1- day sequential period were carried out. The control group consisted of 17 persons of equivalent age, duration of diabetes and insulin dosing.

Following the switch from human regular insulin to insulin analog aspart, HbA1c concentration in blood decreased **Figure 15**, while plasma glucose

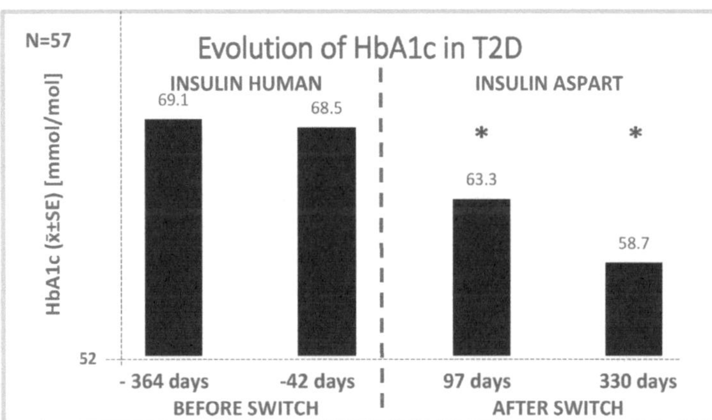


**Figure 15.**
*Impact of insulin aspart (given according the same algorhithms as human insulin) on HbA1c in 57 persons with T2D (* P < 0,05) [44] (2007).*

concentrations in 10-point profiles, daily insulin dose, BMI, and frequency of hypo–/hyperglycemic episodes did not change.

No significant influence of insulin aspart on serum concentrations of triacylglycerols, total cholesterol, and LDL-cholesterol was found. Patients' satisfaction was good. No adverse events were recorded. In the control group, no significant changes of baseline HbA1c, insulin dose and BMI were found.

Hence, insulin analog aspart appears to be more effective than human regular insulin in intensive (complementary) treatment in individuals with T2D.

### 3.3 Trial on effectiveness of Faster (ultrarapid) Insulin ASPart (FIASP)

The benefits of faster insulin aspart (insulin aspart + nicotinamid) were described and discussed. [45, 46]

Aim of our prospective monocentric uncontrolled Real World Evidence study (2017–2019) [47] was to compare the efficacy of FIASP with the efficacy of previous therapy with insulin aspart in people with T1D and T2D on MDI or on insulin pump.

No adverse events appeared in any group. In T2D groups (N < 24) an unsignificant tendency to reduction of PG, MPG, HbA1c, body mass and total daily dose of insulin in the course of FIASP therapy was shown.

So, only the evidence of noninferiority of FIASP versus insulin aspart was demonstrated. Introduction of improved algorithms together with intensive patients´ education appears necessary to improve the expected outcomes of FIASP therapeutic regimen.

## 4. Trial on effectiveness of Continuous Subcutaneous Insulin infusion (CSII) vs. multiple boluses of rapid insulin analog plus once daily basal insulin in T2D

The effectiveness of CSII in T2D was sought for in many previous studies [48–52]. Our (Medtronic supported) prospective single-centre randomized study (2011–2014) [53–55] recruited 36 insulin-resistant, C-peptide-positive, glutamic acid decarboxylase antibodies (GAD Ab)-negative, and CSII-naive patients with T2D (eight screen failures). Insulin treatment was optimized with insulin analogs and metformin. Following the run-in period, patients were randomized into two arms: a CSII arm (n = 11) and an MDI continuation arm (n = 12). HbA1c ≥ 64 mmol/mol, (mean ± standard deviation), age of 57.2 ± 8.0 years, BMI of 36.2 ± 7.0 kg/m$^2$, BM of 106.9 ± 18.3 kg, diabetes duration of 13.3 ± 4.7 years, and HbA1c of 80 mmol/mol). In both arms, at the CSII start the daily insulin dose was reduced by 10% –50% in order not to exceed 80 U/day. After 6 months, persons receiving MDI crossed over to insulin pump and both arms were followed up during consequent 6 months. A total of 10 scheduled visits were carried out in each arm. The final Visit 10 occurred at 12 months. The mean frequency of self-monitoring varied between 3.4 and 5.4 measurements per day.

Patients assigned to the CSII arm (N = 11) achieved a significant HbA1c reduction of 10–12 mmol/mol while reducing their daily insulin dose by 33% of baseline; BMI reduction was 0.86% of baseline. No significant changes were revealed in patients on MDI **Figure 16**.

So, the use of insulin pump (supported with SMBG) in T2D is safe and effective for improving glucose control and reducing daily dose of insulin. Treatment adherence and satisfaction were excellent. All subjects decided to continue using their insulin pumps. On the other hand, an optimum metabolic balance and sustainable reduction in body mass, blood pressure or lipid profile in most of the patients could not be reached.

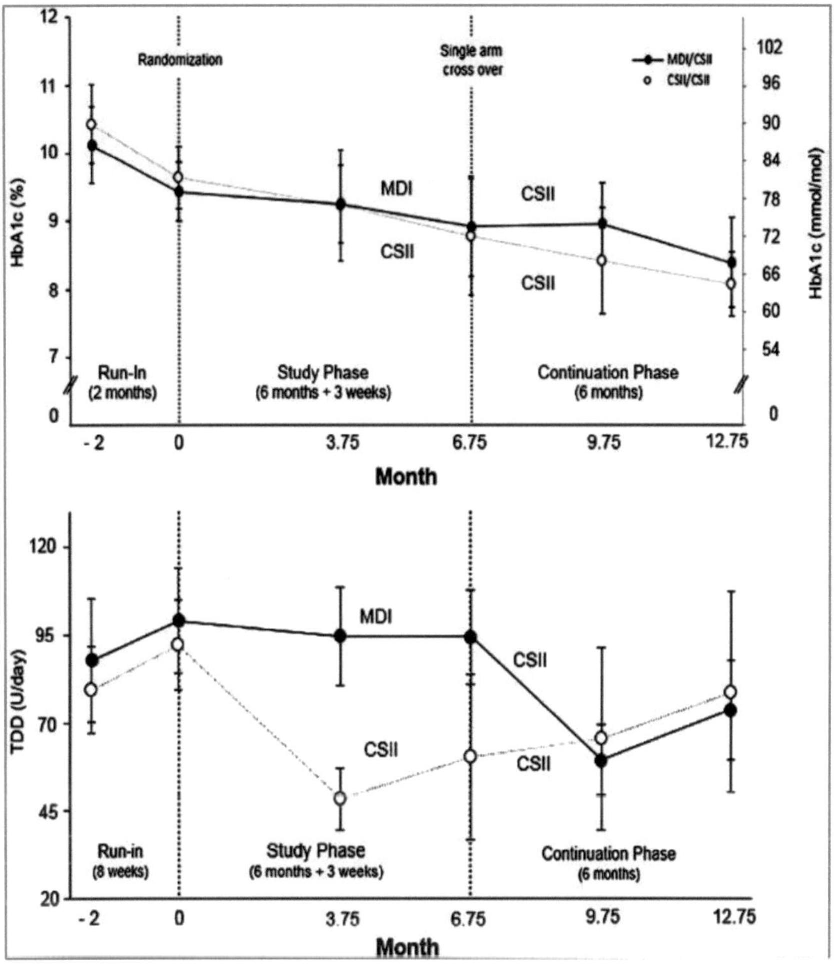


**Figure 16.**
*HbA1c (top) and total daily insulin dose (bottom) in the MDI/CSII arm (N = 11, closed symbols) and in the CSII/CSII arm (N = 11, open symbols). Symbols and bars - mean and 95% CI (confidence interval); CSII - continuous subcutaneous insulin infusion; MDI - multiple daily injections [55] (2017).*

## 5. Case reports targeting incretin analogs/GLP-1 receptor agonists

The first incretin analogs exenatid [56], lixisenatid, liraglutide were used in persons with T2D to improve metabolic control and to reduce body mass - mostly when HbA1c exceeded 60 mmol/mol, BMI was over 35 kg/m2 and oral antidiabetic drugs failed. Their beneficial metabolic and cardiovascular effects were described recently in RCTs LEAD 1 – LEAD 6 [57–62] and LEADER. [63] We had the option to confirm their benefits in several persons.

### 5.1 Effects of liraglutide on body mass and HbA1c

Our case report from the year 2010 [64] demonstrates the benefits of treatment with liraglutide in a 57-year old obese woman (adequately treated for hypothyreosis) with recent evolution of metabolic syndrome. Four-month metformin (M) and liraglutide (L) therapy reduced both body mass index (**Figure 17**), and glycated haemoglobin (**Figure 18**) Even though the previous diabetes control was acceptable, the treatment with high doses of metformin and sitagliptin (S) failed to reach sufficient reduction of body mass and HbA1c.

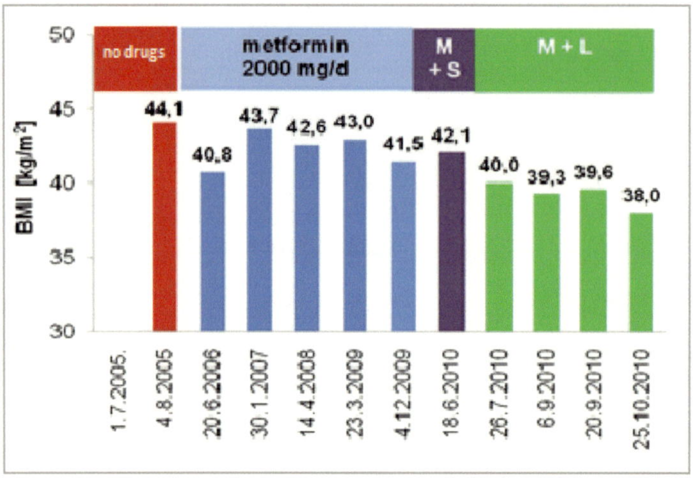


**Figure 17.**
*Lady, age 57. Therapy and evolution of BMI since the detection of T2D in 2006. M-metformin, S-sitagliptin, L-liraglutide (L-start 18.8.2010) [64].*

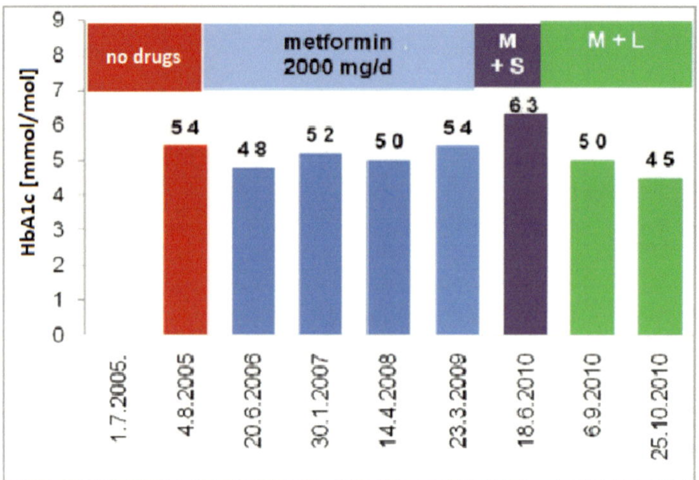


**Figure 18.**
*Lady, age 57. Therapy and evolution of HbA1c since the detection of T2D in 2006. M-metformin, S-sitagliptin, L-liraglutide (L-start 18.8.2010) [64].*

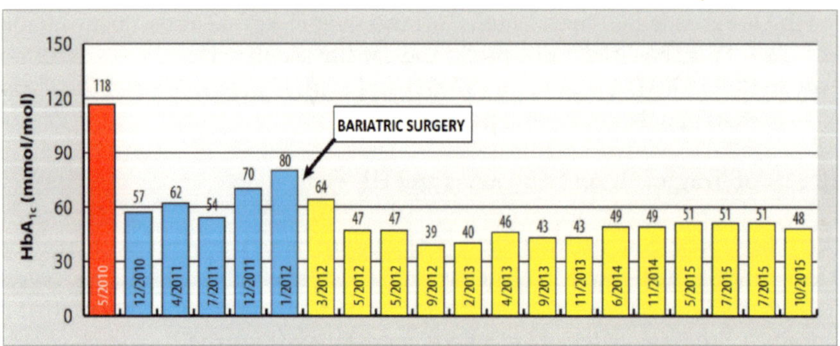


**Figure 19.**
*Man, age 57 y, T2D duration 13 y. Evolution of HbA1c with liraglutide and metformin before (2010–2012, blue) and after (2012–2015) bariatric surgery [65] (2015).*

### 5.2 Effects of liraglutide and bariatric surgery

Our second case report (2010–2016) [65] deals with a temporal positive influence of a 5-year liraglutide therapy on HbA1c (**Figure 19**), BMI and 10-point glyceamic profile in a man with 13-year history of uncontrolled T2D. After one year on liraglutide 1,2 mg/d + metformin 2000–3000 mg/d, the initial decrease of BMI and HbA1c was followed by their slow increase. Following bariatric surgery, the continuing liraglutide and metformin treatment resulted in near-normal HbA1c concentrations not exceeding 51 mmol/mol. The BMI decreased from 39 to 32 kg/m$^2$.

### 5.3 Effects of liraglutide in T2D prevention

The purpose of this case report (2011) [66] is to demonstrate the effects of 5-month off label administration of L and metformin (M) in a 60y old woman with impaired fasting plasma glucose (IFG), BMI 36.4 kg/m$^2$, HbA1c 41 mmol/mol and in excellent physical condition. Since 2005 her body mass increased by 10 kg. Recently diagnosed hypertension was successfully treated by metoprolol and losartan (BP 140/80 mmHg, HF 64/min). She was treated by simvastatin since 2008 (LDL cholesterol 3,4 mmol/l). Proinsulin, C-peptide, TSH. T3, T4 and routine laboratory parameters were found within normal limits. Results of SMPG using glucometer Linus, Agamatrix, USA were slightly abnormal. In August 2010 the therapy with L and M started. First evaluation was made in January 2011 (**Figures 20** and **21**). In 2012 – 2014, L 1.2 mg/d was given only during a 3- month period each year. Then, M 2 g/d continued without L. Food intake was reduced due to lasting satiety. The final check up in February 2021 revealed excellent clinical condition, BM 66.1 kg, BMI 29.4 kg/m$^2$ and HbA1c 39 mmol/mol.

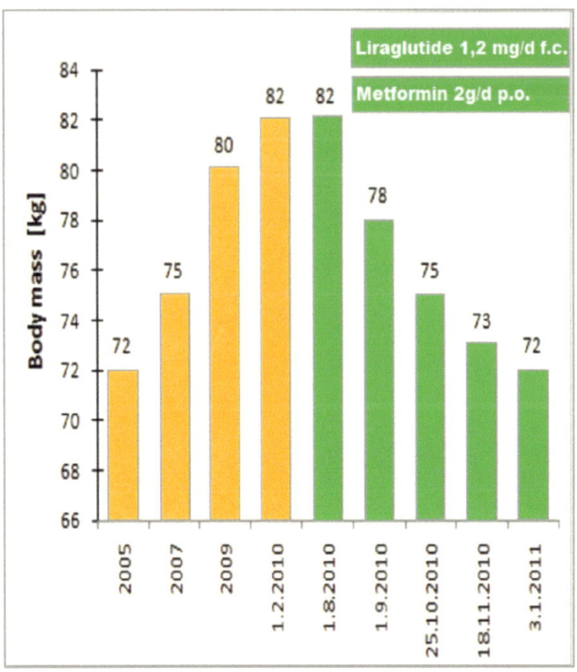


**Figure 20.**
*Lady, age 60 y, prediabetes. Evolution of body mass before and with L + M [66] (2011).*

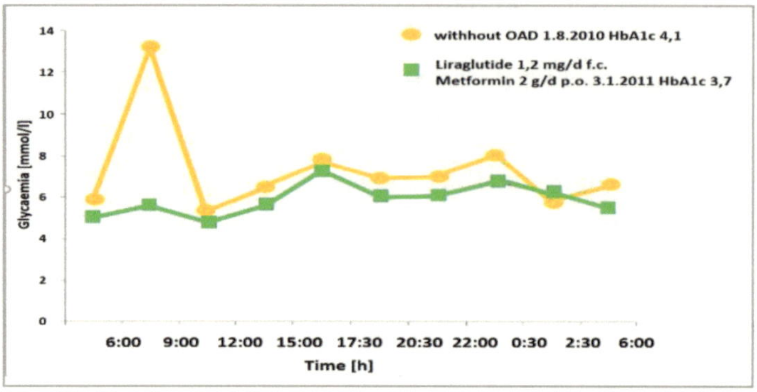


**Figure 21.**
*Lady, age 60 y, prediabetes. 10-point PG profile before and with L + M [66] (2011).*

Independently, 4 of other 6 obese persons with IFG/IGT reduced body mass during L supplementation. So, L therapy appears to be a potentially effective approach to prediabetes conditions and its administration should start rather at an early stage.

## 5.4 Effects of once weekly semaglutide on HbA1c, body mass and well-being

Effects of long-acting incretin analogs (exenatid QW, dulaglutid [67] and semaglutide [68–77] on metabolism, cardiovascular and renal protection were described in clinical studies REWIND and SUSTAIN 1–10, resp.

Our case report (2019–2020) [78] brings insight on benefits of semaglutide in a 79-year-old lady with long-lasting T2D. She has been suffering from both metformin intolerance and insulinofobia. In the course of a long- lasting period of gliptin therapy, the patient's $HbA_{1c}$ concentration increased to 61 mmol/mol. During the following 4-month period with semaglutide, the patient's mean PG concentration

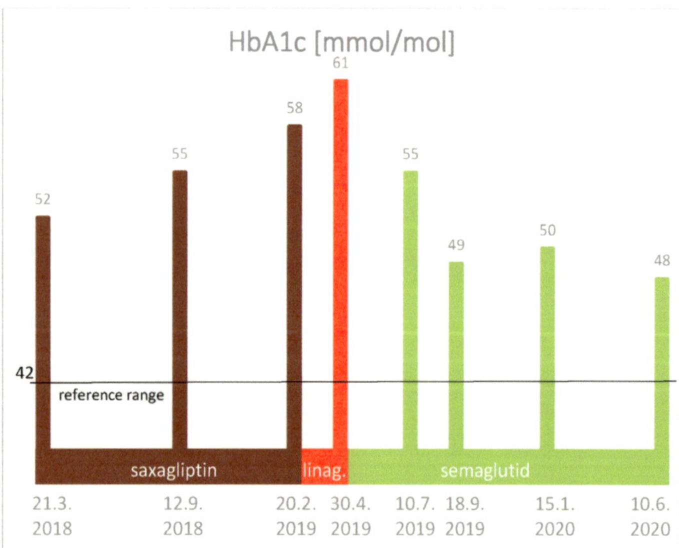


**Figure 22.**
*Lady, age 79 y. Evolution of HbA1c in the course of treatment with saxagliptin, linagliptin and semaglutide, resp., 2018 to 2020 [78].*

of a 10-point daily profile (MPG) decreased from 7.4 mmol/l to 7.0 mmol/l, and her body mass from 80,9 kg to 77,7 kg. One year later, the HbA1c reached 48 mmol/mol (**Figure 22**). No adverse events appeared. We can conclude, the early indication of once-a-week subcutaneously administered semaglutide resulted in improvement of all investigated parameters of saccharide metabolism.

## 5.5 Effects of fixed combination of insulin degludec and incretin liraglutide (IDegLira)

Metabolic and cardiovascular benefits of the fixed combination IdegLira were evaluated in studies DUAL and others. [79–87]

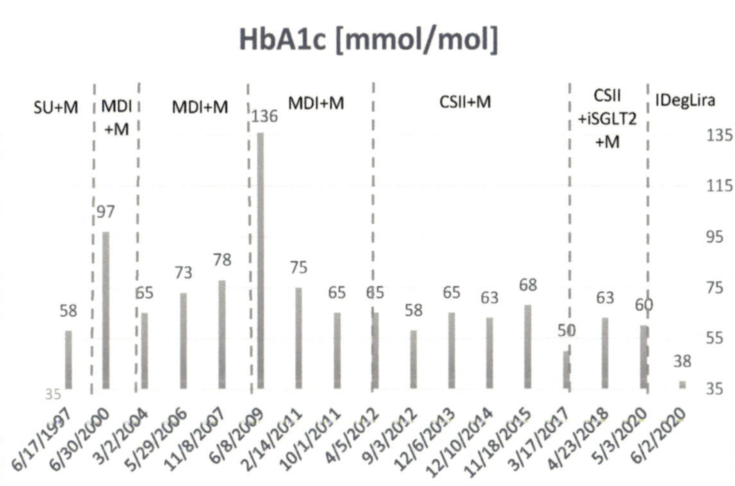


**Figure 23.**
*Lady, age 77 y, T2D since 1985, cast away syndrome. Evolution of HbA1c in the course of different therapy (MDI-CSII-CSII with iSGLT2-IDegLira only) (1997–2020) [88].*

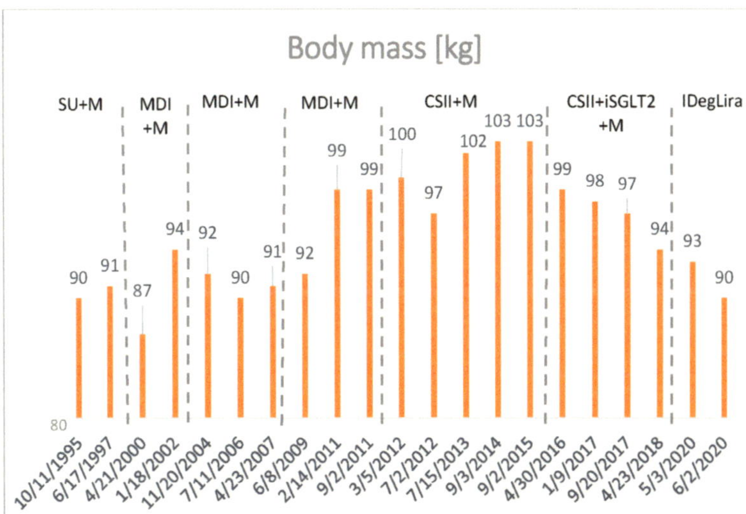


**Figure 24.**
*Lady, age 77 y, T2D since 1985, cast away syndrome. Evolution of BM in the course of different therapy (MDI-CSII-CSII with iSGLT2-IDegLira only) (1995–2020) [88].*

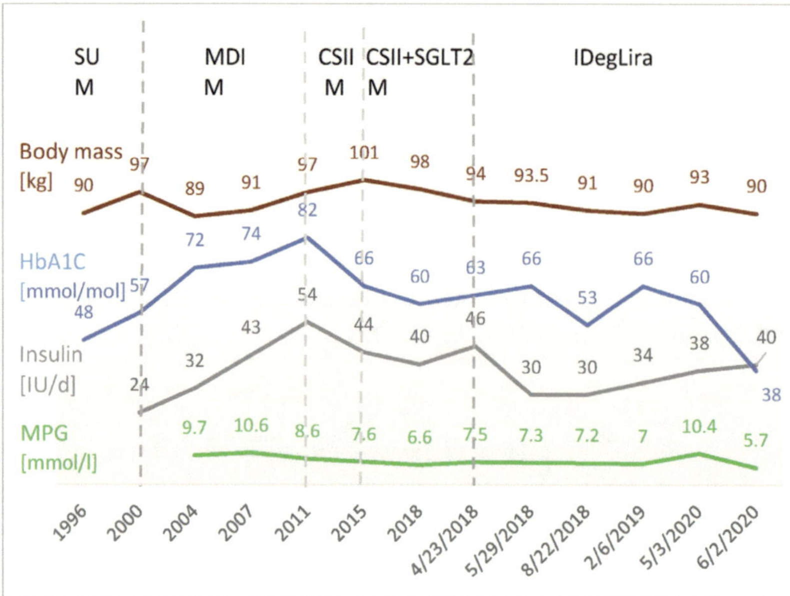


**Figure 25.**
*Lady, age 77 y, T2D since 1985, cast away syndrome. Overview of all parameters (HbA1c, BM, insulin/day, MPG) in the course of different therapeutic regimens (MDI-CSII-CSII with iSGLT2-IDegLira only) (1996–2020) [88].*

We deemed IDegLira could be an option for T2D suffering from impaired cognitive functions. We described this condition as "cast away syndrome".

Our case report (1995–2020) [88] pays attention to IDegLira in a 77-year-old woman with T2D. Her diabetes was treated for 33 years (since 1985) including the last seven- year period of effective insulin pump therapy, finally combined with dapagliflozin. Recently, signs of cognitive deterioration ("cast away syndrome") appeared and the patient was unable to operate her insulin pump. Adding IDegLira to previous metformin and dapagliflozin therapy alongside with support of educated family lead to improvement of patient's condition. The final in-patient period (30. 4. - 1. 7. 2020]) with IDegLira 40 IU/d (no CSII, no metformin, no gliflozin) and specialized diabetes care of nursing staff resulted in reduction of HbA1c to 38 mmol/mol (reference range 20–42 mmol/mol) (**Figures 23–25**).

## 6. Trial on effectiveness of dapagliflozin in uncontrolled T2D using insulin pumps

Gliflozins are inhibitors of sodium glucose co-transporter 2 (SGLT2) in proximal part of renal tubules. Their influence results in lowering of the renal thresholds for glucose and lowering of hyperglycaemia (due to urine excretion of about 70 g glucose per 24 h). Impact of gliflozins (dapagliflozin [89–91], empagliflozin [92] canagliflozin [93–95] and ertugliflozin) on metabolic control and cardiovascular and renal outcomes in T2D was demonstrated in trials EMPAREG, EMPEROR, CANVAS, CREDENCE, DECLARE HF, DECLARE Timi 58 and VERTIS. Benefits were observed in simultaneous therapy with insulin/incretin and gliflozin. [96]

Our pilot prospective trial (2015–2017) [97] aimed to the assessment of effectiveness of dapagliflozin added to people with T2D treated by CSII and metformin (M). A group of 13 T2D on CSII, without serious complications, aged 44.6–70.4 y, diabetes duration 5–26 y, BMI 24.9–57.6 kg/m2, were monitored at 4 visits (before

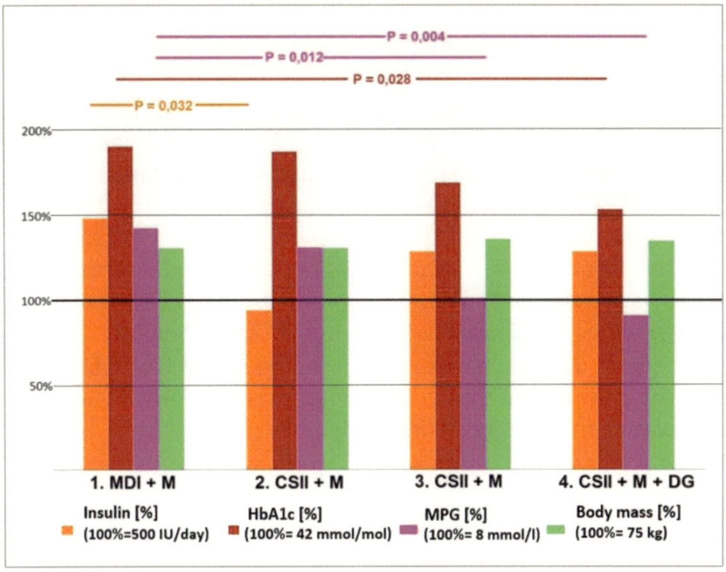


**Figure 26.**
*A group of T2D (N = 13) treated with 3 consequent regimens: 1. MDI + M, 2. CSII+M, 3. CSII+M + DG. Evolution of relative values of INS/d, HbA1c, MPG, BM. Upper border of the reference range of respective parameter was defined as 100% of its value (2015–2017) [97].*

CSII, on CSII + M, on CSII + M shortly before dapagliflozin and finaly on CSII + M after 2.5–11.0 months with dapagliflozin.

CSII appeared to enable reduction of total daily insulin dose with no consequent change of HbA1c and glycaemia. Adding dapagliflozin to CSII resulted in significant reduction of HbA1c. (**Figure 26**) Even though the change in BM was not significant, Spearman analysis revealed correlations between the change of daily insulin dose and change of BM at visit 3 and 4 vs. visit 1.

No side effects appeared. So, dapagliflozin may be considered as a rational therapeutic addition to CSII + M treated people with T2D.

## 7. Conclusions

This chapter summarizes the authors' experience along with outcomes of respected randomized control trials and real world evidence studies. It became clear that the pathophysiologic approach comprising insulin, incretins and gliflozins has created a reliable base to effective treatment of type 2 diabetes. Reduced morbidity and mortality along with other breaking reports [98–101] are offerring some great perspectives.

On the other hand, in everyday practice, hidden clinical inertia, resulting from outdated treatment approach, customs, imbalance between powerty and affluency, should be considered as a dangerous rival.

So, which direction do we take from here?

## Acknowledgements

R.C. was in charge of the selection of cited references and figures and manuscript design, data analysis and critical text review. R.K. and L.H. supervised the performance of therapeutic protocols including HbA1c and 10-point glycaemic profiles, H.Z. was responsible for medical reports, files and IT operations, B.D. took care of laboratory investigations. There is no conflict of interests.

Special thanks to Stanislava Dudová, Emilia Ďurajková, Lenka Kratochvílová, Michaela Nádvorniková, Jana Polcerová, Svatava Tancosová, Jana Ferancová, Pavel Kolčava, Eva Malá, Dana Masnikosová, Hana Peniaková, Jiří Podivínský, Jana Svobodová, Rastislav Šramko and their teams for outstanding neverending support.

Final acknowledgement belongs to specialists, nursing and other staff, students of Palacky University Olomouc, compliant persons with diabetes, as well as to Insurance Companies and pharma industry in the Czech Republic.

Those who found this chapter worthy of reading surely appreciate the support provided by Palacky University, Teaching Hospital Olomouc, Institute of Specialized Treatments Paseka and other important institutions.

## Dedication

Taking into account the dawning observations of Paul Langerhans (1847–1888) [102], Oskar Minkowski (1858–1931) [103], George Ludwig Zülzer (1870–1949) [104], Ernest Lyman Scott (1877–1966) [105] and others in [106, 107], this paper was written in the memory of Nicolae Constantin Paulescu (1869–1931), James Bertram Collip (1892–1965), Frederick Grant Banting (1891–1941), Charles Herbert Best (1899–1978) and John James Rickard Macleod (1876–1935) on the occasion of the 100-year anniversary of insulin (pancrein) discovery (Bucharest, May 1921) [4], and its purification and implementation to human medicine (Toronto, January 1922) [5].

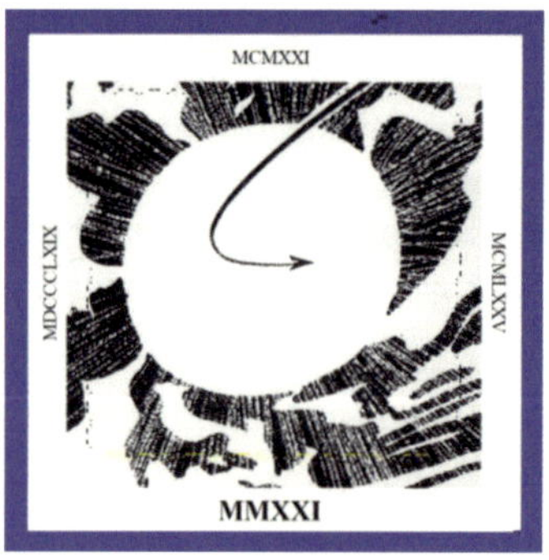

## Author details

Rudolf Chlup[1,2]*, Richard Kaňa[3], Lada Hanáčková[3], Hana Zálešáková[3] and Blanka Doubravová[3]

1 Department of Physiology, Faculty of Medicine and Dentistry, Palacky University Olomouc, Czech Republic

2 2nd Department of Medicine, Teaching Hospital Olomouc, Czech Republic

3 Department of Diabetes Moravský Beroun, Institute of Specialized Treatments, Paseka, Czech Republic

*Address all correspondence to: rudolf.chlup@fnol.cz

## References

[1] DeFronzo RA. From the triumvirate to the ominous octet: a new paradigm for the treatment of type 2 diabetes mellitus. Diabetes 2009;58(4):773-795. https://doi.org/10.2337/db09-9028

[2] Yuan S, Larsson SC. An atlas on risk factors for type 2 diabetes: a wide-angled Mendelian randomisation study. Diabetologia (2020). https://doi.org/10.1007/s00125-020-05253-x

[3] Alonge KM, D'Alessio DA, Schwartz MW. Brain control of blood glucose levels: implications for the pathogenesis of type 2 diabetes. Diabetologia 64, 5-14 (2021). https://doi.org/10.1007/s00125-020-05293-3

[4] Paulescu NC. Action de l'éxtrait pancréatique injecté dans le sang chez un animal diabétique. Comptes rendus des séances de la Société de biologie 1921;85(27):556-559.

[5] Banting FG, Best CH. Pancreatic extracts. J Lab Clin Med 1922;7, 8 (May):3-11.

[6] American Diabetes Association. 9. Pharmacologic approaches to glycemic treatment. Standards of Medical Care in Diabetes-2021. Diabetes Care 2021;44(Suppl.1):S111–S124.

[7] Bruns W, Fiedler H, Altman B, Lundershausen R, Menzel R, Worms F, Kriegstein E. Insulintherapie bei Typ 2 Diabetes Pathophysiologisch begründete Therapie mit Insulin unter besonderer Berücksichtigung der Insulinresistenz und des Inkretineffektes. (Insulin treatment in T2D Pathophysiology-based insulin treatment with particular consideration of insulin resistance and incretins. German.) 2. Auflage; UNIMED Verlag, AG, Bremen, 2010.

[8] Berger M, Jörgens V, Mühlhauser I. Rationale for the use of insulin therapy alone as the pharmacological treatment of type 2 diabetes. Diabetes Care 1999;22(Suppl 3):C71–C75.

[9] Kalfhaus J, Berger M. Supplementäre Insulintherapie (SIT)—wie effektiv und sicher ist die Gabe von praeprandialem Normalinsulin als Therapie-Alternative bei Typ-2-Diabetes? (Supplementary insulin therapy – the effectiveness and accuracy of preprandial regular insulin as a therapeutic alternative for T2D? German.) Diabetes Stoffwechsel 1999;8(Suppl 1):44.

[10] Chlup R, Janů K, Menzel R, Bruns W, Venháčová J. Léčba diabetu pomocí ručního dávkovače inzulinu MADI. (Therapy of diabetes using MAnual Device for Insulin MADI. Czech.) Univerzita Palackého v Olomouci, Olomouc. 1985, p.64.

[11] Pickup JC, Keen H, Parsons JA, Alberti KGMM. Continuous subcutaneous insulin infusion: an approach to achieving normoglycaemia. Brit Med J 1978;1:204-207.

[12] Bode BW, Bailey TS, et al. A 16-week open label, multicenter pilot study assessing insulin pump therapy in patients with type 2 diabetes suboptimally controlled with multiple daily injections. J Diabetes Sci Technol 2011;5:887-893.

[13] Peyrot M, Rubin RR, Chen X, Frias JP. Associations between improved glucose control and patient-reported outcomes after initiation of insulin pump therapy in patients with type 2 diabetes mellitus. Diabetes Technol Ther 2011;13:471-476.

[14] Chlup R. Benefits of intesive selfmonitoring and continuous subcutaneous insulin infusion in persons with type 2 diabetes mellitus. BITs Ist Annual Worlds Congress of Endobolism, 2011; Xiamen, China, Abstract, p.168 (Abstract).

[15] Chlup R, Zapletalova J, Cheng TS, Ramik Z, Slezakova M, Zalesakova H. Impact of incretins in people with type 2 diabetes on insulin pumps. 32nd Congress of the International Danube Symposia on Diabetes Mellitus 12th Congress of Central European Diabetes Association 22.-24. June 2017 Prague, Czech Republic: 20-21 P21 (Abstract).

[16] Chlup R, Zálešáková H. Přínos fixní kombinace dapagliflozin/metformin při léčbě diabetu 2. typu. (Benefits of fixed combination of dapagliflozin/metformin in treatment of type 2 diabetes. Czech.) Farmakoterapie 2016;12(1):30-32.

[17] Chlup R, Payne M, Zapletalová J, Doubravová B, Řezníčková M, Chlupová L, Sečkař P. Results of selfmonitoring on glucometer systems Advance and Optium in daily routine. Biomed Papers 2005;149(1):127-139

[18] Chlup R, Doubravova B, Peterson K, Zapletalova J, Bartek J. Wavesense technology glucometer Linus for routine self-monitoring and clinical practice. Acta Diabetol 2011;48(1):35-40.

[19] Chlup R, Doubravová B, Bartek J, Zapletalová J, Krystyník O, Procházka V. Effective assessment of diabetes control using personal glucometers (Contourlink, Bayer, Germany; Calla, Wellion, Austria; Linus, Agamatrix, USA). Disease Markers 2013;35(6):895-905.

[20] Mlčák P, Fialová J, Trnková K, Chlup R. A continuous glucose monitoring system (CGMS) – a promising aproach for improving metabolic control in persons with type 1 diabetes mellitus treated by insulin pumps. Biomed Papers 2004;148(1):33-38.

[21] Edelman SV, Argento NB, Pettus J, Hirsch IB. Clinical implications of real-time and intermittently scanned continuous glucose monitoring. Diabetes Care 2018;41(11):2265-2274.

[22] Hanas R, John G & On behalf of the International HBA1c Consensus Committee. 2010 Consensus statement on the worldwide standardization of the hemoglobin A1C measurement. Diabetes Care 2010;33:1903-1904.

[23] Davies MJ, D'Alessio DA, Fradkin J et al. Management of hyperglycaemia in type 2 diabetes, 2018. A consensus report by the American Diabetes Association (ADA) and the European Association for the Study of Diabetes (EASD). Diabetologia 2019;62(5): 873.

[24] Škrha J, Pelikanova T, Kvapil M. Doporučeny postup peče o diabetes mellitus 2. typu. (Recommended management of T2D 2020, Czech Diabetes Association) Česka diabetologicka společnost ČLS JEP 2020, online: www.diazpravodaj.cz

[25] ISO/DIS 15197 In Vitro Diagnostic Test Systems—requirements for blood glucose monitoring systems for self-testing in managing diabetes mellitus. ISO/DIS 15197:2013. Geneva: International Standards Organization, 2013.

[26] Maldonato A, Segal P, Golay A. Patient Education and Counseling 2001;44:87-94.

[27] Assal J-Ph, Berger M, Canivet J. History and aims of the diabetes education study group. International Congress Series No. 624. Amsterdam: Excerpta Medica, 1982. p. 3-7.

[28] Chlup R, Navrátilová L, Řehořová J, Bartek J. Efficacy of a 7- day program therapy in insulin-treated diabetic patients in Czech Republic - one center experience. Acta Diabetologica Romana 20 (Abstracts book, 20th National Congress of Romanian Society of Diabetes, Nutrition and Metabolic Diseases, Bucharest, May 26th–29th, 1994):33.

[29] Kudlova P, Chlup R, Zapletalova J. The benefits of postgraduate therapeutic

education in diabetology in the Czech Republic. 3rd icH&Hpsy 2017 International Conference on Health, and Health Psychology 5. - 7. July 2017 Viseu, Portugal. The European Proceedings of Social & Behavioural Sciences EpSBS: XXX, 217-227.

[30] Updike SJ, Shults MC, Cornwell ST et al. Facilitating intensive conventional insulin management using a manually operated syringe injector. Diabetes Res 1984;1:135-141.

[31] Jefferson G, Marteau TM, Smith MA. A multiple injection regimen using an insulin injection pen and prefilled cartridged soluble human insulin in adolescents with diabetes. Diabet Med 1985;2:993-995.

[32] Chlup R, Janů K, Venháčová J, Bartek J. Six models of a new insulin pen (MADI): description and first clinical trial. Practical Diabetes International 1995;12(1):32-35.

[33] Chlup R, Maršálek E, Bruns W. Prospective study of the hazards of multiple use of disposable syringes and needles in intensified insulin therapy. Diabetic Medicine 1990;7:624-627.

[34] Gudiksen N, Hofstätter T, Rønn BB, Sparre T. FlexTouch: an insulin pen-injector with a low activation force across different insulin formulati- ons, needle technologies, and temperature conditions. Diabetes Technol Ther 19, 10: 603-607, 2017.

[35] Menzel R, Chlup R, Jutzi E, Hildmann W. "Catheter-Pens" - an alternative to insulin pump treatment? Exp Clin Endocrinol 1990; 95:157-164.

[36] Peterson K, Zapletalová J, Kudlová P, Matušková V, Bartek J, Novotný D, Chlup R. Benefits of three-month continuous glucose monitoring for persons with diabetes using insulin pumps and sensors. Biomed Papers 2009;153(1):47-52.

[37] Šoupal J, Petruželková L, Flekač M, Pelcl T, Matoulek M, Daňková M, Škrha J, Svačina Š, Prázný M. Ccomparison Of different treatment Modalities for type 1 diabetes, Including Sensor-Augmented Insulin Regimens, In 52 Weeks of follow-up: A COMISAIR Study. Diabetes Technology & Therapeutics 2016;18(9):532-538. 10.1089/dia.2016.0171

[38] Cohen O, Körner A, Chlup R, Zoupas C, Ragozin A, Wudi K, Bartášková D, Pappas A, Niederland T, Taybani Z, Barák L, Vazeou AS. Improved glycemic control through continuous glucose sensor–augmented insulin pump therapy: Prospective results from a community and academic practice patient registry. J Diab Sci Techn. 2009;3(4):804-811.

[39] Poljaková I, Elšíková E, Chlup R, Kalabus S, Hasala O, Zapletalová J. Glucose sensing module – is it time to integrate in into real-time perioperative monitoring? An observational pilot study with subcutaneous sensors. Biomed Pap 2013;157(4):346-357.

[40] Chlup R, Vaverková H, Bartek J. Complementary insulin therapy improves blood glucose and serum lipids parameters in type 2 (non-insulin-dependent) diabetic patients. I. Effects on blood glucose control. Exp Clin Endocrinol Diabetes 1997;105(Suppl 2):70-73.

[41] Vaverková H, Chlup R, Ficker L, Novotný D, Bartek J. Complementary insulin therapy improves blood glucose and serum lipids parameters in type 2 (non-insulin-dependent) diabetic patients. II. Effects on serum lipids, lipoproteins and apoproteins. Exp Clin Endocrinol Diabetes 1997;105(Suppl 2):74-77.

[42] Standl E. Insulin analogues—state of the art. Horm Res 2002;57:40-45.

[43] Home PD, Lindholm A, Hylleberg B, Round P. Improved glycemic control

with insulin aspart. Diabetes Care 1998;21:1904-1909.

[44] Chlup R, Zapletalová J, Seckar P, Malá E, Doubravová B, Táncosová S, Chlupová L, Pukowietz L, Zatloukal P. Benefits of complementary therapy with insulin aspart vs regular human insulin in persons with type 2 diabetes mellitus. Diab Technol Therap 2007; 9(3):223-231.

[45] Bowering K, Case C, Harvey J, Reeves M, Sampson M, Strzinek R, Bretler DM, Bang RB, Bode BW. Faster aspart versus insulin aspart as part of a basal-bolus regimen in inadequately controlled type 2 diabetes: The ONSET 2 Trial. Diabetes Care 2017;40(7):951-957. doi: 10.2337/dc16-1770. Epub 2017 May 8. PMID: 28483786.

[46] Bode BW, Bowering K, Russell-Jones D. Response to Comment on Russell-Jones et al. Diabetes Care 2017;40:943-950. Comment on Bowering et al. Diabetes Care 2017;40:951-957. Diabetes Care 2018;41(3):e29-e30. doi: 10.2337/dci17-0051. PMID: 29463670.

[47] Chlup R, Zapletalová J, Zálešáková H, Kochtová J, Kaňa R. Vliv léčby inzulinem Fiasp na glykemii, HbA1c a tělesnou hmotnost u osob s diabetem 1. a 2. typu: studie z reálné praxe. (Impact of insulin FIASP for glycaemia, HbA1c and body mass in peeople with T1D or T2D: a trial from real practice. Czech.) Diab Obez 2019;19(38):90-97.

[48] Raskin P, Bode BW, Marks JB, et al. Continuous subcutaneous insulin infusion and multiple daily injection therapy are equally effective in type 2 diabetes—a randomized parallel-group, 24-week study. Diabetes Care 2003;26:2598-2603.

[49] Reznik Y, Cohen O, Aronson R, et al. Insulin pump treatment compared with multiple daily injections for treatment of type 2 diabetes (OpT2mise): a randomised open-label controlled trial. Lancet 2014;384:1265-1272.

[50] Conget I, Castaneda J, Petrovski G, et al. for the OpT2MISE Study Group. The impact of insulin pump therapy on glycemic profiles in patients with type 2 diabetes: data from theOpT2mise study. Diabetes Technol Ther 2016;18:22-28.

[51] Aronson R, Reznik Y, Conget I, et al. for the OpT2mise Study Group. Sustained efficacy of insulin pump therapy compared with multiple injections in type 2 diabetes:12-month data from the OpT2mise randomised trial. Diabetes Obes Metab 2016;18(5):500-507.

[52] Pickup JC, Reznik Y, Sutton AJ. Glycemic control during continuous subcutaneous insulin infusion versus multiple daily insulin injections in type 2 diabetes: individual patient data meta-analysis and meta-regression of randomized controlled trials. Diabetes Care 2017;40:715-722.

[53] Chlup R. Insulin pump in people with type 2 diabetes mellitus. Bulletin of the Karaganda University Biology, Medicine, Geography 2016;20/84(4):56-71 ISSN 2518-7201.

[54] Chlup R. Benefits from insulin pump in people with type 2 diabetes. The 42nd National Congress of the Romanian Society of Diabetes, Nutrition and Metabolic Diseases Brasov, Romania 25-28. May 2016 Acta diabetologica Romana 42:28(Abstract).

[55] Chlup R, Runzis S, Castaneda J, Lee S, Nguyen X, Cohen O. Complex assessment of metabolic effectiveness of insulin pump therapy in patients with type 2 diabetes beyond HbA1c reduction. Diabetes Technology and Therapeutics 2018; 20 (2):153-159.

[56] Klonoff DC, Buse JB, Nielsen LL et al. Exenatide effects on diabetes,

obesity, cardiovascular risk factors and hepatic biomarkers in patients with type 2 diabetes treated for at least 3 years. Curr Med Res Opin 24, 1: 275-286, 2008.

[57] Marre M, Shaw J, Brandle M et al. LEAD-1 SU study group. Liraglutide, a once-daily human GLP-1 analogue, added to a sulphonylurea over 26 weeks produces greater improvements in glycaemic and weight control compared with adding rosiglitazone or placebo in subjects with type 2 diabetes (LEAD-1 SU). Diabet Med 2009;26(3):268-278. https://doi.org/10.1111/j.1464-5491.2009.02666.x

[58] Nauck M, Frid A, Hermansen K, Shah NS, Tankova T, Mitha IH, Zdravkovic M, Düring M, Matthews DR. LEAD-2 Study Group. Efficacy and safety comparison of liraglutide, glimepiride, and placebo, all in combination with metformin, in type 2 diabetes: the LEAD (liraglutide effect and action in diabetes)2 study. Diabetes Care 2009 Jan;32(1):84-90. doi: 10.2337/dc08-1355. Epub 2008 Oct 17. PMID: 18931095; PMCID: PMC2606836.

[59] Garber A, Henry R, Ratner R, Garcia-Hernandez PA, Rodriguez-Pattzi H, Olvera-Alvarez I, Hale PM, Zdravkovic M, Bode B. LEAD-3 (Mono) Study Group. Liraglutide versus glimepiride monotherapy for type 2 diabetes (LEAD-3 Mono): a randomised, 52-week, phase III, double-blind, parallel-treatment trial. Lancet. 2009 Feb 7;373(9662):473-481. doi: 10.1016/S0140-6736(08)61246-5. Epub 2008 Sep 24. PMID: 18819705.

[60] Zinman B, Gerich J, Buse JB, Lewin A, Schwartz S, Raskin P, Hale PM, Zdravkovic M, Blonde L. LEAD-4 Study Investigators. Efficacy and safety of the human glucagon-like peptide-1 analog liraglutide in combination with metformin and thiazolidinedione in patients with type 2 diabetes (LEAD-4 Met+TZD). Diabetes Care 2009;32(7):1224-30. doi: 10.2337/dc08-2124. Epub 2009 Mar 16. Erratum in: Diabetes Care. 2010 Mar;33(3):692. PMID: 19289857; PMCID: PMC2699702.

[61] Russell-Jones D, Vaag A, Schmitz O, Sethi BK, Lalic N, Antic S, Zdravkovic M, Ravn GM, Simó R. Liraglutide effect and action in diabetes (LEAD-5 met+SU Study Group). Liraglutide vs insulin glargine and placebo in combination with metformin and sulfonylurea therapy in type 2 diabetes mellitus (LEAD-5 met+SU): a randomised controlled trial. Diabetologia. 2009 Oct;52(10):2046-55. doi: 10.1007/s00125-009-1472-y. Epub 2009 Aug 14. PMID: 19688338; PMCID: PMC2744824.

[62] Buse JB, Rosenstock J, Sesti G, Schmidt WE, Montanya E, Brett JH, Zychma M, Blonde L. LEAD-6 Study Group. Liraglutide once a day versus exenatide twice a day for type 2 diabetes: a 26-week randomised, parallel-group, multinational, open-label trial (LEAD-6) Lancet. 2009 4;374(9683):39-47. doi: 10.1016/S0140-6736(09)60659-0. Epub 2009 Jun 8. PMID: 19515413.

[63] Marso SP, Daniels G H, Brown-Frandsen K et al.: LEADER Steering Committee, LEADER Trial Investigators. Liraglutide and cardiovascular outcomes in type 2 diabetes. N Engl J Med 375, 4: 311-322, 2016.

[64] Chlup, R, Doubravová B, Ďurajková E, Peterson K, Zapletalová J. Léčba liraglutidem u pacientky s metabolickým syndromem a hypotyreózou. (Liraglutide in metabolic syndrom and hypothyreosis.) Kazuistiky v diabetologii (Diabetes Case Reports. Czech.) 2010;8(4):13—17.

[65] Chlup, R. Pětiletá léčba liraglutidem a bariatrický výkon u obézního muže s diabetem 2. typu. (Five- year liraglutide therayand bariatric surgeryin an obese man with T2D.) Kazuistiky v diabetologii (Diabetes Case Reports. Czech.) 2016;14(4):9-12.

[66] Chlup R, Ďurajková E, Peterson K. Reduction of body weight in obese persons with impaired fasting plasma glucose treated with liraglutide and metformin. Diabetes 2011;60(Suppl 1):A699 PO (Abstract).

[67] Gerstein HC, Colhoun HM, Dagenais GR, et al. REWIND Investigators. Dulaglutide and cardiovascular outcomes in type 2 diabetes (REWIND): a double-blind, randomised placebo-controlled trial. Lancet 2019;394: 121-130.

[68] Sorli C, Harashima SI, Tsoukas GM, et al. Efficacy and safety of once-weekly semaglutide monotherapy versus placebo in patients with type 2 diabetes (SUSTAIN 1): double-blind, randomised, placebo-controlled, parallel-group, multinational, multicentre phase 3a trial. Lancet Diabetes Endocrinol 2017;5(4):251-260.

[69] Ahrén B, Masmiquel L, Kumar H, et al. Efficacy and safety of once-weekly semaglutide versus once-daily sitagliptin as an add-on to metformin, thiazolidinediones, or both, in patients with type 2 diabetes (SUSTAIN 2): a 56-week, double-blind, phase 3a, randomised trial. Lancet Diabetes Endocrinol 2017;5(5): 341-354.

[70] Ahmann AJ, Capehorn M, Charpentier G, et al. Efficacy and safety of once-weekly semaglutide versus exenatide ER in subjects with type 2 diabetes (SUSTAIN 3): a 56-week, open-label, randomized clinical trial. Diabetes Care 2018;41(2):258-266.

[71] Aroda, VR, Bain SC, Cariou B, et al. Efficacy and safety of once-weekly semaglutide versus once-daily insulin glargine as add-on to metformin (with or without sulfonylureas) in insulin-naive patients with type 2 diabetes (SUSTAIN 4): a randomised, open-label, parallel-group, multicentre, multinational, phase 3a trial. Lancet Diabetes Endocrinol 2017;5(5): 355-366.

[72] Rodbard HW, Lingvay I, Reed J, et al. Semaglutide added to basal insulin in type 2 diabetes (SUSTAIN 5): a randomized, controlled trial. J Clin Endocrinol Metab 2018;103(6):2291-2301.

[73] Marso SP, Bain SC, Consoli A, et al. SUSTAIN-6 Investigators. Semaglutide and cardiovascular outcomes in patients with type 2 diabetes. N Engl J Med 2016;375(19):1834-1844.

[74] Pratley RE, Aroda VR, Lingvay I, et al. SUSTAIN 7 investigators. Semaglutide versus dulaglutide once weekly in patients with type 2 diabetes (SUSTAIN 7): a randomised, open-label, phase 3b trial. Lancet Diabetes Endocrinol 2018;6(4):275-286.

[75] Lingvay I., Catarig AM, Frias P, et al. Efficacy and safety of once-weekly semaglutide versus daily canagliflozin as add-on to metformin in patients with type 2 diabetes (SUSTAIN 8): a double-blind, phase 3b, randomised controlled trial. Lancet Diabetes Endocrinol 2019;7(11): 834-844.

[76] Zinman B, Bhosekar V, Busch R, et al. Semaglutide once weekly as add-on to SGLT-2 inhibitor therapy in type 2 diabetes (SUSTAIN 9): a randomised, placebo-controlled trial. Lancet Diabetes Endocrinol 2019;7(5):356-367.

[77] Capehorn MS, Catarig AM, Furberg JK, et al. Efficacy and safety of once-weekly semaglutide 1.0 mg vs once-daily liraglutide 1.2 mg as add-on to 1-3 oral antidiabetic drugs in subjects with type 2 diabetes (SUSTAIN 10). Diabetes Metab 2019;5(5):341-354.

[78] Chlup R, Zálešáková H, Šálková V. Účinná indikace semaglutidu. Kazuistika z diabetologické ambulance. (Effective indication of semaglutide. A case report from a diabetes out-patient dept. Czech). Kazuistiky v diabetologii (Diabetes Case Reports) 2019;17(4):16-18.

[79] Becker RHA. In response to: Heise T, Nørskov M, Nosek L, Kaplan K, Famulla S and Haahr HL. Insulin degludec: Lower day-to-day and within-day variability in pharmacodynamic response compared to insulin glargine U300 in type 1 diabetes. Diabetes Obes Metab 2017;19:1032-1039. Diabetes Obes Metab. 2018 Aug;20(8):2043-2047. doi: 10.1111/dom.13308. Epub 2018 May 6. PMID: 29600527.

[80] Gough SC, Bode BW, Woo VC, Rodbard HW, Linjawi S, Zacho M, Reiter PD, Buse JB. One-year efficacy and safety of a fixed combination of insulin degludec and liraglutide in patients with type 2 diabetes: results of a 26-week extension to a 26-week main trial. Diabetes Obes Metab. 2015;17(10):965-73. doi: 10.1111/dom.12498. Epub 2015 Jul 1. PMID: 25980900; PMCID: PMC4744775.

[81] Gough SC, Bode B, Woo V, Rodbard HW, Linjawi S, Poulsen P, Damgaard LH, Buse JB. NN9068-3697 (DUAL-I) trial investigators. Efficacy and safety of a fixed-ratio combination of insulin degludec and liraglutide (IDegLira) compared with its components given alone: results of a phase 3, open-label, randomised, 26-week, treat-to-target trial in insulin-naive patients with type 2 diabetes. Lancet Diabetes Endocrinol. 2014;2(11):885-93. doi: 10.1016/S2213-8587(14)70174-3. Epub 2014 Sep 1. PMID: 25190523.

[82] Linjawi S, Bode BW, Chaykin LB, Courrèges JP, Handelsman Y, Lehmann LM, Mishra A, Simpson RW. The efficacy of IDegLira (Insulin Degludec/Liraglutide combination) in adults with type 2 diabetes inadequately controlled with a GLP-1 receptor agonist and oral therapy: DUAL III Randomized Clinical Trial. Diabetes Ther. 2017 Feb;8(1):101-114. doi: 10.1007/s13300-016-0218-3. Epub 2016 Dec 10. PMID: 27943107; PMCID: PMC5306117.

[83] Lingvay I, Pérez Manghi F, García-Hernández P, Norwood P, Lehmann L, Tarp-Johansen MJ, Buse JB. DUAL V Investigators. Effect of Insulin Glargine Up-titration vs Insulin Degludec/Liraglutide on glycated Hemoglobin levels in patients with uncontrolled Type 2 Diabetes: The DUAL V Randomized Clinical Trial. JAMA. 2016;1;315(9):898-907. doi: 10.1001/jama.2016.1252. Erratum in: JAMA. 2016 May 17;315(19):2125. Tigkas, Stelios [corrected to Tigas, Stelios]. Erratum in: JAMA. 2016 May 17;315(19):2125. Tigkas, Stelios [corrected to Tigas, Stelios]. PMID: 26934259.

[84] Billings LK, Doshi A, Gouet D, Oviedo A, Rodbard HW, Tentolouris N, Grøn R, Halladin N, Jodar E. Efficacy and safety of IDegLira versus Basal-Bolus Insulin Therapy in patients with Type 2 Diabetes ucontrolled on metformin and basal insulin: The DUAL VII Randomized Clinical Trial. Diabetes Care. 2018;41(5):1009-1016. doi: 10.2337/dc17-1114. Epub 2018 Feb 26. PMID: 29483185.

[85] Sofra D. Glycemic control in a real-life setting in patients with Type 2 Diabetes treated with IDegLira at a single Swiss center. Diabetes Ther. 2017;8(2):377-384. doi: 10.1007/s13300-017-0234-y. Epub 2017 Feb 20. PMID: 28220460; PMCID: PMC5380496.

[86] Price H, Blüher M, Prager R, Phan TM, Thorsted BL, Schultes B; EXTRA study group. Use and effectiveness of a fixed-ratio combination of insulin degludec/liraglutide (IDegLira) in a real-world population with type 2 diabetes: Results from a European, multicentre, retrospective chart review study. Diabetes Obes Metab. 2018;20(4):954-962. doi: 10.1111/dom.13182. Epub 2018 Jan 11. PMID: 29205856; PMCID: PMC5873250.

[87] Philis-Tsimikas A, Billings LK, Busch R, Portillo CM, Sahay R,

Halladin N, Eggert S, Begtrup K, Harris S. Superior efficacy of insulin degludec/liraglutide versus insulin glargine U100 as add-on to sodium-glucose co-transporter-2 inhibitor therapy: A randomized clinical trial in people with uncontrolled type 2 diabetes. Diabetes Obes Metab. 2019;21(6):1399-1408. doi: 10.1111/dom.13666. Epub 2019 Apr 4. PMID: 30761720; PMCID: PMC6861. (DUAL IX)

[88] Chlup R, Kaňa R, Polcerová J, Zálešáková H, Ramík Z Možnosti léčby diabetu 2. typu při oslabení kognitivních funkcí. „Syndrom trosečníka (cast away). (Outlook of T2D treatment in patient's cognitive deterioration - „Cast away "syndrome.) Kazuistiky v diabetologii (Diabetes Case Reports. Czech.) 2019;17(2):35-40.

[89] Wiviott SD, Raz I, Bonaca MP, et al. DECLARE–TIMI 58 Investigators. Dapagliflozin and cardiovascular outcomes in type 2 diabetes. N Engl J Med 2019;380:347-357.

[90] McMurray JJV, Solomon SD, Inzucchi SE, et al. DAPA-HF Trial Committees and Investigators. Dapagliflozin in patients with heart failure and reduced ejection fraction. N Engl J Med. 21 November 2019 [Epub ahead of print]. DOI:10.1056/NEJMoa1911303.

[91] Kato ET, Silverman MG, Mosenzon O, et al. Effect of dapagliflozin on heart failure and mortality in type 2 diabetes mellitus. Circulation 2019;139:2528-2536.

[92] Inzucchi SE, Kosiborod M, Fitchett D, et al. Improvement in cardiovascular outcomes with empagliflozin is independent of glycemic control. Circulation 2018;138:1904-1907.

[93] Figtree GA, R°adholm K, Barrett TD, et al. Effects of canagliflozin on heart failure outcomes associated with preserved and reduced ejection fraction in type 2 diabetes mellitus. Circulation 2019;139:2591-2593.

[94] Perkovic V, Jardine MJ, Neal B, et al. CREDENCE Trial Investigators. Canagliflozin and renal outcomes in type 2 diabetes and nephropathy. N Engl J Med 2019;380:2295-2306.

[95] Mahaffey KW, Jardine MJ, Bompoint S, et al. Canagliflozin and cardiovascular and renal outcomes in type 2 diabetes mellitus and chronic kidney disease in primary and secondary cardiovascular prevention groups. Circulation 2019;140:739-750.

[96] Zelniker TA, Wiviott SD, Raz I, et al. Comparison of the effects of glucagon-like peptide receptor agonists and sodium-glucose cotransporter 2 inhibitors for prevention of major adverse cardiovascular and renal outcomes in type 2 diabetes mellitus. Circulation 2019;139:2022-2031.

[97] Chlup R, Zapletalová J, Ramík Z, Tzu Hsuan Cheng, Slezáková M, Zálešaková H. Impact of dapagliflozin on metabolic control in people with type 2 diabetes using insulin pumps. Diabetes 2017;66 (Suppl1):A297–A298 1119-P (Abstract).

[98] Zinman B, Aroda VR, Buse JB, Cariou B, Harris SB, Hoff ST, Pedersen KB, Tarp-Johansen MJ, Araki E. PIONEER 8 Investigators. Efficacy, safety, and tolerability of oral semaglutide versus placebo added to insulin with or without metformin in patients with type 2 diabetes: The PIONEER 8 Trial. Diabetes Care 2019;42(12):2262-2271. doi: 10.2337/dc19-0898. Epub 2019 Sep 17. PMID: 31530667; PMCID: PMC7364672

[99] Šoupal J, Petruželková L, Grunberger G et al. Glycemic outcomes in adults with T1D are impacted more by continuous glucose monitoring than by insulin delivery method: 3 years of follow-up from the COMISAIR study. Diabetes Care 2020;43:37-43.

[100] Rosenstock J, Kjćrsgaard M, Miller D, Hansen M, Goldenberg R. Once-weekly basal insulin icodec offers comparable efficacy and safety vs once-daily insulin glargine U100 in insulin naive patients with type 2 diabetes inadequately controlled on OADs. Virtual EASD annual meeting 21-25. September 2020. Diabetologia 2020.

[101] Cardio-Metabolic Academy Europe East, Expert Panel, Banach M, Gaita D, Haluzik M, Janez A, Kamenov Z, Kempler P, Lalic N, Linhart A, Mikhailidis DP, Nocoń A, Nunes JS, Papanas N, Raposo JF, M. Rizzo M, a Stoian AP. Adoption of the ADA/EASD guidelines in 10 Eastern and Southern European countries: physician survey and good clinical practice recommendations from an international expert panel. Diabetes Research and Clinical Practice 2021; 172, doi: https://doi.org/10.1016/j.diabres.2020.108535

[102] Langerhans P. Beiträge zur mikroscopischen Anatomie der Bauchspeicheldrüse. Wilhelms-Friedrich Wilhelm Universität zu Berlin, printed by G. Lange, 1869.

[103] Mering J, Minkowski O. Diabetes mellitus nach Pankreas extirpation. Zbl Klin Med 1889;10:393-394.

[104] Zülzer G. Über Versuche einer spezifischen Ferment Therapie des Diabetes. Zeitschrift f exp Pathologie u Therapie 1908;5:307-318.

[105] Scott EL. On the influence of intravenous injections of an extract of the pancreas on experimental pancreatic diabetes Am J Phys 1912;9:306-310.

[106] Jörgens V. They got very near the goal: Zülzer, Scott, and Paulescu. In: V Jörgens M Porta, Eds. Unveiling Diabetes Historical Milestones in Diabetology Front Diabetes 2020 Karger p. 58-72.

[107] Porta M. One hundred years ago: the dawning of the insulin era. Acta Diabetologica 2021;58:1-4. https://doi.org/10.1007/s00592-020-01642-1

Chapter 2

# Redox Signaling is Essential for Insulin Secretion

*Petr Ježek, Blanka Holendová, Martin Jabůrek, Jan Tauber, Andrea Dlasková and Lydie Plecitá-Hlavatá*

## Abstract

In this review, we place redox signaling in pancreatic β-cells to the context with signaling pathways leading to insulin secretion, acting for example upon the action of incretins (GLP-1, GIP) and the metabotropic receptor GPR40. Besides a brief description of ion channel participation in depolarization/repolarization of the plasma membrane, we emphasize a prominent role of the elevated glucose level in pancreatic β-cells during glucose-stimulated insulin secretion (GSIS). We focus on our recent findings, which revealed that for GSIS, not only elevated ATP synthesis is required, but also fundamental redox signaling originating from the NADPH oxidase 4- (NOX4-) mediated $H_2O_2$ production. We hypothesized that the closing of the ATP-sensitive $K^+$ channel ($K_{ATP}$) is only possible when both ATP plus $H_2O_2$ are elevated in INS-1E cells. $K_{ATP}$ alone or with synergic channels provides an element of logical sum, integrating both metabolic plus redox homeostasis. This is also valid for other secretagogues, such as branched chain ketoacids (BCKAs); and partly for fatty acids (FAs). Branched chain aminoacids, leucine, valine and isoleucine, after being converted to BCKAs are metabolized by a series of reactions resembling β-oxidation of FAs. This increases superoxide formation in mitochondria, including its portion elevated due to the function of electron transfer flavoprotein ubiquinone oxidoreductase (ETF:QOR). After superoxide conversion to $H_2O_2$ the oxidation of BCKAs provides the mitochondrial redox signaling extending up to the plasma membrane to induce its depolarization together with the elevated ATP. In contrast, experimental FA-stimulated insulin secretion in the presence of non-stimulating glucose concentrations is predominantly mediated by GPR40, for which intramitochondrial redox signaling activates phospholipase iPLA2γ, cleaving free FAs from mitochondrial membranes, which diffuse to the plasma membrane and largely amplify the GPR40 response. These events are concomitant to the insulin release due to the metabolic component. Hypothetically, redox signaling may proceed by simple $H_2O_2$ diffusion or via an SH-relay enabled by peroxiredoxins to target proteins. However, these aspects have yet to be elucidated.

**Keywords:** pancreatic β-cells, insulin secretion, redox signaling, NADPH oxidase 4, branched chain ketoacid oxidation, fatty acid β-oxidation, ATP-sensitive $K^+$ channel, GLP1, GPR40

## 1. Introduction

Recently, we revealed that physiological redox signaling is essential for the first phase of glucose-stimulated insulin secretion (GSIS) in pancreatic β-cells. Elevated

 IntechOpen

glucose intake contributes to the increasing pentose phosphate pathway (PPP) supply of NADPH for NADPH oxidase 4 (NOX4), which directly produces $H_2O_2$. The burst of $H_2O_2$ then represents a redox signal, which fundamentally determines GSIS, while inducing a cooperative induction of plasma membrane depolarization together with ATP elevation (**Figure 1**) [1]. The latter originates from the increased ATP synthesis by oxidative phosphorylation (OXPHOS). Hypothetically, either a closure of the ATP-sensitive $K^+$ channel ($K_{ATP}$) is dependent on both $H_2O_2$ plus ATP; or $H_2O_2$ activates a synergic channel such as transient receptor potential

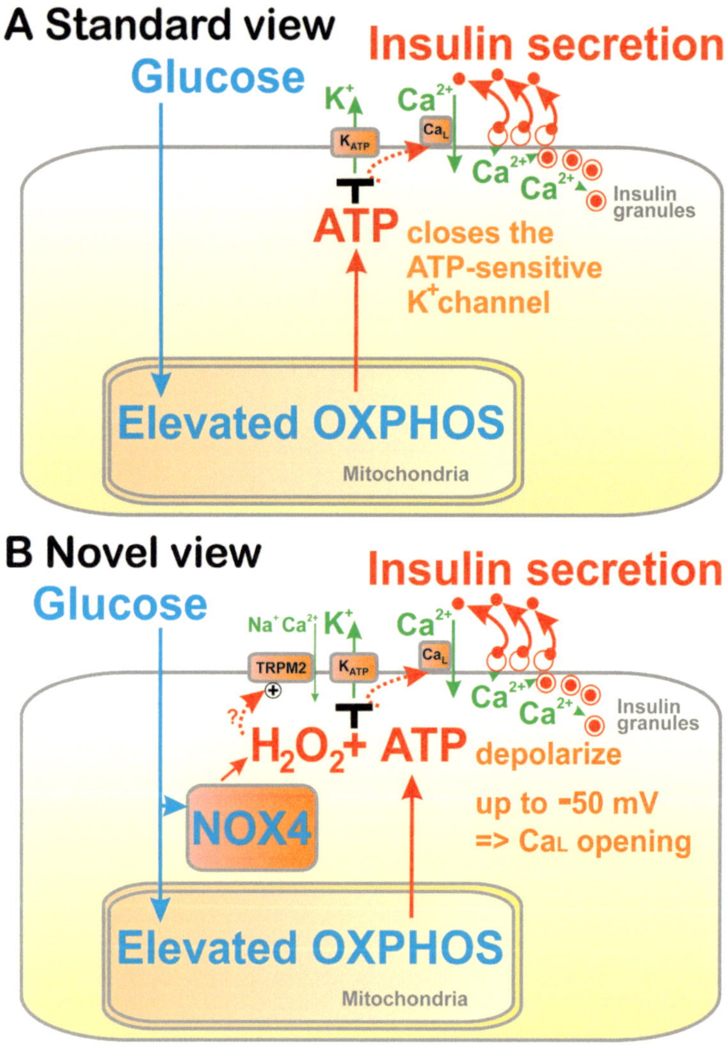


**Figure 1.**

*(A) Traditional ("standard") view of the triggering mechanism of GSIS compared with (B) new paradigm in GSIS mechanism ("novel"), for which the redox signaling by NOX4-produced $H_2O_2$ is essentially required. Upon the glucose intake, PPP and redox shuttles supply cytosolic NADPH to increase NOX4 activity and thus elevate $H_2O_2$ which substantiates redox signaling. Either, the ATP-sensitive $K^+$ channel ($K_{ATP}$) is closed exclusively when both ATP plus $H_2O_2$ are elevated. Alternatively, $H_2O_2$ activates opening of TRPM2 or other nonspecific cation channels required for a depolarization shift to reach a threshold potential of −50 mV, at which the voltage-sensitive $Ca^{2+}$ channels ($Ca_L$) become open, thus starting to fire the action potential. Resulting $Ca^{2+}$ influx into the cell cytosol allows a complex process of exocytosis of the insulin granule vesicles (IGVs), beginning during the so-called 1st phase of GSIS by fusion of pre-attached IGVs with the plasma membrane and exposure of the IGV interior to the extracellular space (capillaries in vivo). $Ca^{2+}$ also promotes the recruitment of distant IGVs towards the plasma membrane as well as ensures the late, so-called 2nd phase of GSIS, lasting about 1 hour in vivo.*

melastin 2 (TRPM2) [2], required for sufficient depolarization. This principle of a logical summation of metabolic plus redox stimulation seems to be universal for other secretagogues (i.e. compounds stimulating insulin secretion), dependent on $K_{ATP}$. However, note that the redox signaling must be distinguished from the oxidative stress [3–6].

## 2. Two phases of GSIS

Two phases exist for GSIS in vivo [7–11]. They are also recognized in isolated pancreatic islets (PIs), but not in insulin-secreting β-cell lines. The consensus became that both $K_{ATP}$-dependent mechanism (also termed „triggering") and $K_{ATP}$-independent mechanisms contribute to both phases [12], while the $K_{ATP}$-independent mechanism still requires the elevation of cytosolic $Ca^{2+}$ [13]. The 2nd phase in vivo was even considered to be independent of the extracellular glucose concentrations [14]. It depends more on the molecular mechanism of the increased sustained mobilization and priming of insulin granule vesicles (IGVs) [15].

The first rapid peak of insulin secretion is observed at 5–10 min after administration of a bolus of glucose in vivo or addition of glucose to the isolated PIs. The 1st phase involves the exocytosis of pre-docked juxtaposed IGVs, residing 100–200 nm from the plasma membrane prior to triggering [16, 17] and also possesses a contribution of deeper localized granules arriving within 50 ms, which were not initially pre-docked [18, 19]. The 2nd phase typically lasts over 1 hr. As a result, a predominant insulin amount is released in this phase. The 2nd phase results most likely from further delayed recruitment of IGVs belonging to the typically excessive reserve. The past hypothesis suggested a main reason for such a delay to involve the restricted passage through the filamentous actin (F-actin) cytoskeleton [20–22], but later a microfilament-independent movement of IGVs was reported [21, 23–25]. However, numerous cytoskeleton components play a more detailed role in the IGV exocytosis, not representing only a simple barrier. Generally, the IGV exocytosis relies on synaptogamin activation by $Ca^{2+}$, syntaxin, SNAP-25, and other target proteins of the SNARE family (SNAp REceptors, where SNAP is soluble NSF attachment proteins and NSF is a N-ethylmaleimide-sensitive fusion factor). They attract IGVs via the IGV-localized synaptobrevins (vesicle-associated membrane proteins), while forming a coiled-coil quarternaly structure [26]. The resulting SNARE core complex relocates the IGV and plasma membrane into proximity, thus facilitating establishment of so-called fusion stalk. Further zippering of coiled-coil structures allows fusion of larger part of the IGV membrane with the plasma membrane until a fusion pore is formed.

However, the recent explanation for the second phase is based on the fact that the two phases of insulin secretion exist when isolated pancreatic islets are studied, but do not exist for isolated primary pancreatic β-cells [27–29]. Hence, the role of inter-cellular contacts is emphasized for the 2nd phase. The inter-cellular contacts allow synchronization of the plasma membrane potential, while paracrine hormone secretion may also contribute to modification and termination of insulin release.

## 3. Mechanisms of the 1st phase of GSIS

GSIS has been consensually described to involve a so-called triggering mechanism accompanied by amplifying mechanism(s) [7, 12, 30–36]. The triggering is exclusively dependent on the $K_{ATP}$ closure and attaining plasma membrane depolarization up to −50 mV. The latter is achieved in a synergy of $K_{ATP}$ with other ion channels. The amplifying mechanisms are given by metabolism or stem from the action of incretins and other hormones. Also, mechanisms concerning other secretagogues, such as branched chain ketoacids (BCKAs) and fatty acids (FAs), were considered as merely amplifying. Nevertheless, we will show below the ambiguity of such a classification. The amplifying mechanisms originate from an incremental increase in $Ca^{2+}$ elevations, not existing within the canonical "triggering" mechanism. Alternatively, they stem from facilitation via numerous proteins of the exocytotic machinery localized either on the IGV or plasma membranes. Therefore, some of these types of events might be $Ca^{2+}$ independent and hence may also proceed at low glucose concentrations.

The traditional explanation of the triggering mechanism of GSIS relied exclusively on the ATP elevation (or elevation of the ATP/ADP ratio) in the cytosol of β-cells. Sole elevated ATP was considered to be sufficient for the $K_{ATP}$ closing [30–33]. Any additional requirement for a parallel redox signaling was not considered, despite the findings that reactive oxygen species (ROS) have been implicated in insulin secretion. This concerned with at least ROS of mitochondrial origin [37], or resulting from mono-oleoyl-glycerol addition [38]. The blockage of PPP, that decreased insulin secretion, also shifted redox homeostasis [39]. An unspecified link of GSIS with the externally added $H_2O_2$ was reported, besides antioxidant effects at decreased glutathione by diethylmaleate [40]. Previously, also an unidentified isoform of NADPH oxidase was implicated in GSIS, since an antisense p47PHOX oligonucleotide [41] or an unspecific NOX inhibitors attenuated GSIS [38, 42, 43].

Recently, we have provided the evidence that the elevated OXPHOS is insufficient to initiate GSIS, despite the increased ATP levels and the elevated ATP/ADP ratio at the peri-plasma- membrane space [1]. We demonstrated that NOX4 is fundamentally required for GSIS [1]. In model rat pancreatic β-cells (INS-1E cells) with silenced NOX4 or in full NOX4 knockout (NOX4KO) mice and in mice with NOX4 knockout, specifically in pancreatic β-cells (NOX4βKO mice), the 1st phase of GSIS was largely blocked [1]. In both studied NOX4 KO mice strains and in their isolated PIs, the 1st phase of GSIS was abolished with NOX4 ablation, while in PIs, either overexpression of NOX4 (achieved at least in the peripheral spheroid layer of islets) or additions of $H_2O_2$ rescued this 1st phase. No effects were found in NOX2 KO mice, although NOX2 has been previously implicated to play an antagonistic role for redox homeostasis [44].

Moreover, using a patch-clamp of INS-1E cells, we demonstrated that the $K_{ATP}$ closure is possible only when NOX4 is intact in INS-1E cells. After showing the well-known closure of $K_{ATP}$ induced by high glucose concentration in cells transfected with scrambled siRNA, we observed no glucose-induced $K_{ATP}$ closure in INS-1E cells silenced for NOX4 [1]. These experiments supported the model, in which $K_{ATP}$ integrates metabolic and redox homeostasis and acts as a logical summation for which both elevated ATP plus elevated $H_2O_2$ exclusively lead to a triggering of GSIS (**Figure 1**). However, since without cation fluxes provided by nonspecific cation channels a threshold depolarization of −50 mV cannot be achieved, despite 100% $K_{ATP}$ ensemble being closed [45, 46], we may also hypothesize that $H_2O_2$ alternatively or in parallel activates the TRPM2 channel [2], known to contain redox-sensitive Met residue [47].

Thus our results set a new paradigm for GSIS, since it had never been considered that the sole ATP increase is insufficient for GSIS and is insufficient particularly for the closing of $K_{ATP}$; as well as it had never been considered that any redox signaling might essentially participate in GSIS.

In further work, we also demonstrated that the redox signaling upon GSIS is provided by elevations of cytosolic $H_2O_2$, whereas ROS in the mitochondrial matrix (both $H_2O_2$ and superoxide release) are diminished due to the enhanced operation of the redox shuttles upon GSIS [48]. One may expect that a portion of cytosolic NADPH as a substrate for NOX4 is provided by the glucose-6-phosphate dehydrogenase and also by 6-phosphogluconate dehydrogenase downstream within the PPP, whereas the second portion is generated due to the operation of redox shuttles. These shuttles become more active at higher glucose concentrations and increasingly produce NADPH. NADPH is particularly produced by isocitrate dehydrogenase 1 (IDH1) and malic enzyme 1 (ME1) in the cytosol upon operation of these redox shuttles [48].

In summary, we describe the revisited mechanism of the 1st phase of GSIS as follows. Elevated glucose metabolism and glycolysis allows an increased branching of the metabolic flux, particularly of glucose-6-phosphate G6P, toward PPP, which acts as a predominant source of NADPH. The essential role of PPP was emphasized elsewhere [49]. Amplification of the cytosolic NADPH is also provided by IDH1 and ME1 due to the elevated operation of the three redox shuttles. Since NOX4 was determined as the only NADPH oxidase producing $H_2O_2$ directly [50, 51], its reaction results in an increase of $H_2O_2$ release into the cell cytosol [1]. Finally, the elevated $H_2O_2$, together with concomitantly elevated ATP from the enhanced OXPHOS, is the only way for plasma membrane depolarization up to −50 mV [1]. This threshold subsequently induces $Ca_L$ opening, followed by the $Ca^{2+}$ influx into the cell cytosol, which in turn induces the exocytosis of insulin granule vesicles. The action potential spikes are then determined by the cycles of $Ca_L$ opening, followed by the opening of voltage-dependent channels ($K_V$) in rodents [52] or calcium-dependent ($K_{Ca}$) $K^+$-channels in humans. Their action deactivates $Ca_L$, which are, however, again activated in the next $Ca_L$-$K_V$ cycle.

Pancreatic β-cells were undoubtedly adapted by phylogenesis to serve as a perfect glucose sensor. The glucose sensing is allowed by several key specific features. At first, specific isoforms of glucose transporters, GLUT2 in rodents and GLUT1 in humans, equilibrate the plasma glucose concentration with the glucose concentration in the cytosol of β-cells [53, 54]. Second, a specific isoform IV of hexokinase (also termed glucokinase) cannot be feed-back inhibited by its product glucose-6-phosphate. As a result, there is an efficient unidirectional flux towards the glycolysis [55, 56] and, most probably, this allows also branching into the PPP [49]. Originally, the PPP was accounted to utilize only 10% of glucose, due to presumably feed-back inhibition by glucose [57, 58]. However, metabolomics studies associated PPP intermediates with GSIS [59], confirming previous studies with various PPP inhibitors [59–62]. These results collectively demonstrated the important PPP contribution to GSIS. This contribution is also reflected by existing patients having a deficiency of glucose-6-phosphate dehydrogenase associated with the impaired 1st phase of GSIS [63].

The third aspect leading to the perfect glucose sensing lays in the virtual absence of lactate dehydrogenase in β-cells and inefficiency in pyruvate dehydrogenase kinases (PDK) [64]. PDKs would otherwise block pyruvate dehydrogenase (PDH). Thus the highly active PDH and other dehydrogenases, activated also by $Ca^{2+}$ influx into the mitochondrial matrix [65], altogether enable that 100% of pyruvate and its equivalents (after pyruvate conversion by transaminases) is utilized by OXPHOS. A minor pyruvate flux ensures anaplerosis of oxaloacetate due to the reaction of pyruvate carboxylase [66]. Its reaction is also important also for the pyruvate/malate redox shuttle.

The fourth aspect reflects the in vivo inhibitory role of the mitochondrial ATPase inhibitory factor, IF1. IF1 adjusts a proper glucose concentration range for GSIS in rat pancreatic β-cells, INS-1E [67, 68]. This is suggested by the demonstration that IF1 silencing allows insulin secretion even at very low glucose approaching to zero in INS-1E cells [67]. In contrast, the IF1 overexpression inhibited GSIS in INS-1E cells [68]. This IF1 role awaits confirmation in vivo.

## 4. Plasma membrane events following $K_{ATP}$ closure

Surprisingly, the plasma membrane of β-cells contains up to 60 channels of 16 ion channel families [69]. Moreover, ion channels are also located on the membrane of IGVs to facilitate fusion with the plasma membrane and insulin exocytosis. Resting plasma membrane potential (*V*p) is created predominantly by the activity of $K^+$-channels due to a higher concentration of $K^+$ inside the β-cell (~150 mM), exceeding that one established outside in capillaries or interstitial fluid (~5 mM). Experimentally, *V*p values are measured to be approximately of – 75 mV [70]. The $K_{ATP}$ closure then induces depolarization [69, 71–73] and activation of $Ca_L$ [74]. The action potential firing is the entity that activates $Ca_L$-$K_V$ cycles (in rodents), however this firing is initiated by more channel types.

Surprisingly, the action potential firing is not induced until >90% of $K_{ATP}$ channels are closed [75, 76]. As a result, only the closure of the remaining ~10% of the $K_{ATP}$ population leads to depolarization [76]. In fact, the activity of the whole $K_{ATP}$ population decreases exponentially with the increasing glucose concentration. Interestingly, 50% of the $K_{ATP}$ population is already closed at 2–3 mM glucose, while *V*p remains steady. However, at about 7 mM glucose, 100% of the $K_{ATP}$ ensemble is closed. This is being reflected by the completely vanished $K_{ATP}$ current, which leads to action potential firing [69, 70]. This event is termed as a supra-threshold depolarization.

Thus, hyperpolarized interburst phases are induced, while a nearly permanent firing exists at high >25 mM glucose [70]. An intermediate depolarization at 10 mM glucose was reported for mouse β-cells, reversed upon withdrawal of $Ca^{2+}$ and $Na^+$, supporting the participation of other channels, such as nonspecific cation channels, contributing to the depolarization (inward) flux [45]. Even an efflux of $Cl^-$ was suggested to fulfil this role [77], including the opening of LRRC8/VRAC anion channels [78, 79]. The participation of TRPM4 and TRPM5 [80] providing inward currents of certain levels seem to be required for induction of sufficient membrane depolarization together with $K_{ATP}$ closing [46]. This is because the measured resting *V*p of – 75 to –70 mV is already depolarized by a some extent from the equilibrium $Vp^{equi}$ of –82 mV (5 mM vs. 130 mM [$K^+$]). The shift is probably due to the opening of nonspecific cation channels, since any of $Na^+$, $Ca^{2+}$ and $K^+$ can penetrate them. The 100% $K_{ATP}$ closing at higher glucose causes only an insufficient depolarization. Without nonspecific cation channels (or $Cl^-$ channels), the established *V*p would only be equal to $Vp^{equi}$, so any shift to –50 mV required for $Ca_L$ would not take place. Contribution by the basal opening of other synergic channels is therefore essential. Open synergic channels always induce the inward shift in *V*p, so to that depolarization given by 100% $K_{ATP}$ closing reaches –50 mV. This allows opening of $Ca_L$ and action potential firing. In summary, besides the heat-activated TRPV1 channel (capsaicin receptor), and TRPV2 or TRPV4, the $H_2O_2$-activated TRPM2 [2], or $Ca^{2+}$-activated TRPM4 and TRPM5 channels belong to the important group of possible synergic channels expressed in β-cells [46].

The same reasoning concerns with anion channels, particularly $Cl^-$ channels. The active $Cl^-$ transport is provided in β-cells by SLC12A, SLC4A, and SlC26A channels. These channels set the cytosolic $Cl^-$ concentration above thermodynamic equilibrium. Besides $GABA_A$, $GABA_B$ and glycine receptor $Cl^-$ channels considered to be part of the insulin secretion machinery, also volume-regulated anion channels (VRAC) were shown to be open at high glucose. VRACs are heteromers of the leucine-rich repeat containing 8 isoform A (LRRC8A) with other LLRC8 isoforms, forming anion channels [79]. Ablation of LRRC8 in mice led to delayed $Ca^{2+}$ responses of β-cells to glucose and diminished GSIS in mice, demonstrating the modulatory role of LRRC8A/VRAC on membrane depolarization leading to $Ca_L$ responses [78, 79].

Upon the action potential firing thus metabolically driven *Vp* oscillations occur due to the initial glucose rising [69, 70]. Cytosolic $Ca^{2+}$ oscillations are superimposed from fast (2–60 s periods) and slow (up to several min) $Ca^{2+}$ oscillations [81], stemming from *Vp* oscillations and an interplay with $Ca^{2+}$ efflux from the endoplasmic reticulum (ER) [82]. Collectively they lead to pulsatile insulin secretion. The ER involvement is given by the phospholipase C (PLC), responding to the glucose-stimulated $Ca^{2+}$ influx. PLC produces inositol triphosphate (IP3), which opens the $Ca^{2+}$ channel of IP3 receptor (IP3R) of ER; plus diacylglycerol (DAG). Importantly, DAG permits the opening of TRPM4 and TRPM5 via the protein kinase C (PKC) pathway. Another ER $Ca^{2+}$ channel, the ryanodine receptor (RyR) may also participate, being activated by ATP, fructose, long-chain acyl-CoAs and cyclic adenosine 5′-diphosphate ribose [81]. Also, the role of other channels was demonstrated for permitting store-operated $Ca^{2+}$ entry from ER, particularly of the ternary complex of TRPC1/Orai1/STIM1 [46, 83]. TRPC1 belongs to the transient receptor potential canonical (TRPC) family with a modest $Ca^{2+}$ selectivity. TRPC1 interacts with Orai1 [84], and in such a functional complex, its channels are activated by STIM1, affecting the amplitude of $Ca^{2+}$ oscillations, and correlating with GSIS.

As mentioned above, deactivation of $Ca_L$ is ensured by the opening of voltage-dependent channels ($K_V$) in rodents [52] or calcium-dependent ($K_{Ca}$) $K^+$-channels in humans. Among the former, tetrameric $K_V2.1$ is the prevalent form in rodent β-cells. A delayed rectifier $K^+$-current is induced at positive *Vp* down to −30 mV [85]. The opening of $K_V2.1$ channels repolarizes *Vp* and thus closes $Ca_L$ channels. Ablation of $K_V2.1$ thus reduces Kv currents by ~80% and prolongs the duration of the action potential, so more insulin is secreted. Mice with ablated $K_V2.1$ possess lower fasting glycemia but elevated insulin and reportedly improved GSIS [86]. In contrast, human β-cells use $K_{Ca}1.1$ channels (i.e. BK channels) for repolarization of *Vp* [70]. Note also that down-regulation of $K_V$ was observed after islet incubation with high glucose for 24 hr [87].

## 5. Possible redox regulations of $K_{ATP}$ and other channels

The structure of $K_{ATP}$ has been resolved and numerous mutagenesis studies of $K_{ATP}$ have been conducted. Amino acid residues that are candidate redox targets are yet to be identified. The $K_{ATP}$ channel is a hetero-octamer consisting of four external regulatory sulfonylurea receptor 1 (SUR1, a product of *Abcc8* gene) subunits and four pore-forming subunits of potassium inward rectifier, Kir6.2 (*Kcnj11* gene) [88, 89]. These Kir6.2 subunits cluster in the middle of ~18 nm size structure with a ~13 nm height [90]. The part exposed to the cytosol contains an ATP binding site, located about 2 nm below the membrane. A single ATP molecule was reported to close the channel, i.e. with the other three binding sites left unoccupied [91]. However, the ATP binding site overlaps with the binding site for phosphatidylinositol 4,5-bisphosphate ($PIP_2$), which stabilizes the open state. Palmitoylation of Cys166 of Kir6.2 was then reported to amplify the responsiveness to $PIP_2$ [92]. Upon the release of $PIP_2$ from the binding site, the open probability becomes decreased [90, 93, 94].

Diazoxide or cromakalim, as well as numerous other openers, set $K_{ATP}$ pharmacologically in the open state even at a high ATP concentration [95]. In contrast, the artificial $K_{ATP}$ closing by sulfonylurea derivatives, such as glibenclamide, takes place independently of ATP. Besides this sulfonylurea binding site, each of the four SUR1 subunits contains MgATP and MgADP binding sites. MgATP is hydrolyzed at the nucleotide binding fold 1 (NBF1) to MgADP. Resulting MgADP subsequently activates $K_{ATP}$ at NBF2. This is indeed reflected by the ATP-sensitive increase in $K^+$ conductance and following lower excitability, accompanied by the lower sensitivity to ATP inhibition [91].

The phosphorylation of $K_{ATP}$ reportedly sets the sensitivity of the $K_{ATP}$ ensemble. The setting is such that transitions upon the glucose rise from 3 or 5 mM to 7 mM or > 10 mM result in the closing of the remaining 10% of the initially open channels by elevations between just the two ATP concentrations falling into the mM range. Any redox component in this was never indicated and should be studied. Nevertheless, phosphorylation mediated by the protein kinase A (PKA) was already reported to act in this unusual setting. Thus Thr224 [96] and Ser372 were reported to be the verified PKA phosphorylation sites. Their phosphorylation increases the open probability of $K_{ATP}$ [97]. This might hypothetically provide closing mechanism acting at higher ATP concentration or even requiring $H_2O_2$. In a longer time scale, phosphorylation also increases the number of channels in the plasma membrane. Also, Thr224 was found to be phosphorylated by $Ca^{2+}$ and calmodulin-dependent kinase II (CaMKII) while interacting with $\beta_{IV}$-spectrin [98]. In vivo, also autonomic innervations and paracrine stimulation ensure sufficient PKA-mediated phosphorylation of $K_{ATP}$.

Since the original discovery of the essential role of $K_{ATP}$ in GSIS [99], only an indirect inhibition of $K_{ATP}$ by $H_2O_2$ was observed in smooth muscle cells [100]. Nevertheless, other redox-sensitive targets have been identified in pancreatic β-cells. But we can exclude the possibility that the IGV exocytosis itself might be directly induced by $H_2O_2$, independently of $Ca^{2+}$ [52], since the ability of exogenous $H_2O_2$ to induce insulin secretion in INS-1E cells was only partially blocked by NOX4-siRNA, but it was completely blocked by a $Ca_L$ blocker nimodipine [1]. Consequently, albeit the used $H_2O_2$ doses exceeded 100 μM, they did not directly stimulate the $K_{ATP}$-independent exocytosis of insulin granules.

A second possibility would be that $Ca_L$ channels themselves may be hypothetically co-activated by $H_2O_2$. Third, the plasma membrane depolarization might be redox sensitive, so that $H_2O_2$ could directly or indirectly inhibit repolarizing $K^+$-channels, such as $K_V$ [101–103]. The fourth plausible redox link with GSIS would concern with the reported redox activation of TPRM2 depolarizing channels [2]. The latter is the most plausible, since it is related to a $Ca^{2+}$-induced [52, 104] or $H_2O_2$-induced exocytosis of insulin granules by the $H_2O_2$-activation of TPRM2 depolarizing channels [2, 105]. Note, our results excluded the $Ca^{2+}$-independent $H_2O_2$-induced exocytosis of IGVs at least in rat pancreatic β-cells [1]. Therefore, if the $H_2O_2$-activated TRPM2-dependent mechanism exists, it must provide the required synergy with $K_{ATP}$, to reach the −50 mV plasma membrane depolarization threshold. Note also, that TRPM2 was already implicated as a significant player in the GLP-1 potentiation of insulin secretion [106].

Finally, a competition for NADPH between NOX4 and a hypothetical NADPH-activated $K^+$-channel could exist. Nevertheless, using patch-clamped INS-1E cells in a whole cell mode, we demonstrated a closure of $K_{ATP}$ by $H_2O_2$ produced by NOX4 at high glucose, since in cells silenced for NOX4, even ATP resulting from the metabolism of high glucose was unable to close the $K_{ATP}$ channel [1].

## 6. Receptor-mediated amplification of insulin secretion

G protein-coupled receptors activating heterotrimeric G proteins ensure pleiades of cell responses, mutually interrelated. G proteins typically regulate production of second messengers. Thus Gαs proteins increase generation of cyclic AMP (cAMP), whereas Gαi/o proteins decrease it [107–109]. The G proteins Gαq/11 initiate PLC-mediated hydrolysis of phosphatidylinositol 4,5-bisphosphate into diacylglycerol (DAG) and IP3 [110, 111]. Gα12/13 proteins promote protein RhoA for remodeling of the cytoskeleton [112]. Class of proteins termed β-arrestins initiates signaling via proximal MAP kinase, IκB, and Akt pathways [113]. The latter two G protein classes rather control long-term effects.

Let us emphasize downstream pathways that are important for acute effects in pancreatic β-cells, which predominantly lead to either modulation of the plasma membrane channels, typically $Ca_L$, $K_{ATP}$ and $K_V$, so to ensure more intensive insulin secretion; or their action evokes stimulation of insulin secretion via ensuring the surplus $Ca^{2+}$ influx to the cytosol from ER or mitochondria; or, else, their action targets proteins of the exocytotic machinery on the IGV or plasma membranes. The latter responses alter the kinetics of IGVs in docking, priming and fusion with the plasma membrane, so to facilitate exocytosis. Interestingly, these events could be independent of $Ca_L$ and theoretically could take place at low glucose concentrations.

Activation of Gαs increases the activity of transmembrane adenylate cyclases (tmAC) producing cAMP from ATP [108, 109]. A number of phosphodiesterases (of 11 families) degrade cAMP (some also or exclusively cGMP). cAMP is a universal 2nd messenger having a specific function in amplifying of GSIS and insulin secretion stimulated with other secretagogues. Also, soluble adenylate cyclases (sACs) exist, notably in the mitochondrial matrix, while their reaction is potentiated by $Ca^{2+}$ and bicarbonate. The major mediators of cAMP effects are cAMP-dependent PKA [114], including PKA tethered to the outer mitochondrial membrane [115, 116], and the parallel pathway of enhanced signaling via exchange proteins directly activated by cAMP 2 (EPAC2) [117–119].

In pancreatic β-cells, the PKA pathway is involved in signaling of incretin (GLP-1 and GIP) receptors [107, 120]. It exerts a minor contribution to signaling from metabotropic receptors, such as GPR40, which is sensing long chain fatty acids [111]. PKA typically amplifies the $Ca^{2+}$-dependent exocytosis of insulin granules. The core pathway involves PKA phosphorylation and hence activation of the $Ca_L$ β2-subunit, in concert with $K_{ATP}$ phosphorylation decreasing the ATP concentration range required for its closure (see above) [121]. In addition, PKA inhibits Kv channels, which otherwise terminate plasma membrane depolarization; hence this prolongs already more intensive $Ca^{2+}$ influx via phosphorylated $Ca_L$ and hence exocytosis of insulin granules [122].

Another PKA target is the exocytosis-modulating protein termed snapin, the phosphorylation of which allows its interaction with the other IGV proteins, which enhances the 1st GSIS phase [123]. Snapin participates in tethering of IGVs to the plasma membrane by coiled-coil interaction with a lipid-anchored protein SNAP-25 [124].

Altogether, the PKA pathway ensures about 50% of cAMP responses in β-cells [125], while the EPAC2 pathway ensures the remaining responses [117–119]. EPAC2 protein possesses a guanine nucleotide exchange activity, thus inducing the $Ca^{2+}$-induced $Ca^{2+}$release from ER via RyR [126] (questioned in [127]), occurring only at high glucose, since it requires the primary $Ca_L$ opening [128], which also partially refills the ER $Ca^{2+}$ stores. The EPAC2 pathway also affects the IGV proteins and thus facilitates the insulin exocytosis. For example, Rim2a protein is a target [129, 130], located on the inner plasma membrane surface and on IGVs, representing a scaffold for IGV exocytosis [131]. Rim2a interacts with Rab3A of IGVs and the resulting Rim2a-Rab3A complex facilitates docking of IGVs into the plasma membrane. This is followed by so-called priming, which is subsequently initiated by the Rim2a interaction with the Munc13–1 protein. Munc13–1 then opens syntaxin 1 from its closed conformation, thus allowing fusion with the plasma membrane. EPAC2 also interacts with NBD1 of SUR1, being released by cAMP [35]. Such locally released EPAC2 induces the release of Rim2 from the α1.2 $Ca_L$ subunit.

The local $Ca^{2+}$ influx within $Ca_L$ ensures EPAC2 binding to Rim2, and subsequent interaction with another $Ca^{2+}$ sensor termed Piccolo. The heterotrimeric complex then interacts with Rab3A and enables IGV exocytosis.

Interestingly, all necessary components of the PKA pathway were identified in the mitochondrial matrix, including sAC, PDE2A2 [132], and also PKA [133]. However, we may also speculate that some proteins can be phosphorylated by cytosolic PKA or by its fraction attached to OMM prior to their import to the mitochondrial matrix. There was also a consensus that cAMP cannot freely diffuse to the matrix [132]. Thus cAMP in the mitochondrial matrix may act as an independent pool [134, 135]. Its source is the matrix-located soluble adenylate cyclase sAC, which is activated by bicarbonate and $Ca^{2+}$ [136, 137]. Since $CO_2$ is increasingly released when the Krebs cycle turnover increases upon GSIS, the matrix localized mtPKA can be activated in this way [138]. In any case, OXPHOS is facilitated in mitochondria of numerous tissues via phosphorylation of Complex I NDUFS4 subunit (facilitating its Hsp70-mediated import), Complex IV COXIV-1 subunit (preventing its inhibition by ATP) [139] as well as via IF1, enhancing ATP synthesis by disabling the inhibitory binding of phosphorylated IF1 dimers to the ATP synthase [140]. A link to redox homeostasis can be viewed in the observed release of the PKA catalytic subunits by the increased ROS [141, 142]. Thus mtPKA can act in parallel to the cytosolic PKA signaling initiated by GPR40 and GLPR or GIPR receptors. PKA targeting of at least IF1, and probably also of Complex I and Complex IV, should contribute to the amplification of insulin secretion by FAs or incretins.

The G protein Gαq/11 initiates signaling through the phospholipase C (PLC-)-mediated hydrolysis of phosphatidylinositol 4,5-bisphosphate into DAG and inositol triphosphate IP3 [110]. The main effector of DAG is protein kinase C (PKC), which is activated by DAG. One of the effectors of IP3 is the IP3 receptor (IP3R; subtypes IP3R1, IP3R2 and IP3R3), which is another important $Ca^{2+}$ channel residing on ER membranes in β-cells [143]. Similarly to the EPAC2-RyR route of $Ca^{2+}$ release from ER $Ca^{2+}$, the opening of this channel amplifies the primary $Ca_L$ mediated $Ca^{2+}$ signaling for insulin release. PKC contributes to the plasma membrane depolarization, while activating TRPM4 and TRPM5 [144]. Besides the canonical plasma membrane effects, PKC and downstream ERK1/2 signaling stimulates OXPHOS, hence mitochondrial ATP synthesis [145].

## 7. GSIS amplification by incretins GLP-1 and GIP

Glucagon-like peptide 1 (GLP-1) and gastric inhibitory polypeptide (GIP) have a prominent impact among other peptides belonging to incretins [107–109]. Oral glucose administration provides a higher insulin secretion response than when administered parenterally [146]. This surplus of potentiation of insulin secretion appears to be about equally ascribed to GLP-1 and GIP [147]. Indeed, diminished insulin secretion response to oral glucose was observed in GLP-1 knock out mice [148, 149] and was even more decreased in double knockout mice (GLP-1 plus GIP) [149].

Incretin-cAMP signaling amplifies GSIS by both PKA-dependent and EPAC2A-dependent pathways. As described above, the EPAC2 pathway is partially dependent on the $Ca_L$ opening, and the PKA pathway enables synergy among actions of $K_{ATP}$, $Ca_L$, and Kv channels, leading again to a more effective $Ca_L$ opening. This knowledge complies with the traditional view, considering that the incretin signaling does not stimulate insulin release in the low glucose conditions [150, 151]. The GLP1R-cAMP-EPAC2-TRPM2 pathway was suggested to be one of the major routes [106].

GLP-1 is secreted by enteroendocrine L-cells, residing predominantly in the distal ileum and colon. Secretion is initiated by postprandial stimuli, i.e. by glucose, fatty acids, or lipids, as well as proteins [152, 153]. Only 10 to 15% of active GLP-1 likely reaches the pancreas via the circulation [154]. Thus concentrations of biologically active GLP-1 in human plasma at fasting account for about 2 pmol/l and maximum10 pmol/l postprandially [155], peaking 30 to 60 min after a carbohydrate or protein intake and 120 min after ingestion of lipids [156]. The most efficient truncated variants are GLP-$1_{(7–37)}$ and variant GLP-$1_{(7–36amide)}$ [152]. The latter is ~80% abundant in humans [157]. Note that full peptide GLP-$1_{(1–37)}$ is much less efficient in GSIS potentiation [150, 151]. Moreover, paracrine GLP-1 signaling acts among the different types of PI cells [150], similarly to the paracrine and endocrine secretion of other hormones. On the systemic level, central control by the brain and nervous system, including GLP-1 secretion in the *nucleus tractus solitarii* of the brainstem [152], further provides an indispensable top level of regulation for the insulin secretion. GLP-1 effects related to β-cell proliferation or apoptosis are beyond the scope of this review.

GLP-1 from the bloodstream acts through its receptor (GLP1R) residing in the plasma membrane of pancreatic β-cells [158]. GLP1R activation stimulates Gαs and Gαq/11 and recruits β-arrestin, depending on biased agonism relative to different agonists, such as exendin-4 and oxyntomodulin [159, 160]. As a scaffold protein, β-arrestin facilitates signaling via Gαs to cAMP but also to CREB [160], extracellular regulated kinase ERK1/2 [161], and insulin receptor substrate 2 (IRS-2), the effects promoting β-cell growth, differentiation, and maintenance [160]. The stimulation of Gαs leads via enhanced cAMP to the initiation of PKA [162] and EPAC2A pathways [163]. Continuous cAMP production and partial potentiation of GSIS was found even for the internalized GLP1R [164].

The PKA pathway provides a surplus intracellular $Ca^{2+}$ above that of the net GSIS without any receptor stimulation. This is ensured by phosphorylation-induced closing among the population of $K_{ATP}$, stimulation of $Ca_L$ opening, and closing of Kv channels [165]. The latter prolongs $Ca^{2+}$ stimulation of IGV exocytosis and hence may also potentiate the 2nd phase of GSIS. In parallel, PKA engages snapin interaction with IGVs, reportedly potentiating the 1st GSIS phase [123, 124]. Simultaneously, the EPAC2 pathway promotes $Ca^{2+}$-induced RyR-mediated $Ca^{2+}$ release from ER, which must be, however, initiated by the ongoing $Ca_L$ opening [163]. The EPAC2 pathway also facilitates docking and priming of IGVs by promoting Rab3A interaction with Rim2a [131] and hypothetically interaction of EPAC2-Rim2-Picollo trimers with Rab3A, enabling IGV exocytosis [152]. Stimulation of GLP1R biased downstream via stimulation of Gαq/11 also contributes by a surplus to intracellular $Ca^{2+}$, while inducing the IP3R-mediated $Ca^{2+}$ release from ER.

When GLP1 effects were simulated and IGV kinetics was monitored using total internal reflection fluorescence microscopy, cAMP and 8-Br-cAMP were found to increase the frequency of fusion events, i.e. IGV fusion with the plasma membrane in both phases of GSIS [25]. EPAC2A was found to interacts also with a small G protein Rap1, affecting its conformation so to release the catalytic region, which subsequently binds and thus activates another G protein Rap113. In EPAC2A knockout mice, most of the potentiation of the 1st GSIS phase vanished [25]. Thus speculatively, the 2nd phase amplification can be due to the PKA pathway.

## 8. Mechanism of insulin secretion stimulated by branched-chain keto-acids

Postprandial response by insulin secretion is also given by substances other than glucose. These substances, which induce the secretion of insulin, are termed secretagogues in general. One important type of secretagogues is branched-chain keto-acids (BCKAs), metabolites of branched-chain amino acids (BCAAs) (**Figure 2**). We found that the alternative to the NOX4-mediated redox signaling exists for some other insulin secretagogues, particularly for BCKAs [1]. For the redox signaling in this case, the mitochondrial redox signaling replaced that one originating from NOX4. Thus we demonstrated that $H_2O_2$ signaling originating from mitochondria is essentially required for insulin secretion stimulated by BCAAs metabolized onto BCKAs, such as 2-ketoisocaproate (KIC; also termed 2-oxoiso-caproate, OIC; leucine metabolite), 2-ketoisovalerate (KIV; valine metabolite) and 2-ketomethylvalerate (KMV; isoleucine metabolite) [166, 167]. This mechanism was evidenced by the effects of mitochondrial-matrix-targeted antioxidant SkQ1. We observed that SkQ1 did not affect GSIS in INS-1E cells, but completely inhibited insulin secretion stimulated by KIC [1]. Thus the NOX4 source of $H_2O_2$ cannot be efficiently inhibited by SkQ1 located within the inner phospholipid leaflet of the inner mitochondrial membrane, whereas the redox signaling originating from mitochondrion must be blocked.

Metabolism of BCKAs begins in the mitochondrial matrix by the reaction of the BCKA dehydrogenase complex (BCKDH), since there is no branched-chain amino acid aminotransferase (BCAT) in the cell cytosol [168]. BCKDH forms isovaleryl-CoA, isobutyryl-Co and methyl-isobutyryl-CoA from KIC, KIV and KMV, respectively. This is followed by a series of reactions resembling β-oxidation of fatty acids. This series, as well as FA β-oxidation, elevates formation of superoxide in the mitochondrial matrix by several ways. The major way is due to the reoxidation of the BCKDH co-factor $FADH_2$ by the electron-transfer flavoprotein (ETF), the one electron carrier. Two electrons from the two ETF molecules are accepted by the electron-transfer flavoprotein: ubiquinone oxidoreductase (ETF:QOR) [169].

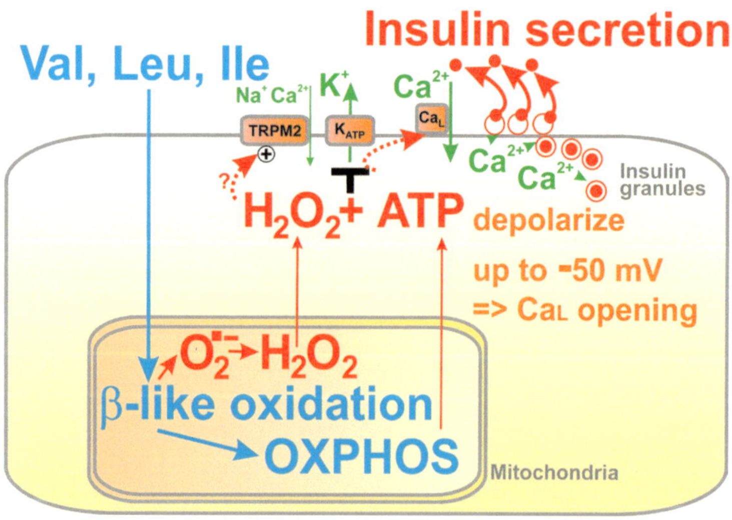


**Figure 2.**
*The mechanism of branched chain keto acid-stimulated insulin secretion involves redox signaling of mitochondrial origin. 2-ketoisocaproate (KIC), 2-ketomethylvalerate (KMV) and 2-ketoisovalerate (KIV) resulting from leucine, isoleucine, and valine, respectively, due to the branched chain aminotransferase reaction in mitochondria (BCAT2), are metabolized by the branched chain ketoacid dehydrogenase (BCKDH) in mitochondria. A series of reactions, BCKA oxidation leads to the electron transfer from the co-factor $FADH_2$ of BCKDH, via ETF towards the ETF:QOR reaction reducing Q to $QH_2$. This effectively retards the competing reaction of the Complex I of the mitochondrial respiratory chain, leading to the superoxide formation. In the mitochondrial matrix, superoxide is transformed to $H_2O_2$ by MnSOD, whereas by CuZnSOD in the intermembrane space and cytosol. The elevated mitochondrial/cytosolic $H_2O_2$ substitutes the redox signal of NOX4 origin. Consequently, such redox signaling, together with elevated ATP, allows the sufficient depolarization of the plasma membrane.*

ETF:QOR reaction is coupled to ubiquinone (Q) oxidation to ubiquinol ($QH_2$). This effectively competes with the Complex I reaction of the respiratory chain, also providing Q oxidation to $QH_2$ driven by NADH. The electron transfer within the Complex I is thus effectively retarded and this results in a higher superoxide formation. Superoxide is then most probably increasingly formed at the $I_Q$ site (i.e. at the proximity of the Q-binding site), similarly as due to the reverse electron transfer.

Alternatively, the Complex I electron transfer is retarded upon the acetyl-CoA entry (propionyl-CoA entry for KIV; through methylmalonyl and Succinyl-CoA) into the Krebs cycle. Also, acetoacetate influences redox homeostasis, as one of the final products of leucine metabolism. After superoxide conversion to the elevated $H_2O_2$ in the mitochondrial matrix, the $H_2O_2$ is elevated in the cytosol and thus represents the mitochondrial retrograde redox signaling. Its target could be again $K_{ATP}$ (or $K_{ATP}$ and TRPM2) which would depolarize the plasma membrane due to this redox signaling ongoing in parallel with the elevated ATP due to concomitantly enhanced OXPHOS.

The BCAA oxidation involves the following sequence of reactions: isovaleryl-CoA dehydrogenase (IVD), methylcrotonyl-CoA carboxylase (MCC), methylglutoconyl-CoA hydratase (MGCoAH) and 3-hydroxy-3-methylglutaryl-CoA lyase (HMGCoAL). The end-products are acetyl-CoA and acetoacetate. Similarly, as for pyruvate metabolism via PDH, the common end-product acetyl-CoA drives the Krebs cycle. This may also increase mitochondrial superoxide formation. Acetyl-CoA is linked to the above acyl-CoA dehydrogenase reaction by the reaction of the ETF:QOR, using ubiquinone (CoQ or Q) to oxidize it to ubiquinol QH. Also, the ETF:QOR itself may produce superoxide.

In summary, independently of the molecular mechanism, BCAA metabolism leads to the increased mitochondrial superoxide formation. After conversion to $H_2O_2$ by the matrix MnSOD and the intermembrane space CuZnSOD, the ongoing $H_2O_2$ efflux from mitochondria can be regarded as redox signaling. We have clearly demonstrated that the absence of such redox signaling, for example, in the presence of the mitochondrial matrix-targeted antioxidants SkQ1 leads to a blockage of insulin secretion, which is otherwise stimulated with BCKAs [1]. Likewise, the silencing of BCKDH led to the inhibition of insulin secretion stimulated with BCKAs.

## 9. Mechanism of fatty acid-stimulated insulin secretion

Fatty acids (FAs) appear in pancreatic islet capillaries either bound to albumin or being part of postprandial chylomicrons resulting from dietary fat lipids. FA pool of lipoproteins can be also considered. The dietary fat lipids are rich in triglycerides, which are cleaved locally in pancreatic islet capillaries by lipoprotein lipase secreted by β-cells. Resulting 2-monoacylglycerol (2MAG) and long chain FAs [170–173] stimulate each own two receptors GPR119 [157] and GPR40/FFA1, respectively. Therefore, fatty acid-stimulated insulin secretion (FASIS) could be defined as the net insulin secretion induced at the low glucose concentration, which itself does not stimulate insulin secretion. It is still controversial, whether such a net FASIS exists, since some previous reports observed that glucose should always be present for fatty acid to induce insulin secretion response. In contrast, the other reports described FASIS at 3 mM glucose, but not at zero glucose. Physiologically, postprandial responses should be due to all secretagogues resulting from major saccharide, fat and protein components. FASIS may dominate late responses upon feeding by fatty meal or an experimental high-fat diet [174].

Theoretically, FASIS must concern with the two components (**Figure 3**). The first one should depend on metabolism and the second one should rely on the stimulation

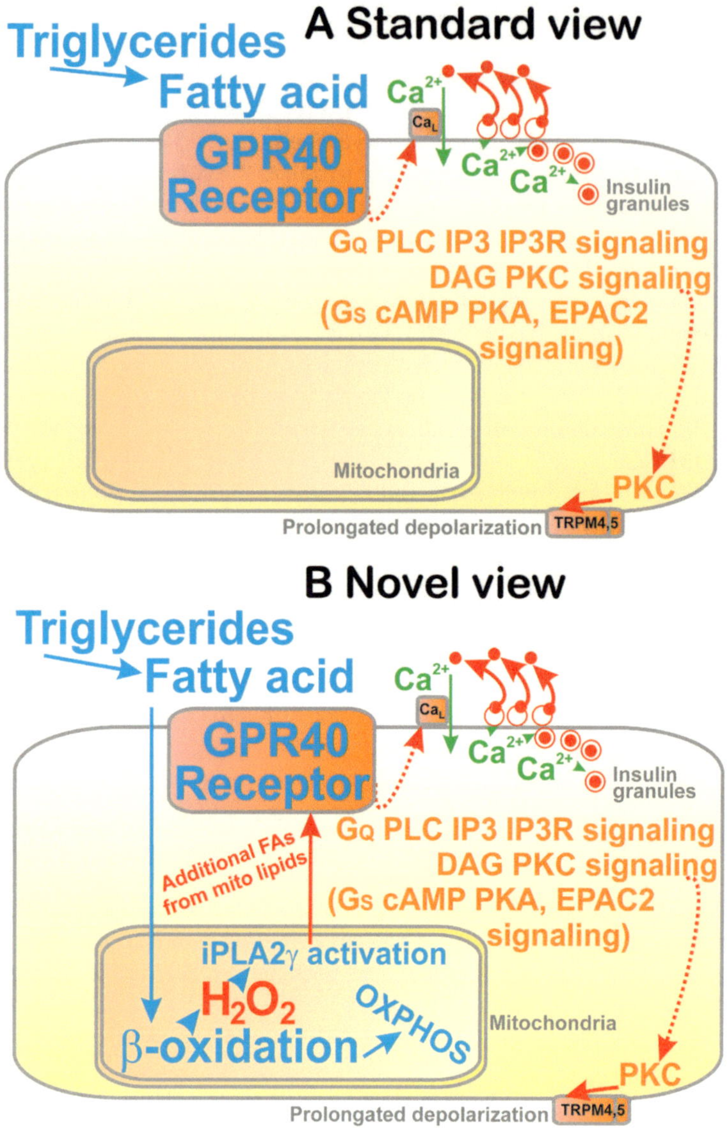


**Figure 3.**
*(A) Traditional ("standard") view of FASIS compared with (B) FASIS with GPR40 receptor supplied by the mitochondrial fatty acids mechanism ("novel view"). The mechanism of FASIS at low glucose appears to be predominantly mediated by GPR40. Its ligands are free long-chain FAs. An excessive supply of GPR40 ligands and hence a substantial amplification of the GPR40 downstream response is given by the redox-activated mitochondrial phospholipase iPLA2γ/PNPLA8. The phospholipase iPLA2γ is directly activated by the elevated $H_2O_2$ in the mitochondrial matrix and cleaves both saturated and unsaturated FAs from the phospholipids of mitochondrial membranes. The cleaved free FAs diffuse up to the plasma membrane, where they activate GPR40.*

of the metabotropic receptor GPR40. In vivo, FASIS-GPR40 axis is paralleled by a portion of insulin secretion stimulated via another metabotropic receptor, GPR119, to which monoacylglycerol (MAG) binds as the second major component of triglycerides. The metabolic component undoubtedly involves fatty acid β-oxidation, providing both ATP from the elevated OXPHOS and $H_2O_2$ from the enhanced superoxide formation by the respiratory chain and ETF:QOR, similarly as for BCKAs [175]. This component is thus directly dependent on $K_{ATP}$, since it leads to its closure and to the canonical downstream events identical to those during GSIS.

The receptor component of FASIS may be at least partly $K_{ATP}$-independent and even $Ca_L$-independent, hence may partly proceed independently of high glucose. In other words, FASIS at low glucose is theoretically possible. The major pathway downstream of GPR40 relies on Gαq/11, which induces PLC-mediated hydrolysis of phosphatidylinositol 4,5-bisphosphate into DAG and IP3 [110, 111]. The latter would amplify the primary $Ca_L$-mediated $Ca^{2+}$ signaling for the insulin release by mediating $Ca^{2+}$ release from ER via the $Ca^{2+}$ channel of the IP3 receptor [143]. However, this would happen provided that some basal $Ca_L$ would be initiated by the metabolic component, i.e. due to partial fatty acid metabolism by β-oxidation followed by $H_2O_2$ plus ATP elevations. Also, PKC could be activated downstream of GPR40 as being the main effector of DAG. The PKC pathway could increase the extent of plasma membrane depolarization since it activates TRPM4 and TRPM5 [144]. Moreover, this may act at low glucose, again providing that the initial triggering is ensured by the metabolic component, and so that certain basal $H_2O_2$ plus ATP elevations exist, leading to the $K_{ATP}$ closure. Also, another route downstream of GPR40 would involve the Gαq/11-PLC-TRPC-induced $Ca^{2+}$ efflux from ER [176]. As mentioned above, the TRPC1-Orai1-STIM1 complex was demonstrated to act during GSIS, while contributing to $Ca^{2+}$ oscillations [46, 83, 84]. The action of such a complex has yet to be studied during experimental FASIS as well as its dependence on $Ca_L$.

Also, biased (promiscuous) pathways of GPR40, i.e., those involving $G\alpha_S$-cAMP initiation of information signaling may exist and contribute to a certain extent to FASIS. Both downstream pathways of GPR40-$G\alpha_S$-cAMP stimulation, i.e. the PKA and EPAC2 pathway, could target components of IGV interactions with the plasma membrane, hence being independent of $Ca_L$. These speculations await experimental evidence.

Our in vitro and in vivo experiments with mice (unpublished) demonstrated that approximately 2/3 of the GPR40 response (amplitude of insulin secretion) is given by the amplifying mechanism due to the mitochondrial phospholipase iPLA2γ/PNPLA8 [175]. This phospholipase cleaves both saturated and unsaturated FAs from the phospholipids of mitochondrial membranes. The cleaved free FAs subsequently diffuse up to the plasma membrane, where they activate GPR40. Moreover, the phospholipase iPLA2γ is directly activated by the elevated $H_2O_2$ in the mitochondrial matrix. The reader may remain that this is just the FA β-oxidation, which via the increased superoxide formation, due to the function of ETF:QOR and respiratory chain, produces $H_2O_2$, while the concomitant OXPHOS provides elevated ATP. As a result, the sufficient plasma membrane depolarization is enabled. The proof of co-existence of the GPR40 receptor component and metabolic component of FASIS is suggested by the experiments when FASIS in iPLA2γ knockout mice or in its isolated islets yielded only ~30% insulin secretion peak in the 1st phase when compared to wt mice (Holendová B., Jabůrek M, et al., unpublished). Incidentally, a similar portion remains when GW1100 antagonist of GPR40 was applied. These results show that in parallel with the GPR40 pathway, a 1/3 portion of FASIS still results from FA β-oxidation, having a similar mechanism as described for ketoacids. The abolished FASIS in the iPLA2γ knockout mice then supports the existence of such an acute mechanism in vivo, when GPR40 is supplied with mitochondrial fatty acids.

## 10. Redox relay as a hypothetical carrier for redox signaling

It has been established that the content of glutathione (GSH) is rather low in pancreatic β-cells [177–180], in contrast to the content of thioredoxins and glutaredoxins [181, 182], peroxiredoxins and other proteins capable of redox relay. Therefore, these proteins are able to conduct and spread the redox signals [183, 184]. From this point of view, the pancreatic β-cell appears to be a well-integrated redox system.

Redox signal spreading may be accomplished either by the direct diffusion of $H_2O_2$ or may be facilitated by the specialized proteins. Redox signals can be traced experimentally as instantly oxidatively modified cysteine residues, which are spread via different sets of proteins in different tissues. However, one may consider their majority as passive targets. For the case of NOX4 residing in the proximity of $K_{ATP}$, undoubtedly, the direct diffusion of $H_2O_2$ would be sufficient. Nevertheless for more distant NOX4 molecules, this would be difficult. Also, for mitochondrial redox signaling towards targets residing in the plasma membrane, a distance over 500 nm must be overcome. Redox signal across such high distances could be conducted through the action of thiol-based proteins capable of redox relay to the target, such as peroxiredoxins (regenerated via thioredoxins and glutaredoxins). The relay would provide a common redox signal transfer. It is yet to be established whether a redox relay exists via an array of peroxiredoxin oligomers.

## Acknowledgment

This chapter is supported by grant No. 20-00408S from the Grant Agency of the Czech Republic (Grantová Agentura České Republiky).

## Author details

Petr Ježek*, Blanka Holendová, Martin Jabůrek, Jan Tauber, Andrea Dlasková and Lydie Plecitá-Hlavatá
Department of Mitochondrial Physiology, No.75, Institute of Physiology of the Czech Academy of Sciences, Prague, Czech Republic

*Address all correspondence to: jezek@biomed.cas.cz

## References

[1] Plecita-Hlavata L, Jaburek M, Holendova B, Tauber J, Pavluch V, Berkova Z, et al. Glucose-Stimulated Insulin Secretion Fundamentally Requires H2O2 Signaling by NADPH Oxidase 4. *Diabetes*. **2020**. DOI: 10.2337/db19-1130

[2] Grupe M, Myers G, Penner R, Fleig A. Activation of store-operated I(CRAC) by hydrogen peroxide. Cell Calcium. **2010**;*48*:1-9. DOI: 10.1016/j.ceca.2010.05.005

[3] Stoian AP, Mitrofan G, Colceag F, Suceveanu AI, Hainarosie R, Pituru S, et al. Oxidative stress in diabetes. A model of complex thinking applied in medicine. Revista de Chimie. **2018**;*69*:2515-2519. DOI: 10.37358/RC.18.9.6566

[4] Picu A, Petcu L, Ştefan DS, Grădişteanu Pîrcălăbioru G, Mitu M, Bajko D, et al. Evolution of Inflammatory and Oxidative Stress Markers in Romanian Obese Male Patients with Type 2 Diabetes Mellitus after Laparoscopic Sleeve Gastrectomy: One Year Follow-Up. Metabolites. **2020**;*10*. DOI: 10.3390/metabo10080308

[5] Pantea Stoian, A.M., G.; Colceag, F.; Serafinceanu, C.; Eftimie Totu, E.; Mocanu, V.; Mănuc, D.; Mihaela Cărăuşu, E. Oxidative Stress Applied in Diabetes Mellitus-A New Paradigm. *Proceedings* **2019**, *11*, doi:10.3390/proceedings2019011007.

[6] Zhang P, Li T, Wu X, Nice EC, Huang C, Zhang Y. Oxidative stress and diabetes: antioxidative strategies. *Frontiers of medicine*. **2020**. DOI: 10.1007/s11684-019-0729-1

[7] Straub SG, Sharp GW. Glucose-stimulated signaling pathways in biphasic insulin secretion. Diabetes/Metabolism Research and Reviews. **2002**;*18*:451-463. DOI: 10.1002/dmrr.329

[8] Hoang DT, Hara M, Jo J. Design Principles of Pancreatic Islets: Glucose-Dependent Coordination of Hormone Pulses. PLoS One. **2016**;*11*:e0152446. DOI: 10.1371/journal.pone.0152446

[9] Kalwat MA, Cobb MH. Mechanisms of the amplifying pathway of insulin secretion in the β cell. Pharmacology & Therapeutics. **2017**;*179*:17-30. DOI: 10.1016/j.pharmthera.2017.05.003

[10] Villard O, Brun JF, Bories L, Molinari N, Benhamou PY, Berney T, et al. The Second Phase of Insulin Secretion in Nondiabetic Islet-Grafted Recipients Is Altered and Can Predict Graft Outcome. The Journal of Clinical Endocrinology and Metabolism. **2018**;*103*:1310-1319. DOI: 10.1210/jc.2017-01342

[11] Henquin JC, Dufrane D, Kerr-Conte J, Nenquin M. Dynamics of glucose-induced insulin secretion in normal human islets. American Journal of Physiology. Endocrinology and Metabolism. **2015**;*309*:E640-E650. DOI: 10.1152/ajpendo.00251.2015

[12] Henquin JC. Regulation of insulin secretion: a matter of phase control and amplitude modulation. Diabetologia. **2009**;*52*:739-751. DOI: 10.1007/s00125-009-1314-y

[13] Gembal M, Detimary P, Gilon P, Gao ZY, Henquin JC. Mechanisms by which glucose can control insulin release independently from its action on adenosine triphosphate-sensitive K+ channels in mouse B cells. The Journal of Clinical Investigation. **1993**;*91*:871-880. DOI: 10.1172/jci116308.

[14] Komatsu M, Takei M, Ishii H, Sato Y. Glucose-stimulated insulin secretion: A newer perspective. Journal of diabetes investigation. **2013**;*4*:511-516. DOI: 10.1111/jdi.12094

[15] Pedersen MG, Tagliavini A, Henquin JC. Calcium signaling and secretory granule pool dynamics underlie biphasic insulin secretion and its amplification by glucose: experiments and modeling. American Journal of Physiology. Endocrinology and Metabolism. **2019**;*316*:E475-e486. DOI: 10.1152/ajpendo.00380.2018

[16] Daniel S, Noda M, Straub SG, Sharp GW. Identification of the docked granule pool responsible for the first phase of glucose-stimulated insulin secretion. Diabetes. **1999**;*48*:1686-1690. DOI: 10.2337/diabetes.48.9.1686

[17] Rorsman P, Renström E. Insulin granule dynamics in pancreatic beta cells. Diabetologia. **2003**;*46*:1029-1045. DOI: 10.1007/s00125-003-1153-1

[18] Nagamatsu S, Ohara-Imaizumi M, Nakamichi Y, Kikuta T, Nishiwaki C. Imaging docking and fusion of insulin granules induced by antidiabetes agents: sulfonylurea and glinide drugs preferentially mediate the fusion of newcomer, but not previously docked, insulin granules. Diabetes. **2006**;*55*:2819-2825. DOI: 10.2337/db06-0105

[19] Ohara-Imaizumi M, Fujiwara T, Nakamichi Y, Okamura T, Akimoto Y, Kawai J, et al. Imaging analysis reveals mechanistic differences between first- and second-phase insulin exocytosis. *The Journal of cell biology*. **2007**;*177*:695-705. DOI: 10.1083/jcb.200608132

[20] Kalwat MA, Thurmond DC. Signaling mechanisms of glucose-induced F-actin remodeling in pancreatic islet β cells. Experimental & Molecular Medicine. **2013**;*45*:e37. DOI: 10.1038/emm.2013.73

[21] Mourad NI, Nenquin M, Henquin JC. Metabolic amplifying pathway increases both phases of insulin secretion independently of beta-cell actin microfilaments. American Journal of Physiology. Cell Physiology. **2010**;*299*:C389-C398. DOI: 10.1152/ajpcell.00138.2010

[22] Wang Z, Thurmond DC. Mechanisms of biphasic insulin-granule exocytosis - roles of the cytoskeleton, small GTPases and SNARE proteins. Journal of Cell Science. **2009**;*122*:893-903. DOI: 10.1242/jcs.034355

[23] Mourad NI, Nenquin M, Henquin JC. cAMP-mediated and metabolic amplification of insulin secretion are distinct pathways sharing independence of β-cell microfilaments. Endocrinology. **2012**;*153*:4644-4654. DOI: 10.1210/en.2012-1450

[24] Mourad NI, Nenquin M, Henquin JC. Amplification of insulin secretion by acetylcholine or phorbol ester is independent of β-cell microfilaments and distinct from metabolic amplification. Molecular and Cellular Endocrinology. **2013**;*367*:11-20. DOI: 10.1016/j.mce.2012.12.002

[25] Shibasaki T, Takahashi H, Miki T, Sunaga Y, Matsumura K, Yamanaka M, et al. Essential role of Epac2/Rap1 signaling in regulation of insulin granule dynamics by cAMP. *Proceedings of the National Academy of Sciences of the United States of America*. **2007**;*104*:19333-19338. DOI: 10.1073/pnas.0707054104

[26] Vakilian M, Tahamtani Y, Ghaedi K. A review on insulin trafficking and exocytosis. Gene. **2019**;*706*:52-61. DOI: 10.1016/j.gene.2019.04.063

[27] Rocheleau JV, Remedi MS, Granada B, Head WS, Koster JC, Nichols CG, et al. Critical role of gap junction coupled KATP channel activity for regulated insulin secretion. PLoS Biology. **2006**;*4*:e26. DOI: 10.1371/journal.pbio.0040026

[28] Idevall-Hagren O, Tengholm A. Metabolic regulation of calcium signaling in beta cells. Seminars in Cell

& Developmental Biology. **2020**;*103*:20-30. DOI: 10.1016/j.semcdb.2020.01.008

[29] Johnston NR, Mitchell RK, Haythorne E, Pessoa MP, Semplici F, Ferrer J, et al. Beta Cell Hubs Dictate Pancreatic Islet Responses to Glucose. Cell Metabolism. **2016**;*24*:389-401. DOI: 10.1016/j.cmet.2016.06.020

[30] Ashcroft FM, Rorsman P. Diabetes Mellitus and the β Cell: The Last Ten Years. Cell. **2012**;*148*:1160-1171. DOI: 10.1016/j.cell.2012.02.010

[31] Maechler P. Mitochondrial function and insulin secretion. *Molecular and Cellular Endocrinology*. **2013**. DOI: 10.1016/j.mce.2013.06.019

[32] Prentki M, Matschinsky FM, Madiraju SRM. Metabolic signaling in fuel-induced insulin secretion. Cell Metabolism. **2013**;*18*:162-185. DOI: 10.1016/j.cmet.2013.05.018

[33] Rutter GA, Pullen TJ, Hodson DJ, Martinez-Sanchez A. Pancreatic β-cell identity, glucose sensing and the control of insulin secretion. Biochemical Journal. **2015**;*466*:203-218. DOI: 10.1042/BJ20141384

[34] Seino S, Sugawara K, Yokoi N, Takahashi H. β-Cell signalling and insulin secretagogues: A path for improved diabetes therapy. Diabetes, Obesity & Metabolism. **2017**;*19*(*Suppl 1*):22-29. DOI: 10.1111/dom.12995.

[35] Shibasaki T, Takahashi T, Takahashi H, Seino S. Cooperation between cAMP signalling and sulfonylurea in insulin secretion. Diabetes, Obesity & Metabolism. **2014**;*16*(*Suppl 1*):118-125. DOI: 10.1111/dom.12343

[36] Seino S. Cell signalling in insulin secretion: the molecular targets of ATP, cAMP and sulfonylurea. Diabetologia. **2012**;*55*:2096-2108. DOI: 10.1007/s00125-012-2562-9

[37] Leloup C, Tourrel-Cuzin C, Magnan C, Karaca M, Castel J, Carneiro L, et al. Mitochondrial Reactive Oxygen Species Are Obligatory Signals for Glucose-Induced Insulin Secretion. Diabetes. **2009**;*58*:673-681. DOI: 10.2337/db07-1056

[38] Saadeh M, Ferrante TC, Kane A, Shirihai O, Corkey BE, Deeney JT. Reactive Oxygen Species Stimulate Insulin Secretion in Rat Pancreatic Islets: Studies Using Mono-Oleoyl-Glycerol. PLoS One. **2012**;*7*:e30200. DOI: 10.1371/journal.pone.0030200

[39] Rebelato E, Abdulkader F, Curi R, Carpinelli AR. Control of the Intracellular Redox State by Glucose Participates in the Insulin Secretion Mechanism. PLoS One. **2011**;*6*:e24507. DOI: 10.1371/journal.pone.0024507

[40] Pi J, Bai Y, Zhang Q, Wong V, Floering LM, Daniel K, et al. Reactive Oxygen Species as a Signal in Glucose-Stimulated Insulin Secretion. Diabetes. **2007**;*56*:1783-1791. DOI: 10.2337/db06-1601

[41] Morgan D, Rebelato E, Abdulkader F, Graciano MFR, Oliveira-Emilio HR, Hirata AE, et al. Association of NAD(P)H Oxidase with Glucose-Induced Insulin Secretion by Pancreatic β-Cells. Endocrinology. **2009**;*150*:2197-2201. DOI: 10.1210/en.2008-1149

[42] Imoto H, Sasaki N, Iwase M, Nakamura U, Oku M, Sonoki K, et al. Impaired Insulin Secretion by Diphenyleneiodium Associated with Perturbation of Cytosolic $Ca^{2+}$ Dynamics in Pancreatic β-Cells. Endocrinology. **2008**;*149*:5391-5400. DOI: 10.1210/en.2008-0186

[43] Syed I, Kyathanahalli CN, Kowluru A. Phagocyte-like NADPH oxidase generates ROS in INS 832/13 cells and rat islets: role of protein prenylation. American Journal of Physiology-Regulatory, Integrative

and Comparative Physiology. **2011**;*300*:R756-R762. DOI: 10.1152/ajpregu.00786.2010

[44] Li N, Li B, Brun T, Deffert-Delbouille C, Mahiout Z, Daali Y, et al. NADPH Oxidase NOX2 Defines a New Antagonistic Role for Reactive Oxygen Species and cAMP/PKA in the Regulation of Insulin Secretion. Diabetes. **2012**;*61*:2842-2850. DOI: 10.2337/db12-0009

[45] Rorsman P, Eliasson L, Kanno T, Zhang Q, Gopel S. Electrophysiology of pancreatic β-cells in intact mouse islets of Langerhans. Progress in Biophysics and Molecular Biology. **2011**;*107*:224-235. DOI: 10.1016/j.pbiomolbio.2011.06.009

[46] Kakei M, Yoshida M, Dezaki K, Ito K, Yamada H, Funazaki S, et al. Glucose and GTP-binding protein-coupled receptor cooperatively regulate transient receptor potential-channels to stimulate insulin secretion [Review]. Endocrine Journal. **2016**;*63*:867-876. DOI: 10.1507/endocrj.EJ16-0262

[47] Sakaguchi R, Mori Y. Transient receptor potential (TRP) channels: Biosensors for redox environmental stimuli and cellular status. Free Radical Biology & Medicine. **2020**;*146*:36-44. DOI: 10.1016/j.freeradbiomed.2019.10.415

[48] Plecitá-Hlavatá L, Engstová H, Holendová B, Tauber J, Špaček T, Petrásková L, et al. Mitochondrial Superoxide Production Decreases on Glucose-Stimulated Insulin Secretion in Pancreatic β Cells Due to Decreasing Mitochondrial Matrix NADH/NAD(+) Ratio. *Antioxidants & redox signaling*. **2020**. DOI: 10.1089/ars.2019.7800

[49] Spégel P, Sharoyko VV, Goehring I, Danielsson AP, Malmgren S, Nagorny CL, et al. Time-resolved metabolomics analysis of β-cells implicates the pentose phosphate pathway in the control of insulin release. The Biochemical Journal. **2013**;*450*:595-605. DOI: 10.1042/bj20121349

[50] Bedard K, Krause K-H. The NOX Family of ROS-Generating NADPH Oxidases: Physiology and Pathophysiology. Physiological Reviews. **2007**;*87*:245-313. DOI: 10.1152/physrev.00044.2005

[51] Serrander L, Cartier L, Bedard K, Banfi B, Lardy B, Plastre O, et al. NOX4 activity is determined by mRNA levels and reveals a unique pattern of ROS generation. Biochemical Journal. **2007**;*406*:105-114. DOI: 10.1042/BJ20061903

[52] MacDonald PE. Signal integration at the level of ion channel and exocytotic function in pancreatic β-cells. American Journal of Physiology-Endocrinology and Metabolism. **2011**;*301*:E1065-E1069. DOI: 10.1152/ajpendo.00426.2011

[53] Leturque A, Brot-Laroche E, Le Gall M. GLUT2 mutations, translocation, and receptor function in diet sugar managing. American Journal of Physiology. Endocrinology and Metabolism. **2009**;*296*:E985-E992. DOI: 10.1152/ajpendo.00004.2009

[54] Kaminski MT, Lenzen S, Baltrusch S. Real-time analysis of intracellular glucose and calcium in pancreatic beta cells by fluorescence microscopy. Biochimica et Biophysica Acta. **2012**;*1823*:1697-1707. DOI: 10.1016/j.bbamcr.2012.06.022

[55] Park JH, Kim SJ, Park SH, Son DG, Bae JH, Kim HK, et al. Glucagon-like peptide-1 enhances glucokinase activity in pancreatic beta-cells through the association of Epac2 with Rim2 and Rab3A. Endocrinology. **2012**;*153*:574-582. DOI: 10.1210/en.2011-0259

[56] Matschinsky FM, Wilson DF. The Central Role of Glucokinase in Glucose Homeostasis: A Perspective 50 Years

After Demonstrating the Presence of the Enzyme in Islets of Langerhans. Frontiers in Physiology. **2019**;*10*:148. DOI: 10.3389/fphys.2019.00148

[57] Schuit F, De Vos A, Farfari S, Moens K, Pipeleers D, Brun T, et al. Metabolic fate of glucose in purified islet cells. Glucose-regulated anaplerosis in beta cells. The Journal of Biological Chemistry. **1997**;*272*:18572-18579

[58] Zhang Z, Liew CW, Handy DE, Zhang Y, Leopold JA, Hu J, et al. High glucose inhibits glucose-6-phosphate dehydrogenase, leading to increased oxidative stress and beta-cell apoptosis. FASEB Journal : Official Publication of the Federation of American Societies for Experimental Biology. **2010**;*24*:1497-1505. DOI: 10.1096/fj.09-136572

[59] Huang M, Joseph JW. Metabolomic analysis of pancreatic β-cell insulin release in response to glucose. Islets. **2012**;*4*:210-222. DOI: 10.4161/isl.20141

[60] Goehring I, Sauter NS, Catchpole G, Assmann A, Shu L, Zien KS, et al. Identification of an intracellular metabolic signature impairing beta cell function in the rat beta cell line INS-1E and human islets. Diabetologia. **2011**;*54*:2584-2594. DOI: 10.1007/s00125-011-2249-7

[61] Ammon HP, Steinke J. 6-Amnionicotinamide (6-AN) as a diabetogenic agent. In vitro and in vivo studies in the rat. Diabetes. **1972**;*21*:143-148. DOI: 10.2337/diab.21.3.143

[62] Verspohl EJ, Händel M, Ammon HP. Pentosephosphate shunt activity of rat pancreatic islets: its dependence on glucose concentration. Endocrinology. **1979**;*105*:1269-1274. DOI: 10.1210/endo-105-5-1269

[63] Monte Alegre S, Saad ST, Delatre E, Saad MJ. Insulin secretion in patients deficient in glucose-6-phosphate dehydrogenase. Hormone and Metabolic Research. **1991**;*23*:171-173. DOI: 10.1055/s-2007-1003644

[64] Akhmedov D, De Marchi U, Wollheim CB, Wiederkehr A. Pyruvate dehydrogenase E1α phosphorylation is induced by glucose but does not control metabolism-secretion coupling in INS-1E clonal β-cells. Biochimica et Biophysica Acta. **2012**;*1823*:1815-1824. DOI: 10.1016/j.bbamcr.2012.07.005

[65] Rutter GA, Hodson DJ, Chabosseau P, Haythorne E, Pullen TJ, Leclerc I. Local and regional control of calcium dynamics in the pancreatic islet. Diabetes, Obesity & Metabolism. **2017**;*19* (*Suppl 1*):30-41. DOI: 10.1111/dom.12990.

[66] Alves TC, Pongratz RL, Zhao X, Yarborough O, Sereda S, Shirihai O, et al. Integrated, Step-Wise, Mass-Isotopomeric Flux Analysis of the TCA Cycle. Cell Metabolism. **2015**;*22*:936-947. DOI: 10.1016/j.cmet.2015.08.021

[67] Kahancová A, Sklenář F, Ježek P, Dlasková A. Regulation of glucose-stimulated insulin secretion by ATPase Inhibitory Factor 1 (IF1). FEBS Letters. **2018**;*592*:999-1009. DOI: 10.1002/1873-3468.12991.

[68] Kahancová A, Sklenář F, Ježek P, Dlasková A. Overexpression of native IF1 downregulates glucose-stimulated insulin secretion by pancreatic INS-1E cells. Scientific Reports. **2020**;*10*:1551. DOI: 10.1038/s41598-020-58411-x

[69] Yang SN, Shi Y, Yang G, Li Y, Yu J, Berggren PO. Ionic mechanisms in pancreatic β cell signaling. Cellular and Molecular Life Sciences. **2014**;*71*:4149-4177. DOI: 10.1007/s00018-014-1680-6

[70] Drews G, Krippeit-Drews P, Düfer M. Electrophysiology of Islet Cells. Advances in Experimental Medicine and Biology. 2010;**654**:115-163

[71] Bennett K, James C, Hussain K. Pancreatic β-cell KATP channels:

Hypoglycaemia and hyperglycaemia. Reviews in Endocrine and Metabolic Disorders. **2010**;*11*:157-163. DOI: 10.1007/s11154-010-9144-2

[72] Szollosi A, Nenquin M, Henquin J. Pharmacological stimulation and inhibition of insulin secretion in mouse islets lacking ATP-sensitive K+ channels. British Journal of Pharmacology. **2010**;*159*:669-677. DOI: 10.1111/j.1476-5381.2009.00588.x

[73] Soty M, Visa M, Soriano S, del Carmen Carmona M, Nadal Á, Novials A. Involvement of ATP-sensitive Potassium ($K_{ATP}$) Channels in the Loss of Beta-cell Function Induced by Human Islet Amyloid Polypeptide. Journal of Biological Chemistry. **2011**;*286*:40857-40866. DOI: 10.1074/jbc.M111.232801

[74] Rorsman P, Braun M, Zhang Q. Regulation of calcium in pancreatic α- and β-cells in health and disease. Cell Calcium. **2012**;*51*:300-308. DOI: 10.1016/j.ceca.2011.11.006

[75] Rorsman P, Braun M. Regulation of insulin secretion in human pancreatic islets. Annual Review of Physiology. **2013**;*75*:155-179. DOI: 10.1146/annurev-physiol-030212-183754

[76] Smith PA, Ashcroft FM, Rorsman P. Simultaneous recordings of glucose dependent electrical activity and ATP-regulated K(+)-currents in isolated mouse pancreatic beta-cells. FEBS Letters. **1990**;*261*:187-190. DOI: 10.1016/0014-5793(90)80667-8

[77] Best L. Glucose-induced electrical activity in rat pancreatic beta-cells: dependence on intracellular chloride concentration. The Journal of Physiology. **2005**;*568*:137-144. DOI: 10.1113/jphysiol.2005.093740

[78] Stuhlmann T, Planells-Cases R, Jentsch TJ. LRRC8/VRAC anion channels enhance β-cell glucose sensing and insulin secretion. Nature Communications. **2018**;*9*:1974. DOI: 10.1038/s41467-018-04353-y

[79] Di Fulvio M, Aguilar-Bryan L. Chloride transporters and channels in β-cell physiology: revisiting a 40-year-old model. Biochemical Society Transactions. **2019**;*47*:1843-1855. DOI: 10.1042/bst20190513

[80] Colsoul B, Schraenen A, Lemaire K, Quintens R, Van Lommel L, Segal A, et al. Loss of high-frequency glucose-induced Ca2+ oscillations in pancreatic islets correlates with impaired glucose tolerance in Trpm5−/− mice. *Proceedings of the National Academy of Sciences of the United States of America*. **2010**;*107*:5208-5213. DOI: 10.1073/pnas.0913107107

[81] Gilon P, Ravier MA, Jonas JC, Henquin JC. Control mechanisms of the oscillations of insulin secretion in vitro and in vivo. Diabetes. **2002**;*51(Suppl 1)*:S144-S151. DOI: 10.2337/diabetes.51.2007.s144

[82] Beauvois MC, Merezak C, Jonas JC, Ravier MA, Henquin JC, Gilon P. Glucose-induced mixed [Ca2+]c oscillations in mouse beta-cells are controlled by the membrane potential and the SERCA3 Ca2+-ATPase of the endoplasmic reticulum. American Journal of Physiology. Cell Physiology. **2006**;*290*:C1503-C1511. DOI: 10.1152/ajpcell.00400.2005

[83] Sabourin J, Allagnat F. Store-operated Ca2+ entry: a key component of the insulin secretion machinery. Journal of Molecular Endocrinology. **2016**;*57*:F35-f39. DOI: 10.1530/jme-16-0106

[84] Sabourin J, Le Gal L, Saurwein L, Haefliger JA, Raddatz E, Allagnat F. Store-operated Ca2+ Entry Mediated by Orai1 and TRPC1 Participates to Insulin Secretion in Rat β-Cells. The Journal of Biological Chemistry. **2015**;*290*:30530-30539. DOI: 10.1074/jbc.M115.682583.

[85] Rorsman P, Trube G. Calcium and delayed potassium currents in mouse pancreatic beta-cells under voltage-clamp conditions. The Journal of Physiology. **1986**;*374*:531-550. DOI: 10.1113/jphysiol.1986.sp016096

[86] Jacobson DA, Kuznetsov A, Lopez JP, Kash S, Ammälä CE, Philipson LH. Kv2.1 ablation alters glucose-induced islet electrical activity, enhancing insulin secretion. Cell Metabolism. **2007**;*6*:229-235. DOI: 10.1016/j.cmet.2007.07.010

[87] Rebelato E, Santos LR, Carpinelli AR, Rorsman P, Abdulkader F. Short-term high glucose culture potentiates pancreatic beta cell function. Scientific Reports. **2018**;*8*:13061. DOI: 10.1038/s41598-018-31325-5

[88] Li N, Wu JX, Ding D, Cheng J, Gao N, Chen L. Structure of a Pancreatic ATP-Sensitive Potassium Channel. *Cell*. **2017**;*168*:101-110.e110. DOI: 10.1016/j.cell.2016.12.028

[89] Martin GM, Yoshioka C, Rex EA, Fay JF, Xie Q, Whorton MR, et al. Cryo-EM structure of the ATP-sensitive potassium channel illuminates mechanisms of assembly and gating. eLife. **2017**;*6*. DOI: 10.7554/eLife.24149

[90] Mikhailov MV, Campbell JD, de Wet H, Shimomura K, Zadek B, Collins RF, et al. 3-D structural and functional characterization of the purified KATP channel complex Kir6.2-SUR1. *EMBO J*. **2005**;*24*:4166-4175. DOI: 10.1038/sj.emboj.7600877

[91] Nichols CG. KATP channels as molecular sensors of cellular metabolism. Nature. **2006**;*440*:470-476. DOI: 10.1038/nature04711

[92] Yang HQ, Martinez-Ortiz W, Hwang J, Fan X, Cardozo TJ, Coetzee WA. Palmitoylation of the K(ATP) channel Kir6.2 subunit promotes channel opening by regulating PIP(2) sensitivity. *Proceedings of the National Academy of Sciences of the United States of America*. **2020**;*117*:10593-10602. DOI: 10.1073/pnas.1918088117

[93] Shyng SL, Nichols CG. Membrane phospholipid control of nucleotide sensitivity of KATP channels. Science. **1998**;*282*:1138-1141. DOI: 10.1126/science.282.5391.1138.

[94] Baukrowitz, T.; Schulte, U.; Oliver, D.; Herlitze, S.; Krauter, T.; Tucker, S.J.; Ruppersberg, J.P.; Fakler, B. PIP2 and PIP as determinants for ATP inhibition of KATP channels. Science **1998**, *282*, 1141-1144, doi:10.1126/science.282.5391.1141.

[95] Shyng S, Ferrigni T, Nichols CG. Regulation of KATP channel activity by diazoxide and MgADP. Distinct functions of the two nucleotide binding folds of the sulfonylurea receptor. *J Gen Physiol*. **1997**;*110*:643-654. DOI: 10.1085/jgp.110.6.643

[96] Lin YF, Jan YN, Jan LY. Regulation of ATP-sensitive potassium channel function by protein kinase A-mediated phosphorylation in transfected HEK293 cells. The EMBO Journal. **2000**;*19*:942-955. DOI: 10.1093/emboj/19.5.942

[97] Béguin P, Nagashima K, Nishimura M, Gonoi T, Seino S. PKA-mediated phosphorylation of the human K(ATP) channel: separate roles of Kir6.2 and SUR1 subunit phosphorylation. *Embo j*. **1999**;*18*:4722-4732. DOI: 10.1093/emboj/18.17.4722

[98] Kline CF, Wright PJ, Koval OM, Zmuda EJ, Johnson BL, Anderson ME, et al. βIV-Spectrin and CaMKII facilitate Kir6.2 regulation in pancreatic beta cells. *Proceedings of the National Academy of Sciences of the United States of America*. **2013**;*110*:17576-17581. DOI: 10.1073/pnas.1314195110

[99] Ashcroft FM, Harrison DE, Ashcroft SJ. Glucose induces closure of single potassium channels in isolated rat pancreatic beta-cells. Nature. **1984**;*312*:446-448. DOI: 10.1038/312446a0

[100] Yasui S, Mawatari K, Morizumi R, Furukawa H, Shimohata T, Harada N, et al. Hydrogen peroxide inhibits insulin-induced ATP-sensitive potassium channel activation independent of insulin signaling pathway in cultured vascular smooth muscle cells. The journal of medical investigation: JMI. **2012**;*59*:36-44

[101] Finol-Urdaneta RK, Remedi MS, Raasch W, Becker S, Clark RB, Strüver N, et al. Block of Kv1.7 potassium currents increases glucose-stimulated insulin secretion. EMBO Molecular Medicine. **2012**;*4*:424-434. DOI: 10.1002/emmm.201200218

[102] MacDonald PE, Salapatek AM, Wheeler MB. Temperature and redox state dependence of native Kv2.1 currents in rat pancreatic beta-cells. The Journal of Physiology. **2003**;*546*:647-653. DOI: 10.1113/jphysiol.2002.035709

[103] Mittal M, Gu XQ, Pak O, Pamenter ME, Haag D, Fuchs DB, et al. Hypoxia induces Kv channel current inhibition by increased NADPH oxidase-derived reactive oxygen species. Free Radical Biology & Medicine. **2012**;*52*:1033-1042. DOI: 10.1016/j.freeradbiomed.2011.12.004

[104] Llanos P, Contreras-Ferrat A, Barrientos G, Valencia M, Mears D, Hidalgo C. Glucose-Dependent Insulin Secretion in Pancreatic β-Cell Islets from Male Rats Requires Ca2+ Release via ROS-Stimulated Ryanodine Receptors. PLoS One. **2015**;*10*:e0129238. DOI: 10.1371/journal.pone.0129238

[105] Kashio M, Tominaga M. Redox Signal-mediated Enhancement of the Temperature Sensitivity of Transient Receptor Potential Melastatin 2 (TRPM2) Elevates Glucose-induced Insulin Secretion from Pancreatic Islets. Journal of Biological Chemistry. **2015**;*290*:12435-12442. DOI: 10.1074/jbc.M115.649913

[106] Yosida M, Dezaki K, Uchida K, Kodera S, Lam NV, Ito K, et al. Involvement of cAMP/EPAC/TRPM2 activation in glucose- and incretin-induced insulin secretion. Diabetes. **2014**;*63*:3394-3403. DOI: 10.2337/db13-1868

[107] Müller TD, Finan B, Bloom SR, D'Alessio D, Drucker DJ, Flatt PR, et al. Glucagon-like peptide 1 (GLP-1). Molecular metabolism. **2019**;*30*:72-130. DOI: 10.1016/j.molmet.2019.09.010

[108] Furman B, Ong WK, Pyne NJ. Cyclic AMP signaling in pancreatic islets. Advances in Experimental Medicine and Biology. **2010**;*654*:281-304. DOI: 10.1007/978-90-481-3271-3_13

[109] Lefkimmiatis K, Zaccolo M. cAMP signaling in subcellular compartments. Pharmacology & Therapeutics. **2014**;*143*:295-304. DOI: 10.1016/j.pharmthera.2014.03.008

[110] Berridge MJ. The Inositol Trisphosphate/Calcium Signaling Pathway in Health and Disease. Physiological Reviews. **2016**;*96*:1261-1296. DOI: 10.1152/physrev.00006.2016

[111] Husted AS, Trauelsen M, Rudenko O, Hjorth SA, Schwartz TW. GPCR-Mediated Signaling of Metabolites. Cell Metabolism. **2017**;*25*:777-796. DOI: 10.1016/j.cmet.2017.03.008

[112] Salloum G, Jaafar L, El-Sibai M. Rho A and Rac1: Antagonists moving forward. Tissue & Cell. **2020**;*65*:101364. DOI: 10.1016/j.tice.2020.101364

[113] Dalle S, Ravier MA, Bertrand G. Emerging roles for β-arrestin-1 in the

control of the pancreatic β-cell function and mass: new therapeutic strategies and consequences for drug screening. Cellular Signalling. **2011**;*23*:522-528. DOI: 10.1016/j.cellsig.2010.09.014

[114] Taylor SS, Ilouz R, Zhang P, Kornev AP. Assembly of allosteric macromolecular switches: lessons from PKA. Nature Reviews. Molecular Cell Biology. **2012**;*13*:646-658. DOI: 10.1038/nrm3432

[115] Zhang F, Zhang L, Qi Y, Xu H. Mitochondrial cAMP signaling. Cellular and Molecular Life Sciences. **2016**;*73*:4577-4590. DOI: 10.1007/s00018-016-2282-2

[116] Ould Amer Y, Hebert-Chatelain E. Mitochondrial cAMP-PKA signaling: What do we really know? Biochimica et Biophysica Acta - Bioenergetics. **2018**;*1859*:868-877. DOI: 10.1016/j.bbabio.2018.04.005

[117] Kang G, Leech CA, Chepurny OG, Coetzee WA, Holz GG. Role of the cAMP sensor Epac as a determinant of KATP channel ATP sensitivity in human pancreatic beta-cells and rat INS-1 cells. The Journal of Physiology. **2008**;*586*:1307-1319. DOI: 10.1113/jphysiol.2007.143818

[118] de Rooij J, Zwartkruis FJ, Verheijen MH, Cool RH, Nijman SM, Wittinghofer A, et al. Epac is a Rap1 guanine-nucleotide-exchange factor directly activated by cyclic AMP. Nature. **1998**;*396*:474-477. DOI: 10.1038/24884

[119] Gloerich M, Bos JL. Epac: defining a new mechanism for cAMP action. Annual Review of Pharmacology and Toxicology. **2010**;*50*:355-375. DOI: 10.1146/annurev.pharmtox.010909.105714

[120] Härndahl L, Jing XJ, Ivarsson R, Degerman E, Ahrén B, Manganiello VC, et al. Important role of phosphodiesterase 3B for the stimulatory action of cAMP on pancreatic beta-cell exocytosis and release of insulin. The Journal of Biological Chemistry. **2002**;*277*:37446-37455. DOI: 10.1074/jbc.M205401200.

[121] Bünemann M, Gerhardstein BL, Gao T, Hosey MM. Functional regulation of L-type calcium channels via protein kinase A-mediated phosphorylation of the beta(2) subunit. The Journal of Biological Chemistry. **1999**;*274*:33851-33854. DOI: 10.1074/jbc.274.48.33851.

[122] MacDonald PE, Wang X, Xia F, El-kholy W, Targonsky ED, Tsushima RG, et al. Antagonism of rat beta-cell voltage-dependent K+ currents by exendin 4 requires dual activation of the cAMP/protein kinase A and phosphatidylinositol 3-kinase signaling pathways. The Journal of Biological Chemistry. **2003**;*278*:52446-52453. DOI: 10.1074/jbc.M307612200.

[123] Song WJ, Seshadri M, Ashraf U, Mdluli T, Mondal P, Keil M, et al. Snapin mediates incretin action and augments glucose-dependent insulin secretion. Cell Metabolism. **2011**;*13*:308-319. DOI: 10.1016/j.cmet.2011.02.002

[124] Somanath S, Partridge CJ, Marshall C, Rowe T, Turner MD. Snapin mediates insulin secretory granule docking, but not trans-SNARE complex formation. Biochemical and Biophysical Research Communications. **2016**;*473*:403-407. DOI: 10.1016/j.bbrc.2016.02.123

[125] Holz GG. Epac: A new cAMP-binding protein in support of glucagon-like peptide-1 receptor-mediated signal transduction in the pancreatic beta-cell. Diabetes. **2004**;*53*:5-13. DOI: 10.2337/diabetes.53.1.5

[126] Holz GG, Leech CA, Heller RS, Castonguay M, Habener JF. cAMP-dependent mobilization of intracellular Ca2+ stores by activation of ryanodine

receptors in pancreatic beta-cells. A Ca2+ signaling system stimulated by the insulinotropic hormone glucagon-like peptide-1-(7-37). The Journal of Biological Chemistry. **1999**;*274*:14147-14156. DOI: 10.1074/jbc.274.20.14147.

[127] Gilon P, Chae HY, Rutter GA, Ravier MA. Calcium signaling in pancreatic β-cells in health and in Type 2 diabetes. Cell Calcium. **2014**;*56*:340-361. DOI: 10.1016/j.ceca.2014.09.001

[128] Kang G, Chepurny OG, Holz GG. cAMP-regulated guanine nucleotide exchange factor II (Epac2) mediates Ca2+–induced Ca2+ release in INS-1 pancreatic beta-cells. The Journal of Physiology. **2001**;*536*:375-385. DOI: 10.1111/j.1469-7793.2001.0375c.xd

[129] Ozaki N, Shibasaki T, Kashima Y, Miki T, Takahashi K, Ueno H, et al. cAMP-GEFII is a direct target of cAMP in regulated exocytosis. Nature Cell Biology. **2000**;*2*:805-811. DOI: 10.1038/35041046

[130] Kashima Y, Miki T, Shibasaki T, Ozaki N, Miyazaki M, Yano H, et al. Critical role of cAMP-GEFII--Rim2 complex in incretin-potentiated insulin secretion. The Journal of Biological Chemistry. **2001**;*276*:46046-46053. DOI: 10.1074/jbc.M108378200.

[131] Yasuda T, Shibasaki T, Minami K, Takahashi H, Mizoguchi A, Uriu Y, et al. Rim2alpha determines docking and priming states in insulin granule exocytosis. Cell Metabolism. **2010**;*12*:117-129. DOI: 10.1016/j.cmet.2010.05.017

[132] Acin-Perez R, Russwurm M, Günnewig K, Gertz M, Zoidl G, Ramos L, et al. A phosphodiesterase 2A isoform localized to mitochondria regulates respiration. The Journal of Biological Chemistry. **2011**;*286*:30423-30432. DOI: 10.1074/jbc.M111.266379.

[133] Zhang F, Qi Y, Zhou K, Zhang G, Linask K, Xu H. The cAMP phosphodiesterase Prune localizes to the mitochondrial matrix and promotes mtDNA replication by stabilizing TFAM. EMBO Reports. **2015**;*16*:520-527. DOI: 10.15252/embr.201439636

[134] DiPilato LM, Cheng X, Zhang J. Fluorescent indicators of cAMP and Epac activation reveal differential dynamics of cAMP signaling within discrete subcellular compartments. Proceedings of the National Academy of Sciences of the United States of America. **2004**;*101*:16513-16518. DOI: 10.1073/pnas.0405973101

[135] Di Benedetto G, Scalzotto E, Mongillo M, Pozzan T. Mitochondrial $Ca^{2+}$ uptake induces cyclic AMP generation in the matrix and modulates organelle ATP levels. Cell Metabolism. **2013**;*17*:965-975. DOI: 10.1016/j.cmet.2013.05.003

[136] Chen Y, Cann MJ, Litvin TN, Iourgenko V, Sinclair ML, Levin LR, et al. Soluble adenylyl cyclase as an evolutionarily conserved bicarbonate sensor. Science. **2000**;*289*:625-628. DOI: 10.1126/science.289.5479.625.

[137] Lefkimmiatis K, Leronni D, Hofer AM. The inner and outer compartments of mitochondria are sites of distinct cAMP/PKA signaling dynamics. The Journal of Cell Biology. **2013**;*202*:453-462. DOI: 10.1083/jcb.201303159

[138] Agnes RS, Jernigan F, Shell JR, Sharma V, Lawrence DS. Suborganelle sensing of mitochondrial cAMP-dependent protein kinase activity. Journal of the American Chemical Society. **2010**;*132*:6075-6080. DOI: 10.1021/ja909652q

[139] De Rasmo D, Micelli L, Santeramo A, Signorile A, Lattanzio P, Papa S. cAMP regulates the functional

activity, coupling efficiency and structural organization of mammalian FOF1 ATP synthase. Biochimica et Biophysica Acta. **2016**;*1857*:350-358. DOI: 10.1016/j.bbabio.2016.01.006

[140] García-Bermúdez J, Sánchez-Aragó M, Soldevilla B, Del Arco A, Nuevo-Tapioles C, Cuezva JM. PKA Phosphorylates the ATPase Inhibitory Factor 1 and Inactivates Its Capacity to Bind and Inhibit the Mitochondrial H(+)-ATP Synthase. Cell Reports. **2015**;*12*:2143-2155. DOI: 10.1016/j.celrep.2015.08.052

[141] Srinivasan S, Spear J, Chandran K, Joseph J, Kalyanaraman B, Avadhani NG. Oxidative stress induced mitochondrial protein kinase A mediates cytochrome c oxidase dysfunction. PLoS One. **2013**;*8*:e77129. DOI: 10.1371/journal.pone.0077129

[142] Rosca M, Minkler P, Hoppel CL. Cardiac mitochondria in heart failure: normal cardiolipin profile and increased threonine phosphorylation of complex IV. Biochimica et Biophysica Acta. **2011**;*1807*:1373-1382. DOI: 10.1016/j.bbabio.2011.02.003

[143] Barker CJ, Berggren PO. New horizons in cellular regulation by inositol polyphosphates: insights from the pancreatic β-cell. Pharmacological Reviews. **2013**;*65*:641-669. DOI: 10.1124/pr.112.006775

[144] Shigeto M, Ramracheya R, Tarasov AI, Cha CY, Chibalina MV, Hastoy B, et al. GLP-1 stimulates insulin secretion by PKC-dependent TRPM4 and TRPM5 activation. The Journal of Clinical Investigation. **2015**;*125*:4714-4728. DOI: 10.1172/jci81975.

[145] Santo-Domingo J, Chareyron I, Dayon L, Núñez Galindo A, Cominetti O, Pilar Giner Giménez M, et al. Coordinated activation of mitochondrial respiration and exocytosis mediated by PKC signaling in pancreatic β cells. FASEB Journal : Official Publication of the Federation of American Societies for Experimental Biology. **2017**;*31*:1028-1045. DOI: 10.1096/fj.201600837R

[146] Elrick H, Stimmler L, Hlad CJ Jr, Arai Y. Plasma insulin response to oral and intravenous glucose administration. The Journal of Clinical Endocrinology and Metabolism. **1964**;*24*:1076-1082. DOI: 10.1210/jcem-24-10-1076

[147] Ebert R, Unger H, Creutzfeldt W. Preservation of incretin activity after removal of gastric inhibitory polypeptide (GIP) from rat gut extracts by immunoadsorption. Diabetologia. **1983**;*24*:449-454. DOI: 10.1007/bf00257346

[148] Scrocchi LA, Brown TJ, MaClusky N, Brubaker PL, Auerbach AB, Joyner AL, et al. Glucose intolerance but normal satiety in mice with a null mutation in the glucagon-like peptide 1 receptor gene. Nature Medicine. **1996**;*2*:1254-1258. DOI: 10.1038/nm1196-1254

[149] Scrocchi LA, Marshall BA, Cook SM, Brubaker PL, Drucker DJ. Identification of glucagon-like peptide 1 (GLP-1) actions essential for glucose homeostasis in mice with disruption of GLP-1 receptor signaling. Diabetes. **1998**;*47*:632-639. DOI: 10.2337/diabetes.47.4.632

[150] Drucker DJ, Philippe J, Mojsov S, Chick WL, Habener JF. Glucagon-like peptide I stimulates insulin gene expression and increases cyclic AMP levels in a rat islet cell line. Proceedings of the National Academy of Sciences of the United States of America. **1987**;*84*:3434-3438. DOI: 10.1073/pnas.84.10.3434

[151] Weir GC, Mojsov S, Hendrick GK, Habener JF. Glucagonlike peptide I (7-37) actions on endocrine pancreas.

Diabetes. **1989**;*38*:338-342. DOI: 10.2337/diab.38.3.338

[152] Teraoku H, Lenzen S. Dynamics of Insulin Secretion from EndoC-βH1 β-Cell Pseudoislets in Response to Glucose and Other Nutrient and Nonnutrient Secretagogues. Journal Diabetes Research. **2017**;*2017*:2309630. DOI: 10.1155/2017/2309630

[153] Graaf Cd, Donnelly D, Wootten D, Lau J, Sexton PM, Miller LJ, et al. Glucagon-Like Peptide-1 and Its Class B G Protein-Coupled Receptors: A Long March to Therapeutic Successes. Pharmacological Reviews. **2016**;*68*:954-1013. DOI: 10.1124/pr.115.011395

[154] Hjøllund KR, Deacon CF, Holst JJ. Dipeptidyl peptidase-4 inhibition increases portal concentrations of intact glucagon-like peptide-1 (GLP-1) to a greater extent than peripheral concentrations in anaesthetised pigs. Diabetologia. **2011**;*54*:2206-2208. DOI: 10.1007/s00125-011-2168-7

[155] Kuhre RE, Wewer Albrechtsen NJ, Hartmann B, Deacon CF, Holst JJ. Measurement of the incretin hormones: glucagon-like peptide-1 and glucose-dependent insulinotropic peptide. Journal of Diabetes and its Complications. **2015**;*29*:445-450. DOI: 10.1016/j.jdiacomp.2014.12.006

[156] Herrmann C, Göke R, Richter G, Fehmann HC, Arnold R, Göke B. Glucagon-like peptide-1 and glucose-dependent insulin-releasing polypeptide plasma levels in response to nutrients. Digestion. **1995**;*56*:117-126. DOI: 10.1159/000201231

[157] Moran BM, Abdel-Wahab YH, Flatt PR, McKillop AM. Activation of GPR119 by fatty acid agonists augments insulin release from clonal β-cells and isolated pancreatic islets and improves glucose tolerance in mice. Biological Chemistry. **2014**;*395*:453-464. DOI: 10.1515/hsz-2013-0255

[158] Moon MJ, Park S, Kim DK, Cho EB, Hwang JI, Vaudry H, et al. Structural and molecular conservation of glucagon-like Peptide-1 and its receptor confers selective ligand-receptor interaction. Frontiers in Endocrinology. **2012**;*3*:141. DOI: 10.3389/fendo.2012.00141

[159] Wootten D, Reynolds CA, Smith KJ, Mobarec JC, Koole C, Savage EE, et al. The Extracellular Surface of the GLP-1 Receptor Is a Molecular Trigger for Biased Agonism. Cell. **2016**;*165*:1632-1643. DOI: 10.1016/j.cell.2016.05.023

[160] Sonoda N, Imamura T, Yoshizaki T, Babendure JL, Lu JC, Olefsky JM. Beta-Arrestin-1 mediates glucagon-like peptide-1 signaling to insulin secretion in cultured pancreatic beta cells. Proceedings of the National Academy of Sciences of the United States of America. **2008**;*105*:6614-6619. DOI: 10.1073/pnas.0710402105

[161] Montrose-Rafizadeh C, Avdonin P, Garant MJ, Rodgers BD, Kole S, Yang H, et al. Pancreatic glucagon-like peptide-1 receptor couples to multiple G proteins and activates mitogen-activated protein kinase pathways in Chinese hamster ovary cells. Endocrinology. **1999**;*140*:1132-1140. DOI: 10.1210/endo.140.3.6550

[162] Light PE, Manning Fox JE, Riedel MJ, Wheeler MB. Glucagon-like peptide-1 inhibits pancreatic ATP-sensitive potassium channels via a protein kinase A- and ADP-dependent mechanism. Molecular Endocrinology. **2002**;*16*:2135-2144. DOI: 10.1210/me.2002-0084

[163] Kang G, Joseph JW, Chepurny OG, Monaco M, Wheeler MB, Bos JL, et al. Epac-selective cAMP analog 8-pCPT-2'-O-Me-cAMP as a stimulus for Ca2+–induced Ca2+ release and exocytosis in pancreatic beta-cells. The Journal of Biological Chemistry.

**2003**;*278*:8279-8285. DOI: 10.1074/jbc.M211682200.

[164] Thompson A, Kanamarlapudi V. Agonist-induced internalisation of the glucagon-like peptide-1 receptor is mediated by the Gαq pathway. Biochemical Pharmacology. **2015**;*93*:72-84. DOI: 10.1016/j.bcp.2014.10.015

[165] MacDonald PE, Salapatek AM, Wheeler MB. Glucagon-like peptide-1 receptor activation antagonizes voltage-dependent repolarizing K(+) currents in beta-cells: a possible glucose-dependent insulinotropic mechanism. Diabetes. **2002**;*51*(*Suppl 3*):S443-S447. DOI: 10.2337/diabetes.51.2007.s443

[166] Panten U, Früh E, Reckers K, Rustenbeck I. Acute metabolic amplification of insulin secretion in mouse islets: Role of cytosolic acetyl-CoA. Metabolism: clinical and experimental. **2016**;*65*:1225-1229. DOI: 10.1016/j.metabol.2016.05.001.

[167] Panten U, Willenborg M, Schumacher K, Hamada A, Ghaly H, Rustenbeck I. Acute metabolic amplification of insulin secretion in mouse islets is mediated by mitochondrial export of metabolites, but not by mitochondrial energy generation. Metabolism: clinical and experimental. **2013**;*62*:1375-1386. DOI: 10.1016/j.metabol.2013.05.006.

[168] Hull J, Hindy ME, Kehoe PG, Chalmers K, Love S, Conway ME. Distribution of the branched chain aminotransferase proteins in the human brain and their role in glutamate regulation. Journal of Neurochemistry. **2012**;*123*:997-1009. DOI: 10.1111/jnc.12044

[169] Brand MD. Mitochondrial generation of superoxide and hydrogen peroxide as the source of mitochondrial redox signaling. Free Radical Biology and Medicine. **2016**;*100*:14-31. DOI: 10.1016/j.freeradbiomed.2016.04.001

[170] Nyrén R, Chang CL, Lindström P, Barmina A, Vorrsjö E, Ali Y, et al. Localization of lipoprotein lipase and GPIHBP1 in mouse pancreas: effects of diet and leptin deficiency. BMC Physiology. **2012**;*12*:14. DOI: 10.1186/1472-6793-12-14

[171] Winzell MS, Ström K, Holm C, Ahrén B. Glucose-stimulated insulin secretion correlates with beta-cell lipolysis. Nutrition, Metabolism, and Cardiovascular Diseases. **2006**;*16*(*Suppl 1*):S11-S16. DOI: 10.1016/j.numecd.2005.11.006.

[172] Cruz WS, Kwon G, Marshall CA, McDaniel ML, Semenkovich CF. Glucose and insulin stimulate heparin-releasable lipoprotein lipase activity in mouse islets and INS-1 cells. A potential link between insulin resistance and beta-cell dysfunction. The Journal of Biological Chemistry. **2001**;*276*:12162-12168. DOI: 10.1074/jbc.M010707200.

[173] Marshall BA, Tordjman K, Host HH, Ensor NJ, Kwon G, Marshall CA, et al. Relative hypoglycemia and hyperinsulinemia in mice with heterozygous lipoprotein lipase (LPL) deficiency. Islet LPL regulates insulin secretion. *The Journal of biological chemistry*. **1999**;*274*:27426-27432. DOI: 10.1074/jbc.274.39.27426.

[174] Itoh K, Moriguchi R, Yamada Y, Fujita M, Yamato T, Oumi M, et al. High saturated fatty acid intake induces insulin secretion by elevating gastric inhibitory polypeptide levels in healthy individuals. Nutrition Research. **2014**;*34*:653-660. DOI: 10.1016/j.nutres.2014.07.013

[175] Ježek J, Dlasková A, Zelenka J, Jabůrek M, Ježek P. H2O2-Activated Mitochondrial Phospholipase iPLA2γ Prevents Lipotoxic Oxidative Stress in Synergy with UCP2, Amplifies Signaling via G-Protein–Coupled Receptor GPR40, and Regulates Insulin Secretion in Pancreatic β-Cells. Antioxidants &

Redox Signaling. **2015**;*23*:958-972. DOI: 10.1089/ars.2014.6195

[176] Yamada H, Yoshida M, Ito K, Dezaki K, Yada T, Ishikawa SE, et al. Potentiation of Glucose-stimulated Insulin Secretion by the GPR40-PLC-TRPC Pathway in Pancreatic β-Cells. Scientific Reports. **2016**;*6*:25912. DOI: 10.1038/srep25912

[177] Lenzen S. Oxidative stress: the vulnerable beta-cell. Biochemical Society Transactions. **2008**;*36*:343-347. DOI: 10.1042/bst0360343

[178] Lenzen S. Chemistry and biology of reactive species with special reference to the antioxidative defence status in pancreatic β-cells. Biochimica et Biophysica Acta - General Subjects. **2017**;*1861*:1929-1942. DOI: 10.1016/j.bbagen.2017.05.013

[179] Lenzen S, Drinkgern J, Tiedge M. Low antioxidant enzyme gene expression in pancreatic islets compared with various other mouse tissues. Free Radical Biology & Medicine. **1996**;*20*:463-466

[180] Welsh N, Margulis B, Borg LA, Wiklund HJ, Saldeen J, Flodström M, et al. Differences in the expression of heat-shock proteins and antioxidant enzymes between human and rodent pancreatic islets: implications for the pathogenesis of insulin-dependent diabetes mellitus. Molecular medicine (Cambridge, Mass.). **1995**;*1*:806-820

[181] Ivarsson R, Quintens R, Dejonghe S, Tsukamoto K, in 't Veld P, Renström E, et al. Redox control of exocytosis: regulatory role of NADPH, thioredoxin, and glutaredoxin. Diabetes. **2005**;*54*:2132-2142

[182] Reinbothe TM, Ivarsson R, Li D-Q, Niazi O, Jing X, Zhang E, et al. Glutaredoxin-1 Mediates NADPH-Dependent Stimulation of Calcium-Dependent Insulin Secretion. Molecular Endocrinology. **2009**;*23*:893-900. DOI: 10.1210/me.2008-0306

[183] Jezek P, Holendova B, Plecita-Hlavata L. Redox Signaling from Mitochondria: Signal Propagation and Its Targets. Biomolecules. **2020**;*10*. DOI: 10.3390/biom10010093

[184] Woo HA, Yim SH, Shin DH, Kang D, Yu DY, Rhee SG. Inactivation of peroxiredoxin I by phosphorylation allows localized H(2)O(2) accumulation for cell signaling. Cell. **2010**;*140*:517-528. DOI: 10.1016/j.cell.2010.01.009

Chapter 3

# Individual Glycation Sites as Biomarkers of Type 2 Diabetes Mellitus

*Alena Soboleva, Natalia Vashurina and Andrej Frolov*

## Abstract

Type 2 diabetes mellitus (T2DM) is a widely spread metabolic disease, the initial stages of which are asymptomatic and have no clinically recognizable manifestation. At the molecular level, T2DM is manifested with essential non-enzymatic structural changes of intra- and extracellular proteins, mostly represented with oxidation and glycation of multiple residues. Protein glycation is one of the most universal markers of T2DM, and is recognized as an indirect, but adequate indicator of plasma glucose levels over prolonged periods of time. Unfortunately, glycated hemoglobin (HbA1c) – the universally accepted T2DM marker, is insensitive for short-term excursions of blood glucose, which are known to precede the onset of disease. Therefore, new generation biomarkers, giving access to the time dimension of Maillard reaction in blood, are desired. In this context, establishment of individual glycation sites of plasma proteins as new T2DM biomarkers might be a promising approach. Indeed, involvement of proteins with different half-life times in such analysis will make the time dimension of protein glycation in blood available and will allow early recognition of blood sugar fluctuations, occurring within few weeks or even days.

**Keywords:** Amadori compounds, biomarkers, glycation, glycation sites, label-free quantification, mass spectrometry, plasma proteins, stable isotope-labeled peptide standards, type 2 diabetes mellitus (T2DM)

## 1. Introduction

T2DM is featured with late onset of the pathology, and represents the form of diabetes which is characterized by insulin resistance, high level of blood sugar, decreased insulin production and pancreatic β-cell deficiency [1]. This state is typically accompanied with suppression of the glucose transport in muscle cells, hepatocytes and adipocytes [2]. Moreover, the increase of blood glucose is accompanied with enhanced degradation of lipids, especially triacylglycerols [3]. Various factors such as hyperglycemia and associated glucotoxicity, lipotoxicity, oxidative stress and mitochondrial dysfunction can induce apoptotic death of ß-cells [4]. As a result of β-cell dysfunction, the fasting-related secretion of the hormone glucagon and the levels of glucose in hepatocytes are not suppressed by subsequent food intake [5]. According to the World Health Organization (WHO), T2DM accounts for 90–95% of the overall number of diabetes cases and its complications are recognized as the important factors causing blindness, kidney failure, heart attacks, stroke and lower limb amputation [1]. The disease is widely distributed in all parts of human population, and occurs in all regions, including rural areas of low- and middle-income countries. China, India, USA, the countries of Middle East and North Africa are in the top of diabetes occurrence rates [6]. The number of diabetes cases is growing steadily. According to the estimations of the International Diabetes Federation, the occurrence of diabetes will increase from approximately 463 million adults (20–79 years) in 2019 to 700 million by 2045 [7].

The onset of T2DM and its early stages are asymptomatic, as well as a period preceding T2DM and characterized with compromised regulation of blood glucose concentration (so-called pre-diabetes) [8]. Because of this, pre-diabetes is asymptomatically changed by T2DM, and this disease is usually diagnosed at relatively advances stages, when therapy is already required. Thus, to date, approximately every second T2DM case (232 million people) remain undiagnosed [7, 8]. Therefore, timely identifying the individuals in the pre-diabetic state, i.e. with the obvious high risk of developing T2DM is critically important, since early interventions can delay or even prevent onset of the full-scale disease manifestation [9].

Glycation, also often referred to as non-enzymatic glycosylation, represents a reversible reaction of amino and guanidino groups in proteins, peptides, and lipids with reducing sugars (aldoses and ketoses) and carbonyl products of their degradation [10]. The process of protein glycation is often referred to as Maillard reaction of proteins, i.e. the knowledge on its chemistry goes back to the works of Louis Camille Maillard in 1912 [11]. In this reaction, the carbonyl groups of reducing sugars interact with amino/guanidino functions of proteins (mainly with lysine, arginine residues and with N-terminal amino acid residues), with lipids and nucleic acids, yielding early glycation products, also known as Amadori [12] and Heyns compounds [13]. These compounds, often referred to as early glycation products, readily undergo rearrangement, cross-linking, oxidative and non-oxidative degradation, forming so-called advanced glycation end products (AGEs), which are known to accompany not only diabetes complications, but also neurodegenerative diseases and aging [14].

Currently, the Maillard reaction of proteins is considered to be the one of the most common pathways in formation of AGEs (**Figure 1**). Thereby, glycoxidation,

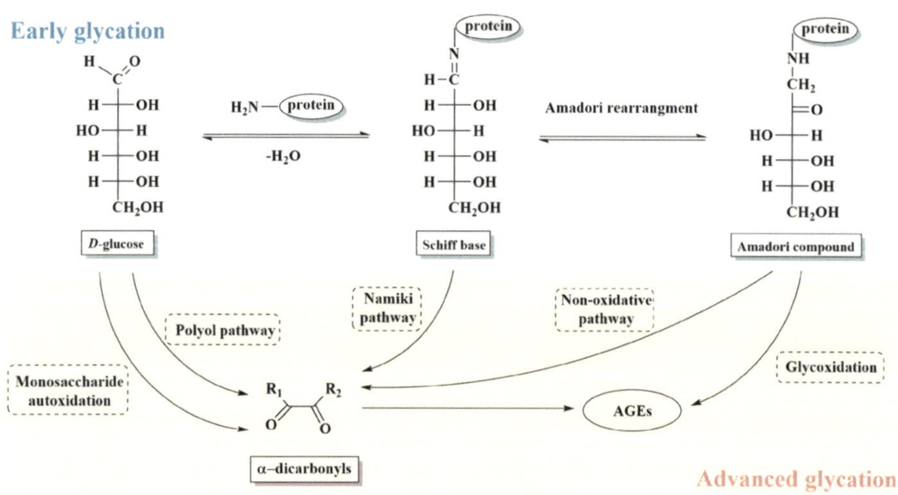


**Figure 1.**
*Formation of early- and advanced glycation in human blood plasma.*

i.e. oxidative degradation of early glycation products [15] represents the main route of AGE formation, at least for such derivatives as CML and pentosidine [16]. Importantly, α-dicarbonyl compounds, such as 3-deoxyglucosone (3-DG), glyoxal (GO), and methylglyoxal (MGO) are the principle intermediates of AGE formation [17]. Besides glycoxidation, these compounds can also appear as intermediates of glucose autoxidation [18], lipid peroxidation [19], polyol pathway [20], and the Namiki pathway [21]. These α-dicarbonyls are highly relevant for diabetes pathology, as increased concentrations of glyoxal, methylglyoxal, and 3-deoxyglucosone have been found in patients with T2DM [22]. Thus, interaction of GO with amino function yields $N^{\varepsilon}$-(carboxymethyl)lysine (CML), which represents one of the major and well-characterized AGE. Further cross-linking of GO-derived AGEs with another lysyl residue yields glyoxal-derived lysine dimer (GOLD) or arginine residue forming glyoxal derived imidazolium cross-link (GODIC) [23]. The GO-derived modification of arginine - glyoxal-derived hydro-imidazolinone (Glarg) slowly hydrolyzes under physiological conditions to yield acid-labile $N^{\delta}$-(carboxymethyl)arginine (CMA) [24]. The interaction of MGO with lysine leads to the formation of $N^{\varepsilon}$-(carboxyethyl)lysine (CEL), and reaction with arginine produced argpyrimidine or methylglyoxal-derived hydro-imidazolone (MG-H1) [17]. The methylglyoxal-lysine dimer (MOLD) is one of the major non-enzymatic cross-links in serum proteins detected during metabolic disorders [25]. Interaction of 3-DG with lysyl residues yields such modifications as pyrraline, pentosidine, imidazolone or CML [26].

In human organism, AGEs exert clearly deleterious effects [27], which are manifested by changes in structure and functions of proteins in human blood. AGEs can interact both with individual proteins *(per se)*, and by direct binding to them through the formation of cross-links. Glycation products are often found in extracellular tissue structures, thus, modified proteins impair matrix–matrix and matrix-cell interactions, leading to reduced cell adhesion, migration and cell death [27]. Intracellular proteins are also readily involved in a broad array of modifications and might lose their functionality at least to some extent [28]. The negative effects of AGEs are summarized on the **Figure 2**.

The term "fructosamine", is a common definition for all ketoamine-containing substances, i.e. Amadori and Heyns compounds, formed during protein glycation [29]. Glycated hemoglobin, which has a lifespan of 90–120 days [29], is routinely used for monitoring of glycemic index in blood of individuals with both T1DM and T2DM. Accumulation of the minor hemoglobin isoform HbA1c, also often referred to as glycated hemoglobin, in blood of diabetic patients was first reported in 1968 [30]. The modification of hemoglobin, underlying this isoform, occurs at the N-terminal valine residue of the β-chain and yields a fructosamine adduct (Amadori product) with high diagnostic value [31].

To date, more than 300 different analytical methods and well-established assays for quantitative determination of HbA1c are reported. The most of these methods rely on ion-exchange chromatography (IEC), high-performance liquid chromatography (HPLC) [32], boronate affinity chromatography (BAC) [33], colorimetry [34], as well as different biosensors, based on amperometric [35], potentiometric [36], impedometric [37] and optical sensing [38] techniques. It needs to be taken into account, however, that in some cases determination of HbA1c may appear to be biased or even unreliable. Such cases include pregnant women and patients with end-stage renal disease or those suffering from heavy alcohol consumption [29]. The other well-recognized limitations of the method are its compromised performance with the individuals characterized with increased red blood cell turnover (the state accompanying, for example, hemolytic anemia and severe blood loss) and interference between different hemoglobin isoforms variants [29].

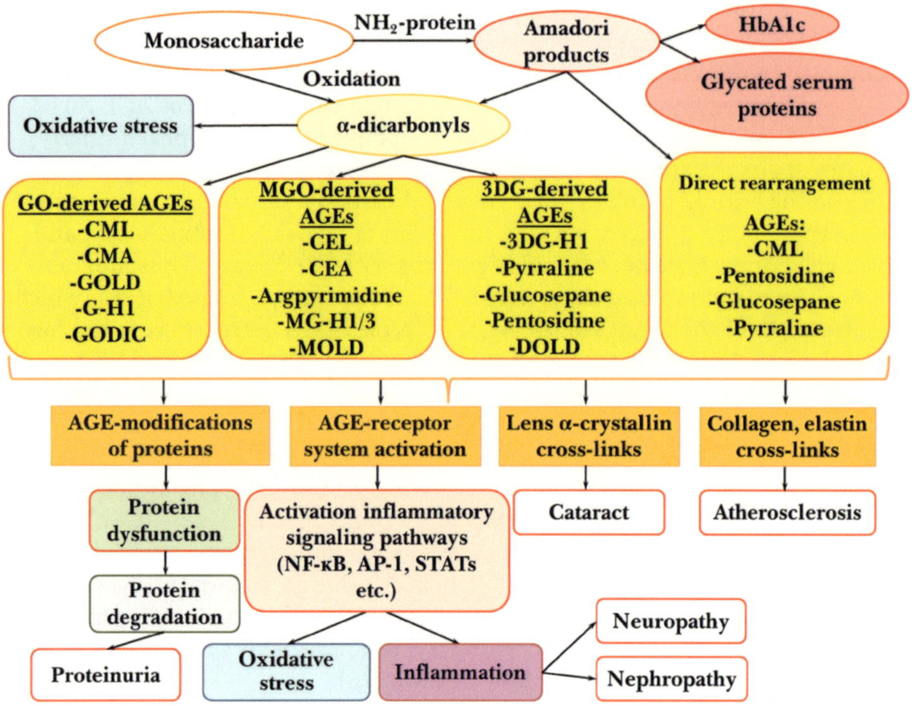


**Figure 2.**
*Pathological role of AGEs in diabetic complications. 3-deoxyglucosone-derived hydroimidazolone 1 (3DG-H1); activator protein-1 (AP-1), $N^{\delta}$-(carboxyethyl)arginine (CEA), 3-deoxyglucosonederived lysine dimer (DOLD); glyoxal-derived hydroimidazolone 1 (G-H1), nuclear factor k-light-chain-enhancer of activated B cells (NF-kB), signal transducer and activator of transcription (STAT).*

To some extent, these limitations can be addressed by implementation of a highly abundant plasma protein as a glycation biomarker supplementary to HbA1c. Human serum albumin (HSA) –the major plasma globular polypeptide with a molecular weight of approximately 67 kDa and a serum half-life of about 20 days, is recognized as the best candidate for such kind of biomarker since decades [39]. HSA constitutes up to 70% of the total serum protein, being the most abundant polypeptide in blood plasma [40]. Thus, glycated HSA (often also referred to as glycated albumin, GA) can be employed in determination of glycemic status when the conventional marker (HbA1c) is not reliable enough [41].

Application of GA can be advantageous in comparison to HbA1c due to lower reagent cost and the ability to automate GA analysis on many common laboratory instruments [29]. To date, multiple methods we proposed for analysis of GA. These include enzymatic assays [42], IEC-HPLC [43] and two-dimensional liquid chromatography including affinity chromatography and separation on reversed phase [44]. Immunoassays also represent a promising approach for assessment of GA contents. This strategy can be implemented by radioimmunoassay [45], ELISA [46], enzyme-linked boronate immunoassays (ELBIA) [47], colorimetry [48] and electrochemical methods [49]. Method characteristics are summarized in the **Table 1**.

Among the strategies of GA analysis, enzymatic method characterized by shorter operational time and easier performance both in manual and automatic mode [54]. This approach relies on exhaustive hydrolysis of GA by albumin specific proteinase with subsequent oxidation of resulted glycated amino acids by ketoamine oxidase to form hydrogen peroxide, which interacts with chromogen. The colored product can be quantified spectrophotometrically at 546/700 nm. The contents of GA are expressed as the percentage of glycated albumin in total

| # | Technique | Protein isolation | Detection | Value of GA | Ref |
|---|---|---|---|---|---|
| 1 | Radioimmuno-assay | Precipitation (ice-cold trichloroacetic acid solution) | Gamma irradiation | Control subjects: 2.0 ± 0.24 nmol/mg, T2DM: 5.3 ± 2.8 nmol/mg | [45] |
| 2 | ELISA | Affinity chromatography | UV: absorbance at 450 nm | Control subjects 2.4 ± 0.22%. Diabetic patients: 4.5 ± 1.2% (1.6–11.6%) | [50] |
| 3 | ELBIA | Affinity chromatography | UV: absorbance at 492 nm | Control and diabetic subjects: 1.1% - 47.8% | [47] |
| 4 | Enzymatic assay | — | UV: absorbance at 546/700 nm | Control subjects 13.4% (range 11.7–16.9%). T2DM 17.4% (14.2–27.0%) in good control and 26.4% (22.6–49.9%) in poor control | [51] |
| 5 | Colorimetry | Fractionation with polyethylene glycol | UV: absorbance at 546/700 nm | Control subjects: 160–222 (μmol/L). Diabetic patients: 424.6 ± 83.6 μmol/L in T1DM and 346.5 ± 61.6 μmol/L in T2DM | [48] |
| 6 | IEC-HPLC | Anion exchange chromatography, boronate affinity chromatography | UV: excitation wavelength 285 nm, emission wavelength 340 nm | Control subjects 20.2 + 1.6% (range 17.2–23.4%). Diabetic patients: 39.6 + 5.4% in T1DM and 39.4 + 5.9% in T2DM | [43] |
| 5 | Electrochemistry | — | Electro-chemical aptasensor | Control subjects 2–4%. Diabetic patients ≥16% | [52] |
| 6 | Lateral flow immunoassay | — | Colori-metric detection | Control subjects 4.59 ± 0.66 mg/mL (2.44–5.55 mg/mL). Diabetic patients 7.16 ± 2.58 mg/mL (3.17–17.21 mg/mL) | [53] |

**Table 1.**
*Overview of analytical techniques employed in analysis of GA. Ultraviolet detector, UV.*

albumin [42]. Although this method was proposed more than 15 years ago, it allows easy and fast quantification of GA with good analytical performance (specificity, accuracy, reproducibility) [55–57]. However, enzymatic assays usually require high concentration of HSA in samples that essentially restricts applicability of the method. Recently, an improved lateral flow immunoassay (LFIA) for simultaneous colorimetric determination of the total HSA and GA, which mostly solves this problem [58].

Due to the wide range of polarities and the different structure of AGEs they can be analyzed by a variety of techniques including spectrofluorimetry, enzyme-linked immunosorbent assays (ELISA), HPLC with UV–VIS detection or coupled on-line to mass spectrometry (MS) [59]. The lack of standardized methods and reference materials increases the risk of analytical errors, negatively affecting accuracy and reproducibility of these methods. Because of this the analysis of AGEs is not widely spread in regular clinical practice [60].

Analysis of total plasma contents of Amadori compounds represents another strategy of glycemic control. Determination of total blood fructosamines provides information on glucose control in the time-frames, mostly limited to the previous two weeks [61]. The total plasma fructosamine content was for the first time used as a diabetes marker in 1983 [62]. The corresponding analytical method relied on the reduction of the dye nitroblue tetrazolium (NBT) to formazan. The level of formazan formation is directly proportional to the fructosamine concentration and can be then assessed by spectrophotometry [62]. The method was significantly improved in 1989 by supplementation of incubation mixtures with a non-ionic detergent in combination with uricase. This made it possible to eliminate the influence of uric acid, lipaemia and polylysine and to provide better sensitivity [63, 64]. Although the method has some disadvantages, such as temperature sensitivity, interference with potential inhibitors of response (such as vitamins and bilirubin) and low standardization, today it remains a valuable tool, which is characterized with ease of handling, low coasts and high potential for automation [29].

Due to a high structural diversity of AGEs their adequate analysis represents a challenging task. In the most easy and straightforward way, analysis of AGEs can rely on their spectral properties, which give access to the total AGE fraction. Indeed, generally, AGEs can be divided into two groups: fluorescent (such as pentosidine or glucosepane) and non-fluorescent AGEs (for example, CML and CEL) as shown on **Figure 3**. Therefore, due to the presence of fluorescent AGEs in the protein structure it is possible to assess AGE-specific fluorescence in serum, urine and saliva using the methods of spectrofluorometry [60]. This AGE-specific fluorescence of cross-linked AGEs can be detected at 440 nm after excitation at 370 nm [65]. For example, using this method, Villa et al. have shown a correlation

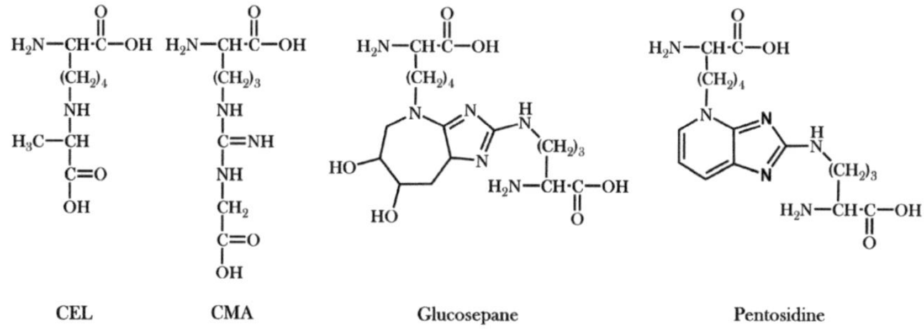


**Figure 3.**
*Fluorescent (glucosepane, pentosidine) and non-fluorescent (CEL, CMA) AGEs; CEL,* $N^{\varepsilon}$*-carboxyethyl lysine; CMA,* $N^{\omega}$*-carboxymethylarginine.*

between *in vitro* glycated BSA, and the levels of circulating and tissue AGE in diabetic rats [66]. Although this method is simple, fast and cheap, there are some serious limitations, such as lack of detection of non-fluorescent AGEs and interference with non-AGE fluorophores [60]. Furthermore, since more than fifteen years a non-invasive method for *in vivo* determination of AGE-specific autofluorescence is established [67]. However, the presence of endogenous fluorescent signals from cutaneous fluorophores (e.g. nicotinamide adenine dinucleotide, NAD) having the same excitation and emission ranges can interfere with the correct measurement of total fluorescence [68].

Unfortunately, such a powerful method as ELISA is also not free from some intrinsic limitations. Thus, as it can rely not only on monoclonal, but also polyclonal primary antibodies [69], ELISA is often featured with insufficient specificity of antibodies. Moreover, it can suffer from such factors, as high background responses due to significant contents of protein glycation adducts [70] and interference with non-glycated modified or non-modified amino acid residues [71] due to heating and alkaline treatment, implemented in the protocol [72]. Enzyme-linked boronate-immunoassay (ELBIA) represents an efficient extension of ELISA, applicable, however, only to analysis of early glycation products. This technique was first established in 1998 as a method based on the interaction of boronic acids and cis-diols of glycated HSA captured by an anti-HSA antibody [47]. A fully automated ELBIA system, giving access to high-throughput, rapid and precise measurements of GA was also developed, which was an essential extension of the method.

It is known since decades, that individual AGEs can be used as biomarkers of different pathologies including diabetes itself. Thereby, individual AGE classes present in biological samples can be assessed by instrumental and immunochemical methods, which need to be more specific due to the targeted character of the analysis. These methods include RP-HPLC, coupled on-line to spectrofluorometry [73], mass spectrometry (MS) [74, 75] or tandem mass spectrometry (MS/MS) [22, 76, 77], as well as gas chromatography - mass spectrometry (GC–MS) [78]. Immunochemical methods are mainly ELISA and Western blotting, using antibodies specific for certain AGE structures [60]. Thus, CML and pentosidine significantly increased in patients with renal failure compared to control subjects [79] and T2DM compared to non-diabetic controls [80].

## 2. Identification of individual glycation sites

Like any chronic pathology, diabetes can be efficiently recognized by a set of reliable well-established methods according universal criteria [81]. However, its first manifestations are often invisible for patients and recognized, therefore, already after onset of the pathology [81]. Thus, early diagnosis of T2DM and timely start of its therapy would allow deceleration of the disease progress and reduction the probability of life-threatening complications. Therefore, it is very important to develop a panel of biomarkers, giving access to the early and reliable discovery of diabetes mellitus.

Although HbA1c, fasting blood glucose and glucose tolerance test are well established and universally recognized diagnostic criteria of DM [81], this setup is usually unable to recognize the short term excursions of blood glucose concentrations, which are characterized the beginning of pre-diabetes [82]. Therefore, it was proposed that the biomarkers based on disease-related structural changes of individual proteins might be more sensitive and, hence, more diagnostically efficient [82]. Among such changes, post-translational modifications (PTMs) represent the most promising source of diagnostic information [82–84]. Thereby, modified peptides, rather than proteins represent the best targets in the search for new T2DM biomarkers of this type. Indeed, under *in vivo* conditions proteins can have multiple modification sites, the patterns of which can be very heterogeneous in terms of diversity of chemical structures (phosphorylation, nitration, carbonylation, glycosylation, methylation, acetylation and many others) and their relative abundances [85]. On the other hand, each individual PTM changes the molecular weight of the target protein, which leads to difficulties in MS analysis [86].

Superior, in comparison to protein analysis, level of precision could provide the fact, that individual lysine and arginine residues in protein molecule are featured with different reactivity with sugars. This effect can be related to both the amino acid environment of the site [87] and its accessibility to the molecule of glycation agent [86, 88]. Moreover, as the blood plasma proteins have different half-lives these markers can potentially cover a broad range of times prior to analysis. Thus, in contrast to HbA1c analysis, this approach might provide a short-term markers, which could successfully address short-term fluctuations in blood glucose, preceding onset of DM [84, 89]. Monitoring of blood protein glycation in this way might provide an opportunity for detection of hyperglycaemia at very early stages of the T2DM [90].

Since decades, the bottom-up proteomics (BUP) approach is the method of choice to address PTMs in proteins [91]. Accordingly, it is efficiently applied to analysis of protein glycation and can be applied to protein mixtures of any composition and complexity [92]. In the most general way it includes several critical steps: (*i*) separation of proteins, (*ii*) limited proteolysis, (*iii*) separation of resulted cleavage peptides, (*iv*) their identification by tandem mass spectrometry (MS/MS) and (*v*) annotation of individual protein sequence tags [79, 83, 89]. In application to sugar-modified proteins, BUP used for detailed information about glycoprotein profile and mapping of specific glycation sites [93].

For the BUP only several microliters of blood plasma are necessarily [83, 84]. The short workflow is present on the **Figure 4**. Plasma proteins can be separated during electrophoresis with further in gel digestion [94], or Amadori-modified proteins can be retained on BAC before digestion *in solution* [89, 92]. Several important aspects need to be continuously considered on this way. Thus, for successful quantitative BUP analysis it is very important to use the same concentration of protein in all samples [79, 80, 95]. Further, tryptic digestion of plasma samples is challenging because of high complexity of sample matrices and needs to be performed in the presence of chaotropic agents like urea [96] or detergents, e.g. sodium dodecyl sulfate (SDS) [83]. Next step is enrichment of glycated peptides on BAC which helps to eliminate chaotropic agents [83, 84, 97]. The BAC method is based on covalent binding of the column-bound ligand (*m*-aminophenyl-boronic acid) to cis-diol groups on the sugar portion of peptides, accompanied with formation of a reversible five-member ring derivative. After washing out non-bound unglycated molecules from the sample by alkaline buffer, the five-member ring can be hydrolyzed under acidic conditions, and glycated peptides can be eluted by acidic (pH 2–3) buffer [98, 99]. Prior to the MS analysis, the obtained peptides need to be desalted by solid phase extraction (SPE) [83, 84, 100, 101]. Several separation steps (on a protein and/or peptide level prior to separation by mass-to-charge ratio) and high specificity of endoproteases used for digestion are provide high proteome discovery rate and sensitivity [85, 87].

The gel-based strategy was implemented for analysis of glycation of apolipoprotein A-I in human plasma samples [94]. For this, blood samples were obtained from ten T2DM patients, affected by end-stage renal disease (ESRD), and ten healthy control individuals. The plasma samples were pooled by mixing the samples of each group of subjects and then applied onto a Centriplus centrifugal concentrator

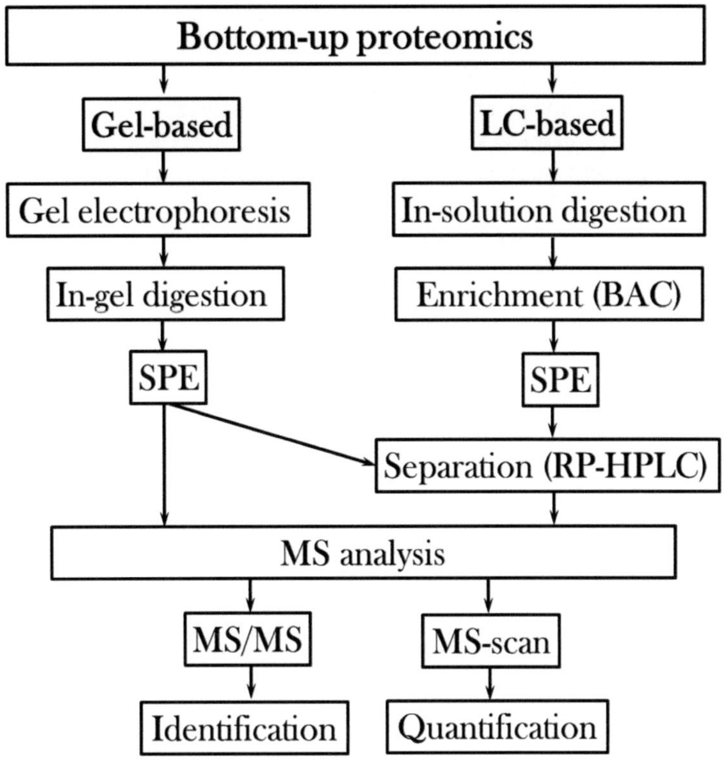


**Figure 4.**
*The short workflow of analysis individual glycation sites.*

membrane with molecular weight cut off (MWCO) 30000. After two-dimensional gel electrophoresis (2-DE) the apolipoprotein A-I spots were cut, digested, and the digests were analyzed by matrix laser desorption ionization time-of-flight (MALDI-TOF) with a standard nitrogen laser (λ = 337 nm). In this study three glycated peptides from apolipoprotein A-I were identified in T2DM and nephropathic patients [94].

One of the first scientific groups started developing methods for analysis of individual glycation sites in proteins of human plasma was the Metz's laboratory. Initially, they investigated *in vitro* glycated proteins in pooled plasma from healthy humans [96]. Glycated proteins were enriched using BAC and then digested by three different proteolytic enzymes (trypsin, Arg-C and Lys-C) to increase sequence coverage. After protein digestion, Amadori-modified peptides were enriched by BAC and analyzed by linear ion trap – orbital trap mass spectrometer (LIT-Orbitrap-MS) with electron-transfer dissociation (ETD) fragmentation option. As a result, 346 unique glycated peptides were identified. It was shown that trypsin was the most applicable enzyme in study of glycated peptides [96].

Alternatively, Zhang et al. performed the first proteomics-based characterization of non-enzymatically glycated proteins in human plasma and erythrocyte membranes from participants with normal glucose tolerance (NGT), impaired glucose tolerance (IGT), and T2DM [102]. In this study one additional step was introduced, and twelve highly-abundant plasma proteins were removed from the samples during immunodepletion procedure. Depletion of such proteins as HSA, immunoglobulin G (IgG), α1-antitrypsin, IgA, IgM, transferrin, haptoglobin, α1-acid glycoprotein, α2-macroglobulin, apolipoprotein A-I, apolipoprotein A-II and fibrinogen from blood plasma enabled the analysis of less abundant plasma proteins. As the result, 260 unique Amadori-modified peptides representing 76 unique glycated proteins from human plasma were identified. Among them 39 unique glycated proteins, represented by 114 unique glycated peptides could be detected in human plasma prior to immunodepletion. On the other hand, further 46 unique glycated proteins (156 unique glycated peptides) were discovered in the low-abundance protein fraction of human plasma. As for the proteins of the erythrocyte membrane, 75 unique glycated peptides corresponding to 31 unique glycated proteins were identified. That means, that under diabetic conditions the functions of major structural proteins, major integral proteins of erythrocyte lipid rafts and GAPDH are affected by glycation. Interestingly that a majority of the identified Amadori-modified proteins appear in all three subject groups, with little variation in terms of the numbers of glycated peptides or glycation sites. In that study no label-free-quantification analysis was performed. However, a roughly estimation showed, that 50 of unique glycated peptides from plasma samples and 14 from erythrocyte membrane were up-regulated in both IGT and T2DM groups compared to the NGT group [102].

The next logical step of the Metz's work was comprehensive identification of glycated peptides in plasma and erythrocytes of control and diabetic subjects performed in 2011 [87]. After a three-step separation by strong cation exchange chromatography (SCX), BAC, nanoHPLC and sub-sequent mass spectrometric analysis with ETD-based fragmentation, a comprehensive database of glycated peptides/glycation sites and corresponding proteins was built to facilitate the discovery of potential novel markers of diabetes. For selective and specific identification of glycated peptides, the authors established a data-dependent neutral loss triggered ETD scan, where the top six most intense ions were first fragmented with and precursor ions producing neutral losses of 3 $H_2O$ and 3 $H_2O$ + HCHO (characteristic neutral losses for Amadori-modified peptides during CID [103]) were further fragmented using ETD. In total, 7749 unique glycated peptides corresponding to 3742 unique glycated proteins were identified [87], that was a massive advantage in sequence coverage in comparison to the previous study. In general, characteristic neutral losses represent a convenient and powerful tool in identification of glycation products: they allow not only identification of involved monosaccharide [99, 100], but also more complex modifications, like ADP-glucose-dependent glycation [104].

In the work of Bai *et al.* [95] the analysis of glycated HSA peptides by liquid chromatography – ion trap – time-of-flight (LC-IT-TOF)-MS revealed 21 glycation sites in the serum samples of healthy persons and only 16 glycation sites in that from the T2DM patients [95]. Here BAC was used for enrichment of glycated proteins. The sub-sequent digestion procedure was carried out by incubation with endoproteinase Glu-C and trypsin. High sequence coverage (88% for GA from healthy person and 78% for GA from T2DM) was achieved by combining the peptide mass fingerprinting mapping results of the digests, obtained by both Glu-C and trypsin [95].

Using capillary flow data-independent acquisition (DIA) proteomics approach, 234 glycation sites in human plasma proteins were characterized [100]. 1508 plasma samples were obtained from overweight/obese non-diabetic adults. For DIA analysis, peptides were loaded on RP-UHPLC coupled on-line to Orbitrap Fusion Lumos MS tribrid. Full MS scan was performed from 350 to 1650 *m/z*, then 33 DIA segments were acquired with higher-energy collisional dissociation (HCD) 27%. For DDA analysis, isolation width was set to 1.6 *m/z*, 3 s method cycle time and 27% HCD for the dependent MS/MS scans. It resulted in identification of 242 glycation sites on 70 proteins. In this study most glycation sites were detected in serum albumin (36 sites), serotransferrin (13) and Ig kappa constant region (7) [100].

AGE-modified sites were also in the focus of research groups working in the field of DM biomarker discovery. Greifenhagen *et al.* [105] optimized the method for identification carboxymethylated (CML-modified) and carboxyethylated (CEL-modified) peptides in tryptic digests of proteins from human plasma, based on the precursor ion approach, earlier established for Amadori compounds [103]. The verification of results and identification of individual glycation sites relied on LIT-Orbitrap-MS analysis. Overall 21CML-modifications sites were identified in 17 proteins including only 2 sites $K_{88}$ and $K_{396}$ in HSA [105]. The same procedure were applied to characterize tryptic peptides (and corresponding glycation sites) with AGE-modified arginine residues [106]. It was shown that 42 plasma proteins are modified by their arginine residues with Glarg, glyoxal-derived dihydroxyimidazolidine (GD-HI), MG-H and methylglyoxal-derived dihydroxyimidazolidine (MGD-HI) [106]. In both strategies [105, 106] were no step of enrichment of AGE-modified peptides which simplifies the analysis and improves the robustness. However, the products can be reliably separated in longer LC gradients, whereas AGE-modified sites can be assigned not only by characteristic mass increments, but also by characteristic fragmentation patterns of in vitro glycated model peptides [24, 107, 108].

Different MS-based methods were developed for characterization of individual glycation sites in plasma proteins.

## 3. Label-free relative quantification of glycation occupancy at individual protein sites

Label-free relative quantification (LFQ) is the widely used method for biomarker discovery. It is based on the relative comparisons of the abundances (expressed as peak areas, heights or spectral counts) of individual analytes in control and experimental samples [109].

The first insight in the potential biomarker value of glycated proteolytic peptides was provided by the Hoffmann's group in 2010 [110]. In their first pilot study the early glycation patterns in HSA in blood samples obtained from five T2DM patients was addressed. The experimental procedure included protein concentration determination, two steps of trypsin digestion, BAC, filtration on Centricon YM-10 cartridges (to remove high molecular mass cleavage products and aggregates), HPLC separation on C18 trap column and C18 nano-column coupled with electrospray ionization - quadrupole-quadrupole-time-of-flight MS (ESI-QqTOF). The MS analysis was performed in the information-dependent acquisition (IDA) mode with CID for fragmentation. Tandem mass spectra were automatically processed with MASCOT (Matrix Science Ltd) against the SwissProt database and also confirmed by manual interpretation [110]. In most fragment ion spectra, the ions of glycated peptides showed intense signals corresponding to consecutive neutral losses of 18 (–H2O), 36 (−2× H2O), 54 (−3× H2O, pyrylium ion) and 84 (−3× H2O–HCHO, furylium ion) units. These patterns of neutral losses are characteristic for peptides, containing a carbohydrate moiety [99, 105]. Quantification relied on integration of specific extracted ion chromatograms (XICs, $m/z \pm 0.02$) at characteristic retention times ($t_R$). The BUP approach revealed 18 fructosamine-modified peptides identified by their fragmentation patterns in the plasma samples. Relative quantification showed that 15 glycated peptides were detected with quite similar intensities of corresponding signals in all T2DM samples, whereas two glycation sites showed dramatically different abundances, which could indicate individual, maybe disease-specific, alteration of glycation patterns [110].

To understand the differences in the levels of site-specific Amadori modifications, observed between healthy individuals and T2DM patients, five blood samples from poor glycemic control (HbA1c ≥ 6.5%) and four non-diabetic participants were used for BUP experiment [83]. The procedure of sample preparation was modified. Filtration step was replaced with SPE on C18-gel loader StageTips, whereas LC–MS analysis followed the procedure of Frolov and Hoffmann [110]. This strategy revealed 52 glycated peptides in T2DM plasma representing 47 glycated lysine residues in12 proteins (HSA, Ig kappa and lambda chain C region, fibrinogen (alpha, beta and gamma chains), complement C3,alpha-2-macroglobulin, serotransferrin, apolipoprotein A-I, and haptoglobin). The Mann–Whitney U-test allowed splitting these peptides into three groups based on the difference of integrated peak area. Five peptides were detected only in T2DM plasma and represented the first group – T2DM-specific sites. The second group included 15 peptides detectable in T2DM plasma at significantly higher levels than in control plasma samples. And third group represented 32 peptides detected inT2DM and control plasma samples at similar intensities, i.e. did not exhibit biomarker properties. It is necessary to take into account that the prevalence of not affected sites could be explained by small size of the cohorts, which could be insufficient for reliable conclusions [83].

Therefore, recently, we extended this approach to larger cohort size and established an integrated biomarker, based on multiple glycation sites [84]. This experiment employed T2DM female patients (n = 20 with the serum levels of HbA1c ≥ 7.5%) and age-matched normoglycemic women (n = 18 with the levels of HbA1c ≤ 6.5%). After nanoLC–MS by the above described workflow, all peptide signals were matched to the most complete glycation site database from Zhang et al. [87, 102] and results of our previous work [83] (in total more than 350 sites in plasma proteins). This approach resulted in identification of 51 Amadori peptides, 42 of which were differentially abundant in diabetic and normoglycemic controls. These peptides represented in total nine plasma proteins (HSA Ig kappa chain C region, complement C4-A, alpha-2-macroglobulin, serotransferrin, apolipoprotein A-I, ceruloplasmin precursor, Vitamin D-binding protein precursor and FLJ00385 protein), with half-lives from 2 to 21 days. Based on these differentially modified sites, we proposed an integrated biomarker based on multiple protein-specific Amadori peptides. The validation of this biomarker relied on linear discriminant analysis (LDA) with random sub-sampling of the training set and leave-one-out cross-validation (LOOCV), which resulted in an accuracy, specificity, and sensitivity of 92%, 100%, and 85%, respectively. In this context, it is logical to assume that a biomarker strategy, based on multiple specific glycation sites in plasma proteins, could essentially increase the efficiency of glycemic control and disease prediction.

Due to a high heterogeneity of AGE structures and relatively low abundances of individual AGEs at specific amino acid residues, label-free analysis of modification sites in advanced glycated proteins is rather challenging [105]. Recently, we reported plasma patterns of amide AGEs in the patients, featured with different obesity status and degree of glycaemic control, i.e. we compared four cohorts represented with hyperglycaemic and normoglycemic lean and obese individuals [111]. Although sample preparation followed our well-established pipeline [105, 106], at the stage of LC–MS analysis we employed gas phase fractionation (18 *m/z* intervals in the overall mass range 100–1400 *m/z*), that allowed higher discovery rates of AGE-modified peptides. As a result, altogether 15 advanced glycated sites in 11 proteins were detected in plasma of hyperglycaemic patients. Thereby, the relative contents of two sites, representing acetylation at $K_{199}$ in HSA ($LK_{acetyl}CASLQK$) and formylation at $K_{51}$ in apolipoprotein A-II ($SK_{formyl}EQLTPLIK$) were significantly ($p < 0.05$) higher in patients with poor glycemic control [111]. Thus, the peptides, representing the sites, can be considered as potential marker of hyperglycemia. The follow-up study, involving larger cohorts and addressing a wider array of

AGEs [112] identified 36 sites in 22 highly abundant proteins in individual plasma samples obtained from T2DM patients with long-term disease. Major modifications were Glarg (11 modification sites), CMA (5), $N^{\varepsilon}$-(formyl)lysine (8), $N^{\varepsilon}$-(acetyl) lysine (7), and CML (7). No significant changes were observed between control and T2DM group [112].

Brede and co-authors [101] established fast and high-throughput analysis of several glycated peptides of HSA. The trypsin digestion was done in 76% acetonitrile. Thereby, the authors skipped BAC enrichment and pre-cleaning with SPE. Before qualitative LC–MS/MS analysis, acetonitrile was evaporated from the samples and tryptic peptides were loaded on a C18 reversed phase trap column and separated on an analytical column coupled on-line to a QqTOF mass spectrometer. Quantitative LC–MS/MS analysis was performed by separation on BEHC18 column coupled with a Xevo TQ-S triple quadrupole tandem mass spectrometer operated in multiple reaction monitoring (MRM) mode. This method allows identification of only several glycated peptides from high abundant plasma protein HSA with the modification sites $K_{525}$, $K_{137}$, $K_{12}$, and $K_{414}$, respectively. Glycated peptide contained $K_{525}$ was used in the quantitative analysis. The level of glycation at $K_{525}$ was strongly correlated with HbA1c (r = 0.84) for patients without ESRD. In theT2DM patients with ESRD had a higher ratio of $K_{525}$/HbA1c on average, provides an excellent incentive for exploring the method as a supplement to HbA1c for detecting increased blood glucose in these patients [101].

In the work of Rathore and co-authors [90], both AGE-modified and Amadori-modified peptides were used for prediction of pre-diabetes in an integrated biomarker approach. Thereby, the authors focused on glycation of the major plasma protein - HSA. Based on HbA1c levels, the patients were categorized as healthy (n = 20) and pre-diabetic (n = 20). The digestion strategy relied on RapiGest – a detergent, which could be removed from the samples by precipitation with strong acids upon digestion and pre-cleaning on C18 zip-tip columns. Tryptic hydrolysates were separated on C18-reverse phase column coupled to Q-Exactive Orbitrap MS operated in parallel reaction monitoring (PRM) mode based on the information about precursor *m/z*, and charge state obtained during DDA (targeted label-fee approach). Normalized peak areas of glycated peptides were used for a two-tailed, unpaired, non-parametric t-test and two way ANOVA to determine the significance of glycation. As consequence, four CML- or Amadori modified peptides corresponding to 3 glucose sensitive lysine residues $K_{36}$, $K_{438}$, and $K_{549}$, respectively showed significantly higher abundance in pre-diabetes than control. Additionally, the abundance of three of these peptides ($K_{Am}$QTALVELVK, $K_{CML}$VPQVSTPTLVEVSR and F$K_{CML}$DLGEENFK) was >1.8-fold in pre-diabetes, which was significantly higher than the differences observed for fasting blood glucose (FBG), 2 h postprandial glucose (PPG), and HbA1c. Further, the four glycated peptides showed a significant correlation with FBG, PPG, HbA1c, triglycerides, very low density lipoproteins (VLDL), and high-density lipoproteins (HDL). It indicates that glycated peptides, containing glucose-sensitive lysine residues $K_{36}$, $K_{438}$ and $K_{549}$ of HSA could be potentially useful markers for prediction of pre-diabetes [90].

As can be seen from the overview, LFQ provides an essential advantage in quantification of relative glycation rates at practically all available modification sites in multiple proteins. Therefore, this approach gives a direct access to combining multiple biomarkers by simultaneous consideration of several proteins with different half-life times. This allows monitoring any long- and short-term fluctuations of blood glucose concentrations, as for any desired duration of the observation period a protein with appropriate half-life can be found.

Currently, accumulation of the information on prospective biomarker sites is necessary. In further studies, this information needs to be verified in large cohorts to assess the predictive potential of these markers. However, on this way, the limitations of label-free approach become critical. Indeed, LFQ is disadvantages for analysis of large cohorts due to sensitivity of electrospray ionization technique (ESI) to multiple factors, which is manifested as matrix effects [113]. Thus, the analysis conditions (e.g. temperature, experimenter, column condition) must be as constant as possible, that is difficult to achieve with big batch sizes. And duration of batch analysis can be rather long, as prolonged gradients are often used to improve peptide separation [114]. To overcome these limitations, absolute quantification strategies can be employed [86].

## 4. Absolute quantification of prospective biomarkers in blood plasma with isotopically labeled internal standards

Absolute quantification of glycation rates at individual modification sites by means of isotopically labeled standards was for the first time proposed by Zhang and co-workers in 2013 [86]. For the early diagnosis of T2DM glycation at the most abundant human plasma protein HSA was monitored by quantitative analysis of its characteristic tryptic peptides. Thereby, all probands were classified into three groups: T2DM (n = 73), IGT (n = 63), and NGT (n = 253). In this study $^{18}O$-labeling was used to screen glucose-sensitive and glucose-insensitive peptides within HSA-derived peptides. Glucose-sensitive peptides tested as biomarker candidates for T2DM in a clinical plasma samples, and glucose-insensitive peptide was selected as the internal standards. Three peptides (LDELRDEGK ($K_{190}$), FKDLGEENFK ($K_{12}$), and KVPQVSTPTLVEVSR ($K_{414}$)) showed significant different in their concentrations in the T2DM group compared with the IGT group. Among them two peptides FKDLGEENFK and KVPQVSTPTLVEVSR exhibited significant differences between both NGT/IGTand IGT/T2DM groups indicating that these peptides could be used as potential biomarkers for the early diagnosis of T2DM. It is important to mention that peptides FKDLGEENFK and KVPQVSTPTLVEVSR showed excellent sensitivities (97.23 and 94.47%, respectively) and specificities (93.65 and 98.41%, respectively) between the NGT/IGT groups. For the NGT/IGT and T2DM groups sensitivity of peptides FKDLGEENFK and KVPQVSTPTLVEVSR was 97.06 and 99.27%, respectively, and specificities was 97.23 and 94.47%. It indicates that these peptides could be prospective biomarkers for the early diagnosis of T2DM [86].

The internal standardization with stable isotope-labeled synthetic peptides and related stable isotope dilution techniques are widely used in glycation research [84, 95, 111, 112]. A stable isotope label can be easily introduced in the step of amino acid building block during the synthesis of Amadori-modified peptides [115]. These peptides can be directly used in the stable isotope dilution approach for absolute quantification (AQUA) [116]. Implementation of synthetic Amadori-modified peptides increases robustness, precision and accuracy of biomarkers analysis [117].

In the classical way this strategy was established for glycated peptides by Spiller and co-workers [118], who applied six standard synthetic peptides containing two isotope-labeled residues (introduced by Fmoc-($^{13}C_6$,$^{15}N$) leucine and Fmoc-($^{13}C_5$,$^{15}N$) proline) along with Amadori modification, introduced by the global post-synthetic glycation approach [119]. The peptides represented six glycation sites in HSA – TCVADESAENCDKSLHTLFGDK ($K_{64}$), SLHTLFGDKLCTVATLR ($K_{73}$), AACLLPKLDELRDEGK ($K_{181}$), ADLAKYICENQDSISSK ($K_{262}$), VFDEFKPLVEEPQNLIK ($K_{378}$) and KLVAASQAALGL ($K_{574}$). The standard mixtures were spiked (25 μL, 1.2 μmol/L) to the tryptic digest, obtained from five T2DM patients and five non-diabetic individuals and, after BAC enrichment and SPE, analyzed by a hybrid quadrupole-linear ion trap MS in the MRM mode with three specific Q1/Q3 *m/z* ranges (transitions) for each analyte [118].

All six analytes and corresponding standard peptides could be detected in all ten plasma samples. The quantities varied from 22.6 ± 3.3 to 180.3 ± 8.8 pmol per mg plasma protein. Also it was shown that content of all six glycated peptides were statistically different between the two cohorts. This study demonstrated the applicability of the AQUA technique to quantification of glycation sites in plasma proteins. In agreement with the results of LFQ studies [83], individual HSA glycation sites responded to hyperglycaemia in different ways. Interestingly, significantly higher, in comparison to others, abundance of glycated sites $K_{64}$ and $K_{378}$ was observed [118].

For absolute quantification of glycated peptides by the standard isotope dilution technique Prof. Stefanowicz and co-workers used bi-labeled peptides that contained stable isotope label, introduced as $^{3}C_6{}^{15}N_2$-lysine, and comprise a dabsyl moiety that cleaves during digestion procedure [115]. Later on we have shown applicability of these bi-labeled glycated peptides for the absolute quantification of individual glycation sites in plasma proteins [120]. Based on the previous label-free quantification [83] the prevalent glycated peptides with biomarker properties were chosen. The Amadori-modified standard peptides DSTYSLSSTLTLSK$_{Am}$ADYE$^{13}C_6{}^{15}N_2$-KK$_{Dab}$K represented the sequence of Ig kappa chain C region protein, ADLAK$_{Am}$YICENQDSISS$^{13}C_6{}^{15}N_2$-KK$_{Dab}$K and VFDEFK$_{Am}$PLVEEPQNLI$^{13}C_6{}^{15}N_2$-KK$_{Dab}$K corresponded to the HSA sequence were synthesized. The mixture of standard stable isotope-labeled peptides (20 pmol each) was added to aliquots of plasma samples (of 5 T2DM patients and 5 non-diabetic individuals). After tryptic digestion, samples were analyzed by QqTOF-MS. Glycated peptides from plasma samples and standards were annotated in MS scans (*m/z* 400–2000) by their $t_R$, *m/z* and isotopic patterns and confirmed by MS/MS analysis using Orbitrap Elite MS. The corresponding MS profiles clearly represented isotopic patterns of both light and heavy peptides with good sensitivities that gave access to reliable quantification by peak areas of analytes and corresponding internal standards. All three potential biomarker peptides demonstrated a significantly higher (in 1.5–1.9-fold) content in diabetic patients, in comparison to that in non-diabetic controls. The obtained results were cross-validated by label-free quantification performed in an independent RP-HPLC-ESI-QqTOF-MS study [120]. The resulting fold changes were close to those observed with the stable isotope dilution approach, proposed by Spiller et al. [118]. It indicates similar power of the both methods for absolute quantification of individual glycation sites in blood plasma proteins [120].

Later Spiller *et al.* [97] studied the glycation degrees of 27 glycation sites representing nine plasma proteins in 48 newly diagnosed male T2DM patients and 48 non-diabetic individuals. After protein digestion with trypsin, samples were spiked with concentration-balanced mixture of synthetic $^{13}C,^{15}N$-labeled glycated peptides (synthesized according Spiller at al [118]) as internal standards. The quantification was based on MRM using specific transitions for each targeted peptide and isotope-labeled internal peptide standards. The samples from two groups of participants were evaluated by different statistical tests (Kolmogorow-Smirnow, Mann–Whitney, and *t* test), classified by a decision tree algorithm using HbA1c in combination with each glycated peptide. Also to find the best feature set for classification, support vector machine-recursive feature elimination (SVM-RFE) method was performed for all glycated peptides and clinical parameters of participants, including HbA1c, fasting plasma glucose (FPG), body mass index (BMI), etc. The most interesting results were obtained for glycated peptide AVGDKLPECEAVCGKPK ($K_{141}$) from haptoglobin which half-life time is 2–4 days. The combination of two biomarkers of T2DM glycated $K_{141}$ of haptoglobin and HbA$_{1c}$provided a sensitivity of 94%, a specificity of 98%, and an accuracy of 96% to identify T2DM.But a set of 15 features considering three glycation sites in HSA, $K_{141}$ in haptoglobin, and 11 routine laboratory measures of T2DM, metabolic syndrome, obesity, inflammation, and insulin resistance provided a sensitivity of 98%, a specificity of 100%, and an accuracy of 99% for newly diagnosed T2DM patients. This study shows great potential of glycation sites in plasma proteins providing an additional diagnostic tool for T2DM and elucidating that the combination of these sites with HbA1c and FPG could improve the diagnosis of T2DM. The combination of both biomarkers HbA1c and glycated haptoglobin with half-life times 2 to 4 days is sensitive to long- and short-term fluctuations of blood glucose concentrations [97].

Selected 27 glycated peptides were tested further in the quality of multiple biomarker set [121]. For this plasma samples from 48 patients with duration of T2DM for more than 10 years, 48 non-diabetic individuals and 20 pre-diabetic persons we examined. The strategy of analysis was the same as described above [97]. In long-term controlled T2DM patients, 27 glycated peptides were detected at significantly higher levels and provided moderate diagnostic accuracies (ACCs) from 61 to 79%, resulting in sub-grouping of patients in three distinct clusters. In this study, a feature set of one glycated peptides from haptoglobin ($K_{141}$) and 6 established clinical parameters provided an ACC of 95%. The same number of clusters was identified in pre-diabetic males (ACC of 95%) using a set of 8 glycation sites (mostly from HSA). Re-examination of all patients present in one cluster showed progression of pre-diabetic state or advanced towards diabetes in the following five years. Overall, the studied glycation sites can play a role of promising biomarkers for sub-grouping pre-diabetic patients to estimate their risk for the development of T2DM [121].

Together with our recent report [84] these work clearly indicate under-explored potential of integrated peptide biomarkers. Moreover, it is well seen, that absolute quantification approaches are preferable, due to their higher precision and lower method-related dispersion. Thus, it is obvious, that after the explorative LFQ-based study, follow-up absolute quantification screening of large cohorts is necessary.

Besides $^{18}O$-labeling and AQUA, tag-based labeling approaches were used for quantification of glycation sites. Thus, Qiu*et al*. proposed the use of isobaric tags for relative and absolute quantification (iTRAQ) to reveal differences in HSA glycation patterns between healthy individuals and diabetic patients [88]. The authors described *in vitro* and *in vivo* experiments have been carried out to evaluate the impact of HSA glycation on the binding to anticoagulant drugs (warfarin and heparin). Plasma samples from 32 diabetic patients and 33 healthy individuals were treated with polyethylene glycol for precipitation of immunoglobulins. After this, the glycated albumin (GA) was separated using BAC. Trypsin digested GA was separated on C18-AQ analytical column and analyzed using a LTQ-Orbitrap Velos Pro MS operated in DDA mode with CID and further with ETD fragmentation. For quantitative analysis, the digested samples were labeled with iTRAQ 8-plex reagents. After labeling, the 8 samples with different mass tags were evenly mixed and glycated peptides with iTRAQ labels were extracted from the pooled samples using BAC. MS analysis was performed on a LTQ-Orbitrap Fusion MS operated in the DDA mode for CID-MS/MS and HCD-$MS^3$. A total of 49 glycation sites (including 43 glycated lysines and six glycated arginines) on GA were successfully identified using this approach. Among them seven glycation sites, $R_{81}$, $R_{117}$, $R_{186}$, $R_{257}$, $K_{313}$, $R_{410}$ and $K_{541}$, were discovered for the first time. It is interesting that glycation at sites $K_4$, $R_{81}$, $R_{117}$, $K_{439}$, $K_{519}$, $K_{538}$, $K_{541}$, $K_{557}$ and $K_{573}$ were specifically present in diabetic patients, while two sites, $R_{410}$ and $K_{436}$, were found only in healthy subjects. Altogether 21 glycation sites were quantified, and 19 of them, including $K_{51}$, $K_{64}$, $K_{93}$, $K_{162}$, $K_{199}$, $K_{233}$, $K_{262}$, $K_{313}$, $K_{323}$, $K_{378}$, $K_{402}$, $K_{414}$, $K_{466}$, $K_{475}$, $K_{525}$, $K_{545}$, $K_{557}$, $K_{564}$ and $K_{574}$, showed statistically enhanced glycation during diabetes [88].

Examples of methods used for absolute quantification of prospective biomarkers in blood plasma with isotopically labeled internal standards are summarized in **Table 2.**

| # | Proteins and sites of glycation | Peptide labeling | MS | Method power | Ref |
|---|---|---|---|---|---|
| 1 | HSA ($K_{414}$) | $^{18}O$-labeling | ESI-QqTOF | Sens. 99.27%, spec. 94.47% | [86] |
| 2 | HSA ($K_{64}$, $K_{73}$, $K_{181}$, $K_{262}$, $K_{378}$, $K_{574}$). | *L*-leucine-$^{13}C_6$,$^{15}N$, *L*-proline $^{13}C_5$,$^{15}N$ | ESI-QqLIT | Statistical difference between control and T2DM: $p < 0.0001$ or $p < 0.05$ | [118] |
| 3 | Ig kappa chain C region protein ($K_{75}$), HSA ($K_{286}$, $K_{402}$) | *L*-lysine-$^{3}C_6$$^{15}N_2$ and dabsyl moiety | ESI-QqTOF | Significantly higher (in 1.5–1.9-fold) content in T2DM | [120] |
| 4 | Haptoglobin ($K_{141}$), HSA ($K_{93}$, $K_{262}$, and $K_{414}$) | $^{13}C$,$^{15}N$-labelling | ESI-QqLIT | Sens. 98%, spec. 100%, accur. 99% | [97] |
| 5 | Haptoglobin ($K_{141}$), HSA ($K_{262}$, $K_{378}$, $K_{73}$, $K_{525}$, $K_{574}$, $K_{359}$, $K_{174}$, $K_{64}$), serotransferrin ($K_{683}$) | $^{13}C$,$^{15}N$-labelling | ESI-QqLIT | Diagnostic accuracy 95% | [121] |
| 6 | HSA ($K_{51}$, $K_{64}$, $K_{93}$, $K_{162}$, $K_{199}$, $K_{233}$, $K_{262}$, $K_{313}$, $K_{323}$, $K_{378}$, $K_{402}$,$K_{414}$, $K_{466}$, $K_{475}$, $K_{525}$, $K_{545}$, $K_{557}$, $K_{564}$ and $K_{574}$) | $^{18}O$-labeling | ESI-LTQ-Orbitrap | Statistical difference between control and T2DM $p < 0.05$ | [88] |

**Table 2.**
*Overview of methods used for absolute quantification of prospective biomarkers in blood plasma with isotopically labeled internal standards. Accuracy (accur.), sensitivity (sens.), specificity (spec.)*

## 5. Conclusions

T2DM is one of the most widely spread metabolic disorders and most often discovered at the step of complications, which makes therapy less efficient and more expensive. HbA1c provides information about changes in glycaemic status over three months, and, hence, is insensitive to short-term glucose fluctuations preceding the disease. In this context, using individual glycation sites as T2DM biomarkers might provide a good solution of this problem. Precise and reliable quantification of glycated peptides is a prerequisite for establishing biomarkers and developing clinical diagnostics of T2DM. Different methods are established and qualified for the quantification of individual glycation sites in plasma proteins using label-free or absolute quantification. Due high precision it is applicable to use in the combination with HbA1c for screening of large patient cohorts for early diagnosis of T2DM, therapy control, sub-typing disease stages, and the prognosis of complication risks. Obviously, the biomarker potential of glycated peptides is still mostly unknown. On one hand, more explorative studies are necessary to discover new biomarker candidates. On the other – these biomarker candidates need to be confirmed in wide-scale screening in large cohorts with reliable absolute quantification methods.

## Acknowledgements

The reported study was funded by Russian Foundation for Basic Research according to the research project #18-34-00927 and Deutsche Forschungsgemeinschaft (DFG, project # FR3117/2-3).

## Conflict of interest

The authors declare no conflict of interest.

## Acronyms and abbreviations

| | |
|---|---|
| 2-DE | Two-dimensional gel electrophoresis |
| 3DG-H1 | 3-deoxyglucosone-derived hydroimidazolone 1 |
| ACC | diagnostic accuracy |
| ACN | acetonitrile |
| AGEs | advanced glycation end products |
| AP-1 | activator protein-1 |
| BAC | boronate affinity chromatography |
| BEH | ethylene bridged hybrid |
| BMI | body mass index |
| BUP | bottom-up proteomic |
| CEA | $N^{\delta}$-(carboxyethyl)arginine |
| CEL | $N^{\varepsilon}$-carboxyethyl lysine |
| CID | collision induced dissociation |
| CMA | $N^{\omega}$-carboxymethylarginine |
| CML | $N^{\varepsilon}$-carboxymethyl lysine |
| DDA | data dependent acquisition |
| DIA | data-independent acquisition |
| DOLD | 3-deoxyglucosonederived lysine dimer |
| ELBIA | enzyme-linked boronate immunoassay |

| | |
|---|---|
| ELISA | enzyme-linked immunosorbent assay |
| ESI | electrospray ionization |
| ESI-QqLIT | electrospray ionization - quadrupole-linear ion trap |
| ESI-QqTOF | electrospray ionization - quadrupole-quadrupole-time-of-flight MS |
| ESRD | end-stage renal disease |
| ETD | electron-transfer dissociation |
| FBG | fasting blood glucose |
| FPG | fasting plasma glucose |
| G-H1 | glyoxal-derived hydroimidazolone 1 |
| GA | glycated albumin |
| GAPDH | glyceraldehyde-3-phosphate dehydrogenase |
| GC–MS | gas chromatography coupled with mass spectrometry |
| GD-HI | dihydroxyimidazolidine |
| Glarg | glyoxal-derived hydro-imidazolinone |
| GODIC | glyoxal derived imidazolium crosslinking |
| GOLD | glyoxal-derived lysine dimer |
| $HbA_{1c}$ | glycated hemoglobin |
| HCD | higher-energy collisional dissociation |
| HDL | high-density lipoproteins |
| HPLC | high-performance liquid chromatography |
| HPLC–MS | high-performance liquid chromatography coupled with mass spectrometry |
| ID | internal diameter |
| IDA | information-dependent acquisition |
| Ig | immunoglobulin |
| IGT | impaired glucose tolerance |
| iTRAQ | isobaric tags for relative and absolute quantification |
| LC-IT-TOF | liquid chromatography – ion trap – time-of-flight |
| LC–MS/MS | liquid chromatography coupled with tandem mass spectrometry |
| LDA | linear discriminant analysis |
| LFQ | label-free relative quantification |
| LFIA | lateral flow immunoassay |
| LIT | linear ion trap |
| LOD | limit of detection |
| LOOCV | leave-one-out cross-validation |
| LOQ | limit of quantification |
| MG-H1 | methylglyoxal-derived hydroimidazolone 1 |
| MGD-HI | methylglyoxal-derived dihydroxyimidazolidine |
| MOLD | methylglyoxal-lysine dimer |
| MRM | multiple reaction monitoring |
| MWCO | molecular weight cut off |
| MS | mass spectrometer |
| MS/MS | tandem mass spectrometry |
| NBT | nitroblue tetrazolium |
| NF-kB | nuclear factor k-light-chain-enhancer of activated B cells |
| NGT | normal glucose tolerance |
| PPG | 2 h postprandial glucose |
| PRM | parallel reaction monitoring |
| SCX | strong cation exchange |
| SDS | sodium dodecyl sulfate |
| SVM-RFE | support vector machine-recursive feature elimination |
| STAT | signal transducer and activator of transcription |

| | |
|---|---|
| T2DM | type 2 diabetes mellitus |
| UHPLC | ultra-high-pressure liquid chromatography |
| UV | ultraviolet detector |
| VLDL | very low density lipoproteins |
| XICs | extracted ion chromatograms |

## Author details

Alena Soboleva[1,2]*, Natalia Vashurina[1] and Andrej Frolov[1,2]

1 Department of Biochemistry, St. Petersburg State University, St. Petersburg, Russia

2 Leibniz Institute of Plant Biochemistry, Halle (Saale), Germany

*Address all correspondence to: asoboleva@ipb-halle.de

## References

[1] Kazi AA, Blonde L. Classification of diabetes mellitus. Clin Lab Med 2001;21:1-13

[2] Chadt A, Al-Hasani H. Glucose transporters in adipose tissue, liver, and skeletal muscle in metabolic health and disease. Pflugers Arch - Eur J Physiol 2020;472:1273-1298. DOI: 10.1007/s00424-020-02417-x

[3] Czech MP, Tencerova M, Pedersen DJ, Aouadi M. Insulin signalling mechanisms for triacylglycerol storage. Diabetologia 2013;56:949-964. DOI: 10.1007/s00125-013-2869-1

[4] Saisho Y. β-cell dysfunction: Its critical role in prevention and management of type 2 diabetes. World J Diabetes 2015;6:109-124. DOI: 10.4239/wjd.v6.i1.109

[5] Lund A, Bagger JI, Christensen M, Knop FK, Vilsbøll T. Glucagon and type 2 diabetes: the return of the alpha cell. Curr Diab Rep 2014;14:1-7. DOI: 10.1007/s11892-014-0555-4

[6] Zheng Y, Ley SH, Hu FB. Global aetiology and epidemiology of type 2 diabetes mellitus and its complications. Nat Rev Endocrinol 2018;14:88-98. DOI: 10.1038/nrendo.2017.151

[7] International Diabetes Federation - Facts & figures. About Diabetes n.d. https://www.idf.org/aboutdiabetes/what-is-diabetes/facts-figures.html (accessed August 19, 2020)

[8] Valdez R. Detecting undiagnosed type 2 diabetes: family history as a risk factor and screening tool. J Diabetes Sci Technol 2009;3:722-726. DOI: 10.1177/193229680900300417

[9] Ambady R, Chamukuttan S. Early diagnosis and prevention of diabetes in developing countries. Rev Endocr Metab Disord 2008;9:193-201. DOI: 10.1007/s11154-008-9079-z

[10] Bilova T, Lukasheva E, Brauch D, Greifenhagen U, Paudel G, Tarakhovskaya E, et al. A snapshot of the plant glycated proteome: structural, functional, and mechanistic aspects. J Biol Chem 2016;291:7621-7636. DOI: 10.1074/jbc.M115.678581

[11] Tamanna N, Mahmood N. Food processing and Maillard reaction products: effect on human health and nutrition. International Journal of Food Science 2015;2015:ID 526762. DOI: 10.1155/2015/526762

[12] Amadori M. The product of the condensation of glucose and p-phenetidine. Atti Reale AccadNazlLincei 1929;9:68-73

[13] Heyns K, Noack H. Die Umsetzung von D-Fructose mit L-Lysin and L-Arginin und dered Beziehung zu nichtenzymatischen Bräunungsreaktion. Chemische Berichte 1962;95:720-727

[14] Chaudhuri J, Bains Y, Guha S, Kahn A, Hall D, Bose N, et al. The Role of Advanced Glycation End Products in Aging and Metabolic Diseases: Bridging Association and Causality. Cell Metabolism 2018;28:337-352. DOI: 10.1016/j.cmet.2018.08.014

[15] Baynes JW. Role of oxidative stress in development of complications in diabetes. Diabetes 1991;40:405-412. DOI: 10.2337/diab.40.4.405

[16] Henning C, Glomb MA. Pathways of the Maillard reaction under physiological conditions. Glycoconj J 2016;33:499-512. DOI: 10.1007/s10719-016-9694-y

[17] Wetzels S, Vanmierlo T, Scheijen JLJM, van Horssen J, Amor S,

Somers V, et al. Methylglyoxal-derived advanced glycation endproducts accumulate in multiple sclerosis lesions. Front Immunol 2019;10. DOI: 10.3389/fimmu.2019.00855

[18] Thornalley PJ, Langborg A, Minhas HS. Formation of glyoxal, methylglyoxal and 3-deoxyglucosone in the glycation of proteins by glucose. Biochem J 1999;344 Pt 1:109-116

[19] Sajithlal GB, Chandrakasan G. Role of lipid peroxidation products in the formation of advanced glycation end products: Anin vitro study on collagen. Proc Indian Acad Sci (Chem Sci) 1999;111:215-229. DOI: 10.1007/BF02869911

[20] Hamada Y, Araki N, Horiuchi S, Hotta N. Role of polyol pathway in nonenzymatic glycation. Nephrol Dial Transplant 1996;11 Suppl 5:95-98

[21] Hayashi T, Namiki M. Role of sugar fragmentation in an early stage browning of amino-carbonyl reaction of sugar with amino acid. Agricultural and Biological Chemistry 1986;50:1965-1970. DOI: 10.1080/00021369.1986.10867692

[22] Scheijen JLJM, Schalkwijk CG. Quantification of glyoxal, methylglyoxal and 3-deoxyglucosone in blood and plasma by ultra performance liquid chromatography tandem mass spectrometry: evaluation of blood specimen. Clin Chem Lab Med 2014;52:85-91. DOI: 10.1515/cclm-2012-0878

[23] Ravichandran G, Lakshmanan DK, Raju K, Elangovan A, Nambirajan G, Devanesan AA, et al. Food advanced glycation end products as potential endocrine disruptors: An emerging threat to contemporary and future generation. Environment International 2019;123:486-500. DOI: 10.1016/j.envint.2018.12.032

[24] Frolov A, Schmidt R, Spiller S, Greifenhagen U, Hoffmann R. Arginine-derived advanced glycation end products generated in peptide-glucose mixtures during boiling. J Agric Food Chem 2014;62:3626-3635. DOI: 10.1021/jf4050183

[25] Odani H, Shinzato T, Usami J, Matsumoto Y, Brinkmann Frye E, Baynes JW, et al. Imidazolium crosslinks derived from reaction of lysine with glyoxal and methylglyoxal are increased in serum proteins of uremic patients: evidence for increased oxidative stress in uremia. FEBS Letters 1998;427:381-385. DOI: 10.1016/S0014-5793(98)00416-5

[26] Jono T, Nagai R, Lin X, Ahmed N, Thornalley PJ, Takeya M, et al. Nepsilon-(Carboxymethyl)lysine and 3-DG-imidazolone are major AGE structures in protein modification by 3-deoxyglucosone. J Biochem 2004;136:351-358. DOI: 10.1093/jb/mvh124

[27] Singh VP, Bali A, Singh N, Jaggi AS. Advanced glycation end products and diabetic complications. Korean J Physiol Pharmacol 2014;18:1-14. DOI: 10.4196/kjpp.2014.18.1.1

[28] Nowotny K, Jung T, Höhn A, Weber D, Grune T. Advanced glycation end products and oxidative stress in type 2 diabetes mellitus. Biomolecules 2015;5:194-222. DOI: 10.3390/biom5010194

[29] Danese E, Montagnana M, Nouvenne A, Lippi G. Advantages and pitfalls of fructosamine and glycated albumin in the diagnosis and treatment of diabetes. J Diabetes Sci Technol 2015;9:169-176. DOI: 10.1177/1932296814567227

[30] Rahbar S. An abnormal hemoglobin in red cells of diabetics. Clin Chim Acta 1968;22:296-298. DOI: 10.1016/0009-8981(68)90372-0

[31] Bunn HF, Haney DN, Kamin S, Gabbay KH, Gallop PM. The biosynthesis of human hemoglobin A1c. Slow glycosylation of hemoglobin in vivo. J Clin Invest 1976;57:1652-1659. DOI: 10.1172/JCI108436

[32] Thevarajah M, Nadzimah MN, Chew YY. Interference of hemoglobin A1c (HbA1c) detection using ion-exchange high performance liquid chromatography (HPLC) method by clinically silent hemoglobin variant in University Malaya Medical Centre (UMMC)--a case report. Clin Biochem 2009;42:430-434. DOI: 10.1016/j.clinbiochem.2008.10.015

[33] Stirk H, Allen KR. Measurement of glycated haemoglobin by boronate-affinity high-pressure liquid chromatography. Ann Clin Biochem 1999;36 ( Pt 2):233-234. DOI: 10.1177/000456329903600217

[34] Erasmus RT, Osotimehin B, Ugbode C, Famuyiwa OO. HbA1C measured by a colorimetric method in normal and diabetic Nigerian subjects. Afr J Med Med Sci 1983;12:177-182

[35] Chawla S, Pundir CS. An amperometric hemoglobin A1c biosensor based on immobilization of fructosyl amino acid oxidase onto zinc oxide nanoparticles-polypyrrole film. Anal Biochem 2012;430:156-162. DOI: 10.1016/j.ab.2012.08.002

[36] Chen P, Pritzker M, Sheikholeslam M. Electrochemical biosensor for glycated hemoglobin (HbA1c). Biosensors for Health, Environment and Biosecurity 2011. DOI: 10.5772/18105

[37] Wang B, Anzai J. Recent progress in electrochemical HbA1c sensors: a review. Materials (Basel) 2015;8:1187-1203. DOI: 10.3390/ma8031187

[38] Wang H-C, Chang F-Y, Tsai T-M, Chen C-H, Chen Y-Y. Development and clinical trial of a smartphone-based colorimetric detection system for self-monitoring of blood glucose. Biomed Opt Express 2020;11:2166-2177. DOI: 10.1364/BOE.389638

[39] Arasteh A, Farahi S, Habibi-Rezaei M, Moosavi-Movahedi AA. Glycated albumin: an overview of the in vitro models of an in vivo potential disease marker. J Diabetes Metab Disord 2014;13:49. DOI: 10.1186/2251-6581-13-49

[40] He XM, Carter DC. Atomic structure and chemistry of human serum albumin. Nature 1992;358:209-215. DOI: 10.1038/358209a0

[41] Zendjabil M. Glycated albumin. Clin Chim Acta 2020;502:240-244. DOI: 10.1016/j.cca.2019.11.007

[42] Kouzuma T, Usami T, Yamakoshi M, Takahashi M, Imamura S. An enzymatic method for the measurement of glycated albumin in biological samples. Clin Chim Acta 2002;324:61-71

[43] Shima K, Ito N, Abe F, Hirota M, Yano M, Yamamoto Y, et al. High-performance liquid chromatographic assay of serum glycated albumin. Diabetologia 1988;31:627-631. DOI: 10.1007/BF00264772

[44] Pepaj M, Thorsby PM. Analysis of glycated albumin by on-line two-dimensional liquid chromatography mass spectrometry. Journal of Liquid Chromatography & Related Technologies 2015;38:20-28. DOI: 10.1080/10826076.2013.864980

[45] Kato M, Nakayama H, Makita Z, Aoki S, Kuroda Y, Misawa K, et al. Radioimmunoassay for non-enzymatically glycated serum proteins. Horm Metab Res 1989;21:245-248. DOI: 10.1055/s-2007-1009204

[46] Irshad S, Riaz R, Ghafoor F. Value of serum glycated albumin in

prediction of coronary artery disease in type 2 diabetes mellitus. Public Health Research 2012;2:37-42

[47] Ikeda K, Sakamoto Y, Kawasaki Y, Miyake T, Tanaka K, Urata T, et al. Determination of glycated albumin by enzyme-linked boronate immunoassay (ELBIA). Clin Chem 1998;44:256-263

[48] Mashiba S, Uchida K, Okuda S, Tomita S. Measurement of glycated albumin by the nitroblue tetrazolium colorimetric method. Clin Chim Acta 1992;212:3-15

[49] Attar AM, Richardson MB, Speciale G, Majumdar S, Dyer RP, Sanders EC, et al. Electrochemical quantification of glycated and non-glycated human serum albumin in synthetic urine. ACS Appl Mater Interfaces 2019;11:4757-4765. DOI: 10.1021/acsami.8b16071

[50] Cohen MP, Hud E. Measurement of plasma glycoalbumin levels with a monoclonal antibody based ELISA. J Immunol Methods 1989;122:279-283. DOI: 10.1016/0022-1759(89)90275-5

[51] Paroni R, Ceriotti F, Galanello R, Battista Leoni G, Panico A, Scurati E, et al. Performance characteristics and clinical utility of an enzymatic method for the measurement of glycated albumin in plasma. Clin Biochem 2007;40:1398-1405. DOI: 10.1016/j.clinbiochem.2007.08.001

[52] Bunyarataphan S, Dharakul T, FucharoenS,PaiboonsukwongK,JaprungD. Glycated albumin measurement using an electrochemical aptasensor for screening and monitoring of diabetes mellitus. Electroanalysis 2019;31:2254-2261. DOI: https://doi.org/10.1002/elan.201900264

[53] Ki H, Jang H, Oh J, Han G-R, Lee H, Kim S, et al. Simultaneous detection of serum glucose and glycated albumin on a paper-based sensor for acute hyperglycemia and diabetes mellitus. Anal Chem 2020;92:11530-11534. DOI: 10.1021/acs.analchem.0c02940

[54] Freitas PAC, Ehlert LR, Camargo JL, Freitas PAC, Ehlert LR, Camargo JL. Glycated albumin: a potential biomarker in diabetes. Archives of Endocrinology and Metabolism 2017;61:296-304. DOI: 10.1590/2359-3997000000272

[55] Ciaccio M. Introduction of glycated albumin in clinical practice. Journal of Laboratory and Precision Medicine 2019;4. DOI: 10.21037/jlpm.2019.08.02

[56] Kohzuma T, Yamamoto T, Uematsu Y, Shihabi ZK, Freedman BI. Basic performance of an enzymatic method for glycated albumin and reference range determination. J Diabetes Sci Technol 2011;5:1455-1462. DOI: 10.1177/193229681100500619

[57] Freitas PAC, Ehlert LR, Camargo JL. Comparison between two enzymatic methods for glycated albumin. Anal Methods 2016;8:8173-8178. DOI: 10.1039/C6AY02350A

[58] Ki H, Oh J, Han G-R, Kim M-G. Glycation ratio determination through simultaneous detection of human serum albumin and glycated albumin on an advanced lateral flow immunoassay sensor. Lab Chip 2020;20:844-851. DOI: 10.1039/C9LC00967A

[59] Putta S, Kilari EK. A Review on methods of estimation of advanced glycation end products. WJPR 2015;4:689-699

[60] Perrone A, Giovino A, Benny J, Martinelli F. Advanced Glycation End Products (AGEs): Biochemistry, Signaling, Analytical Methods, and Epigenetic Effects. Oxidative Medicine and Cellular Longevity 2020;2020:e3818196. DOI: https://doi.org/10.1155/2020/3818196

[61] Roohk HV, Zaidi AR. A review of glycated albumin as an intermediate

glycation index for controlling diabetes. J Diabetes Sci Technol 2008;2:1114-1121. DOI: 10.1177/193229680800200620

[62] Johnson RN, Metcalf PA, Baker JR. Fructosamine: a new approach to the estimation of serum glycosylprotein. An index of diabetic control. Clin Chim Acta 1983;127:87-95. DOI: 10.1016/0009-8981(83)90078-5.

[63] Schleicher ED, Vogt BW. Standardization of serum fructosamine assays. Clin Chem 1990;36:136-139

[64] Kruse-Jarres JD, Jarausch J, Lehmann P, Vogt BW, Rietz P. A new colorimetric method for the determination of fructosamine. Journal of Laboratory Medicine 1989;13:245-253. DOI: 10.1515/labm.1989.13.7-8.245

[65] Sell DR, Monnier VM. Structure elucidation of a senescence cross-link from human extracellular matrix. Implication of pentoses in the aging process. J Biol Chem 1989;264:21597-21602

[66] Villa M, Parravano M, Micheli A, Gaddini L, Matteucci A, Mallozzi C, et al. A quick, simple method for detecting circulating fluorescent advanced glycation end-products: Correlation with in vitro and in vivo non-enzymatic glycation. Metab Clin Exp 2017;71:64-69. DOI: 10.1016/j.metabol.2017.03.004

[67] Meerwaldt R, Graaff R, Oomen PHN, Links TP, Jager JJ, Alderson NL, et al. Simple non-invasive assessment of advanced glycation endproduct accumulation. Diabetologia 2004;47:1324-1330. DOI: 10.1007/s00125-004-1451-2

[68] Yuan Y, Sun H, Sun Z. Advanced glycation end products (AGEs) increase renal lipid accumulation: a pathogenic factor of diabetic nephropathy (DN). Lipids Health Dis 2017;16:126. DOI: 10.1186/s12944-017-0522-6

[69] Takeuchi M, Takino J, Furuno S, Shirai H, Kawakami M, Muramatsu M, et al. Assessment of the concentrations of various advanced glycation end-products in beverages and foods that are commonly consumed in Japan. PLoS One 2015;10. DOI: 10.1371/journal.pone.0118652

[70] Thornalley PJ. Measurement of protein glycation, glycated peptides, and glycation free adducts. Perit Dial Int 2005;25:522-533

[71] Miki Hayashi C, Nagai R, Miyazaki K, Hayase F, Araki T, Ono T, et al. Conversion of Amadori products of the Maillard reaction to Nε-(carboxymethyl)lysine by short-term heating: possible detection of artifacts by immunohistochemistry. Laboratory Investigation 2002;82:795-808. DOI: 10.1097/01.LAB.0000018826.59648.07

[72] Perkins RK, Miranda ER, Karstoft K, Beisswenger PJ, Solomon TPJ, Haus JM. Experimental hyperglycemia alters circulating concentrations and renal clearance of oxidative and advanced glycation end products in healthy obese humans. Nutrients 2019;11. DOI: 10.3390/nu11030532

[73] Sun Z, He J, Qiu S, Lei C, Zhou Y, Xie Z, et al. Using serum advanced glycation end products-peptides to improve the efficacy of World Health Organization fasting plasma glucose criterion in screening for diabetes in high-risk Chinese subjects. PLOS ONE 2015;10:e0137756. DOI: 10.1371/journal.pone.0137756

[74] Ehrlich H, Hanke T, Born R, Fischer C, Frolov A, Langrock T, et al. Mineralization of biomimetically carboxymethylated collagen fibrils in a model dual membrane diffusion system. Journal of Membrane Science 2009;326:254-259. DOI: 10.1016/j.memsci.2008.10.003

[75] Antonova K, Vikhnina M, Soboleva A, Mehmood T, Heymich M-L, Leonova T, et al. Analysis of chemically labile glycation adducts in seed proteins: case study of methylglyoxal-derived hydroimidazolone 1 (MG-H1). International Journal of Molecular Sciences 2019;20:3659. DOI: 10.3390/ijms20153659

[76] Smuda M, Henning C, Raghavan CT, Johar K, Vasavada AR, Nagaraj RH, et al. Comprehensive analysis of maillard protein modifications in human lenses: effect of age and cataract. Biochemistry 2015;54:2500-2507. DOI: 10.1021/bi5013194

[77] Ahmed N, Thornalley PJ. Quantitative screening of protein biomarkers of early glycation, advanced glycation, oxidation and nitrosation in cellular and extracellular proteins by tandem mass spectrometry multiple reaction monitoring. Biochem Soc Trans 2003;31:1417-1422. DOI: 10.1042/

[78] Pamplona R, Naudí A, Gavín R, Pastrana MA, Sajnani G, Ilieva EV, et al. Increased oxidation, glycoxidation, and lipoxidation of brain proteins in prion disease. Free Radic Biol Med 2008;45:1159-1166. DOI: 10.1016/j.freeradbiomed.2008.07.009

[79] O'Grady KL, Khosla S, Farr JN, Bondar OP, Atkinson EJ, Achenbach SJ, et al. Development and application of mass spectroscopy assays for Nε-(1-carboxymethyl)-L-lysine and pentosidine in renal failure and diabetes. J Appl Lab Med 2020;5:558-568. DOI: 10.1093/jalm/jfaa023

[80] Ghanem AA, Elewa A, Arafa LF. Pentosidine and N-carboxymethyl-lysine: biomarkers for type 2 diabetic retinopathy. Eur J Ophthalmol 2011;21:48-54. DOI: 10.5301/ejo.2010.4447

[81] Standards of medical care in diabetes-2016: Summary of revisions. Diabetes Care 2016;39 Suppl 1:S4-5. DOI: 10.2337/dc16-S003.

[82] Kohnert K-D, Heinke P, Vogt L, Salzsieder E. Utility of different glycemic control metrics for optimizing management of diabetes. World J Diabetes 2015;6:17-29. DOI: 10.4239/wjd.v6.i1.17

[83] Frolov A, Blüher M, Hoffmann R. Glycation sites of human plasma proteins are affected to different extents by hyperglycemic conditions in type 2 diabetes mellitus. Anal Bioanal Chem 2014;406:5755-5763. DOI: 10.1007/s00216-014-8018-y

[84] Soboleva A, Mavropulo-Stolyarenko G, Karonova T, Thieme D, Hoehenwarter W, Ihling C, et al. Multiple glycation sites in blood plasma proteins as an integrated biomarker of type 2 diabetes mellitus. Int J Mol Sci 2019;20:E2329. DOI: 10.3390/ijms20092329

[85] Karve TM, Cheema AK. Small changes huge impact: the role of protein posttranslational modifications in cellular homeostasis and disease. Journal of Amino Acids 2011;2011:ID 207691. DOI: 10.4061/2011/207691

[86] Zhang M, Xu W, Deng Y. A new strategy for early diagnosis of type 2 diabetes by standard-free, label-free LC-MS/MS quantification of glycated peptides. Diabetes 2013;62:3936-3942. DOI: 10.2337/db13-0347

[87] Zhang Q, Monroe ME, Schepmoes AA, Clauss TRW, Gritsenko MA, Meng D, et al. Comprehensive identification of glycated peptides and their glycation motifs in plasma and erythrocytes of control and diabetic subjects. J Proteome Res 2011;10:3076-3088. DOI: 10.1021/pr200040j

[88] Qiu H, Jin L, Chen J, Shi M, Shi F, Wang M, et al. Comprehensive glycomic

analysis reveals that human serum albumin glycation specifically affects the pharmacokinetics and efficacy of different anticoagulant drugs in diabetes. Diabetes 2020;69:760-770. DOI: 10.2337/db19-0738

[89] Zhang Q, Ames JM, Smith RD, Baynes JW, Metz TO. A perspective on the Maillard reaction and the analysis of protein glycation by mass spectrometry: probing the pathogenesis of chronic disease. J Proteome Res 2009;8:754-769. DOI: 10.1021/pr800858h

[90] Rathore R, Sonwane BP, Jagadeeshaprasad MG, Kahar S, Santhakumari B, Unnikrishnan AG, et al. Glycation of glucose sensitive lysine residues K36, K438 and K549 of albumin is associated with prediabetes. J Proteomics 2019;208:103481. DOI: 10.1016/j.jprot.2019.103481

[91] Soboleva A, Schmidt R, Vikhnina M, Grishina T, Frolov A. Maillard proteomics: opening new pages. International Journal of Molecular Sciences 2017;18:2677. DOI: 10.3390/ijms18122677

[92] Zhang Y, Fonslow BR, Shan B, Baek M-C, Yates JR. Protein analysis by Shotgun/Bottom-up proteomics. Chem Rev 2013;113:2343-2394. DOI: 10.1021/cr3003533

[93] Pan S, Chen R, Aebersold R, Brentnall TA. Mass spectrometry based glycoproteomics--from a proteomics perspective. Mol Cell Proteomics 2011;10:R110.003251. DOI: 10.1074/mcp.R110.003251

[94] Lapolla A, Brioschi M, Banfi C, Tremoli E, Cosma C, Bonfante L, et al. Nonenzymatically glycated lipoprotein ApoA-I in plasma of diabetic and nephropathic patients. Ann N Y Acad Sci 2008;1126:295-299. DOI: 10.1196/annals.1433.005

[95] Bai X, Wang Z, Huang C, Wang Z, Chi L. Investigation of non-enzymatic glycosylation of human serum albumin using ion trap-time of flight mass spectrometry. - PubMed - NCBI. Molecules (Basel, Switzerland) 2012;17:8782-8794

[96] Zhang Q, Schepmoes AA, Brock JWC, Wu S, Moore RJ, Purvine SO, et al. Improved methods for the enrichment and analysis of glycated peptides. Anal Chem 2008;80:9822-9829. DOI: 10.1021/ac801704j

[97] Spiller S, Li Y, Blüher M, Welch L, Hoffmann R. Glycated lysine-141 in haptoglobin improves the diagnostic accuracy for type 2 diabetes mellitus in combination with glycated hemoglobin HbA1c and fasting plasma glucose. Clin Proteomics 2017;14:10. DOI: 10.1186/s12014-017-9145-1

[98] Pieroni L, Iavarone F, Olianas A, Greco V, Desiderio C, Martelli C, et al. Enrichments of post-translational modifications in proteomic studies. Journal of Separation Science 2020;43:313-336. DOI: 10.1002/jssc.201900804

[99] Frolov A, Hoffmann R. Analysis of amadori peptides enriched by boronic acid affinity chromatography. Ann N Y Acad Sci 2008;1126:253-256. DOI: 10.1196/annals.1433.060

[100] Bruderer R, Muntel J, Müller S, Bernhardt OM, Gandhi T, Cominetti O, et al. Analysis of 1508 plasma samples by capillary flow data-independent acquisition profiles proteomics of weight loss and maintenance. Molecular & Cellular Proteomics 2019. DOI: 10.1074/mcp.RA118.001288

[101] Brede C, Hop B, Jørgensen K, Skadberg Ø. Measurement of glycated albumin in serum and plasma by LC-MS/MS. Scand J Clin Lab Invest 2016;76:195-201. DOI: 10.3109/00365513.2015.1129671

[102] Zhang Q, Tang N, Schepmoes AA, Phillips LS, Smith RD, Metz TO.

Proteomic profiling of nonenzymatically glycated proteins in human plasma and erythrocyte membranes. J Proteome Res 2008;7:2025-2032. DOI: 10.1021/pr700763r

[103] Frolov A, Hoffmann P, Hoffmann R. Fragmentation behavior of glycated peptides derived from D-glucose, D-fructose and D-ribose in tandem mass spectrometry. J Mass Spectrom 2006;41:1459-1469. DOI: 10.1002/jms.1117

[104] Fedorova M, Frolov A, Hoffmann R. Fragmentation behavior of Amadori-peptides obtained by non-enzymatic glycosylation of lysine residues with ADP-ribose in tandem mass spectrometry. J Mass Spectrom 2010;45:664-669. DOI: 10.1002/jms.1758

[105] Greifenhagen U, Nguyen VD, Moschner J, Giannis A, Frolov A, Hoffmann R. Sensitive and site-specific identification of carboxymethylated and carboxyethylated peptides in tryptic digests of proteins and human plasma. J Proteome Res 2015;14:768-777. DOI: 10.1021/pr500799m

[106] Schmidt R, Böhme D, Singer D, Frolov A. Specific tandem mass spectrometric detection of AGE-modified arginine residues in peptides. J Mass Spectrom 2015;50:613-624. DOI: 10.1002/jms.3569

[107] Zhang Q, Frolov A, Tang N, Hoffmann R, van de Goor T, Metz TO, et al. Application of electron transfer dissociation mass spectrometry in analyses of non-enzymatically glycated peptides. Rapid Commun Mass Spectrom 2007;21:661-666. DOI: 10.1002/rcm.2884

[108] Greifenhagen U, Frolov A, Hoffmann R. Oxidative degradation of N(ε)-fructosylamine-substituted peptides in heated aqueous systems. Amino Acids 2015;47:1065-1076. DOI: 10.1007/s00726-015-1940-2

[109] Al Shweiki MR, Mönchgesang S, Majovsky P, Thieme D, Trutschel D, Hoehenwarter W. Assessment of label-free quantification in discovery proteomics and impact of technological factors and natural variability of protein abundance. J Proteome Res 2017;16:1410-1424. DOI: 10.1021/acs.jproteome.6b00645

[110] Frolov A, Hoffmann R. Identification and relative quantification of specific glycation sites in human serum albumin. Anal Bioanal Chem 2010;397:2349-2356. DOI: 10.1007/s00216-010-3810-9

[111] Greifenhagen U, Frolov A, Blüher M, Hoffmann R. Plasma proteins modified by advanced glycation end products (AGEs) reveal site-specific susceptibilities to glycemic control in patients with type 2 diabetes. J Biol Chem 2016;291:9610-9616. DOI: 10.1074/jbc.M115.702860

[112] Greifenhagen U, Frolov A, Blüher M, Hoffmann R. Site-specific analysis of advanced glycation end products in plasma proteins of type 2 diabetes mellitus patients. Anal Bioanal Chem 2016;408:5557-5566. DOI: 10.1007/s00216-016-9651-4

[113] Taylor PJ. Matrix effects: the Achilles heel of quantitative high-performance liquid chromatography-electrospray-tandem mass spectrometry. Clin Biochem 2005;38:328-334. DOI: 10.1016/j.clinbiochem.2004.11.007

[114] Sandin M, Chawade A, Levander F. Is label-free LC-MS/MS ready for biomarker discovery? Proteomics Clin Appl 2015;9:289-294. DOI: 10.1002/prca.201400202

[115] Modzel M, Płóciennik H, Kielmas M, Szewczuk Z, Stefanowicz P.

A synthesis of new, bi-labeled peptides for quantitative proteomics. J Proteomics 2015;115:1-7. DOI: 10.1016/j.jprot.2014.12.001

[116] Chen Q, Jiang Y, Ren Y, Ying M, Lu B. Peptide selection for accurate targeted protein quantification via a dimethylation high-resolution mass spectrum strategy with a peptide release kinetic model. ACS Omega 2020;5:3809-3819. DOI: 10.1021/acsomega.9b02002

[117] Edwards SH, Stribling SL, Pyatt SD, Kimberly MM. Reference measurement procedure for total glycerides by isotope dilution GC-MS. Clin Chem 2012;58:768-776. DOI: 10.1373/clinchem.2011.177063

[118] Spiller S, Frolov A, Hoffmann R. Quantification of specific glycation sites in human serum albumin as prospective type 2 diabetes mellitus biomarkers. Protein Pept Lett 2017. DOI: 10.2174/0929866524666170202124120

[119] Frolov A, Singer D, Hoffmann R. Site-specific synthesis of Amadori-modified peptides on solid phase. J Pept Sci 2006;12:389-395. DOI: 10.1002/psc.739

[120] Soboleva A, Modzel M, Didio A, Płóciennik H, Kijewska M, Grischina T, et al. Quantification of prospective type 2 diabetes mellitus biomarkers by stable isotope dilution with bi-labeled standard glycated peptides. Anal Methods 2017;9:409-418. DOI: 10.1039/C6AY02483A

[121] Spiller S, Li Y, Blüher M, Welch L, Hoffmann R. Diagnostic accuracy of protein glycation sites in long-term controlled patients with type 2 diabetes mellitus and their prognostic potential for early diagnosis. Pharmaceuticals (Basel) 2018;11. DOI: 10.3390/ph11020038

Chapter 4

# The Mechanistic and Pathophysiological Role of Adiponectin and Resistin towards Regulation of Food Intake and Appetite in Cardiovascular Associated Risk Factor of Metabolic Syndrome

*Mimie Noratiqah Jumli and Muhammad Ilyas Nadeem*

## Abstract

Insulin resistance syndrome or syndrome X is also known as metabolic syndrome (MetS). It is an emerging problem globally with the surge of increasing prevalence among urban population of developing countries. The etiology of pathophysiology of metabolic syndrome includes the inflammatory pathways of insulin resistance, deregulated appetite, diet-induced, inflammation-induced obesity, and cardiovascular diseases (CVD). Adipose tissue is an endocrine organ that secrets adipokines like adiponectin and resistin during physiological and pathological states. Moreover, the adipokines associated with diet-induced and inflammation-induced obesity have secondary deteriorating effects on cardiovascular system. Although, the adiponectin and resistin were potentially found in regulating food intake and appetite but their mediating effect on pathophysiology of CVD still needs future investigations. However, the prior studies reported the association of adiponectin and resistin levels with CVD complications related to food intake but still there is need to understand its multifactorial heterogeneity. Therefore, literature suggests figuring out potential target mechanistic and therapeutic approaches of adiponectin and resistin hormone towards food intake and appetite involvement in metabolic syndrome and CVD.

**Keywords:** cardivascular disease, metabolic syndrome, food intake, adiponectin, resistin

## 1. Introduction: cardiovascular associated with metabolic syndrome

Syndrome X or Insulin resistance syndrome is also known as metabolic syndrome (MetS). It is defined as the concurrence of obesity-associated cardiovascular risk factors inclusive of abdominal obesity, impaired glucose tolerance,



IntechOpen

hypertriglyceridemia and hypertension [1]. Meanwhile, CVD is a heart and circulatory system disease that is currently one of the main causes of morbidity and mortality worldwide. They are the series of heterogeneous diseases, like most commonly caused by CVD atherosclerosis and chronic diseases that evolve progressively over a lifetime, and are asymptomatic for a long period of time [2]. It is world leading cause of death worldwide, and 17.9 million people died every year with high record from developed and developing countries. In 2017, World Health Organization (WHO) list out diseases related to CVD such as coronary heart disease (CHD), cerebrovascular disease, peripheral arterial disease, rheumatic heart disease, congenital heart disease, deep vein thrombosis, and pulmonary embolism [3].

In addition, Ford et al. [4] stated that MetS is a syndrome had a link with 3–5 coronary heart disease (CHD) risk factors and increases the incidence of cardiovascular events especially among the elderly population. Some studies have shown that MetS is 1.50–2.00 times more common in individuals with CHD and significantly increases frequency of cardiovascular events, progress and risk of consequences [5, 6]. The risk of CHD is 7 times higher among individuals with MetS and diagnosed diabetes mellitus [7]. On the other hand, obesity plays a major role as an underlying risk factor for cardiovascular disease and changes in cardiac function associated with obesity have been described as "obesity cardiomyopathy".

Besides that, the relation between obesity and metabolic risk factors is growing rapidly. Across the globe, obesity and related metabolic disorders are becoming significant health care issues. Obesity pathogenesis involves the balance between consumed calories and energy expenditure, followed by body weight maintenance. The complex process of weight loss involves the interaction of diet, physical activity, environmental, behavioral and physiological factors, as there are several hormones and peptides involved in the regulation of appetite, eating behavior and energy expenditure [8]. In addition, chronic increase in body weight and adiposity in the cardiovascular system can lead to significant neuro-hormonal changes and adaptations.

These alterations include renin-angiotensin-aldosterone system activation, altered adipocytokine and pro-inflammatory cytokine levels, and sympathetic nervous system activation. These inflammatory products are produced in abnormal quantities in the event of obesity. Any of these items has been involved in affecting one of the metabolic risk factors or another related to MetS. Activation of the sympathetic nervous system can contribute to the commonly described increase in heart rate, retention of renal sodium, circulating blood volume, end-diastolic ventricular volume, cardiac output, and blood pressure. More generally, vascular and cardiac function abnormalities (vasoconstriction, tachycardia) and metabolic balance abnormalities (excess lipolysis driving the level of fatty acids, peripheral and hepatic insulin resistance induced by catechol) can be simultaneously driven by activation of the sympathetic nervous system [1].

## 2. Regulation of food intake and appetite

Food intake plays a role as a transportation for food supply which modulated by metabolic drive generated for energy requirement. While appetite is a psychological desire to eat which related to the energy balance model of weight regulation by involving in various aspects of eating pattern such as frequency of eating, serving portion, type of food and palatability of food [9]. The complex interactions between hormones from gastrointestinal tract and the hypothalamus involve particular regions where hormones interact to create feelings of appetite and satiety that can lead to the food intake or a feeling of fullness beyond the metabolic needs [10]. Meanwhile, homeostatic system plays an important role in balance the energy expenditure and food intake that contribute to the stability of body fat content over time [11].

Generally, ingestion of food started in the oral cavity and taste receptor. The taste of sour, sweet, salty, bitter and savory will be validated by G-protein-coupled receptors by sending the information via blood circulation to the brain. In the stomach, Brain-derived neurotrophic factor (BDNF) and neurotrohin-3 are known as neurotrophic factor helping in innervating of the stomach wall during nutrient storing. Ghrelin is a hormone sending an important signal during empty stomach and rapidly suppressed upon the ingestion of food. Bloodstream is a major route of ghrelin to the brain to control the appetite. In the intestine area, fat, protein and glucose from food intake will enhance enteroendocrine cells and adipocyte to release hormones for the digestion and absorption process with various signaling pathways involved [12]. Enterendocrine cells produced the gut hormones such as glucagon-like peptide 1 (GLU-1), cholecystokinin (CCK) and glucose-dependent insulinotropic polypeptide which rapidly secreted into bloodstream or distributed as local messengers [13].

There are many theories to explain about appetite mechanism such as Glucostat theory, Dual-centre theory, Aminostatic theory and Lipostat theory [14]. In 1950 [15], Mayer proposed the Glucostat theory which states that the drop in blood glucose level below than the threshold regulates the neuronal activity for the food intake. This theory regulates short-term control over appetite. However, this theory had been largely abandoned in 1970 due to the failure of finding any correlation between arteriovenous blood glucose concentration with hunger rate and food intake [16–18].

Next, dual-centre theory involved with two centre of brain known as Ventro medial hypothalamus (VMH) and Lateral hypothalamus (LH) which related to blood glucose level (**Figure 1**). Hunger state will be induced by LH in producing ghrelin hormone which trigger by the drop of blood glucose level while after taking meal blood glucose level will be raise and activate VMH to initiate satiety state. In addition, VMH is potentially found to develop over eating which can lead to obesity [14, 19].

In 1956, Mellinkoff [20] proposed the aminostatic theory involving the production of amino acid after protein stores breakdown sends signals to the brain for energy balance. Muscle catabolism activities caused high amino acid production and stimulate eating behavior while satiety will be reached by diminished level of amino acids [14]. However, it should be noted that evidence of such regulation or the existence of "protein-stat" is not extensive; mainly because of the concept has not been a target for investigation [21].

Lipostat theory explains the activity of adipose tissues undergo lipolysis in generate fatty acids and glycerol. Both lipolysis products will be circulated in the blood and brain for energy expenditure maintenance. High rate of lipolysis will lead to increase in food consumption and post prandial will decrease lipolysis as resulted in its termination [14]. Adipocytokines play an important role in orexigenic pathway which enhance the food intake and anorexigenic pathway which inhibit the food intake. In 1994, Zhang et al. [22] had discovered leptin as primary adipose tissue-derived factor secreted from white adipose tissue and acts on hypothalamus to induce satiety in regulating food intake and energy expenditure [23] while adiponectin have opposite functions of leptin. Various experiments have done and accepted that leptin is a signal that conveys information from the periphery to the brain regarding the long-term state of the body's energy stores [21, 24, 25]. Lipostat is not limited to leptin mechanism only but it is involved with all type of adipose tissue hormones.

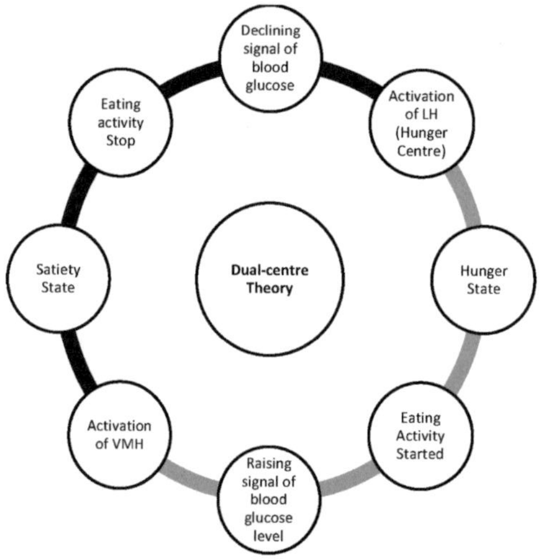


**Figure 1.**
*The circulation of dual-Centre theory related to blood glucose on hunger and satiety.*

Energy balance requires an ability of the brain to detect the status of energy stores and match energy intake with expenditure. Dysregulation of appetite and impaired energy expenditure causes excessive food consumption and disrupt the energy balance. In addition, it will cause repeated sense of hunger which contributes to the development of visceral obesity and metabolic syndrome. Frequent intakes of food expose body to store extra calorie which will turn into fat and distribute in different parts of body. There are few hunger hormones known for generating hunger state such as resistin, leptin and ghrelin involve in this process [26]. Previous study mentioned that uncontrolled eating habits like diminishing the frequency of eating, repeated fasting and recurrent over eating were link with obesity-related disorder such as cardiovascular disease, insulin resistance and inflammation [26].

## 3. Cardiovascular effects on adipocytokines

Over the last two decades adipose tissue had established as a dynamic organ that carries out several important physiological processes. It is considered one of the largest endocrine organs in the body as well as an active tissue for cellular reactions and metabolic homeostasis [27]. It also secretes numerous peptide hormones such as leptin, adiponectin, resistin and many others [28, 29]. Generally, there are three types of adipose tissue in humans which are white adipose tissue (WAT), brown adipose tissue (BAT) and beige/brite/brown-like adipose tissue (bAT). Different types of adipose tissue have distinct morphologies in reflecting their distinct functions [30] (**Figure 2**).

WAT is a major component of body's adipose tissue that provides most of the total body fat and source of fatty acids which are used as energy substrates for the generation of energy through oxidative phosphorylation of adenosine triphosphate (ATP) high-energy bond [31, 32]. Excess accumulation of WAT is potential in developing obesity and obesity-related diseases. There are three types of obesity which are android obesity, central obesity and gynoid obesity. Android or Central obesity is related to the accumulation of WAT at the upper part of body which is potentially related to some inflammatory pathologies. Meanwhile, gynoid obesity is related to the accumulation of WAT at lower part of body which does not affect any metabolic complication (**Figure 2**) [31, 32].

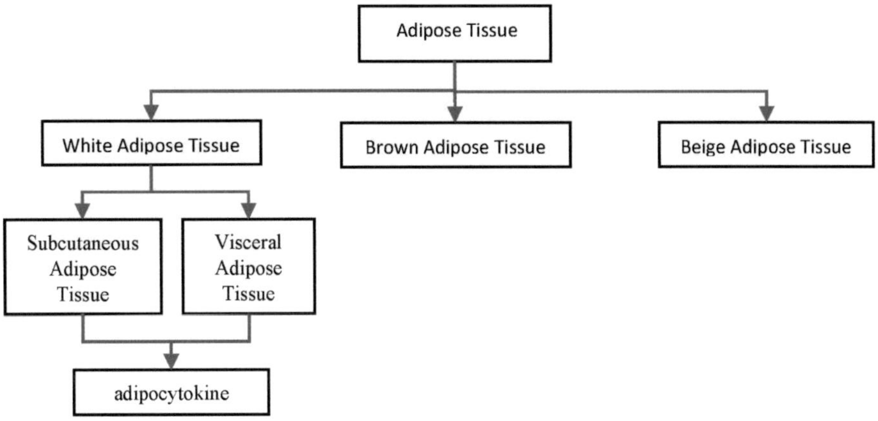


**Figure 2.**
*Types of adipose tissue.*

Anatomically, WAT contains two main depots around internal organs which are subcutaneous WAT (SAT) and visceral WAT (VAT). WAT contributes to the whole body insulation and endocrine functions including secretion of leptin, TNF-$\alpha$, adiponectin, resistin, and other compounds related to the degree of obesity and insulin sensitivity. It is located in the peritoneal cavity, where it forms a compact tissue, or as single adipocytes. Adipocytes contain a single lipid droplet which is known as univacuolar adipocytes. It can be measured between 40 and 120 μm because the size of the lipid droplet may differ significantly [33]. WAT exhibits many essential physiological roles, including the triglyceride accumulation of postprandial glucose and the secretion of signaling factors to control appetite and energy homeostasis. In periods of energy demand by the body, WAT plays role to store excess lipids in the form of triglycerides (TG) and releasing free fatty acids (FFA). It often synthesizes and releases adipokines that control metabolic homeostasis.

The general term for a bioactive substance formed by adipose tissue is known as adipocytokine or adipokine. It is a type of peptide that link the function of adipose tissue to the brain and other target organs [34]. Adipocytokine are hormones formed by fat tissues and play a role in energy homeostasis, the metabolism of sugar and fat, regulation of thermogenesis, reproduction and immunity. They also affect cardiovascular function, either through direct action by paracrine effects on the vascular wall or by influencing endothelial function through altered adipokine plasma and tissue levels relative to the total mass of adipose tissue in the body [34, 35].

### 3.1 Role of adiponectin

Adiponectin is an abundant circulating hormone present in at least three multimeric forms: trimers, hexamers, and high-molecular-weight (HMW) complexes. Among them, the HMW oligomer is major active form mediating the insulin-sensitizing and cardiovascular protective effects of the adipokine [36–38]. Adiponectin is a protein hormone with 244 amino acids derived from adipose tissue and mainly target adiponectin receptors in regulating energy metabolism and exerts functions such as antiatherogenic, anti-inflammatory, anti-diabetic and cardioprotective effect [39]. It is primarily found in WAT and also could be found in osteoblast, skeletal muscle and cardiomyocytes [40]. Adiponectin's activity is contrary to the function of leptin and resistin. It has two widely expressed receptors (AdipoR1 and AdipoR2) which cross the cerebrospinal fluid in the brain [41].

Plasma protein contains 0.01% of adiponectin and in normal human subjects it is found about 3 to 30 ug/ml [42, 43].

In order to regulate the metabolism of fatty acids, carbohydrates, cholesterol and amino acids, as well as mitochondrial function, autophagy and the growth of cells, both receptors are critical in inducing AMP-activated protein kinase (AMPK) activity. In addition, both receptors are also important in energy balance and energy expenditure as these processes activate CNS and peripheral metabolic system to trigger metabolic processes. The brain suppresses feeding activity in the event of elevated energy consumption or induces the accumulation of surplus energy in other tissues, such as glycogen in liver or triglycerides in adipose tissue [44].

On the other hand, when energy expenditure is greater than energy intake, it increases appetite and reduces energy expenditure through different metabolic pathways, including metabolism of fatty acids and activation of the AMP-activated protein kinase nutrient sensor (AMPK) [44]. Besides that, AdipoR2 contrarily enhances glucose consumption by regulating their gene expression via PPAR-α signaling pathway. Therefore, adiponectin improves hepatic insulin resistance by making balance via reducing glycogenesis and lipogenesis and increase glucose consumption [45]. Besides that, adiponectin receptors also ameliorate vascular dysfunction via activation of endothelial nitric oxide (NO) production and anti-atherogenic effects by inhibiting the inflmmtion in the various vasculature [46–50].

The administration of adiponectin via intracerebroventricular showed increase in energy consumption and decrease in food intake. It has also been suggested as a mediator of the fasting metabolic response. Previous research has shown that food intake rises, energy expenditure decreases and weight increases occur when adiponectin is administered peripherally to mimic rising levels during fasting. These results were associated with increases in hypothalamus of AMP kinase activity expression [41, 51]. Other than that, an elevation of adiponectin in plasma by either pharmacological or genetic approaches alleviates obesity-induced endothelial dysfunction and also prevents atherosclerosis, myocardial infarction and diabetic cardiomyopathy [36].

At the chromosome 3q27, there is a gene that codes the human adiponectin has been reported by Genom-wide association studies (GWAS), and is linked with susceptibility to diabetes and CVD [36, 52]. Meanwhile, Al Khadli [53] reported that human adiponectin gene exists on chromosome 3q26 which associated with type 2 diabetes mellitus and metabolic syndrome susceptibility [40]. The hypertrophic cardiomyopathy studies show that overexpression of adiponectin had reduced the hyperthrophy by activating the AMPK and inhibits the hypertrophic response to α-adrenergic receptor stimulation [21, 54]. The AMPK activation has been shown to inhibit protein synthesis in cardiac myocytes, which is mediated by decrease in phosphorylation of p70S6 kinase and increase in eukaryotic elongation factor-2 phosphorylation [21, 55]. Adiponectin's anti-hypertrophic activities on AMPK are thought to occur via the receptors of AdipoR1 and R2 [21, 56].

Besides a study reported that adiponectin gene mutation causes cellular secretion impairment by preventing trimer assemblage and is clinically associated with hypoadiponectinemia. Hypoadiponectinemia is a condition referred as low concentration of adiponectin as compare to the baseline [40, 57, 58]. In vivo study found that high fat diet causes adiponectin resistance by inhibiting the receptor expression which impacts on the reduction of adiponectin concentration. Adiponectin resistance in skeletal muscle and liver tissue causes development of systemic hyperglycemia and hyperlipidemia consequently causes vascular injury and cardiovascular complications. Cytokine production such as Tumor Necrosis Factor-alpha (TNFα) plays a critical pathogenic role in cardiovascular complication and it is significantly higher in obese or diabetic individuals [59]. There are many in-vivo studies which supported that decrease level of adiponectin significantly the obesity status, hypertension and type-2 diabetes.

However, diet high in polyunsaturated fatty acids (PUFAs) especially omega-3 potentially increases the gene expression and plasma level of adiponectin [60]. PUFAs are simply fat molecules that have more than one unsaturated carbon bond in the molecule. Omega and omega-6 are the type of PUFAs which cannot be made by the body and should be obtained via dietary sources. Fish oil consumption presented an association to increase the concentration of adiponectin. Generally, omega-3 PUFAs are perceived as a beneficial dietary intervention to enhance the adiponectin levels for the prevention and treatment of CVDs [61].

### 3.2 Role of resistin

In 2001, resistin was firstly discovered in mice with abundantly found in WAT and has ability to act on insulin resistance actions which link between obesity and diabetes. In mice, studies found that resistin is expressed in several cell types such as intestinal epithelium, skeletal muscle cells, astrocytes and adipocytes. Human resistin is a 12.5 kDa cysteine-rich peptide with a mature sequence consisting of 108 amino acids and located at chromosome 19. It is primarily produced by peripheral blood mononuclear cells (PBMCs), macrophages, bone marrow and adipocytes [62, 63].

Resistin exists in three forms which are trimer, hexamer and a monomer, with lower molecular weight form being the most active [64, 65]. Decorin is a functional receptor for resistin and was identified on the surface of adipose tissue progenitor cells [64, 66]. The normal serum concentration of resistin in human is between 7 to 22 ng/mL$^{-1}$ [62, 63]. While in obese and diabetic patient, resistin was reported higher than normal reading. A few studies mentioned that, there is a correlation shown between resistin expression with inflammatory markers, coronary artery disease and CVDs in patients with Mets [62, 67, 68]. Jonas [69] mentioned that participant who is suffered from hypertension and diagnosed with metabolic syndrome shows high level of resistin.

Resistin is emerging as an important biomarker and therapeutic target for coronary artery disease and others. It also appears to be involved in angiogenesis, thrombosis and vascular smooth muscle cell (VSMC) migration and proliferation which contribute to atherosclerosis [62]. Toll Like receptor 4 (TLR-4) is the earliest confirmed resistin receptor which is known as a major mediator in innate and adaptive immune responses stimulated by lipopolysaccharide (LPS) [70, 71] while Adenylyl Cyclase-Associated Protein 1 (CAP1) is also a resistin receptor which selected out by immunoglobulin assay [70, 72]. TLR-4 and CAP1 play a role in atherogenesis from endothelial dysfunction to diverse terminal outcome with various pathways.

A study done by Gencer [73] found that there was an association between resistin and increased risk of CVD events independently of clinical variable. Resistin promotes expression of pro-atherogenic molecules such as Intracellular Adhesion molecule –1 (ICAM-1), Vascular cell adhesion molecule-1 (VCAM-1), Monocyte chemo-attractant protein-1 (MCP-1) and Endothelial-1 (ET-1), down regulates anti-atherogenic molecules and implicated in the first stage of the atherosclerosis process via endothelial cell activation.

On the other hand, high fat diet will cause body fat mass increment which can influence the level of resistin and cause insulin resistance and inflammation. Low High Density Lipoprotein (HDL), high triglyceride and high Low Density Lipoprotein (LDL) are characterize as atherogenic dyslipidemia while resistin will induce dyslipidemia to accelerate atherogenesis [70]. A study done by Leon et al. [74]

reported that food rich in saturated fat and triglyceride were found to have positive relationship on the increment of resistin concentration. Atherogenesis is a process of forming plaques in the intima layer of arteries. It developed progressively with inflammation and lipid accumulation varying significantly among individuals [75]. Thus, resistin provide macrophages with overly large lipid fractions inducing dyslipidemia and result in the progress of atherosclerosis plaques.

## 4. Conclusions and future direction

As a summary, this chapter has explained on the relationship of food intake pathway and adipocytokine hormone effecting CVD in MetS. Adiponectin and resistin were found to have good correlation in the condition of high fat intake. High fat intake such as saturated fat and LDL food sources would potentially induce the level of resistin while polyunsaturated fatty acids and HDL food type potentially increase the level of adiponectin. High level of resistin and low level of adiponectin would contribute to the cardiovascular disease via AMPK and TLR4 pathways, respectively.

There were many studies done in investigating the action of adiponectine and resistin related to MetS and suggested various signaling pathways and mechanisms supporting effect of both protein hormones on CVD. Study believes that food intake would play a huge role in adjusting the level of adiponectin and resistin at various levels such as gene modification. Therefore, there is a scope for future studies to investigate narrowly on the mechanisms affecting adiponectin and resistin single nucleotide polymorphisms (SNPs) towards the development of Mets at cellular level.

## Acknowledgements

The authors would like to thank the Faculty of Medicine, Universiti Sultan Zainal Abidin (UniSZA) and Faculty of Health and Life Sciences, Management and Science University (MSU) for providing the facilities and support.

## Conflict of interest

The authors declare no conflict of interest.

## Author details

Mimie Noratiqah Jumli[1] and Muhammad Ilyas Nadeem[2*]

1 Faculty of Medicine, Universiti Sultan Zainal Abidin (UniSZA), Kuala Terengganu, Terengganu, Malaysia

2 Faculty of Health and Life Sciences (FHLS), Management and Science University (MSU), Shah Alam, Selangor, Malaysia

*Address all correspondence to: muhd_ilyas@msu.edu.my

## References

[1] Tune JD, Goodwill AG, Sassoon, DJ, Mather KJ. Cardiovascular Consequences of Metabolic Syndrome. Journal of Laboratory and Clinical Medicine. 2017; 183: 57-70. DOI:10.1016/j.trsl.2017.01.001

[2] Frančula-Zaninović S, Nola, IA. Management of measurable variable cardiovascular disease risk factors. Curr Cardiol Rev. 2018; 14(3): 153-163. DOI: 10.2174/1573403X1466618 0222102312

[3] World Health Organization (WHO). Cardivascular Disease (CVDs) [Internet]. 2017. Available from: https:// www.who.int/news-room/fact-sheets/ detail/cardiovacular-disease-(cvds)

[4] Ford ES, Giles WH, Dietz WH. Prevalence of the Metabolic Syndrome among US Adults Findings from the Third National Health and Nutrition Examination Survey. Journal American Medical Association. 2015; 287(3): 356-359. DOI: 10.1001/jama.287.3.356

[5] Suh S, Baek J, Bae C, Kim K, Park MK, Kim DK, Cho NH, Lee M. Sex factors in the metabolic syndrome as a predictor of cardiovascular disease. Endocrinology and Metabolism 2014; 29(4):522-529. DOI: 10.3803/ EnM.2014.29.4.522

[6] Espinola-Klein C, Rupprecht H, Bickel C, Post F, Genth-Zotz S, Lackner K, Munzel T, Blankenberg S. Impact of metabolic syndrome on atherosclerotic burden and cardiovascular prognosis. Am J Cardiol. 2007; 99(12): 1623-1628. DOI: 10.1016/j. amjcard.2007.01.049

[7] Kazlauskienė L, Butnorienė J, Norkus A. Metabolic syndrome related to cardiovascular events in a 10-year prospective study. Diabetology & Metabolic Syndrome. 2015; 7(1): 1-7. DOI: 10.1186/s13098-015-0096-2

[8] Cercato C, Fonseca FA. Cardiovascular risak and obesity. Diabetology & Metabolic syndrome. 2019: 11(74): 1-15. DOI: 10.1186/ s13098-019-0468-0

[9] Hopkins M, Blundell JE, Halford J, King N, Finlayson G. The regulation of food intake in humans. 2016. In: Feingold KR, Anawalt B, Boyce A, et al. editors. Endotext[Internet], South Dartmouth (MA); MD Tect.com, Inc 2020.

[10] Yeung AY, Tadi P. Physiology, Obesity Neurohormonal appetite and satiety control. Treasure Island: StatPearls Publishing. 2020.

[11] Mortan GJ, Meek TT, Schwartz MW. Neurobiology of Food Intake in Health and Disease. Nat Rev Neurosci.2015. 15(6): 367-378. DOI: 10.1038/nrn3745

[12] Lenard NR, Berthoud HR. Central and peripheral regulation of food intake and physical activity: pathways and genes. Obesity (Silver Spring). 2008. 16(3): 11-22. DOI: 10.1038/oby.2008.511

[13] Gribble FM, Reimann F. Function and mechanisms of enteroendocrine cells and gut hormones in metabolism. Nat Rev Endocrinol. 2019. 15:226-237. DOI:10.1038/s41574-019-0168-8

[14] Jain S, Singh SN. Regulation of food intake: A complex Process. Defence Life Science Journal. 2018. 3(2): 182-189. DOI: 10.14429/dlsj.3.12401

[15] Mayer J. Regulation of enery intake and the body weight, the glucostatic theory and the lipostatic hypothesis. Ann NY Acad Sci. 1955. 63:15-43

[16] Chaput JP, Tremblay A. The glucostatic theory of appetite control and the risk of obesity and diabetes. Int J Obes. 2009. 33: 46-53. DOI: 10.1038/ ijo.2008.221

[17] Stunkard AJ, Van Itallie TB, Reiss BB. Effect of glucagon on gastric hunger concentration in man. Proc Soc Exp Biol Med. 1955. 89:258-261

[18] Van Itallie TB, Beaudoin R, Mayer J. Arteriovenous glucose differences, metabolic hypoglycemia and food intake in man. J Clin Nutr. 1953. 1:208-216

[19] Lashley KS. The experimental analysis of instinctive behavior. Psychol Rev. 1938. 45(6):445-471. DOI: 10.1037/h0060183

[20] Mellinkoff SM, Frankland M, Boyle D, Greipel M. Relationship between serum amino acid concentration and fluctuations in appetite. J Appl Physiol. 1956. 8(5):535-538. DOI:10.1152/jappl.1956.8.5.535

[21] Hopkins M, Blundell JE. Energy metabolism and appetite control: Separate roles for fat-free mass and fat mass in the control of food intake in humans. In: Hariss RBS editors. Appetite and food intake: Central control. 2nd edition. Boca Raton (FL):CRC Press/Taylor & Francis;2017. Chapter 12.DOI: 10.1201/9781315120171-12.

[22] Zhang Y, Proenca R, Maffei M, Barone M, Leopold L, Friedman JM,. Positional cloning of the mouse obese gene and its human homologue. Nature. 1994. 372: 425-432. DOI: 10.1038/372425a0

[23] Henry BA, Clarke IJ. Adipose tissue hormones and the regulation of food intake. Journal of Neuroendocrinology. 2008. 842-849. DOI: 10.1111/j.1365-2826.2008.1730.x

[24] Woods SC, Ramsay DS. Food intake, metabolism and homeostasis. Physiol Behav. 2011. 104(1): 4-7. DOI: 10.1016/j.physbeh.2011.04.026

[25] Badman MK, Flier JS. The gut and energy balance: Visceral allies in the obesity wars. Science. 2005. 307 (5717);1909-1914. DOI: 10.1126/science.1109951

[26] Han JM, Kim HG, Lee JS, Chai MK, Kim YA, Son CG. Repeated sense of hunger leads to the development of visceral obesity and metabolic syndrome in a mouse model. pLOS One. 2014; 9(5). DOI: 10.1371/journal.pome.0098276

[27] Unamuno X, Fruhbeck G, Catalan V. Adipose Tissue. Encyclopedia of Endocrine Disease. 2019; 1: 370-384.

[28] Roumaud P, Martin LJ. Roles of leptin, adiponectin and resistin in the transcriptional regulation of steroidogenic genes contributing to decreased leydig cells function in obesity. Horm Mol Biol Clin Invest. 2015. 24(1): 25-45. DOI: 10.1515/hmbci-2015-0046

[29] Pardo M, Roca-Rivada A, Seoane LM, Casanueva FF. Obesidomics; contribution of adipose tissue secretome analysis to obesity research. Endocrine. 2012. 41:374-383. DOI:10.1007/s12020-012-9617-z

[30] Choe SS, Huh JY, Hwang IJ, Kim JI, Kim JB. Adipose tissue remodeling: Its role in energy metabolism and metabolic disorder. Front. Endocrinol. 2016; 7(30):1-16. DOI: 10.3389/fendo.2016.00030

[31] Balistreri CR, Caruso C, Candore G. The role of adipose tissue and adipokines in obesity-related inflammatory disease. Mediators of Inflammation. 2010. 1-19. DOI: 10.1155/2010/802078

[32] Gesta S, Tseng YH, Kahn CR. Development origin of fat: tracking obesity to its source. Cell. 2007. 131(2): 242-256. DOI:10.1016/j.cell.2007.10.004

[33] Pavelka M, Roth J. White Adipose Tissue. Functional Ultrastructure. 2010;

290-291. DOI: 10.1007/978-3-211-99390-3_149

[34] Smekal A, Vaclavik J. Adipokines and cardiovascular disease: A comprehensive review. Biomed Pap Med Fac Univ Palacky Olomouc Czech Repub. 2017; 161(1): 31-40. DOI: 10.5507/bp.2017.002

[35] Gualillo O, González-Juanatey JR, Lago F. The emerging role of adipokines as mediators of cardiovascular function: physiologic and clinical perspectives. Trends Cardiovasc Med 2007; 17:275-283. DOI: 10.1016/j.tcm.2007.09.005

[36] Hui X, Lam KS, Vanhoutte PM, Xu A. Adiponectin and cardiovascular health: an update. British Journal Pharmacology. 2012. 165():574-590. DOI: 10.1111/j.1476-581.20.01395.x

[37] Kobayashi H, Ouchi N, Kihara S, Walsh K, Kumada M, Abe Y, Funahashi T, Matsuzawa Y. Selective suppression of endothelial cell apoptosis by the hig molecular weight form of adiponectine. Circ Res. 2004. 94: 27-31. DOI: 10.1161/01.RES.000019921.86460.37

[38] Pajvani UB, Hawkins M, Combs TP, Rajala MW, Doebber T, Berger JP, Wagner JA, Wu M, Knopps A, Xiang AH, Utzschneider KM, Kahn SE, Olefsky JM, Buchanan TA, Scherer PE. Complex distribution, not absolute amount of adiponectin, correlates with thiazolidinedione-mediated improvement in insulin sensitivity. J Biol Chem. 2004a. 279(13): 12152-12162. DOI: 10.1074/jbc.M311113200

[39] Xiang L, Wu q, Cheng L, Sun K, Li J, Yoshida M, Qi J. Leptin and adiponectin signaling pathways are involved in the antiobesity effects of peanut skin extract. Oxidatve medicine and cellular longevity.2019. DOI: 110.1155/2019/2935315

[40] Wang Y, Ma XL, Lau WB. Cardiovascular adiponectin resistance: the critical role of adiponectin receptor modification. Trends Endocrinol Metab. 2017. 28(7): 519-530. DOI: 10.1016/j.tem.2017.03.004

[41] Ahima RS, Antwi DA. Brain regulation of appetite and satiety. Endocrinol Metab Clin North Am. 2008. 37(4): 811-823. DOI: 10.1016/j.ecl.2008.08.005

[42] Hopkins TA, Ouchi N, Shibata R, Walsh K. Adiponectin action in the cardiovascular system. Cardiovascular research. 2007. 74(1):11-18. DOI: 10.1016/j.cardiores.206.10.009

[43] Arita Y, Kihara S, Ouchi N, Takahashi M, Maeda K, Miyagawa J, Hotta K, Shimomura I, Nakamura T, Miyaoka K, Kuriyama H, Nishida M, Yamashita S, Okubo K, Matsubara K, Muraguchi M, Ohmoto Y, Funahashi T, Matsuzawa Y. Paraoxical decrease of an adipose-specific protein, adiponectin, in obesity. Biochem Biophys Res Commun. 1999. 257(1):79-83. DOI; 10.1006/bbrc.1999.0255

[44] Huynh MKQ, Kinyua AW, Ynag DJ, Kim KW. Hypothalamic AMPK as a Regulator of Energy Homeostasis. Neural Plasticity. 2016. 1-12. DOI: 10.1155/2016/2754078

[45] Ilyas MN, Atif AB, Al-Hatamleh MAI, Al-Shajrawi OM, Ariff TM, Simbak N. Rising trend of obesity in Malaysia; Role of inflammation and inflammatory marker's in obesity related insulin resistance: A nuclear Factor Kappa B (Nfkb) Perspective. Curr Trends Biomedical Eng & Biosci. 2017. 10(4);1-3. DOI;10.19080/CTBEB.2017.10.555793

[46] Lee S, Kwak HB. Role of adiponectin in metabolic and cardiovascular disease. J Exerc Rehabil. 2014. 10(2): 54-59. DOI: 10.12965/jer.140100

[47] Omae T, Nagaoka T, Tanano I, Yoshida A. Adiponectin-induced dilation

of isolated porcine retinal arterioles via production of nitric oxide from endothelial cells. Invest Ophthalmol Vis Sci. 2013. 54(7): 4586-4594. DOI: 10.1167/iovs.13-11756

[48] Yamauchi T, Kamon J, Ito Y, Tsuchida A, Yokomizo T, Kita S, Sugiyama T, Miyagishi M, Hara K, Tsunoda M, Murakami K, Ohteki T, Uchida S, Takekawa S, Waki H, Tsuno NH, Shibata Y, Terauchi Y, Froguel P, Tobe K, Koyasu S, Taira K, Kitamura T, Shimizu T, Nagai R, Kadowaki T. Cloning of adiponectin receptors that mediate antidiabetic metabolic effects. Nature. 2003. 423: 762-769. DOI: 10.1038/nature01705

[49] Okamoto Y, Kihara S, Ouchi N, Nishida M, Arita Y, Kumada M, Ohashi K, Sakai N, Shimomura I, Kobayashi H, Terasaka N, Inaba T, Funahashi T, Matsuzawa Y. Adiponectin reduces atherosclerosis in apolipoprotein E-deficient mice. Circulation. 2002. 106: 2767-2770. DOI: 10.1161/01.cir.0000042707.50032.19

[50] Yamauchi T, Kamon J, Minokoshi Y, Ito Y, Waki H, Uchida S, Yamashita S, Noda M, Kita S, Ueki K, Eto K, Akanuma Y, Froguel P, Foufelle F, Ferre P, Carling D, Kimura S, Nagai R, Kahn BB, Kadowaki T. Adipoenctin stimulates glucose utilization and fatty-acid oxidation by activating AMP-activated protein kinase. Nat Med.2002. 8: 1288-1295. DOI: 10.1038/nm788

[51] Kubota N, Yano W, Kubota T, Yamauchi T, Itoh S, Kumagai H, Kozono H, Takamoto I, Okamoto S, Shiuchi T, Suzuki R, Satoh H, Tsuchida A, Moroi M, Sugi K, Noda T, Ebinuma H, Ueta Y, Kondo T, Araki E, Ezaki O, Nagai R, Tobe K, Terauchi Y, Ueki K, Minokoshi Y, Kadowaki T. Adiponectin stimulates AMP-activated protein kinase in the hypothalamus and increases food intake. Cell Metab. 2007. 6(1):55-68. DOI: 10.1016/j.cmet.2007.06.003

[52] Stumvoll M, Tschritter O, Fritsche A, Staiger H, Renn W, Weisser M, Machicao F, Haring H. Association of the T-G polymorphism in adiponectin (exon 2) with obesity and insulin sensitivity: Interaction with family history of type 2 diabetes. Diabetes. 2002. 51(1):37-41.

[53] Al Khaldi R, Mojiminiyi O, Almulla F, Abdella N. Associations of TERC Single Nucleotide Polymorphisms with human leukocyte telomere length and the risk of type 2 diabetes mellitus. PLoS One. 2015. 10(12). DOI; 10.1371/journal.pone.0145721

[54] Shibata R, Ouchi N, Kihana S, Sato K,Funahashi T, Walsh K. Adiponectin stimulates angiogenesis in response to tissue ischemia through stimulation of amp-activated protein kinase signalling. J Biol Chem. 2004. 279(27):28670-28674. DOI: 10.1074/jbc.M402558200

[55] Chan AY, Soltys CL, Young ME, Proud CG, Dyck JR. Activation of AMP-activated protein kinase inhibits protein synthesis associated with hyperthrophy in the cardiac myocyte. J Biol Chem. 2014. 279(31): 32771-32779. DOI: 10.1074/jbc.M403528200

[56] Fujioka D, Kawabata K, Saito Y, Kobayashi T, Nakamura T, Kodama Y, Takano H, Obata JE, Kitta Y, Umetani K, KugiyamaK. Roleofadiponectinreceptors in edothelin-induced cellular hypertrophy in cultured cardiomyocytes and their expression in infarcted heart. Am J Physiol Heart Circ Physiol. 2006. 290(6): 2409-2416. DOI: 10.1152/ajpheart.00987.2005

[57] Liu M, Chen H, Wei L, Hu D, Dong K, Jia W, Dong LQ, Liu F. Endoplasmic reticulum (ER) localization is critical for DsbA-L protein to suppress ER stress an adiponectin downregulation in adipocyte. J Biol Chem. 2015. 290(16);10143-10148. DOI: 10.1074/jbc.M115.645416

[58] Waki H, Yamauchi T, Kamon J, Ito Y, Uchida S, Kita S, Hara K, Hada Y, Vasseur F, Froguel P, Kimura S, Nagai R, Kadowaki T. Impaired multimerization of human adiponectin mutants associated with diabetes. Molecular Structure abd Multimer formation of adiponectin. J Biol Chen. 2003. 287(41):40352-40363. DOI: 10.1074/jbc.M300365200

[59] Li R, Xu M, Wang X, Wang Y, Lau WB, Yuan Y, Yi W, Wei X, Lopez BL, Christopher TA, Wang XM, Ma XL. Reduced vascular responsiveness to adiponectin in hyperlipidemic rats-mechanism and significance. J Mol Cell Cardiol. 2010. 49(3):508-515. DOI: 10.1016/j.yjmcc.2010.03.002

[60] Reis CEG, Bressan J, Alfenas RCG. Effect of the diet components on adiponectin levels. Nutr Hosp. 2010. 25(6): 881-888. DOI: 10.3305/nh.2010.256.4760

[61] Ander BP, Dupasquier CMC, Prociuk MA, Pierce GN. Polyunsaturated fatty acids and their effects on cardiovascular disease. Exp Clin Cardoil. 2003. 8(4): 164-172.

[62] Jamaluddin MS, Weakley SM, Yao Q, Chen C. Resistin; functional roles and therapeutic considerations for cardiovascular disease. Br J Pharmacol. 2012. 165(3):622-632. DOI: 10.111/j.1476-5381.2011.01369.x

[63] Steppan CM, Brown EJ, Wright CM, Bhat S, Banerjee RR, Dai CY, Enders GH, Silberg DG, Wen X, Wu GD, Lazar MA. A family of tissue-specific resistin-like molecules. Proc Natl Acad Sci U.S.A. 2001. 98(2): 502-506. DOI: 10.1073/pnas.98.2.502

[64] Rashid S. Mechanism by which elevated resistin level accelerate atherosclerotic cardiovascular disease. Rheumatol Curr Res. 2013. 3(115):1-6. DOI: 10.4172/2162-1149.1000115

[65] Patel SD, Rajala MW, Rossetti L, Scherer PE, Shapiro L. Disulfide-dependentmultimericassembly of resistin family hormones. 2004. 304(5674): 1154-1158. DOI: 10.1126/science.1093466

[66] Daquinag AC, Zhang Y, Amaya-Manzanares F, Simmons PJ, Kolonin MG. An isoform of decorin is a resistin receptor on the surface of adipose progenitor cell. Cell Stem Cell. 2011. 9(1):74-86. DOI: 10.1016/j.stem.2011.05.017

[67] Ohmori R, Momiyama Y, Kato R, Taniguchi H, Ogura M, Ayaori M, Nakamura H, Ohsuzu F. Associations between serum resistin levels and insulin resistance, inflammation and coronary artery disease. J Am Coll Cardiol. 2005. 19(46): 379-380. DOI: 10.1016/j.jacc.2005.04.022

[68] Reilly MP, Lehrke M, Wolfe ML, Rohatgi A, Lazar MA, Rader DJ. Resistin is an inflammatory marker of atherosclerosis in humans. Circulation. 2005. 111(7): 932-939. DOI:10.1161/01.CIR.0000155620.10387.43

[69] Jonas MI, Kurylowicz A, Bartoszewicz Z, Lisik W, Jonas M, Domienik-Karlowic J, Puzianowska-kuznicka M. Adiponectin/resistin interplay in serum and in adipose tissue of obese and normal-weight individuals. Diabetol Metab Syndr. 2017. 9(95): 1-9. DOI: 10.1186/s13098-017-0293-2

[70] Zhou L, Li JY, He PP, Yu XH, Tang CK. Resistin: potential biomarker and therapeutic target in atherosclerosis. Clinica Chimica Acta. 2021. 512: 84-91. DOI: 10.1016/j.cca.2020.11.010

[71] Marangui I, Gornati I, Artuso I, Zanoni I, Granucci F. Below the surface: The inner lives of TLR4 and TLR9. J Leukoc Biol. 106(1): 147-160. DOI:10.1002/JLB.3MIR1218-483RR

[72] Lee S, Lee HC, Kwon YW, Lee SE, Cho Y, Kim J, Lee S, Kim JY, Lee J, Yang HM, Mook-Jung I, Nam KY, Chung J, Lazar MA, Kim HS. Adenylyl cyclase-associated protein 1 is a receptor for human resistin and mediates inflammatory actions of human monocytes. Cell Mtab. 2014. 19(3):484-497. DOI: 10.1016/j.cmet.2014.01.013

[73] Gencer B, Auer R, RekeneireND, ButlerJ, KalogeropoulosA, Bauer DC,Kritchevsky SB, Miljkovic I, Vittinghoff E, Harris T, Rodondi N. Association between resistin levels and cardiovascular disease events in older adults: The health, aging and body composition study. Atherosclerosis. 2016. 245:181-186. DOI: 10.1016/j.atherosclerosis.2015.12.004

[74] Leon ACD, Gonzalez DA, Hernandez AG, Coello SD, Marrugat J, Sanchez JJA, Diaz BB, Rodriguez IM, Perez MDCR. Relationships between serum resisttin and fat intake, serum lipid concentration and adiposity in the general population. J Atheroscler Thromb. 2014. 21: 454-462. DOI: 10.5551/jat.22103

[75] Athanasiou LS, Fotiadis DI, Michalis LK. Atheroslerotic plaque characterization methods based on Coronary Imaging. 2017. 1-21. DOI: 10.1016/B978-0-12-804734-7.00001-4

Section 2

# Screening Diabetes

Chapter 5

# Oral Glucose Tolerance Test (OGTT): Undeniably the First Choice Investigation of Dysglycaemia, Reproducibility can be Improved

*Dahiru Saleh Mshelia, Sani Adamu and Rebecca Mtaku Gali*


## Abstract

Type 2 diabetes mellitus accounts for ≈90–95% of those with diabetes, about 50% of those with type 2 diabetes are unaware and it can remain undiagnosed for up to 12 years, ≥25% of people have evidence of microvascular complications at diagnosis. The consequences of diabetes can be reduced by screening and early interventions. Urinalysis as a screening test is limited by its low sensitivity ranging from 21% and 64%, though has high specificity (>98%), it has a place where no other procedure is available. Fasting plasma glucose though recommended as a universal screening and diagnostic test for diabetes mellitus, a changed in the diagnostic criteria was made when this did not give corresponding hyperglycaemic impact compared to the OGTT results, bringing a complex and variable effect on the prevalence of diabetes and on subjects diagnosed. To date the searching to finding the corresponding FPG to what is normal or IGT is still ongoing. FPG testing poorly identify early signs of dysglycaemia. This is due to the difficulty ensuring compliance with instructions about fasting, FPG represents glucose handling during the moment of fasting period only and is affected easily by short-term lifestyle changes, FPG has diurnal variation, higher in the morning than in the afternoon, these may cause serious misclassifications. OGTT do indicates the pathophysiology responsible for diabetes better as it provides information on what happens in the postprandial state when the functional capacity of pancreatic β-cell is crucial. It accurately detects changes in post-prandial glycaemia that tend to precede changes in fasting glucose. OGTT is the gold standard for the diagnosis of GDM and the only means of identifying people with IGT and WHO placed emphasis on the OGTT as the "gold standard", in diagnosis of dysglycaemia. Reproducibility can be improved remarkably when patient preparation, a forvarable atmosphere during the procedure, standardized sampling protocol, sample handling, and analysis are given high attention. Measurement of A1c equals the assessment of hundreds of FPG levels and also captures postprandial glucose peaks. Regrettably, it has been shown that 44% of people with newly diagnosed diabetes with OGTT had A1c <6.0% and that a stronger correlations with plasma glucose is better in subjects with known diabetes, but not in the general population. A1C values just above the upper limits of normal require OGTT to be correctly interpreted; it is not available in many part of the world. Finally, A1c can not diagnose IFG and IGT to disclose high-risk subjects for



IntechOpen

diabetes. In conclusion an OGTT is undeniably the best test in investigation of dysglycaemia, either with the intention of testing for pre-diabetes, type 2 diabetes, or for gestational diabetes mellitus.

**Keywords:** Dysglycaemia, T2DM, GDM, Screening, Urinalysis, Fasting Plasma Glucose, OGTT, A1c

## 1. Introduction

The term diabetes mellitus describes a metabolic disorder of multiple aetiology characterised by chronic hyperglycaemia with disturbances of carbohydrate, fat and protein metabolism resulting from defects in insulin secretion, insulin action, or both.

The diabetes epidemic is accelerating in the developing world and Type 2 diabetes has been recently reported in children and adolescents [1]. This is likely to increase further the burden of chronic diabetic complications worldwide. Diabetes is associated with reduced life expectancy, significant morbidity due to specific diabetes related microvascular complications, increased risk of macrovascular complications (ischaemic heart disease, stroke and peripheral vascular disease), and diminished quality of life. These can be reduced by screening and early interventions (prevention or treatment).

## 2. Classification of diabetes mellitus

Several distinct types of diabetes mellitus exist and are caused by a complex interaction of genetic and environmental factors, however, assigning a type of diabetes to an individual often depends on the circumstances present at the time of diagnosis, and many diabetic individuals do not easily fit into a single class. Therefore understanding the pathogenesis of the hyperglycaemia and to treat it effectively is more important. It can therefore simply be classified as presented below [2–4].

**Type 1 diabetes** (β-cell destruction, either immune-mediated or Idiopathic), accounts for only 5–10% of those with diabetes mellitus, usually leading to absolute insulin deficiency. The immune-mediated has strong HLA associations, linkage to DQA and DQB genes and is influence by DRB genes, while the idiopathic has no known aetiology, have permanent insulinopaenia, prone to ketoacidosis, has no evidence of autoimmunity, strongly inherited and is not HLA associated.

**Type 2 diabetes** (ranging from predominantly insulin resistance with relative insulin deficiency to predominantly an insulin secretory defect with insulin resistance), accounts for ≈90–95% of those with diabetes, and most patients are obese and/or have an increased percentage of body fat with predominant abdominal region distribution, ketoacidosis seldom occurs spontaneously. Patients may have normal or elevated insulin levels, though still less with respect to degree of hyperglycaemia, thus insulin secretion is defective and insufficient to compensate for insulin resistance. This type of diabetes is frequently associated with a high genetic predilection compared to the autoimmune form of type 1 diabetes, yet the genetics are complex and not obviously defined.

**Gestational diabetes mellitus (GDM)** [4]**:** Defined as any magnitude of glucose intolerance with onset or first recognition during pregnancy, whatever modalities of treatment use or whether the condition lingers after index pregnancy. It include unrecognized glucose intolerance antedating or begun in the index pregnancy. It complicates ≈4% of all pregnancies in the USA, with prevalence ranging from 1 to 14% of pregnancies, depending on the population studied. GDM represents nearly 90% of all pregnancies complicated by diabetes. Deterioration of glucose tolerance occurs normally during pregnancy, particularly in the 3rd trimester.

**Other specific types of diabetes** [4]:

a. **Genetic defects of the β-cell:** Fair numbers of diabetes are affiliated with monogenetic defect in β-cell function, referred to maturity onset diabetes of the young (MODY) and are characterised by impaired insulin secretion with minimal or no defects in insulin action. Inherited in an autosomal dominant pattern

b. **Genetic defects in insulin action:** These are rare causes of diabetes sequel to genetic abnormalities of insulin action. The metabolic flaws amalgamated with mutations of the insulin receptor may traverse from hyperinsulinaemia and modest hyperglycaemia to severe diabetes and some may have acanthosis nigricans, women may be virilized and have enlarged, cystic ovaries. Leprechaunism and Rabson-Mendenhall syndromes are two paediatric syndrome with mutations in the insulin receptor gene

c. **Diseases of the exocrine pancreas:** Any process that diffusely injures the panaceas can causes diabetes, ranging from infections, trauma, metabolic, and rarely neoplasm

d. **Endocrinopathies:** Several hormones (growth hormone, cortisol, glucagon, epinephrine) antagonize insulin action. Excess amounts of these hormones as noted in acromegaly, Cushing's syndrome, glucagonoma, Phaeochromocytoma, respectively can cause diabetes

e. **Drugs or chemical-induced diabetes**: Many drugs can impair insulin secretion. These drugs may not cause diabetes by themselves but they may precipitate diabetes in individuals with insulin resistance

f. **Infections:** Certain viruses have been associated with β-cell destruction; eg. Congenital rubella, Coxsackievirus B, cytomegalovirus, adenovirus, and mumps have been implicated in inducing certain cases of the diabetes

g. **Unknown forms of immune-mediated diabetes:** In this variety, two conditions are known, others may occur. The stiff-man syndrome distinguished by inflexible axial muscles with painful spasms. Patients routinely present with high titers of the GAD autoantibodies, and roughly one-third will develop diabetes

h. **Other genetic syndromes sometimes associated with diabetes:** Many genetic syndromes are accompanied by an increased incidence of diabetes mellitus, eg., Down's syndrome, Klinefelter's syndrome, and Turner's syndrome. Wolfram's syndrome is an autosomal recessive disorder characterised by insulin-deficient diabetes and the absence of β-cells at autopsy

**Prevalence and burden of diabetes mellitus, Table 1.**

Diabetes burden goes beyond individual but extends to families and society as a whole. It has huge consequences affecting both national productivity and economies particularly in the low- and middle-income countries when considering the projection for the year 2025.

| |
|---|
| a. The prevalence is increasing and is projected to reach pandemic proportions over the next 10–20 years. |
| b. By the year 2025, diabetes population will reach 333 million –90% will have Type 2 diabetes. |
| c. There will be disproportionate in the developed and developing countries, 42% (increase from 51 to 72 million) and 170% (increase from 84 to 228 million), respectively |
| d. Thus, >75% of all people with diabetes will be in the developing countries, as compared to 62% in 1995, over a period 30 years |
| e. Without interventions to halt the increase in diabetes, there will be at least 629 million people living with diabetes by 2045. |
| f. In most Western societies, the overall prevalence has reached 4–6%, and is as high as 10–12% among 60–70-year-old people. |
| g. High blood glucose causes almost 4 million deaths each year, and the IDF estimates that the annual global health care spending on diabetes among adults was US$ 850 billion in 2017. |
| h. The annual health costs caused by diabetes and its complications account for around 6–12% of all health-care expenditure. |
| i. The ADA estimated the national costs of diabetes in the USA for 2002 to be $US 132 billion, increasing to $US 192 billion in 2020. |

**Table 1.**
*The BURDEN of Diabetes Mellitus [5–8].*

Determinates of increasing prevalence of diabetes mellitus may be summarized as: Rising levels of overweight/obesity; increasing age of life expectancy in the general population; decreasing age of onset of type 2 diabetes; increasing number diagnosed due to decreased level of fasting plasma glucose; improved methods of health records; and increasing number of detection by practice-based screening and greater public awareness.

## 3. Need for screening for dysglycaemia

About 50% of those who have diabetes are unaware since the most prevalent form [9], Type 2 diabetes, can remain undiagnosed for many years, up 12 years [10], ≥25% of people have evidence of microvascular complications at diagnosis [11–13] and individuals with undiagnosed T2DM are at significantly higher risk for macrovascular complications than the nondiabetic population. Therefore, the magnitude of the epidemic increase in diabetes, particularly among younger age group including children, its serious long-term consequences, the high prevalence of undiagnosed diabetes and the proportion of cases with evidence of complications at diagnosis, coupled with complex treatment requirements that are difficult and costly to implement, undoubtedly create a strong imperative for screening, making the prevention of diabetes a critical public health goals. Since 1997 some major clinical trials examined whether lifestyle changes or pharmacologic interventions would prevent or delay the development of diabetes in populations at high risk [14–16]. These trials achieved 25–60% reduction in development of diabetes and the largest reduction by lifestyle modification and thiazolidinediones [14–16], though a lesser reduction (25—30%) were achieved with other drugs [16]. These must be emphasized particularly in the developing countries where the expected increase is disproportionately higher.

### 3.1 Considerations in screening of a disease in general

The term screening should be based on the WHO principles of screening document [17]. Screening is offered to individuals at sufficiently high risk of a particular disorder to be informed for further directives. These are usually carried out on asymptomatic individual and are often initiated by medical personnel or authorities. Screening will not only benefit the individual but the society at large.

Although it is desirable to have a test that is both highly sensitive and highly specific, this is usually not possible. Only a valid, reliable and reproducible test in a population is recommended. This requires uniform procedures and methods, standardized techniques, properly functioning equipments, well trained personnel, and quality assurances are necessary to achieve these properties. Screening for dysglycaemia requires three-stages: (a) selection from the general population using practice registers or self-completed questionnaires amongst at high risk; (b) Testing blood glucose, eg OGTT; and (c) confirmation (or not) of raised blood glucose noted in stage (b) above using the same method of glucose testing. The biochemical tests currently available are blood glucose (Fasting blood glucose or OGTT), blood HbA1c or blood fructosamine measurements or urine glucose measurements. Each screening test needs a designated and pre-determined threshold or "cut point" that defines high risk.

WHO adapted 10 criteria that still serve as foundation for much of the discussions surrounding screening programs and are as indicated in **Table 2** [17].

The above criteria is not focus on the test itself but the disease and every criterion should be present for a given screening test to improve the health of the population.

### 3.2 Applying these qualities to dysglycaemia screening

The main reasons for the current interest in screening for T2DM can be summarized as follows [18]; which undauntedly fulfills the WHO principles of screening" document [17]

a. Type 2 diabetes is becoming more common and many with the condition, about ≥30%, are undiagnosed [19]

b. The rising prevalence of T2DM world-wide [18], the seriousness of the immediate effects and long-term complications of T2DM are alarming

c. That there is a long, latent, asymptomatic period in which the condition can be detected [20]

d. Many of newly referred cases of T2DM already have evidence of the microvascular complications of diabetes

| | |
|---|---|
| a. The prevalence of disease to be screened for must be high in that particularly population to increase sensitivity of the test | e. There should be a suitable test or otherwise that is acceptable to the population |
| b. There must be an acceptable treatment for patient with the disease | f. The natural history of the disease should be adequately understood |
| c. Methods for diagnosis and treatment should not only be available but affordable | g. There should be an agreed policy on whom to screen and treat as a patient |
| d There must be a recognized latent or early symptomatic period | h. The cost of case-finding should be economically balance with attended objective of treatment |
| | i. Screening should be a continuous process for that particular population |

**Table 2.**
*The following criteria should available for disease to qualify for screening [17].*

e. There have been advances in risk scoring, screening methods and more convenient methods of blood testing using HbA1c in non-fasting state

f. Diabetes care is advanced, including screening for detection of complications early enough and a wider range of treatments for glycaemia and its complications

g. Evidence supporting the efficacy of intensive blood glucose control [20, 21], blood pressure control [22], blood lipid control [23], and these development of CVD in T2DM

h. Increasing pressure from professional organisations, lay groups and from some of the members associations of IDF to institute screening for type 2 diabetes if only to further highlight the increasing prevalence and public health importance of the condition

i. Individuals with IGT have increased risk of CVD and on average, 11% of people with pre-diabetes develop type 2 DM each yr. (1.5–4%) and in 10 yrs. and 50% higher risk of CVD, this can be prevented or delayed by Life style and/or pharmacologic interventions.

### 3.3 However not everybody is convinced that it is worthwhile screening for type 2 DM and their views are

a. Some of the NSC criteria for screening programme are not met [18]

b. A 13-year follow-up in health measures or cardiovascular morbidity showed no advantage after screening for diabetes

c. The ADDITION trial did not show any benefit after applying intensified management

d. Up to now there is yet to be a perfect screening test for dysglycaemia

e. If other cardiovascular risk factors are assessed and addressed, the benefits of screening for hyperglycaemia are modest in terms of further reducing cardiovascular risk

f. The proportion of undiagnosed diabetes has probably been reduced by opportunistic screening

Although there are advances in screening for and treatment of type 2 diabetes, the policies and practices do have profound consequences for individuals, health systems and society in general [18].

### 3.4 Consequences for individuals' include

a. The time and other resources necessary to undergo the screening and diagnostic tests may not be there particularly for the poor [18]

b. The fair of unknown on both the test outcome, the reflection on societal views, the cost of treatment and what is said about the disease in the society is grave. These may include occupational discrimination and/or increased costs or difficulty in obtaining insurance

### 3.5 The consequences on the health system and society as a whole are

1. The costs and other consequences particularly on primary health care system of carrying out screening and confirmatory test may be huge and unattainable [18]

2. The additional costs of starting treatment early of diabetes and preventions and/or its complication

3. Since there is no perfect screening test yet, consequences of false negative and false positive results are inevitable and is grave

4. Any loss of production as a result of the earlier diagnosis of the condition(from absence from work or reduced job opportunities, for example)

### 3.6 The potential benefits of early detection of T2DM are

a. Not only boost life span but also the quality resulting from a diminish severity and occurrence of instantaneous effects or prevention or slow diabetes long-term complications [18]

b. Increase savings and allow redistribution by reduced levels of care required for diabetes complications (reduction in hospital admissions and length of stay)

## 4. Methods use for screening of dysglycaemia

### 4.1 Urinalysis

The usefulness of urinary glucose as a screening test is limited because of the low sensitivity ranging from 21% and 64% with specificity >98% in studies which included performing OGTT in the entire study population or a random sample of negative screeners. Despite this, urine glucose testing may have a place in low resource settings where no other procedure is available. This is particularly so when the prevalence of undiagnosed diabetes is likely to be high [23, 24]. Urine should be protected from direct sunlight, add 5 ml glacial acetic acid to preserve glucose in the urine otherwise up to 40% may be lose after 24-hr storage at room temperature [25]. Keeping samples on ice-water slurring during collection is also recommended [26]. However, this may not be feasible in rural areas of developing countries; it is therefore recommended that urinalysis should be done immediate after urine collection in such situations.

### 4.2 Blood glucose estimation

Plasma glucose estimation has high intraindividual biological variability (4–14%). This is accounted for by method of sample collection and storage, lifestyle measures while preparing for sample collection like exercise, calorie restriction and difficulty in ensuring fasting state. About 3-8 mg/dl/hr. of glucose is lose in a sample kept at room temperature. Therefore, in interpreting blood glucose test result, the need to be conversant with causes of intraindividual and interindividual variation of blood glucose is necessary. Such variability can be grouped as

a. The biological variability is substantially greater than analytical variability

b. Analytical imprecision <3.3%

c. Bias <2.5%

d. Total error < 7.9%

e. Glucose assay ~4%

f. Biological CV 6.9%

On the basis of biological variation, glucose analysis having analytical imprecision 3.3%, bias 2.5%, and total error 7.9%, may produce classification errors, although imprecision is usually low at the diagnostic decision limits. It is also believed generally that glucose assay is highly reproducible across laboratories, however, a recent survey conducted in 6,000 US laboratories clearly documented a significant bias in glucose assessment in as many as 41% of them, yielding a misclassification of glucose tolerance in 12% of subjects [27]. The coefficients of variation of A1c, FPG, and 2-h PG were demonstrated to be 3.6%, 5.7%, and 16.6% respectively [28], reflecting both biological and analytical variability.

Preanalytical processing of blood samples can markedly affect the results of plasma glucose readings because ongoing glycolysis by erythrocytes and leukocytes prior to centrifugation lowers its concentration [29, 30]. A study reported 5–7% [0.6 mmol/L (10 mg/dl)] an average rate of glycolysis per hour [31]. This varies with the glucose concentration, temperature, white blood cell count and other factors [32], *for example,* it has been estimated that pre-analytical variability of FPG is 5–10% and the within day-day variability is 12–15%. Glycolysis can be attenuated by inhibition of enolase with sodium fluoride (2.5 mg fluoride/ml of blood) or, less commonly, lithium iodoacetate (0.5 mg/ml of blood). A citrate tubes should be use if a delay in centrifugation is expected because citrate more rapidly inhibits glycolysis [30]. It should be noted that although fluoride maintains long-term glucose stability, the rates of decline of glucose in the first hour after sample collection in tubes with and without fluoride are virtually identical [31]. Currently, both WHO and ADA recommend that for preanalytical processing for plasma glucose measurements involves venous blood collection into sodium fluoride (NaF) tubes with placement in ice-water slurry prior to centrifugation within 30 min of sample collection [33, 34]. The benefit of this policy is demonstrated in the following studies: An observed increase rate of GDM from 11.6% to 20.6% on changing to a protocol of centrifuging blood collected into NaF tubes within 10 min of venipuncture compared to delayed centrifugation was noted [35]. A study in Ireland showed a 2.7-fold higher (38.1% compared with 14.2%) when the ADA preanalytic protocol was followed compared with the previous standard practice of collecting blood into NaF tubes, leaving them at room temperature, and centrifuging after collection of all three samples [36]. Similarly, the impact of long delays in centrifugation for OGTT samples collected in NaF tubes on GDM diagnosis in Western Australia was estimated to be an under diagnosis rate of 62% [37]. In HAPO, a reference study for GDM, blood samples for all glucose measurements were collected into NaF tubes, placed in ice-water slurry immediately after phlebotomy, and kept that way until they could be centrifuge and separated [38].

### 4.3 Specimen for glucose estimation

Glucose can be measured in whole blood, serum, or plasma, but plasma is recommended for diagnosis. It can also be measured in capillary, venous or arterial blood. It is essential that in a repeat sampling for confirmation of blood glucose result, the same type of sampling used previously must be use. The molality of glucose (i.e., amount of glucose per unit water mass) in whole blood and plasma is identical. Although red blood cells are essentially freely permeable to glucose, the concentration of water (kg/L) in plasma is 11% higher than that of whole blood depending on the haematocrit, increasing to 15% at a haematocrit of 0.55 and decreasing to 8% at a haematocrit of 0.30 [39]. Therefore, glucose concentrations in plasma are 11% higher than whole blood if the hematocrit is normal. Glucose concentrations in heparinized plasma are reported to be 5% lower than in serum [40]. This may be caused by water shifting from red blood cells to plasma sequel to effect of anticoagulants. In feed (OGTT) state capillary glucose is higher by about [mean of 1.7 mmol/L (30 mg/dL), equivalent to 20–25%*]* than in venous blood*, but the* mean difference in fasting samples is only 0.1 mmol/L (2 mg/dL) [41].

### 4.4 Fasting plasma glucose (FPG): a tool in screening for dysglycaemia

In 1997, ADA Expert Committee on the Diagnosis and Classification of Diabetes Mellitus [42] recommended universal use of FPG for screening and diagnosis of diabetes mellitus because of its ease of administration, convenience, acceptability to patients, and lower cost in comparison to the OGTT and also based on assumption that the measurement reproducibility would be better. Since the goal and premise of diabetes management is the prevention of diabetes-associated complications, and this goal is best achieved when the disease is diagnosed at an early stage, the committee lowered the diagnostic threshold of FPG from 7.8 mmol/L to 7.0 mmol/L and also created a new category, defined as individuals exhibiting FPG levels between 6.1 and 6..9 mmol/L, called impaired fasting glucose (IFG) to describe the zone between the upper limit of normal FPG and the lower limit of the diabetic FPG. The IFG was believed at that time to be analogous to the zone between the upper limit of a normal 2-hr plasma glucose and the lower limit of the diabetic 2-hr plasma glucose described by IGT and was adapted by WHO in 1999 [43]. The FPG of 6.1 mmol/L was adopted by both ADA [44] and WHO [43] as the upper limit of "normoglycaemia" because this is the level above which first-phase of insulin secretion is lost in response to intravenous glucose and is also the level at which there is associated progressively greater risk of developing micro- and macrovascular complications.

In 2003, the ADA reviewed its diagnostic criteria when it found out that the FPG stated in the earlier classifications does not give corresponding hyperglycaemic impact compared to the OGTT results. The threshold for IFG was lowered from 6.1 mmol/L to 5.6 mmol/L [44] dependent on ROC curve analysis indicating that a cut-point of 5.4–5.5 mmol/L gives the best combination of sensitivity and specificity for predicting future diabetes, and this consequently increased the overall prevalence of IFG approximately three- to four-fold, though WHO and IDF maintained this as FPG 6.1–6.9 mmol/L. To date the searching to finding the corresponding FPG to what is normal or IGT is still ongoing.

Although both IGT and IFG are associated with resistance to insulin and increased insulin secretion, they do not identify identical patient populations and are not equivalent in predicting development of T2DM or cardiovascular events [45]. People with isolated IFG predominantly have hepatic insulin resistance and normal muscle insulin sensitivity, whereas individuals with isolated IGT have normal to slightly reduced hepatic insulin sensitivity and moderate to severe muscle insulin resistance [46]. Individuals with isolated IFG have reduction in both first-phase (0–10 min) during IVGT and early phase (first 30 min) during OGTT insulin secretion but maintained the late-phase (60–120 min) response during OGTT, while Isolated IGT apart from having defect in early-phase insulin secretion in response to OGTT also has a severe deficit in late-phase insulin secretion [47].

The prevalences of IFG and IGT varies widely, varied considerably among different ethnic groups [48], differ significantly in their age and sex distribution; and increase with advancing age. IGT is more frequent in women than in men [49]. A study of 1,245 Italian telephone company employees followed for 11.5 years found that, unlike baseline IGT, baseline IFG did not predict progression to DM, and the categories only overlapped 40% of the time [48]. The natural history of both IFG and IGT is variable, with approx 25% progressing to diabetes, 50% remaining in their abnormal glycaemic state, and 25% reverting to NGT over an observational period of 3-5 years [50, 51].

### 4.5 Advantages of using FPG in screening for dysglycaemia

American Diabetes Associated did not recommend OGTT to be used commonly in the diagnosis of type 1 and 2 diabetes because it was thought that if FPG is appropriately use it will identify almost the same number of dysglycaemia in the population as the OGTT, and that OGTT is not practicable in routine practice and in many studies OGTT is found to be poorly reproducible, with an estimated rate of only about 50–66% [52].

### 4.6 Disadvantages of FPG in screening for dysglycaemia

The fasting blood glucose testing in nondiabetic persons poorly identify early signs of dysglycaemia because high postprandial glucose marks the journey of first signs of abnormal glucose regulation and this best predict cardiovascular outcome. Fasting is not really the central issue and it seems to be overemphasized in diagnosing dysglycaemia.

One problem well known in the measurement of FPG in population studies is the difficulty in ensuring that all the participants have complied with the instructions about fasting [53]. Consequently, some participants with completely normal glucose homeostasis might have been misclassified into impaired fasting glucose category or, more rarely, even into a diabetes category. More so, FPG represents glucose handling during the moment of fasting period only (particularly so, of that moment of blood sampling), and this is affected easily by short-term lifestyle changes such as over activity, stress and drug ingestions. Therefore under these conditions subjects may be classified wrongly if only FPG is used. Knowledge of intraindividual variability of FPG concentrations is essential for meaningful interpretation of patient values. A study of healthy individuals [mean glucose, 4.9 mmol/L (88 mg/dL)] exhibited within- and between-subject CVs of 4.8–6.1% and 7.5–7.8%, respectively [34]. Recent evidence revealed a diurnal variation in FPG, with mean FPG higher in the morning than in the afternoon, indicating that many cases of undiagnosed diabetes would have been missed in patients seen in the afternoon [54]. A study with repeated OGTT in 31 nondiabetic adults at 48-hr intervals, demonstrated FPG varied by 10% in 22 participants (77%) and by 20% in 30 participants (97%) [44]. Similarly, in population studies of subjects with newly diagnosed diabetes showed a wide distribution of FPG, ranging in one study from <5.0 mmol/1 to >30.0 mmol/L [55]. As a consequence, the sensitivity of the OGTT is naturally higher, given the current criteria.

The change in the diagnostic procedure has brought a complex and variable effect on the prevalence of diabetes and on subjects diagnosed. Many studies have reported that FPG and 2-hr plasma glucose do not identify the same people as having diabetes. The difference between the prevalence of diabetes based on the FPG and 2-hr criteria varied from −4.0% to 13.2% in the 16 European survey in the DECODE study. In that study [56], of the 1517 people with newly diagnosed diabetes, 40% met only the FPG criterion, 31% met only the 2-hr criterion and 29% met both criteria. In the DECODA study [49], of 1215 subjects with diabetes by either criterion, only 449 (37%) met both criteria, of the 995 subjects with 2-hr ≥11.1 mmol/L, 546 (55%) had non-diabetes FPG value, and of the 669 subjects with FPG ≥7.0 mmol/L, 220 (33%) had non-diabetes 2-hr value. In the two studies the concordance rate ranges between 29–37%. In the NHANES study data cited in the 1997 ADA report showed 38% of subjects with newly diagnosed diabetes using only ADA criteria were missed when OGTT was carried out in the same population [42]. An even larger discrepancy was observed for the categories of IFG and IGT. In DECODA study, more than three quarter (≥3/4) of the subjects with IGT would be classified as normal if only the FPG criteria is used. Degree of hyperglycaemia, age, sex, BMI and ethnicity influence the concordance. The severer the hyperglycaemia the better the agreement between the two criteria. It might therefore be appropriate to use the FPG alone in subjects with clinical symptoms of diabetes to confirm. It is inappropriate to use it as the only test in the general population for epidemiological purposes, or in cohort with slightly higher glycaemia but without any symptoms because a large proportion of subjects diagnosed by 2-hr criteria would not be identified by the FPG particularly in Asians. In 1999, WHO recommended retaining the use of OGTT for epidemiological purposes, and this appears to be particularly important for the Asian population. The 2-hr criterion is more sensitive in the elderly and fasting criterion in the mid-aged. Barrett-Conner, et al. [57] reported that 70% of women and 48% of men aged 50–89 years had new diabetes diagnosed solely by elevated 2-hr plasma glucose. Similarly, in the Early Diabetes Intervention Program study [58], 24% and 50% of subjects with OGTT-confirmed diabetes had FPG levels between 5.5 and 6.0 and 6.1–6.9 mmol/L, respectively. Still in a further study, an isolated elevation of 2-hr glucose (2-hr glucose ≥11.1 mmol/L and FPG <7.0 mmol/L) identified as high as 65%(61/94) of those with newly diagnosed diabetes while 76%(644/845) who were normal by fasting blood glucose were identified with IGT and these individuals carry high risk of cardiovascular disease events [59]. A recent report showed that even if the concordance between the WHO and ADA criteria increased with this lower cutoff of IFG, 29% of patients with diabetes revealed by an OGTT and 57% with IGT would still have remained undiagnosed using FPG [59]. All individuals with IFG should have an OGTT, as a significant number (approximately 5%, but up to 20%, in some populations) will already have diabetes by 2-hr post challenge criteria [60], so why delaying diagnosis, why not start with OGTT in the first place.

Impaired glucose tolerance (IGT), not diagnosed with FPG estimation, is associated with risk of cardiovascular events almost as high as in subjects with diabetes which is not similarly observed in people with IFG necessitating ADA to lowered the threshold for IFG from 6.1 mmol/L to 5.6 mmol/L in order to detect more subjects with pre-diabetes [61]. Consequently, with regards to the assessment of the risk of mortality and cardiovascular disease events, these discrepancies are crucially important. Therefore, in screening programs, clinical research, and population-based epidemiological studies, where participants often lack diabetes symptoms or complications, an OGTT is commonly used to detect diabetes, thus adding to the diabetic "pool" an equal-sized group of subjects with unrecognized diabetes and it is misleading trying to assess glucose homeostasis without information on post-prandial glucose metabolism.

In conclusion, although in clinical practice the OGTT is often regarded as a cumbersome, time-consuming, and patient-unfriendly procedure, for a more detailed and sensitive assessment of the glucose dysmetabolism, the oral glucose tolerance test (OGTT) is the best.

## 5. Oral glucose tolerance test (OGTT): undeniably the best choice investigation for dysglycaemia

The OGTT is a non-physiological procedure required to unveil a highly compensated derangement in insulin's handling of glucose metabolism [62]. It requires administration of glucose solution to a patient who has indication for investigation of glucose dysmetabolism. Although more sensitive diagnostic test than FPG, the OGTT is affected by a number of factors that result in less acceptable reproducibility. Therefore OGTT requires that any influence in glucose handling must be eliminated or minimize where result should reflect patient's internal milieu, to increase reproducibility. Subsequently, patient preparation, a forvarable atmosphere during the procedure, standardized sampling protocol, sample handling, and analysis are paramount. OGTT or 2-hr post-glucose levels do indicates the pathophysiology responsible for diabetes better than any other glycaemic parameter as it provides information on what happens in the postprandial state, when glucose is high in the system and when the functional capacity of pancreatic β-cell is crucial. Normal blood glucose levels 2-hr after glucose load indicates a good β-cell capacity, whereas high levels document an impairment of β-cell function [63]. This means that only 2-hr OGTT PG can provide reliable information on the key pathophysiological defect of dysglycaemia or providing advice regarding the correct therapy to overcome it.

### 5.1 Advantages of OGTT in screening for dysglycaemia

The oral glucose tolerance test has a long history [64] but from time to time had to endure considerable criticism. One review pointed out that the considerable number of variables involved results in both poor reproducibility and difficulties in interpretation [65]. In spite of this the oral glucose tolerance test survives and for routine use in the diagnosis of diabetes mellitus it is not replaceable (Undeniably). The OGTT detects changes in post-prandial glycaemia that tend to precede changes in fasting glucose. In fact, inability to respond appropriately to a glucose challenge, i.e., glucose intolerance, represents the fundamental pathologic defect in diabetes mellitus and OGTT is currently the gold standard for the diagnosis of diabetes. The OGTT is vital for the characterization of metabolic syndrome, the metabolic actions of cardiovascular and metabolic drugs, and natural progression from prediabetes to T2DM. OGTT is extensively used as a sensitive indicator of GDM. Therefore, OGTT is an important Lab tool in preclinical studies as it provides an indication of the relative roles of insulin secretion and insulin resistance in the progression of glucose intolerance.

The OGTT allows all of the normal stages of insulin secretion and glucose processing to take place in sequence without causing stress or trauma to the subject. The OGTT is the most robust means of establishing the diagnosis of diabetes and provides a more comprehensive assessment of dynamic glucose handling. Thus, the OGTT more accurately mirrors daily life. OGTT is much more sensitive in identifying the loci of insulin resistance and its modulation by different interventions. Thus, the OGTT is useful as a research tool, yields laboratory data with greater relevance to the prevention and treatment of human disease. It is the reference method for the assessment of glucose tolerance, despite the notoriously poor reproducibility of the test (CV = 50%) for 2 h blood glucose. Some of these cause of variations can be minimized with adequate attention to physical activities, dietary preparation and taking care of sample collection at the 2-hr sample (sampling must be done within 5 minutes of 120 minute [66]. The WHO (1999) placed emphasis on the OGTT as the "gold standard", with both fasting and 120-min values being taken into consideration [67]. This is by no means a mistake. Only when an OGTT cannot be performed should the diagnosis rely on fasting levels. Other hormones and metabolites can be measured during OGTT, not just glucose and insulin, eg., the OGTT is the primary test used for the diagnosis of GH hypersecretion.

OGTT is the only means of identifying people with IGT, and IGT is an essential diagnostic step, especially when FPG is within the normal range, as these subjects are at high risk not only for type 2 diabetes, but in particular for cardiovascular disease. The main clinical significance of IGT are [68]: (1) It is a risk factor for type 2 diabetes, about 20–50% of subjects with IGT develop type 2 diabetes over 10 years; (2) It predisposes individual to cardiovascular disease (CVD); and (3) It is a component of the metabolic syndrome and its consequences. IGT when identified and subsequently managed will prevent or delayed progression to type 2 diabetes mellitus. It has been indicated by recent studies [69–71] that persons classified with IGT using WHO criteria have increased risk of cardiovascular disease, however many of these subjects do not have impaired fasting glucose (IFG) by the new ADA criteria. Furthermore, the OGTT by WHO criteria identifies diabetes in 2% more individuals than does FPG using ADA criteria [70], although diabetic individuals who are identified by both abnormal FPG and 2-h OGTT have a higher risk of premature death than those with only an increased FPG concentration [71]. More so, fasting plasma glucose alone fails to diagnose in about 30% of cases of diabetes diagnosed by OGTT. OGTT establishes whether an IFG subjects has normal 2hPG and only the simultaneous information obtained from 2hPG (OGTT) allows the screening to become effective. An important matter here is that people with IGT who cannot be identified by either FPG or A1c have ≈40% increased mortality compared with normoglycaemic subjects and lifestyle intervention in these individuals can prevents progression to type 2 diabetes and may reduce their mortality risk to the level observed among normoglycaemic population. These prevention benefits do not exist for A1c or FPG, and this evidences should not be forgotten when deciding the approaches to identify intermediate dysglycaemia. We should therefore make OGTT a priority in an attempt to diagnose hyperglycaemia as early as possible.

Thus, using solely FPG, would deceitfully reassure a large proportion of individuals as having NGT, without warning them on the benefits of preventive treatment. Epidemiological studies showed that A1c and plasma glucose (FPG and/or 2-hr OGTT) identify partially different groups of diabetic subjects. While A1c ≥6.5% identifies only ≈30–40% newly diagnosed patients with diabetes [72], a larger percentage was detected by FPG (≈50%), and more so by 2-hr PG(≈90%).

These findings are based on several recent studies, including the 2003–2006 NHANES study demonstrating only 30% of diabetic individuals were detected by A1c ≥6.5%, 46% by PFG ≥126 mg/dl, and the IRAS demonstrated 32%, 45%, and 87%, respectively) [73] indicating OGTT is superior. However, the pivotal issue on OGTT is its low reproducibility which is significantly represented by physiologic contexts of the test. The plasma glucose during OGTT are influenced by both insulin sensitivity and secretion, however, impact of other factors particularly incretins, neural responses to nutrient ingestion, gastrointestinal motility and gastric emptying are also important. These factors differ significantly between individuals and are part of non-modifiable factors that govern post-load glucose metabolism and plasma glucose concentration, and are difficult to measure in every individual undergoing OGTT. Finally, all trials aimed at type 2 diabetes prevention included IGT subjects [74, 75], who could not be possibly recognised without OGTT, seems therefore evident that the routine execution of OGTT is presently the one and only possible answer (Undeniably) [76].

## 5.2 Disadvantages of OGTT

### *5.2.1 Factors why OGTT may not be the first choose in screening for dysglycaemia*

a. Biological variation which may account for about 5.7% of available blood glucose value

b. Variable effects of administration of hyperosmolar glucose solution on gastric emptying, eg, nausea, vomiting, osmotic diarrhea, abdominal distension. Flavoring with sugar-free lemon and chilling increases palatability and may reduce nausea.

c. More cost and time, Cumbersome, unfriendly procedure for patients

d. Because of the OGTT's high variability and low sensitivity, epidemiological studies based on a single OGTT may overestimate the prevalence of diabetes by as much as 16%

Due to the number of limitations, the OGTT should be undertaken on two separate occasions before the results are considered abnormal (unless the initial results are grossly abnormal). It has high intra-and interperson variability. This may be due to a number of factors, including diet and exercise during the days before the test, caffeine use, smoking, medications, and stress. However, with careful patient preparation the impact of these modifiable factors can be markedly reduced resulting in improved reproducibility. These modifiable factors can be placed into three categories:

a. When preparing patient for test: duration of fast; prior carbohydrate intake; medications (e.g. thiazide, oral contraceptives and corticosteroids); trauma; intercurrent illness; age; physical activity.

b. Glucose given: quantity of glucose ingested; volume of administration; and rate of ingestion.

c. Fasting sample: posture; anxiety; caffeine; smoking; physical activity; stress, and time of the day

This shows that with proper patient preparations spanning through history taking and physical examination and appropriate patient education will highly improve the reproducibility of OGTT, hence care must be taken of the factors [65, 77] in **Table 3** during patient preparation.

An increase in the volume or decrease in the osmolality of a meal may result in an increase in the rate of gastric emptying and in a subsequent increase in glycaemia. Gastric emptying has implications for the reproducibility of the OGTT. It was twice observed that the faster an OGTT meal is emptied from the stomach, the higher the resulting postprandial glycaemia level. About 30%, 19.8% and 14% differences in postprandial glucose after the dilution of 75-g (present study), 50-g and 25-g tolerance tests was noted, respectively [77]. The dilution effect is noted

| | |
|---|---|
| a. The OGTT is a non-physiological procedure and the interperson variability is rather high.<br>b. Analytical and biological variability<br>c. Use of different samples(eg; venous and capillary for a repeat or during same procedure<br>d. Biological variation is been found to be up to 20–35%—these can be minimized by stringent careful attention to the protocol | e. Other factors are: Lack of adequate patient preparations, Diet<br>f. Exercise during the days before the test<br>g. Caffeine use, Smoking, Medications, Stress<br>h. Changed in ambient temperature<br>i. Volume of the glucose solution<br>j. Others are: gastric emptying, Intestinal absorption, the gastrointestinal hormonal stimulus to insulin release, the liver, and the pancreatic islets. |

**Table 3.**
*Causes of variability in OGTT results.*

more between 90 and 180 minutes post-glucose solution ingestion. It is possible therefore that some of the earlier reports of poor reproducibility of the test may be attributable to a volume effect. The gastric emptying falls as the glucose concentration rises and this was demonstrated over a wide range of glucose concentrations [77]. It has been suggested that this is due to the stimulation of receptors in the duodenum sensitive to the osmotic pressure of the duodenal contents. The rate for gastric emptying in normal individuals lies between 40 and 80 minutes. Chronic pancreatitis does, however, causes overt diabetes in some patients, and most patients with this condition have impaired insulin secretion [78] even if this is not sufficiently severe to produce disturbances in carbohydrate tolerance. The liver, situated between the portal and systemic circulation, is in a position to influence oral glucose tolerance profoundly. Reproducibility can be improved by drawing Blood at the stipulated time or at least within $\pm 5$ minutes and centrifuge sample within 45 minutes of drawing it to obtain plasma.

To improve the reliability of a test it should be conducted in the individual that appropriately require the test, hence OGTT reproducibility can be improved when it is conducted in the selected individuals noted in **Table 4**.

### *5.2.2 Patient's preparation for conduct of OGTT, improving reproducibility*

Interaction with patients before procedure is very important because one of the conditions leading to spurious result in patient investigation is lack of patient's

| | |
|---|---|
| 1. Age > 45 yrs. (type 2 among 40-70 yr —7%, IGT—20%. In general pop—4.3%<br>2. Body Mass Index(BMI) >27 kg/m$^2$<br>3. High risk ethnic groups—Africans, Carribeans, Asians<br>4. Family history(first-degree relatives (increase risk by 2–4 fold<br>5. High waist circumference(>92 cm, >80 cm)<br>6. Sedentary lifestyle<br>7. History of gestational diabetes mellitus<br>8. Previous evidence of IGT or IFG<br>9. Dyslipidaemia(decrease HDL and increase TGs)<br>10. Patient with Cardiovascular disease | 11. Women with polycystic ovarian disease<br>12. Woman who delivered a macrosomic baby(>4 kg)<br>13. Have other clinical conditions associated with insulin resistance<br>14. Hypertension<br>15. Recurrent infections<br>16. It also helps determine if there is other condition that affects blood glucose levels (e.g., Cushing's syndrome, celiac disease, cystic fibrosis, acromegaly, pheochromocytoma, hemochromatosis, or Wilson's disease). |

**Table 4.**
*Indications for OGTT.*

education and preparation. Interacting with patient is important in improving reproducibility of test for the following reasons:

a. Enable the caregiver know about the patient—classify patient according to the three categories of tests mentioned earlier

b. Educate patient about why he/she is coming for the tests, and emphasize on what to avoid during pre-test period, and make patient to understand his/her role in obtaining good result

c. Know types of medications patient is on and withdraw those possible and record those which cannot be withdrawn

d. Emphasize the importance of patient's compliance and the result outcome

e. This interaction will prepare patient's mind and will alleviate fears and stress

## 6. Instructions to patient before the procedure: improving reproducibility

The OGTT results can be affected by carbohydrate intake and duration of fasting preceding the test, time of day for the test to be performed or activity during the test, sample collection, and medications. Instructions are as follows:

1. Patient must be on meal containing >150 g carbohydrate (approximately ten 40 g slices of bread per day) in the last three days before the test, and in the night before the test should take 30-50 g of carbohydrate containing meal

2. No strenuous exercise three days prior to test, but normal work is allowed. Patient should not rush when coming for the test (avoid stress). Need to rest before for minimum of 15 minutes before conducting test

3. No alcohol or Caffeine use 48 hrs before the test and during the test

4. Overnight fast (8-14 hr) water is allow—for patients convenience

5. Time for the test (morning hour is preferred, convenience of overnight fast, and fluctuation in FPG-higher in the morning and lower in the evening)

6. Maximum 75 g, anhydrous (82 g monohydrate) glucose dissolved in 250–300 ml of water

7. Glucose solution ingestion within the shortest possible time—usually within 5 minutes. Intolerance for sweet taste—patient may come with lemon juice, sometimes lucozide (375 ml) can be used instead.

8. Others are Glucola (224 ml) equivalent of 75 g anhydrous glucose. Polycal liquid (previously called Fortical) is used as the glucose load. 61.4 g maltodextrin/100 ml. Oral glucose solutions come in 10 US fluid ounces

a. Once patient arrived, confirm compliance with preparations, with emphasis on duration of fasting
b. You may wish to put in place an indwelling drip for sampling to avoid the stress of repeated needle pricking during sampling
c. Ensure patient is comfortable before starting the procedure
d. Take sample for fasting and any other investigations intended, before ingestion of glucose solution
e. Constitute the glucose solution—75 g(anhydrous) and 82 g(monohydrous)—10% more of anhydrous glucose, in 250–300 ml
f. Ask the patient to take the solution within 5 minutes
g. Time 0 minute of the test is when patient start taking the glucose solution and not when fasting sample is taken
h. Take samples at 30 minutes interval for 2 hr.(3, 5 hrs) or at 2 hr. only
i. Same type of sample must be taken throughout the procedure(, venous or capillary)
j. No smoking, caffeine, alcohol or any exercise during the waiting period
k. Monitor patient especially when approaches convenience—patient may vomit
l. Should the patient sit, lie, stand, walk, talk, etc.(seating is preferred—minimal activity)
m. Only minimal activity is allow but ensue that patient remain comfortable throughout the period of the test
n. Label samples appropriately, place sample ice-water slurry and ensure separation within 30 min of sampling

**Table 5.**
*Conduct of OGTT in a non-pregnant adult.*

(296 ml) bottles containing 50, 75, or 100 g of glucose (5, 7.5, and 10 g per fluid ounce)

9. If patient is under unavoidable stress, the test should be postponed

10. Patient should be aware of being seated in waiting area for a minimum of 2 hrs for the test

11. Failure to comply with all instructions will invalidate result

Ensure that all staff involved in undertaking any elements of the test have been provided with suitable training and are assessed to be competent (**Table 5**).

## 7. Interpreting OGTT result: improving reproducibility

### 7.1 Considerations when interpreting OGTT result

When interpreting the result remember that OGTT has variable reproducibility and care should be taken not to over-interpret the results. Use only one criterion, eg WHO criteria, to indicate a diagnosis of IFG, IGT or diabetes. In most cases the results of fasting and 2-hr post-glucose load are enough. Always look for help from local diabetes serves in uncertainty. Refer cases you can not evaluate to endocrinologist for further for assessment. Usually there are no causes of false-positive result when processes are strictly followed. These arts will improve the reproducibility.

### 7.2 While interpreting OGTT result you will not get information concerning

a. Patient preparation for and how the glucose was administrated.

b. The result shows assessment of glucose tolerance at the time of the test only and cannot provide any other information.

c. Results give only a qualitative idea of the average 24-hr blood glucose

d. Nor will result predict response to hypoglycaemic therapy or the current or future risk of diabetes complications

Therefore result will be better interpreted with the cognition of the above in mind.

**7.3 Result interpretation**

a. Normal response has the following characteristics:

1. Initial fasting glucose within normal limits

2. The highest value does not exceed the renal threshold (160-180 mg/dl (8.8-10 mmol/L))

3. The fasting level is again reached by 2–2.30 hours

4. No glucose or ketone bodies are detected in any urine specimen

b. Response of diabetic patient

1. Fasting blood glucose may raise above normal usually in the impaired range

2. The peak is reached between 1 and 1.30 hours

3. Glucosuria is usually present because the highest value exceeds the renal threshold

4. Plasma glucose does not return to fasting level within 2.30 hours, the most characteristic feature of DM response

c. LAG curve for oxyhyperglycaemia

1. Normal Fasting glucose level

2. Plasma glucose rises rapidly within 30 minutes to 1-hr post glucose ingestion exceeds renal threshold with corresponding glucosuria

3. Return to normal quickly and completely

4. This is usually noted in Hyperthyroidism, post gastroenterostomy, during pregnancy, early diabetes

d. Response for renal glycosuria

1. Glucose appears in the urine at normal plasma glucose much below renal threshold

2. Usually no glucosuria during fasting but mainly post-prandial

3. It may be physiological, in pregnancy or in renal disease or early diabetes

e. A flat glucose tolerance curve can be a normal finding and is as a result of rapid metabolism and not of either deficient absorption or slow gastric emptying.

Under certain pathological conditions such as hyper- and hypothyroidism changes in the gastric emptying rate may significantly alter the shape of the glucose tolerance curves [79]. Rapid gastric emptying associated with duodenal ulcer and partial gastrectomy where plasma glucose rises rapidly within 30 minutes of glucose ingestion stimulating hyperinsulinaemia and resultant reactive hypoglycaemia though measurement of serum insulin levels does not reveal evidence of such direct relationship.

In a healthy young adult with increase physiologic activities, there is associated rapid metabolism and when venous rather than capillary blood is analyzed, a flat curve can be a normal findings and not of either deficient absorption or slow gastric emptying. Hypoglycaemia in a fasting subject is normally prevented by hepatic gluconeogenesis. This stopped after glucose ingestion when blood glucose rises, and begun when plasma glucose is falling preventing fasting hypoglycaemia Reactive hypoglycaemia in either normal healthy young adult, patient with peptic ulcer or partial gastrectomy might, therefore, be due to the failure of the liver to resume glucose production sufficiently and rapidly. The normal exponential pattern of gastric emptying results in a very gradual decline of the rate at which glucose enters the intestine and this should provide ideal conditions for the liver gradually to resume glucose production. The absorption of glucose by the small intestine is highly efficient. After ingestion of a concentrated solution, a combination of slow gastric emptying, dilution within the duodenum, and active peristalsis ensure that within the jejunum the glucose solution no longer remains hypertonic. The small intestine is efficient in glucose absorption.

Every dynamic test requiring appropriate patient preparation and procedure for the conduct of the test will not be without contraindication if result is to be reliable. Such contraindications for conduct of OGTT are shown in **Table 6**. The primary objective is to demonstrate presence of dysglycaemia in a condition that has long latent period, except when monitoring success of treatment in secondary causes of hyperglycaemia. Subject must be conscious and alert to obey order (in both preparation and conduct of the test), in a no stressful condition, physically or otherwise. Patient should be able to take the stated amount or an equivalent and under influence of no other condition except what is being investigated for.

| | |
|---|---|
| a. Diagnosed diabetes mellitus<br>b. Suspected Type 1 DM<br>c. Unconscious patient<br>d. Patient who can not obey instructions<br>e. Refusal to follow instructions<br>f. Not for diabetes follow-up except during treatment of secondary diabetes; eg acromegaly, glucagonoma, Cushing's syndrome, Phaeochromocytoma<br>g. Hospitalized, acutely ill or immobile patients | h. Vomiting during the procedure<br>i Patient who could not consumed the glucose solution<br>j. Patient who developed moderate to severe hypoglycaemia during the test<br>k. Do not perform the test on patients with uncontrolled thyroid dysfunction, under physical stress, eg post surgery, trauma, infection or extreme psychological stress or in patient with hypokalaemic periodic paralysis |

**Table 6.**
*Conditions under which OGTT should not be conducted or when procedure should be stopped.*

### 7.4 Testing of children for type 2 diabetes mellitus

Until recently, type 1 diabetes was the most frequent form of diabetes among young people [80]. Recently however, there are increasing reports of T2DM, previously a disorder of middle-aged or elderly persons among children and adolescents. In the 1990s, various reports indicated that the incidence of childhood type 2 diabetes was increasing and this trend continues at present. The ADA and the American Academic of Paediatrics approved screening for T2DM in children because T2DM can be asymptomatic at diagnosis and requires tight glycaemic control to delay the onset of chronic vascular complications. Several studies have shown an increased risk of microvascular complications among young adolescents with T2DM compared to those with T1DM. Therefore, screening for IGT and T2DM in children at risk of glucose intolerance is necessary.

#### *7.4.1 Criteria/indications*

a. Overweight (BMI ≥ 85th percentile for age and sex, weight for height ≥ 85th percentile, or weight >120% of ideal for height)

    1. Plus any two of the following risk factors

    2. Family history of Type 2 DM, 1° or 2°

    3. Native American, black, Asian, Latino

b. Signs of insulin resistance (acanthosis nigricans, hypertension, dyslipidaemia)

c. Age of initiation: 10 years or onset of puberty

d. Frequency: every two years

e. Test: FPG preferred

The dose of glucose is weight dependent-1.75 g/kg body weight. The maximum load is 75 g. Lucozade may be given instead which is more palatable. Formulation 73 kcal carbohydrate/100 ml, gives 75 g glucose in 419 ml Maximum dose is 75 g. Apply ametop gel 45 minutes prior to cannulations to ensure the area is numbed. Utilize a member of the play team to prepare the child for the procedure and provide distractive techniques throughout. Give full explanations to the child and family about the procedure and answer any questions they may ask.

## 8. OGTT in gestation diabetes mellitus, an undeniably the only test for dysglycaemia of GDM

### 8.1 Gestational Diabetes Mellitus (GDM)

Normal pregnancy is characterized by approximately 50% decrease in insulin-mediated glucose disposal in humans and a 200–250% increase in insulin secretion to maintain euglycaemia in the mother [81]. Women with adequate insulin secreting capacity overcome this insulin resistance of pregnancy by secreting more endogenous insulin to maintain normal blood glucose. In a study involving non-GDM pregnancies, plasma glucose levels during late pregnancy (mean ± 1 SD) were noted to be fasting 3.9 ± 0.4 mmol/L, 1 hour postprandial 6.1 ± 0.7 mmol/L, and 2 hours postprandial 5.5 ± 0.6 mmol/L with a mean glucose of 4.9 ± 0.6 mmol/L [82]. The HAPO study reported a mean fasting glucose of 4.5 ± 0.4 mmol/L, derived from 23316 pregnant women [38]. But women with diabetes or those who have tendency to develop GDM, endogenous insulin secretion is inadequate to compensate for the insulin resistance (IR), hence their hyperglycaemia worsen or they development hyperglycaemia.

Numerous factors such as placental hormones, obesity, inactivity, an unhealthy diet, genetic and epigenetic contributions influence IR in pregnancy, but the causal mechanisms are complex and still not completely elucidated [83]. Placental derived hormones are believed to be a major factor in reprogramming maternal physiology to achieve an I-R state. Human placental lactogen (hPL) and human placental growth hormone (hPGH) are the major player in pregnancy induced IR [84]. Prolactin, progesterone, estradiol and cortisol are increased during pregnancy and may contribute to the development of IR in pregnancy [85]. Recently, studies have implicated adiponectin from adipocytes and secreted factors, such as TNF-α, leptin, IL-6, resistin in mediating IR of pregnancy [86]. Most women who develop GDM have increased IR caused by alteration in insulin signaling pathway, abnormal subcellular localization of GLUT4 transporters, increased expression of the membrane glycoprotein PC-1 or reduced insulin-mediated glucose transport. GDM is usually diagnosed after 20 weeks' gestation when placental hormones are increase substantially as the placental size increases.

In 2014, the WHO has defined hyperglycaemia in pregnancy (HIP) as diabetes first detected at any time during pregnancy, along with pre-existing diabetes and is further sub-classified as diabetes in pregnancy (DIP) and gestational diabetes mellitus (GDM) [87]. Nowadays type 2 diabetes is frequently found in young women due to ongoing epidemics of obesity therefore the number of undiagnosed (before pregnancy) is increasing. Screening for GDM earlier than 24-28 weeks in identifying these young women and address perinatal risks that may be particular to their greater degree of hyperglycaemia is becoming more important because of the following [87]:

1. Rise chances of congenital malformations in offsprings

2. Risk of diabetes complications requiring treatment during early part pregnancy

3. Early treatment Prompt or frequent follow-up to maintain normoglycaemia

4. Post-pregnancy screening ensuring confirmation and appropriate treatment of diabetes after pregnancy

How then do we identify these women? Early glucose testing is important. Usually in early part of pregnancy (e.g. first trimester and first half of second trimester) fasting and postprandial glucose concentrations are normally lower than in normal due to less effect of placental hormone and decreased appetite, compared to non–diabetes women. Elevated fasting or postprandial plasma glucose levels at this time in pregnancy may reflect diabetes antedating pregnancy. In this regards there was a uniform agreement during IADPSG Pasadena meeting that this assessment should be made during the initial visit for prenatal care. However, there is variability in time of enrollment for prenatal care beyond the control of health care providers. Accordingly, no limit can be place on the timing of initial assessment for detection of overt diabetes in pregnancy. It was advised that selective, stepwise screening particularly in the low- and mid-income countries is more cost effective. This entail: (a) Categorizing all women at first antenatal visit into low, moderate and high risk of GDM; (b) Those in moderate to high risk groups should have glucose challenge test with 50 g anhydrous glucose diluted in 150 ml of water to drink and venous sample is taken at 1-hr. If result is 7.8 (7.2) mmol/L, at first visit, proceed to diagnostic OGTT. If result is negative repeat glucose challenge test at 24–28 weeks of gestation; (c) Those in low risk group should be screening only at 24–28 weeks of gestation. However, if enrollment is at 24 weeks gestation or later and overt diabetes is not found, the initial test should be either 50 g glucose challenge first or the 75-g OGTT. Although IAFPSG Consensus Panel members favored use of A1c at first visit, this is not feasible in most low- and mid-income countries. It was also recommended that an FPG value in early pregnancy ≥5.1 mmol/L (92 mg/dl) also be classified as GDM.

Determining prevalence of GDM is difficult due to inconsistencies in screening methods. Because the IADPSG's is stricter when applied by IDF about 14% of 18 million live births were affected by gestational diabetes mellitus, where South-East Asia had the highest prevalence of GDM at 24.2% and the lowest was in Africa at 10.5% [88]. Almost 90% of cases of hyperglycaemia in pregnancy occurred in low- and middle-income countries, where access to maternal healthcare is limited. In Nigeria, the prevalence of HIP is projected to be 13.9%, and age-adjusted prevalence of 37.5% (crude 41.0%) in the United Arab Emirates is note [89]. The incidence of GDM has increased over the past decades in parallel with the increase in rates of obesity and type 2 diabetes mellitus, and this trend is expected to continue. GDM affects 7% of all pregnancies worldwide, 1.1% to 14.3% in USA, 3.8% to 6.5% in Canada, 6–9% in India. It is diagnosed at 16.3% in ≤16 weeks of gestation, 22.4% between 17 and 23 weeks and 61.3% after 23 weeks of gestation [90]. It occurs more frequently among African Americans, Hispanic/Latino Americans, and American Indians. It is also more common among obese women and women with a family history of diabetes. After delivery, GDM will follow 1 of 3 clinical courses [91, 92]:

a. Approximately 10% continue to have markedly abnormal glucose metabolism and fulfill criteria for diabetes in the nonpregnant adult these patients are reclassified as having diabetes (Hyperglycaemia in pregnancy).

b. Approximately 5–10% of patients continue to exhibit abnormal glucose metabolism that is below diabetic levels. These patients are reclassified as having IFG or IGT, as appropriate.

c. The remainder exhibit normal glucose metabolism.

GDM has about 20–50% chance of developing type 2 diabetes in about 5–10 years even when there is lack of signs and symptoms of diabetes. The enormity defers among different ethnic groups, ranging from 9% in Caucasians, 11.9% in Latinos, and 25% in women of Mediterranean or east-Asian descent [93]. When GDM women were followed for a longer period, higher incidence of type 2 diabetes after index pregnancies was noted in 40% while there are evidence rates as high as 70% in Canadian Aboriginal women [93].

### 8.2 Should we then screen for GDM

Screening and diagnosis of GDM and treating it effectively not only prevent adverse maternal and perinatal outcome but also future diabetes in both mother and child. The goal of screening therefore is to reduce maternal and fetal complications such as preeclampsia, caesarean delivery, congenital malformations, macrosomia, shoulder dystocia, nerve palsy, bone fracture, hyperbilirubinaemia and infant death, or later childhood/adolescent overweight as demonstrated in some studies. The Australian Carbohydrate Intolerance Study in Pregnant Women (ACHOIS) [94], showed a 4% reduction in the composite outcome of severe perinatal complications (death, shoulder dystocia, bone fracture, nerve palsy) among women randomized to routine care compared with 1% among the intervention group, while in the National Institute of Child Health and Human Development (NICHD) study, though there was no reduction in the composite primary outcome (perinatal mortality, birth trauma and neonatal hypoglycaemia, hyperbilirubinaemia, or hyperinsulinaemia), there was reductions in fetal overgrowth, shoulder dystocia, caesarean section delivery and pre-eclampsia. During pregnancy, gestational diabetes requires treatment to normalize maternal blood glucose levels to avoid complications in both the infant and the mother. Untreated hyperglycaemia in pregnancy may result into either or all of the following complications in **Table 7**.

About 10–25% of infants born of GDM pregnancies are macrosomic; maternal euglycaemia in labour reduces the risk of hypoglycaemia, hypocalcaemia, hyperbilirubinaemia and polycythemia in the baby. In addition, the maternal metabolic milieu was identified as a key determinant for the susceptibility to obesity, metabolic syndrome and T2DM in the offspring, a phenomenon often described as 'fetal programming'. A study showed that infant of GDM were followed biennially from the age of 5 years using 75 g 2-hr OGTT among the Pima Indians in Arizona, USA, and Diabetes developed in the next generation in 6.9% and 30.1% of breast-fed offspring of non-diabetic and diabetic women, respectively and in 11.9% and 43.6% of bottle-fed offspring, respectively. Shoulder dystocia (SD) occurs in 1–2% of pregnancies, with majority of cases occurring in non-macrosomic fetuses, however, it increased for all birth weights, with a three-fold increase when birth weight is >4000 g. Brachial plexus injury (BPI) occurs in 0.06%–0.26% of normal deliveries but occurs in 16–23% of births complicated by shoulder dystocia. GDM is an independent risk factor for BPI with a relative risk of 1.9–3.19 but in only 6–10%% of BPI is maternal GDM documented. It can be inferred therefore that the incidence of adverse perinatal outcomes increases as glucose intolerance increases, that identification of women with hyperglycaemia in pregnancy has clinical significance. As hyperglycaemia in pregnancy is an asymptomatic condition, diagnosis is dependent on some form of screening.

| | |
|---|---|
| a. Placenta abruption<br>b. Premature delivery<br>c. Shoulder dystocia and Brachial plexus injury<br>d. Macrosomic baby (weight ≥ 4 kg) or weight of >90th centile for gestational(according to ethnicity)<br>e. Baby is prone to hypoglycaemia<br>f. Hyperbilirubinaemia<br>g. Increase tendency of assisted delivery, Caesarean section, or induction of labour | a. Respiratory distress in the baby, and associated feeding problems<br>b. Pregnancy induced hypertension, Pre-eclampsia and eclampsia<br>c. The risk of developing diabetes later in life or in a future pregnancy is increased<br>d. Haemorrhage and preterm delivery<br>e. Sevenfold higher risk of the mother developing T2DM after pregnancy<br>f. Increase chances of death in both mother and the baby |

**Table 7.**
*Complications of GDM if it is not diagnosed or properly managed [95].*

### 8.3 What is the optimal method of screening for GDM?

a. The optimal method of screening for GDM depends on the location, the strength of the health facility, the principle of practicing Physician and affordability of the patients. Screening is therefore either universal based or risk factor based [96].

b. In order to reduce the burden of screening on women and the health care system, the concept of selective (risk factor based) screening was introduced.

c. The goal of risk factor based screening would be to ideally identify through historical and clinical factors those patients who would benefit most from biochemical screening while allowing those at lower risk to avoid the screening processes. This is preferred particular in the low-income and mid-income nations

d. Selective screening originally consisted of taking a personal and family history in order to identify a high-risk population in need of further directed testing. With this method, women are categorized into low-risk, moderate-risk and high-risk. Women with any of the risk factors below were advised to perform a 50 g glucose challenge test.

e. High risk women should undergo diagnostic test as early in pregnancy as possible and that testing should be repeated at 24–28 weeks if initial results are negative

f. Screening by risk factors alone has a sensitivity of 63% and a specificity of 56%. In other words, 37–50% of women with GDM may go undiagnosed using this approach.

g. Hence universal screening was considered and is widely practices. Universal screening for GDM is practiced by 84% of Canadian obstetricians, 94–97% of US obstetricians; however in recent survey only 17% of physicians in the UK practiced universal screening while 11% did not screen for GDM and 72% screened in the presence of maternal risk factors.

Routine screening of women at 24–28 weeks of gestation may be recommended with 50 g glucose challenge test (GCT), using a threshold of 7.8 mmol/L (140 mg/dl), except in those who fulfill the criteria for low risk and may not need screening for GDM at all. Properties used in categorizing a woman to at low-risk are [95, 96] (**Table 8**).

Women at moderate risk: women who do not meet all low risk criteria but lack two or more risk factors for GDM. Average-risk patients (all patients who fall between low and high risk) should be tested at 24–28 weeks of gestation. High risk

| |
|---|
| a. Caucasian or member of other ethnic group with low prevalence of diabetes |
| b. Pregnancy with body mass index(BMI) ≤27 kg/m$^2$ |
| c. No previous history of GDM or glucose intolerance or adverse pregnancy outcome associated with GDM |
| d. No family history of diabetes in first-degree relative |
| e. No history of GDM-associated adverse pregnancy outcome |

**Table 8.**
*Low-risk group.*

| |
|---|
| a. Obesity(BMI ≥ 30 kg/m$^2$ |
| b. Previous macrosomic baby weighing ≥4.5 kg |
| c. Previous GDM |
| d. Glucosuria(1+ on two occasion or 2+ on one occasion) |
| e. Family history of T2DM(first degree relative with T2DM) |
| f. Ethnic family origin with a high prevalence of DM |
| g. Clinical conditions associated with insulin resistance like PCOS, acanthosis nigricans |
| h. History of hypertension or hypercholesterolaemia |

**Table 9.**
*Feature indicators of women at high-risk for GDM.*

criteria are: This category of women needs to be screened at first antenatal visit and repeat at 24–28 week if they were negative at early screening. Women with these features are categorized as high-risk [95, 96] (**Table 9**).

The most common method of screening is with stepwise 50 g OGTT at 24 to 28 weeks of gestation, followed by an OGTT as the diagnostic test if a certain threshold has been surpassed. The procedure for glucose challenge test (GCT), is that 50 g anhydrous glucose load dissolve in 150 ml fluid to be ingested within 5 minutes irrespective of time of the day or last meal. Blood is collected 1-hr post ingestion of glucose solution Views diverge on the optimal cutoff value for the 50 g GCT. 90% of women with GDM will be identified if 7.2 mmol/L (130 mg/dl) is used, however, as high as 20–25% of those screened will to undergo 100 g OGTT for diagnosis. Increasing the cutoff value to 7.8 mmol/L (140 mg/dl) will identify only 80% of women with GDM but decrease to 14–18% of women will do 100 g diagnostic testing [97]. A cutoff value of 7.2 mmol/L is advice in those with FPG level is <140 mg/dl (<7.8 mmol/L) and manifests symptoms compatible with complications of diabetes. Finally, at 24 to 28 weeks of gestation, every women should undergo 50 g challenge test and those with values between 7.2 to 7.8 mmol/L (130–140 mg/dl) should proceed to 100 g OGTT for diagnosis of GDM and sampling over 3-hrs.

As women with negative GCT do not undergo the diagnostic OGTT, it is possible that they could have undiagnosed GDM or GIGT. In a study involving 202 pregnant women with a negative GCT screening test that underwent subsequent OGTT, the only positive predictor noted is the average glucose value in those with normal and those with GDM/GIGT. Therefore, false negative GCTs cannot be readily predicted by risk factors. However, their clinical implications at delivery may be benign [98]. During pregnancy, some women have a low glucose level on the 75 g OGTT. These women tend to have more booking weight and higher rate of congenital anomaly; however their pregnancy outcome was shown not to be significantly different from those with normal screening OGTT results [99]. The performance of the GCT as a screening test depends on the cutoff values used, the criteria for diagnosis of GDM and the prevalence of GDM in the screened population. A study conducted in China where 422 gravidas [100] were screened with 50-g glucose and those with a positive results (≥135 mg/dl (7.5 mmol/L)), underwent additional glucose testing. GDM was defined using National Diabetes Data Group (NDDG) standards for the 3-h GTT. When Carpenter and Coustan was used for comparison, any woman with elevated 50-g value and no 3-hr OGTT was performed, a fasting serum glucose ≥140 mg/dl (7.8 mmol/L) were considered evidence of gestational diabetes. One hundred twenty four (29.4%) had GDM as defined by the NDDG criteria; this increased to 161 (38%) when the diagnosis was based on Carpenter and Coustan's criteria. As expected, the prevalence of GDM increased in relation to an increasing 50-g value. All subjects with a 50-g screen >216 mg/dl (>12.0 mmol/L) had evidence of gestational diabetes and required insulin for glycemic control. Patients with a 50-g screen ≥220 mg/dl (12.2 mmol/L) do not require a 3-h GTT. Those with fasting serum

| | |
|---|---|
| a. Previous pregnancy with gestational diabetes | h. A family history of diabetes (first degree relatives) |
| b. Previous 'big' baby (at or over 4.5kgs – 10lbs) | i. A previous still-birth |
| c. Frequent loss of pregnancy or premature delivery | j. Long usage of steroids |
| d. Large for gestational age | k. Women with PCOS (Polycystic ovary syndrome) |
| e. Positive glycosuria(1+ on 2 occasions or 2 + on one occasion) | l. Polyhydramnios |
| f. BMI ≥30 kg/m$^2$ | m. High risk ethnic groups |
| g. Maternal age ≥ 40 years old | |

**Table 10.**
*Indications for OGTT in pregnancy [101].*

glucose of ≥140 mg/dl (7.8 mmol/L) may begin diet therapy, glucose monitoring, and insulin as indicated. If the fasting serum glucose is <140 mg/dl (7.8 mmol/L), a 3-h GTT should be performed for confirmation of GDM. This approach will facilitate rapid therapeutic intervention and reduce the cost of care in this subset of patients. This findings need to be validated at different places using different ethnic groups. What should be considered an indication for screening for gestation diabetes mellitus (GDM) (**Table 10**).

Polycystic ovary syndrome (PCOS) is the most common endocrine disorder of women of reproductive-aged and is the most common endocrine-associated cause of infertility. Approximately 6.5% of women of reproductive age have PCOS. Women with PCOS are known to be at increased risk for IR, IGT, and type 2 diabetes mellitus though often present with normal FPG [102]. The current guideline of Androgen Excess Society is that a 2-hour OGTT be performed on all obese women with PCOS [102]. Though screening for GDM is considered compulsory in affluent countries and highly recommended in low- and middle-income countries, the administering the required amount of glucose in pregnancy is not without side effects. The recognised disadvantages are as noted in **Table 11**, ranging from mild to moderate consequences.

However, advantage almost always surpasses the disadvantages. The advantages are as shown in **Table 12**.

## 8.4 Diagnosis of GDM is only done using OGTT

The gold standard for the diagnosis of GDM is OGTT irrespective of how it is performed, using 100 g as recommended by ACOG, or 75 g, according to the ADA criteria.

In 1964, O'Sullivan and Mahan first developed the two-step method OGTT for the diagnosis of GDM [103] and this is based on the risk of maternal type 2 diabetes later in life [104]. As explained earlier, those with glucose levels meeting screening limit undergo a 100 g, 3 hours or 75 g, 2-hour diagnostic OGTT and by Carpenter and Coustan (C-C) criteria, GDM is diagnosed in women with two or more abnormal values (5.3–10.0-8.6 mmol/L at fasting, 1-hr and 3-hour (2 hour) post glucose [104]. This with some modifications was adapted by many organizations, NDDG

| |
|---|
| 1. There are no serious direct risks to the GTT, however, some women reported dizziness, fainting, vomiting, due to fasting and/or the use of a high glucose drink on an empty stomach |
| 2. Fasting for 8–12 hrs in pregnancy can be difficult |
| 3. Soreness, bruise, swelling or infection at site of needle insertion |
| 4. More cost burden in a patient with positive or borderline result who has be closely monitor |
| 5. Patient may not be eligible for midwifery led care options such as homebirth or MLU |
| 6. Induction of delivery may be recommended before date is due |

**Table 11.**
*Disadvantages of the OGTT in a pregnant woman.*

| |
|---|
| a. The GTT is considered the most effective way to determine if you have GDM<br>b. Early detection of GDM gives a better chance of monitoring glucose levels<br>c. Managing glucose levels early decreases the risks to the baby<br>d. Managing the glucose levels early decreases the chances of macrosomic baby and its complications<br>e. Managing glucose levels decreases the risk of interventions in labour and delivery |

**Table 12.**
*Advantages of OGTT for a pregnant woman.*

[105], ADA [106], as the standard method for diagnosis of GDM for more than two decades.

In 2008, the HAPO study [39] demonstrated presence of unfavourable neonatal outcomes even in those with mild hyperglycaemia which did not meet the old criteria of GDM [107]. Based on this notion the International Association of Diabetes and Pregnancy Study Group (IADPSG) recommended a one-step 75 g OGTT testing but lowered the diagnostic cut-point of the OGTT to (5.1–10.0-8.5 mmol/L, fasting, 1-hour and 2 hours postprandial) in 2010 [108] and only one abnormal value was enough to make a diagnosis. This was adopted by ADA [109], WHO [110] and FIGO [111] by recommending a one-step 75 g glucose OGTT between 24 and 28 gestational weeks and diagnosis of GDM is made with only one abnormal value equal to or exceeding 5.1–10.0-8.5 mmol/L, due to the result of the HAPO study regarding mild hyperglycaemia and adverse clinical outcome, including LGA, primary caesarean, clinical neonatal hypoglycaemia, and C-protein cord blood [108] where a more strict strategy may help reduce the frequency of these potential complications. However, several guidelines including the ACOG [112], NIH [113] and SOGC [114] did not support the IADPSG criteria and their guidelines still recommend the two-step strategy and the C-C or NDDG criteria for the OGTT, the reasons provided are:

a. The benefit from the treatment of mild GDM in women is not well established

b. Additional healthcare costs will be generated by increased prevalence

c. Caesarean delivery and intensive newborn assessment will increase

d. Life disruptions and psychosocial burdens will be developed in a patients with GDM

Current ADA guidelines recommended selective screening of high risk women for GDM, where ACOG guideline advice universal screening and NICE guideline recommended screening all women of South Asians ethnicity. In the HAPO study risk of adverse outcomes were very low when FPG was ≤4.4 mmol/L (80 mg/dl). In Chinese women with FPG value ≥5.1 mmol/L, one can make a diagnosis of GDM (specificity 100% and, in those with value ≤4.4 mmol/L one can exclude GDM (87.8%, sensitivity). These results are similar to those reported by Agarwal, et al. in the HAPO cohort. In HAPO and two other studies, the incidence of selected adverse maternal and fetal outcomes increases along a continuum of increasing maternal hyperglycaemia, with no outcome-associated glycaemic thresholds were identified that could be used to define internationally accepted criteria for the diagnosis of GDM. In 2010, IADPSG [108] consensus panel using HAPO study primary outcomes (birthweight >90%, primary caesarean section rate, neonatal hypoglycaemia and cord C-peptide levels >90%) and threshold for 75-g OGTT reached odds ratio 1.75. These arbitrary thresholds, when applied to the HAPO cohorts, led to a GDM incidence of 17.8%. In 2013 Canadian Diabetic Association expert committee conceded the dispute and chosen sequential screening with a 50 g GCT followed by 75 g OGTT using the glucose thresholds that result in an Odds Ratio (OR) of 2.00 (fasting ≥5.3 mmol/L, 1 hour ≥10.6 mmol/L, 2 hours ≥9.0 mmol/L).

Hyperglycaemia first detected at any time during pregnancy should be classified as either:

- Diabetes mellitus in pregnancy
- Gestational diabetes mellitus

When glucose abnormalities persist postpartum in a woman with GDM, her diabetes is re-categorized as overt diabetes, especially if the diagnosis of GDM occurred before 20 weeks' gestation and glucose levels were markedly elevated in pregnancy. The 2006 WHO criteria should be used in diagnosis of Diabetes mellitus in pregnancy when one or more of the following criteria are met:

- FPG ≥ 7.0 mmol/L (126 mg/dl), demonstrated on two occasions
- 2hPG ≥ 11.1 mmol/L (200 mg/dl) following a 75 g oral glucose load
- RPG ≥ 11.1 mmol/L (200 mg/dl) in presence of diabetic symptoms

The diagnosis of GDM at any time during pregnancy should be based on any one of the following values:

- FPG 5.1–6.9 mmol/l (95–125 mg/dl)
- 1hPG 75 g OGTT ≥10.0 mmol/L (180 mg/dl)
- 2-hPG 75 g OGTT 8.5–11.0 mmol/L (153-199 mg/dl)

There are no established criteria for the diagnosis of diabetes based on the 1-hour post-load value. At least one of these thresholds must be equaled or exceeded to make a diagnosis of GDM.

## 9. A1c, Can it replace OGTT?

The measurement of A1c equals the assessment of hundreds (virtually thousands) of fasting glucose levels and also capture postprandial glucose peaks; therefore, it is a more and reliable measurement than FPG and/or 2-hr OGTT plasma glucose (PG) oscillates above and below the cut point of 200 mg/dl.

FPG of 6.7 mmol/L to 7.2 mmol/L (120 or 130 mg/dl) or having a 2-h PG of 10.3 mmol/L to 11.9 mmol/L (185 or 215 mg/dl) are considered similar because they define a point where physiological disturbance is apparent, however from other angles it makes a lot of difference. Therefore, an appliance evaluating chronic rather than spot hyperglycaemia is unquestionably more desirable. A1c assay is now the preferred test not only for chronic management of diabetes but also for its diagnosis. However, the cost of assay in some parts of the world rules out its typical use. In such instances, clinicians should continue using glucose measurements for both diagnosis and monitoring of diabetes.

A1c assay may not be reliable under the underlisted conditions [115]

a. First, some haemoglobin traits, such as HbS, HbC, HbF, and HbE, interfere with some A1c assay method. These are common among blacks

b. Second, conditions causing changes in red cell turnover: haemolytic anaemias, chronic malaria, major blood loss, or blood transfusions,

c. Third, A1c levels appear to increase with age [116], though this is not sufficiently clear

d. Similarly, racial disparities in A1c, the etiology and significance are unclear [117]

e. Finally, in rapidly evolving type 1 diabetes, no time to "catch-up" with the sudden elevations in glucose levels; diagnosis should be relied on plasma glucose in association with typical symptoms

The glycated haemoglobin (HbA1c) test has been suggested as an alternative screening test for type 2 diabetes. HbA1c overcomes many of these difficulties as fasting state is not required, analytical variability is less than 2% and gives glycaemic status over past 2–3 month. The coefficient of variation is usually 2–3% for the same day analysis, while the inter-assay variation is 4–5%. HbA1c values are relatively stable after collection, and the recent introduction of a new reference method to calibrate all HbA1c assay instruments should further improves HbA1c assay standardization.

Advantages of HbA1c assay are:

a. better indicator of overall glycemic exposure

b. less variability, unaffected by outside factors like stress

c. not a timed test, requires no fasting; more convenient

d. Better at predicting complications

Regrettably, at variance with that report, the New Hoorn Study [118] showed that 44% of people with newly diagnosed diabetes with OGTT had A1c $< 6.0\%$ and that a stronger correlations between plasma glucose and A1c is better in subjects with known diabetes, but not in the general population. Moreover, in the Rancho Bernardo Study [119], 85% of the participants with A1c $\geq 6.5\%$ were not classified as diabetes by ADA criteria and a 1/3rd of people with diabetes on OGTT had A1c

| |
|---|
| 1. Assay is normalized and aligned to the DCCT/UKPDS |
| 2. Better summary of overall glycaemic exposure and risk for long-term complications |
| 3. It has significantly less biologic fluctuation |
| 4. No need for fasting or timed samples |
| 5. Relatively unaffected by acute(eg stress or illness related) perturbations in glucose levels |
| 6. Currently used to guide management and adjust therapy |

**Table 13.**
*The beauty of A1c testing compared to blood glucose for diagnose of diabetes mellitus.*

< 6.0%. Thus, this study demonstrated that 30% of subjects who are already diabetic or pre-diabetic would have been missed if A1c had been used instead of OGTT. In conclusion, the data confirmed, in agreement with an Australian study, that an A1C ≤5.5% or ≥ 7% can predict the absence or presence of diabetes respectively, while intermediate values are inconclusive (**Table 13**).

A1C values just above the upper limits of normal, depend upon post-prandial glycaemias (ie 2hPG), still requiring the OGTT to be correctly interpreted. Although in certain cases A1c gives equal or almost equal sensitivity and specificity to glucose measurement, it is not available in many part of the world and it is not well enough standardised for its use to be recommended at this time particularly in low- and mid-income countries.

Finally, although ADA recommended the use of A1c, by emphasizing the importance of IFG and IGT, which cannot be diagnosed without OGTT, to disclose high-risk subjects for diabetes, obviously shows that A1c would be of minute use without OGTT and that pre-diabetes includes different entities. OGTT is the only test that can efficiently disclose obscure diabetes when FPG<7.0 mmol/L and screen competently within the range of rather heterogeneous pre-diabetic values [120].

In conclusion an OGTT is undeniably the best test in investigation of dysglycaemia, either with the intention of testing for pre-diabetes, type 2 diabetes, or for gestational diabetes mellitus.

## Author details

Dahiru Saleh Mshelia[1*], Sani Adamu[2] and Rebecca Mtaku Gali[3]

1 Chemical Pathology, Faculty of Basic Clinical Sciences, College of Medical Sciences, University of Maiduguri, Maiduguri, Nigeria

2 Chemical Pathology, Faculty of Basic Clinical Sciences, College of Medical Sciences, Gombe State University, Gombe, Nigeria

3 Medical Laboratory Science, Faculty of Allied Health Science, College of Medical Sciences, University of Maiduguri, Maiduguri, Nigeria

*Address all correspondence to: dsmkinging@gmail.com

## References

[1] Wild S, Roglic G, Green A, Sicree R, King H. Global Prevalence of Diabetes: Estimates for the year 2000 and projections for 2030. Diabetes Care2004; 27:1047-1053

[2] Kasper DL, Fauci AS, Hauser SL, Lango DL, Jameson JL, Loscalzo J. Harrison's Principles of Internal Medicine. 17th ed. USA: The McGraw-Hill Companies, Inc; 2015. Chapter 338: Diabetes Mellitus; Cla

[3] Classification and Diagnosis of Diabetes: Standards of Medical Care in Diabetes-2020. American Diabetes Association. Diabetes Care 2020; 43 (suppl 1):S14-S31

[4] Diagnosis and Classification of Diabetes Mellitus. American Diabetes Association position statement. Diabetes Care; 32(suppl 1):S62-S67

[5] Ramachandran A, Snehalatha C and Viswanathan V. Burden of type 2 diabetes and its complications-The Indian scenario. Current Science 83; 2002: 1471-1476

[6] IDF Diabetes Atlas. 88th Edition. Brussels: International Diabetes Federation. 2017

[7] Global report on diabetes. Geneva: World Health Organization; 2016

[8] American Diabetes Association. Economic costs of diabetes in the US in 2002. Diabetes Care 2003; 26:917-932

[9] Harris MI. Undiagnosed NIDDM: Clinical and public health issues. Diabetes Care 1993; 16: 642-652

[10] Harris MI, Klein R, Wellborn TA, Kruiman MW. Onset of NIDDM occurs at least 4-7 years before clinical diagnosis. Diabetes Care 1992; 15: 815-819

[11] Zimmet P, Alberti KG, Shaw J. Global and societal implications of the diabetes epidemic. Nature. 2001; 414: 782-787

[12] Ruigomez A and Garcia Rodriguez LA. Presence of diabetes related complication at the time of NIDDM diagnosis: An important factor. European Journal of Epidemiology 1998; 14:439-445

[13] UK Prospective Diabetes Study Group, UK prospective diabetes study 6. Complications in newly diagnosed type 2 diabetic patients association with different clinical and biochemical risk factors. Diabetes Res 1990;13:1-11

[14] Tuomilehto J, Lindstrom J, Eriksson JG, Valle TT, Hamallainen H, Ilanne-Pariikka, et al. The Finnish Diabetes Prevention Study Group: Prevention of type 2 diabetes mellitus by changes in lifestyle among subjects with impaired glucose tolerance. N. Engl. J Med 2001; 344: 1343-1350

[15] The Prevention or Delay of Type 2 Diabetes. American Diabetes Association National Institute of Diabetes, Digestive and Kidney Diseases. Diabetes Care 2003;26: S62-S69

[16] Knowler WC, Barrett-Conner E, Fowler SE, Hammon RF, Lachin JM, Walker EA and Nathan DM. The Diabetes Prevention Program Research Group: Reduction in the incidence of type 2 diabetes with lifestyle intervention or metformin. N Engl J Med 2002; 346: 393-403

[17] World Health Organization. Principles of Screening (draft). Geneva: World Health Organization, 2001

[18] Screening for Type 2 Diabetes. Report of a World Health Organization

and International Diabetes Federation meeting. WHO/NMH/MNC/03.1 Original: English. World Health Organization Department of Noncommunicable Disease Management Geneva. © World Health Organization 2003

[19] UK Prospective Diabetes Study (UKPDS) Group. The UK Prospective Diabetes Study 30. Diabetes retinopathy at diagnosis of non-insulin-dependent diabetes mellitus and associated risk factors. Archives of Ophthalmology 1998; 116:670-677

[20] King H, Aubert RE, Herman WH. Global Burden of diabetes, 1995-2025. Diabetes Care 1998; 21: 1414-1431

[21] Ohkubo Y, Kishikawa H, Araki E, Miyyata T, Isami S, Motoyoshi S, et al. Intensive insulin therapy prevents the progression of diabetic microvascular complications in Japanese patients with non-insulin-dependent diabetes mellitus: a randomized prospective 6-year study. Diabetes Research and Clinical Practice 1995; 28: 103-117

[22] UKPDS Group. Intensive blood glucose control with sulphonylureas or insulin compared with conventional treatment and risk of complications in patients with type 2 diabetes (UKPDS 33).Lancet 1998; 352: 837-853

[23] UK Prospective Diabetes Study Group. Tight blood pressure control and risk of macrovascular complications in type 2 diabetes: UKPDS 38. BMJ 1998; 317: 703-713

[24] Englelgau MM, Narayan VKM, Herman WH. Screening for Type 2 diabetes. Diabetes Care 2000; 23: 1563-1580

[25] Sacks DB. Carbohydrates. In: Burtis CA, Ashwood ER, eds. Tietz Textbook of Clinical Chemistry. 3rd ed. Philadelphia: WB Saunders 1999: 750-785

[26] Tietz NW, ed. Clinical Guide to Laboratory Tests, 4th ed. Philadelphia. WB Saunders Company, 2006: 444-451

[27] Milller WG, Myers GL, Ashwood ER, Killeen AA, Wang E, Ehlers GW, et al. State of the art in trueness and Interlaboratory harmonization for 10 analytes in general clinical chemistry. Arch Pathol Lab Med 2008; 132: 838-846

[28] David BS, David EB, David EGG, Noel KM, Jay MM, Marian P. Guidelines and Recommendations for Laboratory Analysis in the Diagnosis and Management of Diabetes Mellitus. Clinical Chemistry 2002; 48: 3436-3472

[29] Bonetti G, Cancelli V, Coccoli G, et al. Which sample tube should be used for routine glucose determination? Prim Care Diabetes 2016; 10: 227-232

[30] Norman M, Jones I. The shift from fluoride/Oxalate to acid citrate/fluoride blood collection tubes for glucose testing-the impact upon patient results. Clin Biochem 2014; 47: 683-685

[31] Chan AYW, Swaminathan R, Cockram CS. Effectiveness of sodium fluoride as a preservative of glucose in blood. Clin Chem 1989; 35:315-315

[32] Ladenson JH, Non-analytical sources of variation in clinical chemistry results. In: Sonnenwirth A, Jarett L, eds Clinical Laboratory methods and diagnosis. St. Louis, MO: CV Mosby 1980: 149-192

[33] Sack DB, Arnold M, Bakris GL, et al. National Academy of Clinical Biochemistry. Position Statement executive summary: guideline and recommendations for laboratory analysis in the diagnosis and management of diabetes mellitus. Diabetes Care 2011; 34: 1419-1423

[34] Sacks DB, Arnold M, Bakris GL, Bruns DE, Korvath AR, Kirkman MS, et al. Guidelines and Recommendations for

Laboratory Analysis in the Diagnosis and management of Diabetes Mellitus. Clinical Chemistry 2011; 57(6): E1-E47

[35] Strict Preanalytical Oral Glucose Tolerance Test Blood Sample Handling Is Essential for Diagnosing Gestational Diabetes Mellitus. Diabetes Care 2020; 43: 1438-1441

[36] Daly N, Flunn I, Carroll C, Farren M, McKeating A, Turner MJ. Impact of implementing preanalytical laboratory standards on the diagnosis of gestational diabetes mellitus: a prospective observational study. Clin Chem 2016; 62: 387-391

[37] Jamieson EL, Spry EP, Kirke AB, Atkinson DN, Marley JV. Real-world gestational diabetes screening: problems with the oral glucose tolerance test in rural and remote Australia. Int J Environ Res Public Health 2019; 16: E4488

[38] Metzger BE, Lowe LP, Dyer AR, et al. HAPO Study Cooperative Research Group. Hyperglycaemia and adverse pregnancy outcome. N Engl J Med 2008; 358: 1991-2002

[39] Fodh-Anderson N, Wimberley PD, Thode J, Siggaard-Andersen O. Direct reading glucose electrodes detect the molality of glucose in plasma and whole blood. Clin Chem Acta 1990; 189:33-38

[40] Ladenson JH, Tsai LM, Michael JM, Kessler G, Joist JH. Serum versus heparinized plasma for eighteen common chemistry tests: is serum the appropriate specimen? Am J Clin Pathol 1974; 62: 545-552

[41] Larsson-Cohn U. Differences between capillary and venous blood glucose during oral glucose tolerance tests. Scand J Clin Lab Invest 19976;36: 805-808

[42] The Expert Committee on the Diagnosis and classification of Diabetes Mellitus: Report of the expert committee on the diagnosis and classification of diabetes mellitus. Diabetes Care 1997; 20: 1183-1197

[43] World Health Organization: Definition, Diagnosis and Classification of Diabetes Mellitus and its Complications: Report of a WHO Consultation, Part 1: Diagnosis and Classification of Diabetes Mellitus. Geneva, World Health Org., 1999

[44] The Expert Committee on the Diagnosis and Classification of Diabetes Mellitus. Follow-up Report on the Diagnosis of Diabetes Mellitus. Diabetes Care 2003; 26:3160-3167

[45] John LP, Darren KM. Impaired glucose tolerance and impaired fasting glucose-a review of diagnosis, clinical implications and management. Diabetes Vasc Dis Res 2005; 2: 9-15

[46] Abdul-Ghani MA, Tripathy D, DeFronzo RA: Contributions of β-cell dysfunction and insulin resistance to the pathogenesis of impaired glucose tolerance and impaired fasting glucose. Diabetes Care 2006; 29: 1130-1139

[47] David MN, Mayer BD, Ralph AD, Robert JH, Robert RH, Richard P, Bernard Z. Impaired fasting glucose and impaired glucose tolerance: implications for care. Diabetes Care 2007; 30:

[48] CDC: National Diabetes Fact Sheet, 2005

[49] Qiao Q, Nakagami T, Tuomilehto J, Borch-Johnsen K, Balkau B, Iwamoto Y, Tajima N. International Diabetes Epidemiology Group, DECODA Study Group on behalf of the International Diabetes Epidemiology Group: Comparison of the fasting and the 2-h glucose criteria for diabetes in different Asian cohorts. Diabetologia 2000; 43: 1470-1475

[50] Shaw JE, Zimmet PZ, de Courten M, Dowse GK, Chitson P, Gareeboo H,

Hemraj F, Fareed D, Tuomilehto J, Alberti KG.. Impaired fasting glucose or impaired glucose tolerance: what best predicts future diabetes in Mauritius? Diabetes Care 1999; 22: 399-402

[51] Gabir MM, Hanson RL, Dabetea D, Imperatore G, Roumain J, Bennett PH, Knowler WC: The 1997 American Diabetes Association and 1999 World Health Organization criteria for hyperglycaemia in the diagnosis and prediction of diabetes. Diabetes Care 2000; 23: 1108-1112

[52] Ko GT, Chan JC, Woo J, Lau E, Yeung VT, Chow CC, et al. The reproducibility and usefulness of the oral glucose test in screening for diabetes and other cardiovascular risk factors. Ann Clin Biochem 1998; 35: 62-67

[53] Qiao Q, Pyorala K, Pyorala M, Nissinen A, Lindstrom J, Tilvis R, Tuomilehto J. Two-hour glucose is a better risk predictor for incident coronary heart disease and cardiovascular mortality than fasting glucose. European Heart Journal 2002; 23: 1267-1275

[54] Rebecca MI, Catherine CC, Maureen IH. Diurnal Variation in Fasting Plasma Glucose: Implications for Diagnosis of Diabetes in Patients Examined in the Afternoon. JAMA 2000; 284:3157-3159

[55] Modan M, Harris MI. Fasting plasma glucose in screening for NIDDM in the US and Israel. Diabetes Care 1994; 17: 436-439

[56] DECODE Study Group. Will new diagnostic criteria for diabetes mellitus change phenotype of patients with diabetes? Reanalysis of European Epidemiological Data. BMJ 1998; 317: 371-375

[57] Barrett-Connor E, Ferrara A. Isolated post challenge hyperglycaemia and the risk of fatal cardiovascular disease in older women and men: The Rancho Bernardo Study. Diabetes Care 1998; 21: 1236-1239

[58] Perry RC, Shankar RR, Fineberg N, McGill J, Baron AD. HbA1c Measurement Improves the Detection of Type 2 Diabetes in High-Risk Individuals with Nondiagnostic Levels of Fasting Plasma Glucose. The Early Diabetes Intervention Program (EDIP). Diabetes Care 2001; 24: 465-471

[59] Bartnik M, Ryden L, Malmberg K, Ohrvik J, Pyorala K, Standl E, Ferrari R, Simoons M, Soler-Soler J. Oral glucose tolerance test is needed for appropriate classification of glucose regulation in patients with coronary artery disease: a report from the Euro Heart Survey on Diabetes and the Heart. Heart 2007; 993: 72-77

[60] Unwin N, Shaw J, Zimmet P, Albert KGMM. Impaired glucose tolerance and impaired fasting glycaemia: the current status on definition and intervention: Writing committee. © 2002 Diabetes UK. Diabetes Medicine 2002; 19: 708-723

[61] Gimero SGA, Ferreira SRG, Franco LJ, Iunes M. The Japanese-Brazilian Diabetes Study Group: Comparison of glucose tolerance categories according to World Health Organization and American Diabetes Association diagnostic criteria in a population-based study in Brazil. Diabetes Care 1998; 21: 1889-1892

[62] Stolk RP, Orchard TJ, Grobbee DE. Why Use The Oral Glucose Tolerance Test? Diabetes Care 1995; 18:1045-1049

[63] Abdul-Ghani MA, Lyssenko V, Tuomi T, Defronzo RA, Groop L. The shape of plasma glucose concentration curve during OGTT predicts future risk of type 2 diabetes. Diabetes Metab Res Rev 2010; 26: 280-286

[64] McIntyre N. Oral glucose tolerance: the role of the liver and small intestine. M.D. Thesis, University of London 1967

[65] Baird JD, Duncan LJP. The glucose tolerance test. Postgrad. Med J 1959; 35: 308-314

[66] Kanedo T, Wang PY, Tawata M, Sato A. Low carbohydrate intake before oral glucose tolerance tests. Lancet 1998; 352: 289

[67] World Health Organization. Definition, diagnosis and classification of diabetes mellitus and its complication. Part 1: Diagnosis and Classification of Diabetes Mellitus. Geneva: World Health Organization, 1999

[68] George K, Alberti MM. Impaired glucose tolerance: what are the clinical implications? Diabetes Res Clin Pract 1998; 40: S3-S8

[69] De Vegt F, Dekker JM, Stehouwer CDA, Nijpels G, Bouter LM, Heine RJ. The 1997 American Diabetes Association criteria versus the 1985 World Health Organization criteria for the diagnosis of abnormal glucose tolerance: poor agreement in the Hoom Study. Diabetes Care 1998; 21: 1686-1690

[70] Fornengo P, Bruno A, Grassi G, Vineis P, Pagano G. Concordance between American Diabetes Association and World Health Organization criteria in a northwestern Italian population (Letter). Diabetes Care 1999; 22: 652-653

[71] Sainaghi PP, Castello L Limoncini AM, Bergamasco L, Bartoli E, Schianca GPC. Poor specificity of fasting plasma glucose cut-off values in ruling out glucose intolerance: the complementary usefulness of OGTT. Exp Clin Endocrinol Diab 2007; 115: 112-117

[72] Carson AP, Reynolds K, Fonseca VA, Muntner. Comparison of A1c and fasting glucose criteria to diagnosis diabetes among US adults. Diabetes Care 2010; 33: 95-97

[73] Lorenzo C, Wagenknecht LE, Hanley AJG, Rewers MJ, Karter AJ, Haffner SM. A1c between 5.7 and 6.4% as a marker for identifying pre-diabetes, insulin sensitivity and secretion, and cardiovascular risk factors: the Insulin Resistance Atherosclerosis Study(IRAS). Diabetes Care 2010; 33: 2104-2109

[74] Tuomilehto J, Lindstrom J, Eriksson JG, Valle TT, Hamalainen H, Ilanne-Parikka P, et al. Prevention of type 2 diabetes mellitus by changes in lifestyle among subjects with impaired glucose tolerance. N Engl J Med 2001; 344: 1343-1350

[75] Perreaolt L, Kahn SE, Cristophi CA, Knowler WC, Hamman RF. Regression from prediabetes to normal glucose regulation in the diabetes prevention program. Diabetes Care 2009; 32: 1583-1588

[76] Bartoli E, Fra GP, Carnevale GP, Schianca. The oral glucose tolerance test (OGTT) revisited. European Journal of Internal Medicine 2011; 22: 8-12

[77] Sievenpiper JL, Jenkins DJA, Josse RG, Vuksan V. Dilution of the 75-g oral glucose tolerance test increases postprandial glycaemia: implications for diagnostic criteria. CMAJ 2000; 162(7): 993-996

[78] Yanling Wu, Ding Y, Tanaka Y, Zhang W. Risk Factors Contributing to Type 2 Diabetes and Recent Advances in the Treatment and Prevention. Int J Med Sci 2014; 11(11): 1185-1200

[79] Holdsworth CD. The gut and oral glucose tolerance. Gut 1969; 10: 422-427

[80] Kim MS, Jo DS, Lee D-Y. Comparison of HbA1c and OGTT for the diagnosis of type 2 diabetes in

children at risk of diabetes. Pediatrics and Neonatology 2019; 60: 428-434

[81] Barbour LA, McCurdy CE, Hernandez TL, Kirwan JP, Catalano PM, Friedman JE. Cellular Mechanisms for Insulin Resistance in Normal Pregnancy and Gestational Diabetes. Diabetes Care 2007;30:

[82] Hernandez TL, Friedman JE, Van Pelt RE, Barbour LA. Patterns of glycaemia in normal pregnancy: should the current therapeutic targets be challenged?. Diabetes Care 2011; 34: 1660-1668

[83] Kampmann U, Knorr S, Fuglsang J, Ovesen P. Determinations of Maternal Insulin Resistance during Pregnancy: An Updated Overview. J Diabetes Res 2019; Article ID 5320156,9

[84] Barbour L, Shao J, Qiao L, Pulawa L, Jensen D, Bartke A, et al Human placental growth hormone causes severe IR in transgenic mice. Am J Obstet Gynecol 2002; 186: 512-517

[85] Stanley JL, Baker PN, Reynolds CM, Vickers MH. The Pathophysiology of Gestation Diabetes Mellitus. J Mol Sci 2018; 19: 3342; doi:10.3390/ijms 19113342

[86] Kirwan J, De Mouzon S, Lepercq J, Challier J, Presley L, Friedman J, et al. TNF-α is a Predictor of IR in Human Pregnancy. Diabetes 2002; 51: 2207-2213

[87] World Health Organization. Diagnostic criteria and classification of hyperglycaemia first detected in pregnancy: a World Health Organization Guideline. Diabetes Res and Clin Pract 2014; 103: 341-363

[88] International Diabetes Federation. IDF Diabetes Atlas, 8th ed; IDF: Brussels, Belgium, 2017

[89] Macaulay S, Dunger DB, Norris SA. Gestational diabetes mellitus in Africa: review. PLoS One 2014; 9: e978871

[90] Kios SL, Buchanan TA, Greenspoon JS, et al. Gestational diabetes mellitus: the prevalence of glucose tolerance and diabetes mellitus in the first two months postpartum. Am J Obstet Gynecol 1990; 33: 562-568

[91] Dacus JV, Meyer NL, Muram D, et al. Gestational diabetes: postpartum glucose tolerance test. Am J Obstet Gynecol 1994; 171: 927-931

[92] Emancipator K. Laboratory Diagnosis and Monitoring of Diabetes Mellitus. Am J Clin Pathol 1999; 112: 665-674

[93] Crowther CA, Hiller JE, Moss JR, McPhee AJ, Jeffries WS, Robinson JS. The effect of gestational diabetes mellitus on pregnancy outcomes. N Engl J Med 2005; 352: 2477-2486

[94] Virjee S, Robinson S, Johnson DG. Screening for diabetes in Pregnancy. JR Soc Med 2001; 94: 502-509

[95] Howard B, Toronto ON JC, St. John"s DF, Toronto ON. Screening for Gestational Diabetes Mellitus. J Obstet Gynaecol Can 2002;24(11): 894-903

[96] Chang Y, Mathew S, Philip WC, Anthony JH, Bernard Z, Ravi R. Obstetrics Predictors and Clinical Implications of a False Negative Glucose Challenge Test in Pregnancy. J Obstet Gynaecol Can 2013; 35: 889-898

[97] Bonomo M, Gandini ML, Mastropasqua A, et al. Which cutoff level should be used in screening for glucose intolerance in pregnancy? Am J Obstet Gynecol 1998; 179: 179-185

[98] Lili Y, Sara B, Vincent WW, Hamish R. Hypoglycaemia on an oral glucose tolerance test in pregnancy-Is it clinically significant? Diabetes Research and Clinical Practice 2019; 147: 111-117

[99] © 1996 Willey-Liss, Inc. Gravidas with a very high 50-g screen are at

significant risk of requiring insulin to maintain euglycaemia during pregnancy

[100] Rani PR, Begum J. Screening and Diagnosis of Gestational Diabetes Mellitus, Where Do We Stand? J Clin and Diagnostic Res 2016; 10(4): QE01-QE04.1-4

[101] Stovall DW, Bailey AP, Pastore LM. Assessment of Insulin Resistance and Impaired Glucose Tolerance in Lean Women with Polycystic Ovary Syndrome. J Women's Health 2011; 20 (1): 37-43

[102] Salley KE, Wickham EP, Cheang KL, et al. Glucose intolerance in polycystic ovary syndrome-A position statement of the Androgen Excess Society. J Clin Endocrinol Metab 2007; 92: 4556-4556

[103] O'Sullivan JB, Mahan CM. Criteria for the oral glucose tolerance test in pregnancy. Diabetes 1964; 13: 278-285

[104] O'Sullivan JB, Mahan CM, Charles D, et al. Screening criteria for high-risk gestational diabetic patients Am J Obstet Gynecol 1973; 116: 895-900

[105] Classification and diagnosis of diabetes mellitus and other categories of glucose intolerance. National Diabetes Data Group. Diabetes 1979; 28: 1039-1057

[106] American Diabetes Association. Gestational diabetes mellitus. Diabetes Care 2000; 23(1): S77-S79

[107] Liao L-z, Xu Y, Zhuang X-D, Hong S-b, Wang Z-l, Dobs AS, Liu B. Evaluation of guidelines on the screening and diagnosis of gestational diabetes mellitus: systemic review. BMJ Open 2019; 9: e023014. Doi:10.1136/bmjopen-2018-023014

[108] Metzger BE, Gabbe SG, Persson B, et all. International association of diabetes and pregnancy study groups recommendations on the diagnosis and classification of hyperglycaemia in pregnancy. Diabetes Care 2010; 33: e98-82.

[109] American Diabetes Association. Diagnosis and classification of diabetes mellitus. Diabetes Care 2011; 34(1): S62-S69

[110] WHO Guidelines Approved by the Guidelines Review Committee. Diagnostic criteria and classification of hyperglycaemia first detected in pregnancy. Geneva, 2013

[111] Hod M, Kapur A, Sacks DA, et al. The International Federation of Gynecology and Obstetrics(FIGO) Initiative on gestational diabetes mellitus: A pragmatic guide for diagnosis, management, and care. Int J Gynaecol Obstet 2015; 131(3): S173-S211

[112] Committee on Practice Bulletins-Obstetrics. Practice Bullcin No. 137: Gestational diabetes mellitus. Obstet Gynecol 2013; 122(2Pt1): 406-416

[113] National Institute of Health consensus development conference statement: diagnosing gestational diabetes mellitus. 2013; 122(2Pt 1): 358-369

[114] Berger H, Gagnon R, Sermer M, et al. Diabetes in pregnancy. J Obstet Gynaecol Can 2016; 38: 667-679

[115] Roberts WL, Safa-Pour S, De BK, Rohlfing CL, Weykamp CW, Little RR. Effects of hemoglobin C and S traits on glycohemoglobin measurements by eleven methods. Clin Chem 2005; 51: 776-778

[116] Pani LN, Korenda L, Meigs JB, Driver C, Chamany S, Fox CS, Sullivan LD, Agostino RB, Nathan DB. Effects of aging on A1c levels in individuals without diabetes. Diabetes Care 2008; 31: 1991-1006

[117] Herman WH, Ma Y, Uwaifo G, Haffner S, Kahn SE, Horton ES, Lachin JM, Montez MG, Brennman T, Barrett-Conner E. The Diabetes Prevention Program Research Group. Differences in A1c by race and ethnicity among patients with impaired glucose tolerance in the Diabetes Prevention Program. Diabetes care 2007;30:2756-2758

[118] Van't Riet E, Marjan Alssema M, Rijkelijkhuizen JM, Kostense PJ, Nijpels G, Dekker JM. Relationship between A1c and glucose levels in the general Dutch population: the new Hoorn study.. Diabetes Care 2010; 33:61-66

[119] Kramer CK, Araneta MRG, Barrett-Connor E. A1c and diabetes diagnosis: The Rancho Bernado Study. Diab Care 2010; 33: 101-103

[120] Padala RK, Anil B, Nuthuswamy R, Shobhit B, Pinaki D, Thakur JS, Naresh S, Sanjay KB, Rama Walia. Utili of Glycated Hemoglobin in Diagnosing Type 2 Diabetes Mellitus: A Community-Based Study. Endocrine Care. J Clin Endocrinol Metab 2010; 95: 2832-2835

Chapter 6

# Organic Volatile Compounds Used in Type 2 Diabetes

*Mioara Petrus, Cristina Popa and Ana-Maria Bratu*

## Abstract

Analysis of volatile organic compounds (VOCs) in exhaled breath is non-invasive method and appears as a promising tool for metabolic monitoring. Diabetes is a complex syndrome, metabolic diseases that is characterized by hyperglycemia associated with major changes in lipids and proteins. The pathophysiology of the link between diabetes, hypertension, inflammatory syndrome and oxidative stress is complex. We conducted a study and applied quantitative analysis of exhaled ethylene and ammonia in patients with type 2 diabetes mellitus (T2DM) and a healthy control group. For breath gas analysis, a very sensitive $CO_2$ laser photoacoustic spectroscopy ($CO_2$LPAS) was applied. The concentration of exhaled VOCs differed between T2DM patients and healthy group, in particular, T2DM patients exhaled significantly higher amounts of ethylene and ammonia compared to healthy control group. The data obtained by the $CO_2$LPAS system revealing that the increased breath VOCs has a close relationship with high glucose levels and with healthy complications.

**Keywords:** type 2 diabetes, exhaled breath, volatile organic compounds, ethylene, ammonia, $CO_2$ laser photoacoustic spectroscopy

## 1. Introduction

The analysis of volatile organic compounds (VOCs) represents a rapid and non-invasive method of early diagnosis. Some of the detected VOCs can be used as biomarkers for certain diseases or can reflect the metabolic profile of an organism and are presented in the exhaled breath, skin secretions, saliva, blood, urine and feces [1]. Breath analysis is considered to be a promising tool for noninvasive analysis of biochemical processes in the human body [2–5]. Exhaled breath contains both exogenous VOCs that come from environmental exposures as the ingestion of food, smoking cigarettes or/and air pollution, or endogenous VOCs that are produced by biological processes in the human body like oxidative stress (OS), inflammation, infectious disease. Breath analysis is currently used in the diagnosis of different pathologies, including gastrointestinal and liver disease, renal failure, lung disorders, cancer, and diabetes [6–8].

Diabetes Mellitus (DM) affects millions of people worldwide, and the incidence is increasing every year. Diabetes is a chronic condition characterized by hyperglycemia caused by a defect in insulin secretion or insulin action. Diabetes is a heterogeneous syndrome, characterized by a complex disorder in the regulation of the body's energy metabolism, which affects the use of carbohydrates, lipids and proteins, as well as other metabolisms [1–3]. The most prevalent type of DM is:

type 2 diabetes mellitus (T2DM), type 1 diabetes mellitus (T1DM) and gestational diabetes mellitus (GDM). According to International Diabetes Federation (IDF) 1 of 11 adults (20–79 years) have diabetes (463 million people), 1 in 2 adults with diabetes are undiagnosed (232 million people) and 2 in 3 people with diabetes lives in urban areas (310.3 million) [9, 10].

Individuals with T2DM presents increased risk for microvascular and macrovascular complications due to hyperglycemia. The complications related to diabetes are: eye disease (diabetic retinopathy), cardiovascular disease (one-third do half of all are diabetes related deaths), kidney disease, oral, nerve and/or vascular damage and diabetic foot complications (diabetic foot and lower limb complications affect between 40 and 60 million people with diabetes globally), diabetes-related complications of pregnancy (approximately 20.4 million of live births were affected by hyperglycemia in pregnancy in 2019) [9–14].

Studies over time have shown that oxidative stress contributes to the development and progression of diabetes, in T2DM particularly [15]. In diabetics, through hyperglycemia, hyperlipidemia, and hypertension is induced oxidative stress that affects multiple organs, leading to various complications including coronary artery disease, stroke, neuropathy, nephropathy, retinopathy [16, 17].

The aim of this chapter is showing the role of breath analysis in the evolution of type 2 diabetes mellitus by measuring ethylene and ammonia as oxidative stress breath biomarkers at T2DM and healthy subjects, using a $CO_2$ laser photoacoustic spectroscopy ($CO_2$LPAS) system. At the same time, it was determined the glycated hemoglobin HbA1c and blood glucose levels. Breath tests were compared between the two groups (healthy and with T2DM) to see if the breath analysis can discriminate between diabetic and healthy subjects, and if the breath tests are in accordance with blood tests.

## 2. Oxidative stress in diabetes mellitus

When the human's cells are perturbed by nutritional imbalance, infections, bacteria, toxins or disease reactive oxygen species (ROS) and reactive nitrogen species (RNS) are formed. ROS molecules are highly reactive and, the pathological consequence is damage to proteins, lipids and DNA [18, 19]. This oxidative damage may lead cell death and disease such as cancer or diabetes. Thus, oxidative stress may fi define as an imbalance between production of such reactive species and the body's ability to detoxify.

Diabetic subjects tend to have an increase in ROS generation and a decrease in antioxidant defenses [18–24], in this case oxidative stress is a response to glucose and/or lipid overload. Thus, oxidative stress is involved in the occurrence of complications in subjects with T2DM [20–24], and also affect the two major mechanisms failing during diabetes: insulin resistance and insulin secretion [25–28].

According to Giugliano et al. patients with diabetes present a high level of oxidative stress leads to the appearance of atherosclerosis [29]. Also, according to Ceriello, hyperglycemia generates oxidative stress, which leads to endothelial dysfunction in blood vessels [30]. Atherosclerotic disease is the most important and frequent macrovascular complication in diabetics and it means the chronic inflammation and injury to the arterial. Oxidized lipids accumulate in the endothelial wall of the arteries, and this accumulation can lead to acute vascular infarction [20].

The link between diabetes and oxidative stress was conducted by measuring certain biomarkers such as lipid peroxidation products, biomarker for protein oxidation or DNA damage biomarker. These biomarkers are the result of free radical's damage on lipids, proteins and DNA [18–20].

Responsible for oxidative stress is the attack on proteins induce by the reaction between ROS and some amino acids [24]. Proteins are the principal target of ROS causing protein glycation and oxidative degeneration. Therefore, glycated hemoglobin HbA1c measure the protein alteration and is considered as biomarker of oxidative stress [31]. Ammonia is a biomarker of protein metabolism, and at subjects with T2DM, insulin deprivation is associated with an increase in amino acids and by an accelerated protein catabolism.

In diabetes the lipid profile is modified thus leading to the occurrence of lipid peroxidation. Another target of free radicals are the polyunsaturated fatty acids in cell membranes [32]. The end-products of LP that can be used to measure the effects of free radicals on lipids are malondialdehyde (MDA) measured in blood and ethylene as breath biomarker [33].

## 3. VOCs biomarkers in exhaled breath

### 3.1 Overview of breath analysis

Breath analysis can be considered as a potentially tool for the diagnosis and study of medical diseases. Respiratory analysis has been used in medicine since ancient times, from the time of Hippocrates (460–370 BC), when ancient Greek doctors assessing human health using human breath aroma [34–39]. The first breath analysis was conducted by Lavoisier in 1782, this showing that carbon dioxide from breathing is a product of combustion produced in the body [2, 38–40]. Respiratory studies continued later, when it was shown that human respiration contains VOCs, important in assessing human health [3–5]. The first invention that use gaseous compounds exhaled breath to assess human health was made in 1931 by Dr. Rolla N. Harger. He invented the 'drunkometer a breath-alcohol test, used to determine the alcohol concentration and has been widely used since 1938. An important step in breath analysis was conducted by Pauling et al. in 1971 when using a gas chromatograph were able to detect more than 200 VOCs in human breath [40]. Many studies on exhaled breath have been carried aiming to characterize these VOCs, and the studies carried out of Phillips estimated 1259 compounds in normal subjects in 1997 [41], and over 3000 compounds in 1999 [42]. The analysis of exhaled air is under investigation as a promising tool for express and noninvasive analysis of biochemical processes in the human body. The techniques currently used are promising to translate into clinics not for a specific disease diagnostic but more for providing information about biochemical processes that arise from underlying diseases. Nowadays, there are several commercially available devices for monitoring of breath biomarkers, such as $^{13}C$ used to diagnose Helicobacter pylori [43], $CH_4$ in breath accompanied by electrochemical sensors to detect $H_2$ and $O_2$ for diagnosis of gastrointestinal disorders [44], asthma detection by exhaled nitric oxide, breath alcohol testing [45], lung cancer detection [46], fructose malabsorption with hydrogen breath test, monitoring uptake of disinfection by-products following swimming [47] chronic kidney disease (CKD) and diabetes mellitus [48].

### 3.2 Exhaled breath

Human respiration is a gaseous mixture, and the main compounds are nitrogen, oxygen, carbon dioxide, inert gases, water vapor. In addition to these compounds that are found in high concentration in respiration, VOCs and inorganic molecules can also be found [49]. The presence of the latter in the composition of respiration depends on several external or internal factors. Thus, the composition of human respiration is influenced both by exogenous compounds from exposure of the human body to various external environmental factors, and from endogenous compounds resulting from biological processes produced in the human body (in the lung tract, blood or peripheral tissues) [50].

Humans breath is a mixture of nitrogen, oxygen, carbon dioxide, inert gases, water vapor and thousands of VOCs traces and inorganic molecules [49]. The composition of breath contains exogenous compounds that originate from environmental exposures, and endogenous compounds that are produced by biological processes in the human body (in the pulmonary tract, blood, or peripheral tissues) [50]. The complex matrix of breath varies from each person both quantitatively and qualitatively. The development of different methods for gas samples analysis has allowed the detection of gaseous compounds traces from respiration, and research has shown that the most common VOCs in human respiration are nitric oxide (10–50 ppb), 1–20 ppb), ammonia (0, 5–2 ppm), carbon monoxide (0–6 ppm), hydrogen sulfide (0–1.3 ppm), acetone (0.3–1 ppm), methane (2–10 ppm), pentane (0–10 ppb) etc. [51–56].

### 3.3 Breath biomarkers

Biomarkers are chemicals, usually VOCs, which indicate the normal or abnormal process that take place in the human body and can suggest the presence of a disease or a recent exposure to a drug or an environmental pollutant. The most important breath biomarkers are ammonia, acetone, isoprene, nitic oxide, hydrogen sulphide, methane, ethane and pentane [30–42, 51–58].

#### *3.3.1 Ammonia*

Ammonia ($NH_3$) is very important for the human body and is involved in many physiological processes. The ammonia originates from the catabolism of the amino acids (which are produced mainly by degradation of proteins), can penetrate the blood-lungs and appears in the exhaled breath. Ammonia is absorbed into the portal circulation, taken up by the liver and converted to urea by the urea cycle. Urea cycle is the metabolic pathway that converts urea nitrogen excretion from the body.

Ammonia ($NH_3$) is highly toxic to humans, it is converted into urea which is non-toxic, highly soluble and easily excreted by the kidney. Urea is formed in the urea cycle from $NH_4^+$, $CO_2$, and the nitrogen of aspartate [59, 60]. The cycle occurs mainly in the liver. Ammonia travels to the liver from other tissues, mainly in the form of alanine and glutamine and is released from amino acids in the liver by a series of transamination and deamination reactions. Urea cycle enzyme deficiency will result in insufficient elimination of $NH_4^+$ or hyperammonemia which leads to central nervous system deterioration in the form of mental retardation, seizure, coma, and death [60]. The deamination of amino acids, transamination of most amino acids with $\alpha$-ketoglutaric acid to form glutamic acids, and operation of glutaminase enzyme in the kidney represent the main source of ammonia in the human body. In addition to these sources of ammonia, this can be produced during purine and pyrimidine catabolism, by the action of intestinal bacteria on the non-absorbed dietary amino acids, or by the action of monoamine oxidase enzyme. Therefore, ammonia can be considered to be an important biomarker monitored in the blood, urine, saliva or breath [57–65]. The ammonia concentration is dependent on a range of factors including the health status of the patient, the route of sampling (nasal or oral), contribution from oral bacteria, diet, pharmaceutical use, physical activity and levels of metabolic activity. High levels of ammonia are associated with a variety of pathological conditions, such as hepatic and renal dysfunction, Reye's syndrome, errors in the metabolism of urea cycle (urea cycle disorders, UCD) and is also a potential biomarker in exercise physiology and studies of drug metabolism. Normal concentration of ammonia in exhaled breath is 50–2000 ppb (parts per billion) [61–66].

### *3.3.2 Ethylene*

Ethylene ($C_2H_4$) is produced by the oxidation of cellular lipids [67, 68]. The relation among ethylene, free radicals, and diabetes can be explained by the oxidative stress. The free radicals attack cellular biomembranes causing cell damage and even cell death [69, 70]. A free radical is an unstable and highly reactive molecular species with an unpaired electron that can donate or accept an electron from other molecules [71, 72].

There are many types of radicals, but the species highly unstable and concern in biological systems are derived from oxygen and known as reactive oxygen species (ROS), such as superoxide radicals, $O_2^{\cdot}$-, hydrogen peroxide, $H_2O_2$, and hydroxyl radicals, $HO^{\cdot}$ [70–72]. Under stress, ROS levels increase and this can lead to significant cell damage, damage known as oxidative stress. The term "oxidative stress" (OS) is defined as the imbalance between the production of free radicals and the body's ability to defend itself [18, 19]. This process is kept in balance by the antioxidant defense system. Certain chronic diseases such as atherosclerosis, cancer, diabetes, rheumatoid arthritis, post-ischemic perfusion injury, myocardial infarction, cardiovascular disease, chronic inflammation, stroke and septic shock, aging and other degenerative diseases in humans can be caused or their process it can be accelerated by the appearance of oxidative lesions at the biomolecular level in (lipids, proteins or DNA) when there is an imbalance in the production of free radicals [18, 19, 69–72]

The human body contains a high percentage of lipids (including polyunsaturated fatty acids - PUFA) vulnerable to free radical attack. Lipid peroxidation (LP) occurs as a result of oxidative degradation of polyunsaturated fatty acids induced by free radicals. Therefore, in LP process a peroxidative sequence is initiated by the attack of any free radical species which can extract a hydrogen atom from the group of methylene ($CH_2$), together with an electron on the carbon atom (•CH). By molecular rearrangement the resulting carbon radical is stabilized and is produce a conjugated diene that formed a lipid peroxyl radical (LOO•). But, the propagation of LP continues because these radicals can still extract hydrogen atoms from other lipid molecules to form the lipid hydroperoxides (LOOH). The LP process is finished with the end products that includes malondialdehyde, 4-hidroxinonenal and hydrocarbons, such as pentane, ethane and ethylene [18, 19, 68–74]. The stable end-products of LP, such as ethane, ethylene and pentane are suitable for the estimation of cell damage, because these species are excreted in the breath within a few minutes of their formation in tissues. Excess ethylene in the exhaled breath is associated with biochemical events around LP and can be considered a direct measurement of oxidative stress [67–69, 74]. Ethylene was one of the first breath compounds studied, being reported to range between 3 and 100 ppb [75, 76].

## 4. Laser photoacoustic spectroscopy as a method for breath VOCs detection

The analysis of trace gases from human breath for medical monitoring and diagnostics and require gas sensors characterized by high sensitivity and selectivity (to avoid interference from other potential interfering species), multi-component capability, real time measurements, large dynamic range, in situ measurements, ease to use. Laser photoacoustic spectroscopy (LPAS) is sufficiently sensitive and rapid to allow the simultaneous analyses of several trace gas metabolites in single breath exhalations. Over the years, the LPAS technique has demonstrated its ability to detect traces of gas in fields such as biology and medicine due to several factors, such as: real-time detection of one or more volatile compounds, detection limits ranging from ppm (parts-per-million) to ppb (parts-per-billion), high sensitivity and selectivity, use of a single breath collection from a small sampling volume (few 100 ml) without the need for further preparation [66–68, 75–82].

### 4.1 Laser photoacoustic spectroscopy: basic principles

Laser photoacoustic spectroscopy is based on the photoacoustic effect that occurs at the interaction between light and matter with the generation of a sound wave. In 1880, Alexander Graham Bell discovered these phenomena [83] while trying to find wireless communication. Thus, he discovered that certain optically absorbing solids emit a sound when illuminated by a modulated light. In 1881, Bell [84] Tyndall [85], Röntgen [86] and Preece [87] have demonstrated that the photoacoustic (PA) effect occurs not only in solid but also in liquid and gas. They found also, that the sound was stronger when the sample was placed in a cavity called photophone or spectrophone. With the appearance of sensitive microphones, increased interest in this technique. Afterwards, techniques based on this phenomenon have been known a continuous development, and today can be applied in almost all disciplines of Science and Technology.

An instrument based on the PA effect and which uses a laser as a radiation source, has important advantages for the analysis of gas traces such as high sensitivity ppb or even ppt (parts per trillion) concentrations and selectivity, high dynamic range, high accuracy and precision, good time resolution, versatility, reliability, robustness and is easy to use.

Over the years, photoacoustic spectroscopy (PAS) has proven its ability to detect traces of gas and has been used successfully as a gas sensor in biological and medical applications [88–93].

In gases, the PA effect is produced as a result of the following sequences (see **Figure 1**) [76]: absorption of incident laser radiation modulated in frequency or amplitude by the target gas molecules; local heating due to non-radiative relaxation; the extension and contraction of the gas sample that determines the pressure variation, which is an acoustic wave; detection of acoustic waves using microphones.

### 4.2 Experimental section for VOCs breath analysis

Exhaled breath was analyzed using a LPAS system and we have measured ammonia and ethylene concentration from the exhaled breath in subjects with T2DM and healthy subjects [66, 75, 76]. The block diagram of the laser PA spectrometer is presented in **Figure 2**.

LPAS main components of the system are: a $CO_2$ laser (home-built) emitting in the 9.2–10.8 μm range (area where ammonia and ethylene shows a high

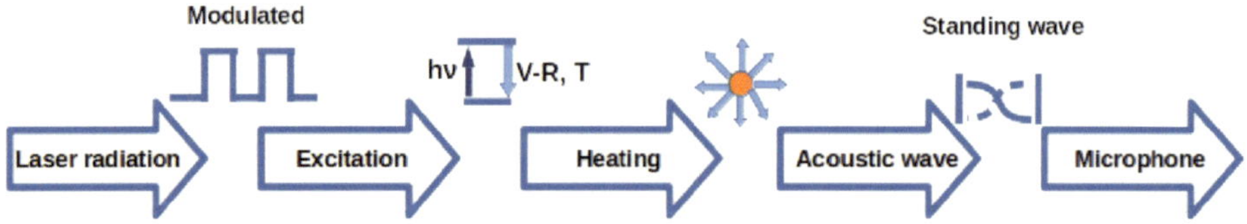


**Figure 1.**
*Schematic of the physical processes occurring in PAS [76].*

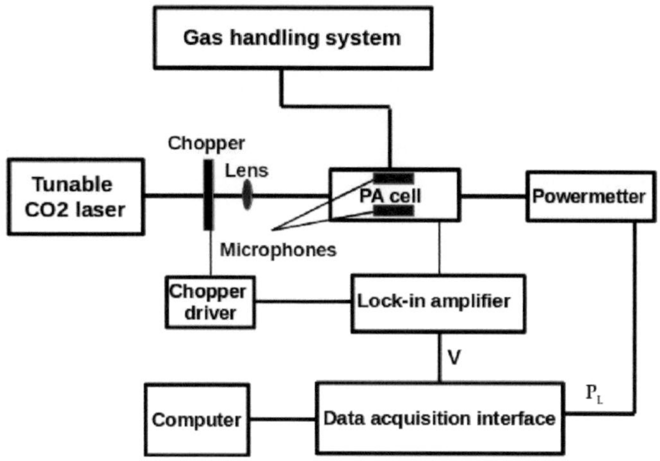


**Figure 2.**
*$CO_2$LPAS system.*

absorption), frequency-stabilized and an output power between 2 and 5 W, and an external PA cell (the external resonator home-build), inside it being mounted four microphones (sensitivity of 20 mV/Pa each), connected in series are mounted flush with the internal surface of the resonator tube. Before entering into the PA cell, the cw laser beam is modulated by a mechanical chopper that operate at the resonant frequency of the PA cell (564 Hz) and focused by a ZnSe lens. The laser beam power after passing through the PA cell is measured by a radiometer connected to a data acquisition interface module together with a lock-in amplifier. The acquisition interface is connected to a computer where all experimental data are processed in real-time and stored. The software allows the display of several parameters, such the values for the PA voltage, average laser power after chopper, and the trace gas concentration, and the response of the PA system is based on the formula:

$$V = \alpha C P_L S_M c.$$

Where:
$V$ (V)—photoacoustic signal (peak-to-peak value);
$\alpha$ ($cm^{-1}$ $atm^{-1}$)—gas absorption coefficient at a given wavelength;
$C$ (Pa cm $W^{-1}$)—cell constant;
$P_L$ (W)—cw laser power before chopper;
$S_M$ (V $Pa^{-1}$)— microphone responsivity;
$c$ (atm)—concentration or partial pressure of the trace gas.

Another important part of the $CO_2$LPAS system is represented by the gas handling system. It has the role to ensure the purity of the PA cell, to introduce the sample gas into the PA cell at a controlled flow rate, to pump out the sample gas from the PA cell, and to monitor the total and partial pressures of mixture gas sample. This several functions can be performed by the gas handling system without being necessary any disconnections.

### 4.3 Breath collection

In breath analysis, depending on the desired result, is required a knowledge and understanding of respiratory physics. In the individual, normal, resting breathing is about 0.5 L, breathing known as tidal volume. The total volume of the lung is about

6 L, of which 4.8 L is called the vital capacity and the remaining 1.2 liters is called the residual volume and remains in the lungs [77–79].

Exhaled breath is an inhomogeneous gas mixture composed of "dead space" (roughly 150 milliliters) and the gas part represented by the "alveolar" respiration coming from the lungs (about 350 milliliters). Human exhalation contains both gas molecules resulting from the exchange of blood, but also compounds from the atmosphere. In the process of breath gases collection, there are three basic approaches [79, 80]:

1. Dead-space gas collection (or upper airway collection), which is the volume of air in the conducting airways where gas exchange cannot take place, where no exchange of oxygen or carbon dioxide occurs. There is also an alveolar dead space, which is the air in those alveoli that are ventilated but not perfused, where gas cannot be exchanged.

2. Alveolar collection (pure alveolar gas is collected), refers at the portion of exhaled breath that contain gases that have exchanged with blood. In the lungs there is a great flow of blood and the exhaled breath that contains both gas molecules resulting from the exchange of blood, but also compounds from the atmosphere. More specifically, excluding the dead-space from the analysis are excluded the chemicals that originate from the atmosphere. Most respiratory tests use this type of test because it contains VOCs resulting from endogenous activity and the influence of exogenous VOCs is eliminated.

3. Mixed breath collection means that total breath, dead-space air and alveolar gas, is collected.

For the desired results must be taken into account different factors such as the type of breath collected, single or multiple exhalation, and the technique used for sample analysis.

### 4.4 Protocols and procedures for breath analysis

Our measurement procedure to determine the concentrations of gases involves the following basic steps: cleaning the cell, calibration of the cell or measurement of the cell responsivity, and acquiring spectra of ethylene and ammonia [45, 56, 57].

For the measurement and detection of the gases from breath, the laser is kept tuned where ethylene and ammonia exhibit the strongest and most characteristic peaks. The cleaning of the cell must be carried out by successive washing with nitrogen of purity 6,0 (99,9999%) at atmospheric pressure, cleaning performed each time the contents of the cell are changed. An adequate degree of cell clearance is considered to be obtained if the PA signal measured in the nitrogen atmosphere has a rather low level, usually 30 μV. Absorption measurements are performed at room temperature, in the range 20° C - 22°C.

Exhaled breath samples are collected in aluminized bags (750 ml aluminum-coated bags) consisting of: a disposable mouthpiece, a tee-mouthpiece assembly (including a plastic tee and a removable one-way flutter valve), a bag with the role of collecting "dead air" (the first part of expired breath), while the alveolar air in the collection bag and a discard multi-patient collection bags are designed to collect multiple. The breath sample can be kept in multi-patient collection bags for up to 6 hours.

Ammonia is a highly adsorbed compound and the ammonia molecules adhere very well to the walls of the PA cell, so that to ensure the quality of each measurement, an intense $N_2$ washing cycle of the PA cell is performed. In this way the PA signal measured is due exclusively to the absorption of ammonia or ethylene molecules. Before measurements the PA cell is filled with pure nitrogen and the background signal detected, and we started from a background signal ~25 μV.

After collecting the breath sample, the gas sample is transferred from the bag to the PA cell at a controlled flow rate 36 l $h^{-1}$ (600 standard cubic centimeters per minute (sccm)). Before the PA cell is found a trap filled (with a volume > 100 $cm^3$) with KOH (potassium hydroxide) pellets replaced after each measurement, pellets used to retain interfering gases such as carbon dioxide (~4% in exhaled breath sample) and water vapor [94].

All of the collected samples were analyzed over a period of three months. To remove any residual contaminants, all of these bags were thoroughly cleaned by flushing with nitrogen gas (purity 99.9999%) and subsequently evacuated for breath sample collection. Following the procedure, the breath samples was introduced in the PA cell, the PA cell closed and used for measurements. The measurements were performed on the 10P (14) laser line (where ethylene exhibits a strong absorption with an absorption coefficient of 30.4 $cm^{-1}$ $atm^{-1}$) and 9R (30) (where ammonia exhibits a strong absorption with an absorption coefficient of 57 $cm^{-1}$ $atm^{-1}$). In this way the signal measured by microphones in PA cell is quantified and is proportional to the ethylene and to the ammonia concentrations.

## 5. VOCs measurement from the exhaled breath in type 2 diabetes

Oxidative damage was quantified by measuring breath ethylene and ammonia concentrations using $CO_2$LPAS system. PA detection provides necessary selectivity for analyzing multicomponent mixtures by the use of line-tunable $CO_2$ lasers. Breath samples were collected in special sample bags, aluminized multi-patient collection bags from QuinTron (750 mL aluminum-coated bags). All samples were given between 09:00 and 11:00 a.m. and analyzed using the $CO_2$LPAS system. Measurements of HbA1c and glucose were done using standard procedure. The subjects involved in this study are persons diagnosed with T2DM (n = 16), recruited from the family doctor, age between 42 and 71 years, body mass index BMI = 31.4–35.3, known stable cases of T2DM whose medical therapy had been unaltered over the last 12 months, and a healthy control group (n = 9), age between 29 and 42 years, non-smokers, non-diabetics and body mass index BMI = 19.8–23.4. From T2DM subjects, 7 present hypertension and inflammatory syndrome. No patients were on supplements with antioxidants. Informed consent was obtained from all individuals. The participants with hormonal disorders, benign or malignant disorders, renal failure, central nervous system disorders, and also smokers were excluded from the study.

As an observation of the results obtained, it can be seen that the average ethylene of T2DM subjects is higher than the average ethylene healthy subjects (see **Figure 3**). The ethylene values in healthy subjects are normal and in the range 10.73 ppb and 57.13 ppb, but at the subjects with T2DM the ethylene concentrations range was between 78 ppb and 444 ppb. The differences in exhaled breath ammonia concentration are presented in **Figure 4**, where the mean values of breath ethylene concentrations in healthy control group and subjects with T2DM are presented. The ammonia values in healthy subjects are normal and in the range 0.832 ppm and 1.76 ppm, but at the subjects with T2DM the ammonia concentration range was between 2.74 ppm and 10.16 ppm. Our measurements showed a significantly increase of ammonia concentrations in the exhaled breath at diabetic subjects compared to healthy subjects.

For the subjects involved in this study, among the exhaled breath analyses, were determined blood analyses such as blood glucose levels and glycated hemoglobin HbA1C. **Table 1** shows the values of HbA1c and glucose blood tests, as well as the values of the respiration results obtained with the $CO_2$LPAS system.

Among subjects with T2DM, 7 have hypertension and inflammatory syndrome. In those subjects averages of all analyzes, both blood tests and the breathing are

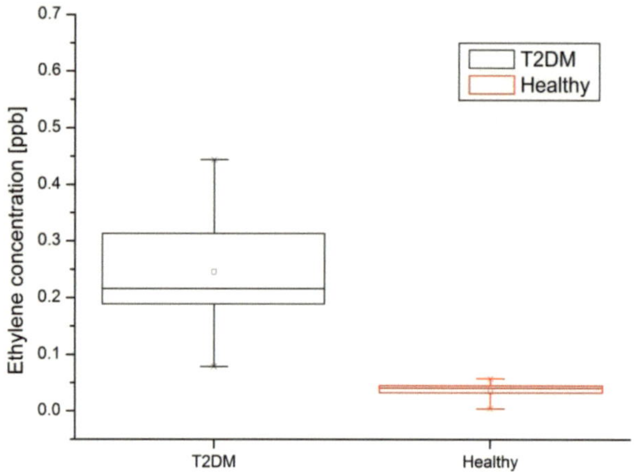


**Figure 3.**
*Mean breath ethylene concentrations in healthy subjects and T2DM.*

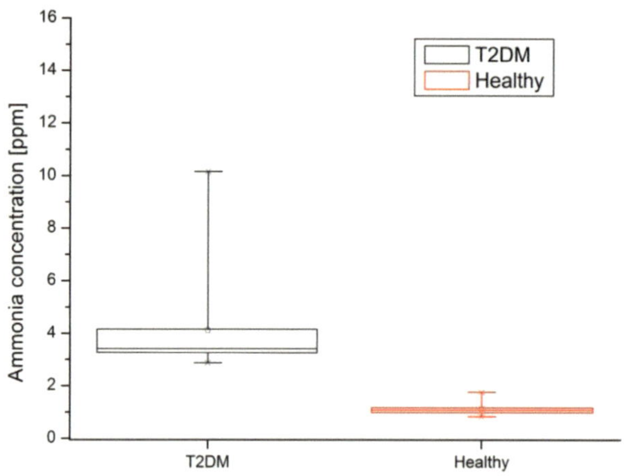


**Figure 4.**
*Mean breath ammonia concentrations in healthy subjects and T2DM.*

| Parameters | Healthy subjects | T2DM | T2DM with hypertension and inflammatory syndrome |
|---|---|---|---|
| Blood glucose (mg $dL^{-1}$) | 83.94 ± 9.2 | 200.17 ± 44.01 | 200.17 ± 44.01 |
| HbA1C [%] | 4.79 ± 0.52 | 7.88 ± 0.66 | 8.21 ± 1.1 |
| $C_{C2H4}$ [ppb] | 24 ± 3.35 | 238 ± 92 | 246 ± 59 |
| $C_{NH3}$ [ppm] | 1.296 ± 0.18 | 3.96 ± 0.85 | 5.16 ± 1.12 |

**Table 1.**
*Mean values for subjects involved with standard deviations (SD).*

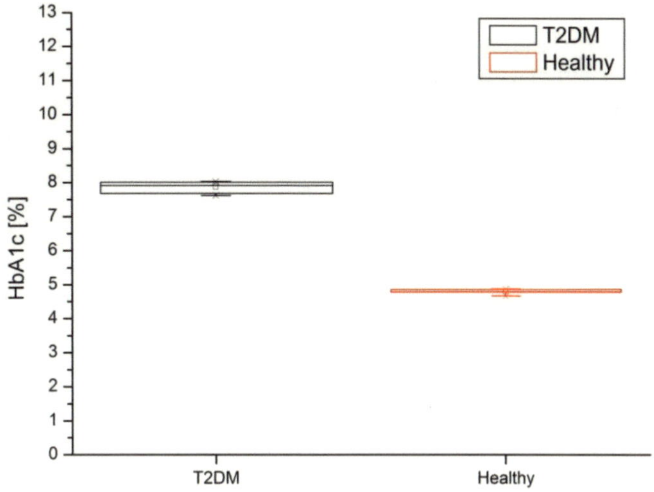


**Figure 5.**
*Mean values of HbA1C in n healthy subjects and T2DM.*

higher in subjects with T2DM who have hypertension and inflammatory syndrome compared to those who have no health complications.

Our results show a high difference in the HbA1c mean value of healthy group and the and the mean values obtained in subjects with T2DM. These differences are presented in **Figure 5**. In diabetes, impaired detoxification of free radicals and this degree of damage can be seen in HbA1c, which is a biomarker of oxidative stress.

## 6. Discussions

Damage to proteins and lipids due to oxidation has been implicated in the pathogenesis of type diabetes. Previous studies on oxidative stress are based on invasive blood samples analysis, and these studies found significant high level of LP product such as malondialdehyde [25, 26, 95, 96]. Through this research, Nour Eldin et al. 2014 shows that malondialdehyde concentration in blood as LP biomarker was elevated in T2DM compared to healthy control group, and that there is an association between hyperglycemia and oxidative stress [27].

Diabetes mellitus and hypertension are interrelated diseases, and hypertension is about twice as frequent in individuals with diabetes as in those without diabetes. Breath ammonia concentrations in subjects with diabetes can be a consequence of oxidative stress after ROS attack on proteins, accelerated catabolism of proteins due to insulin deprivation and hepatic glucose production [28]. According to Erejuwa, 2012, ROS are involved in insulin signaling, and goes to development of insulin resistance [97]. Therefore, oxidative stress increased insulin resistance and increase the free radical's formation in diabetes, which leads to damage in proteins and lipids. Hyperglycemia generates an increased level of free radicals which can lead to dysfunctions [98, 99] and increases oxidative damage which cause in development of health complications in diabetes, complications associated with inflammation [100] or vascular disorders [100, 101].

Some of the subjects with T2DM involved in this study, present complications such as hypertension and/or inflammatory syndrome. T2DM is an inflammatory disease, and inflammation is caused by insulin resistance correlated with obesity, or by hyperglycemia and hyperlipidemia.

Breath ethylene concentrations in subjects with T2DM was found in higher level compared with healthy subjects. Breath ethylene is considered a marker of oxidative stress, being an end-product of LP, caused by the attack of free radicals on polyunsaturated fatty acids. The damage related to free radical's action increase and a direct measurement of the damage can be achieved by quantitative determination of ethylene concentrations.

Ammonia is a biomarker of protein metabolism, and at subjects with T2DM, insulin deprivation is associated with an increase in amino acids and by an accelerated protein catabolism. Moreover, we found that breath ethylene and ammonia concentrations are higher in T2DM subjects that present hypertension and/or inflammatory syndrome than in those without complications. It is known that T2DM lead to complications like kidney failure, heart disease, cerebrovascular disease, but there is a lack of information of ammonia level in subjects with T2DM and the relationship between ammonia level and diabetes complications.

In subjects with T2DM by measuring the percentage of HbA1c, clinicians are able to get an overall picture of the average blood sugar levels have been for the past 2–3 months. Through our measurements, the diabetics present a high level of glycated hemoglobin HbA1c. An increased level of HbA1c reflect a poor metabolic control of the patients with diabetes in uncontrolled T2DM [102–106].

The relation between level of ammonia and ethylene in the exhaled breath and T2DM could be explained by the inadequate insulin control with disease progression by development of complications such as oxidative stress, inflammatory syndrome, and hypertension. The studies show a relation between hyperglycemia, oxidative stress and inflammation coexist in pathological processes but also that hyperglycemia and free radicals increase the oxidative stress which will then activate the inflammatory processes [97, 107].

Future studies are needed to understand the relationship between them and the importance of breath ammonia and ethylene biomarkers.

## 7. Conclusions

Real-time breath ethylene and ammonia monitoring in subjects with type-2 diabetes using a $CO_2$LPAS system was realized.

This paper has presented accurate measurement of breath ethylene and ammonia concentrations and the results obtained in comparison with the blood samples analysis have demonstrated the suitability of the experimental PA system for trace gas detection.

This study shows a high level of oxidative stress in people with diabetes through a high level of glycated hemoglobin HbA1c, and high concentrations of ethylene and ammonia in respiration.

Our study suggests that sensitive, noninvasive, real-time analysis of oxidative stress, using ethylene and ammonia as breath biomarkers, distinguishes healthy subjects from those with type 2 diabetes and controlled by uncontrolled diabetes.

The breath analysis may also bring opportunities in molecular monitoring for other research fields by using an LPAS system.

Despite these advances, there is a continuing need for miniaturized devices, in addition to a precise and easy to use instrument, which should provide a quick response, preferably in real time.

Further research is therefore required to expand the applicability of breath analysis in clinical diagnosis.

## Funding

This work was supported by Romanian Ministry of Education and Research, under Romanian National Nucleu Program LAPLAS VI – contract n. 16 N/2019.

## Author details

Mioara Petrus*, Cristina Popa and Ana-Maria Bratu
National Institute for Laser, Plasma and Radiation Physics, Laser Department, Magurele, Romania

*Address all correspondence to: mioara.petrus@inflpr.ro

## References


[1] Cicolella A. Volatile organic compounds (VOC): Definition, classification and properties. Revue des Maladies Respiratoires. 2008;25(2): 155-163.

[2] Phillips M. Breath tests in medicine. Sci. Am. 1992; 267: 74-79, doi:10.1038/scientificamerican0792-74.

[3] Risby TH. Volatile organic compounds as markers in normal and diseased states. In Disease Markers in Exhaled Breath; Marczin, N., Yacoub, M.H., Eds.; IOS Press: Amsterdam, The Netherlands, 2002; p. 113-122.

[4] Amann A, Poupart G, Telser S, Ledochowski M, Schmid A., Mechtcheriakov S. Applications of breath gas analysis in medicine. Int. J. Mass Spectrom. 2004; 239: 227-233. doi:10.1016/j.ijms.2004.08.010.

[5] Pauling L, Robinson AB, Teranish R, Cary P. Quantitative analysis of urine vapor and breath by gas-liquid partition chromatography. Proc. Natl. Acad. Sci. USA. 1971; 68: 2374.

[6] Probert CSJ, Ahmed1I, Khalid T, Johnson E, Smith S, Ratcliffe N. Volatile organic compounds as diagnostic biomarkers in gastrointestinal and liver diseases. Journal of Gastrointestinal and Liver Diseases. 2009;18(3):337-343.

[7] Horvath I, Lázár Z, Gyulai N, Kollai M, Losonczy G. Exhaled biomarkers in lung cancer. European Respiratory Journal. 2009; 34(1):261-275.

[8] Chambers ST, Scott-Thomas A, Epton M. Developments in novel breath tests for bacterial and fungal pulmonary infection. Current Opinion in Pulmonary Medicine. 2012; 18(3):228-232.

[9] International Diabetes Federation, https://idf.org/ [Accessed: 2020-08-13]

[10] International Diabetes Federation, https://www.idf.org/aboutdiabetes/what-is-diabetes.html [Accessed: 2020-08-13]

[11] ADA. (2009). Diagnosis and classification of diabetes mellitus. Diabetes Care. 2009; 32(1): 62-67.

[12] Shaw JE, Sicree RA, Zimmet PZ (2010). Global estimates of the prevalence of diabetes for 2010 and 2030. Diabetes Res Clin Pract. 2010; 87(1): 4-14.

[13] King H, Aubert RE, Herman WH. Global burden of diabetes 1995-2025: prevalence, numerical estimates, and projections. Diabetes Care. 1998; 21(9): 1414-1431.

[14] International Diabetes Federation, https://www.idf.org/aboutdiabetes/type-2-diabetes.html [Accessed: 2020-08-13]

[15] Pham-Huy LA, He H, Pham-Huy, C. Free radicals, antioxidants in disease and health. IJB. 2008; 4(2): 89-96.

[16] Asfandiyarova N, Kolcheva N, Ryazantsev I, Ryazantsev V. Risk factors for stroke in type 2 diabetes mellitus. Diab. Vasc. Dis. Res. 2007; 3: 57-60.

[17] Phillips M, Cataneo RN, Cheema T, Greenberg J.Increased breath biomarkers of oxidative Oxidative stress in diabetes mellitus and the role of vitamins with antioxidant actions. stress in diabetes mellitus. Clin. Chim. Acta. 2004; 344 (1-2): 189-194.

[18] Lazo-de-la-Vega M-L, Fernandez-Mejia C. In: Morales-Gonzalez, J.A. (ed.) Oxidative Stress and Chronic Degenerative Diseases—A

Role for Antioxidants. IntechOpen. 2013. doi:10.5772/51788 (2013).

[19] Ullah A, Khan A, Khan I. Diabetes mellitus and oxidative stress—A concise review. Saudi Pharmaceutical Journal. 2016; 24: 547-553.

[20] Fowler JM. Microvascular and macrovascular complications of diabetes. Clin. Diabetes. 2011; 29: 116-122.

[21] Jialal I, Devaraj S, Venugopal SK. Oxidative stress, inflammation, and diabetic vasculopathies: the role of alpha tocopherol therapy. Free Radic. Res. 2002; 36: 1331-1336.

[22] Pickup JC. Inflammation and activated innate immunity in the pathogenesis of type 2 diabetes. Diabetes Care. 2004; 27: 813-823.

[23] Johansen JS, Harris AK, Rychly DJ, Ergul A.:Oxidative stress and the use of antioxidants in diabetes: linking basic science to clinical practice. Cardiovasc. Diabetol. 2005. doi:10.1186/1475-2840-4-5

[24] Nishigaki I, Hagihara M, Tsunekawa H, Maseki M, Yagi K. Lipid peroxide levels of serum lipoprotein fractions of diabetic patients. Biochem. Med. 1981; 25(3): 373-378.

[25] Mahreen R, Mohsin M, Nasree Z, Siraj M, Ishaq M. Significantly increased levels of serum malonaldehyde in type 2 diabetics with myocardial infarction. Int. J. Diabetes Dev. Ctries. 2010; 30:49-51.

[26] Volpe VM, Abreu L, Gomes PS, Gonzaga RM, Veloso C, Nogueira-Machado JA. The production of nitric oxide, IL-6, and TNF-alpha in palmitate-stimulated PBMNCs is enhanced through hyperglycemia in diabetes. Oxid. Med. Cell. Longev. 2014; ID 479587.

[27] Nour Eldin EEM, Almarzouki A, Assiri AM, Elsheikh OM, Mohamed BEA, Babakr AT. Oxidized low density lipoprotein and total antioxidant capacity in type-2 diabetic and impaired glucose tolerance Saudi men. Diabetol. Metab. Syndr. 2014; 6: 94-103.

[28] Stanley WJ, Litwak SA, Quah HS, Tan SM, Kay TWH, Tiganis T, de Haan JB, Thomas HE, Gurzov EN, Inactivation of Protein Tyrosine Phosphatases Enhances Interferon Signaling in Pancreatic Islets. Diabetes. 2015; 64: 2489-2496.

[29] Giugliano D, Ceriello A, Paolisso G. Diabetes mellitus, hypertension, and cardiovascular disease: which role for oxidative stress? Metabolism. 1995; 44 (3): 363-368.

[30] Ceriello A. Oxidative stress and diabetes-associated complications. Endocr. Pract. 2006; 12 (1): 60-62.

[31] Maritim AC, Sanders RA, Watkins JB. Diabetes, oxidative stress, and antioxidants: a review. J. Biochem. Mol. Toxicol. 2003; 17 (1):24-38.

[32] Butterfield DA, Koppal T, Howard B, Subramaniam R, Hall N, Hensley K, Yatin S, Allen K, Aksenov M, Aksenova M, Carney J. Structural and functional changes in proteins induced by free radical-mediated oxidative stress and protective action of the antioxidants N-tert-butyl-alpha-phenylnitrone and vitamin E. Ann N Y Acad Sci. 1998; 854:448-462.

[33] Esterbauer H, Schaur RJr, Zollner H. Chemistry and biochemistry of 4-hydroxynonenal, malonaldehyde and related aldehydes. Free Rad. Biol. Med. 1991; 11(1): 81-128.

[34] Francesco FD, Fuoco R, Trivella MG, Ceccarini A. Breath analysis: Trends in techniques and

clinical applications. Microchem. J. 2005; 79: 405-410.

[35] Miekisch W, Schubert JK, Noeldge-Schomburg GFE. Diagnostic potential of breath analysis—Focus on volatile organic compounds. Clin. Chim. Acta. 2004; 347: 25-39.

[36] Dent AG, Sutedja TG, Zimmerman PV. Exhaled breath analysis for lung cancer. J. Thorac. Dis. 2013; 5: S540. doi:10.3978/j.issn.2072–1439.2013.08.44.

[37] Kim KH, Jahan SA, Kabir E. A review of breath analysis for diagnosis of human health. Trends Anal. Chem. 2012; 33: 1-8.

[38] Righettoni M, Amann A, Pratsinis SE. Breath analysis by nanostructured metal oxides as chemo-resistive gas sensors. Mater. Today. 2015; 18: 163-171.

[39] Mazzatenta A, Giulio CD, Pokorski M. Pathologies currently identified by exhaled biomarkers. Respir. Physiol. Neurobiol. 2013; 187: 128-134.

[40] Phillips M. Method for the collection and assay of volatile organic compounds in breath. Anal. Biochem. 1997; 247: 272-278.

[41] Phillips M, Gleeson K, Hughes JM, Greenberg J, Cataneo RN, Baker L, McVay PW. Volatile organic compounds in breath as markers of lung cancer: A cross-sectional study. Lancet. 1999; 353: 1930-1933.

[42] Popov TA. Human exhaled breath analysis. Ann. Allergy Asthma Immunol. 2011; 106: 451-456. doi:10.1016/j.anai.2011.02.016.

[43] Kearney DJ, Hubbard T, Putnam D. Breath ammonia measurement in helicobacter pylori infection. Dig. Dis. Sci. 2002; 47: 2523-2530, doi:10.1023/A:1020568227868.

[44] Rezaie A, Buresi M, Lembo A, et al. Hydrogen and Methane-Based Breath Testing in Gastrointestinal Disorders: The North American Consensus. Am J Gastroenterol. 2017;112(5):775-784. doi:10.1038/ajg.2017.46

[45] Hlastala MP: The alcohol breath test—a review Archived 2011-06-26 at the Wayback Machine. Journal of Applied Physiology. 1998; 84 (2): 401-408.

[46] "NASA's electronic nose could sniff out cancer". New Scientist. 27 Aug. 2008; 13: 1325-1336. doi:10.4155/bio-2016-0045. PMID 27277875.

[47] Heaney LM, Lindley MR. Translation of exhaled breath volatile analyses to sport and exercise applications. Metabolomics. 2017; 13 . doi:10.1007/s11306-017-1266-z.

[48] Saidi T, Zaim O, Moufid M, El Bari N, Ionescu R, Bouchikhi B: Exhaled breath analysis using electronic nose and gas chromatography–mass spectrometry for non-invasive diagnosis of chronic kidney disease, diabetes mellitus and healthy subjects. Sensors and Actuators B: Chemical. 2018; 257: 178-188.

[49] Pleil JD, Stiegel MA, Risby TH, Clinical Breath Analysis: Discriminating Between Human Endogenous Compounds and Exogenous (Environmental) Chemical Confounders. J. Breath Res. 2013; 7: 017107.

[50] Agapiou A, Amann A, Mochalski P, Statheropoulos M, Thomas CLP. Trace detection of endogenous human volatile organic compounds for search, rescue and emergency applications. Trends Anal. Chem. 2015; 66: 158-175.

[51] Risby TH, Pleil JD. Breath analysis—Past, present and future: A special issue in honour of Michael Phillips' 70th birthday. J. Breath Res. 2013; 7: 010201.

[52] Horváth I, Hunt J, Barnes PJ. Exhaled breath condensate: Methodological recommendations and unresolved questions. Eur. Respir. J. 2005; 6: 523-548. doi:10.1183/09031936.05.00029705.

[53] Mochalski P, Wiesenhofer H, Allers M, Zimmermann S, Güntner AT, Pineau NJ, Lederer W, Agapiou A, Mayhew CA, Ruzsanyi V. Monitoring of selected skin- and breath-borne volatile organic compounds emitted from the human body using gas chromatography ion mobility spectrometry (GC-IMS). J. Chromatogr. B. 2018; 1076: 29-34.

[54] Gaugg MT, Gomez DG, Barrios-Collado C, Vidal-de-Miguel G, Kohler M, Zenobi R, Sinues PML. Expanding metabolite coverage of real-time breath analysis by coupling a universal secondary electrospray ionization source and high resolution mass spectrometry-a pilot study on tobacco smokers. J. Breath Res. 2016; 10: 9.

[55] Mathew TL, Pownraj P, Abdulla S, Pullithandathil B. Technologies for clinical diagnosis using expired human breath analysis. Diagnnostics. 2015; 5: 27-60.

[56] Spagnolo V, Lewicki R, Dong L, Tittel FK. Quantum-cascade-laser-based optoacoustic detection for breath sensor applications. In: Proceedings of the IEEE International Symposium on Medical Measurements and Applications; 30—31 May 2011; Bari Italy; 2011. doi:10.1109/MeMeA.2011.5966773.

[57] Harvey RA, Ferrier DR. Lippincott's Illustrated Reviews:Biochemistry. 5th ed., Wolters Kluwer Lippincott Williams &Wilkins Health. Philadelphia; 2011.

[58] Bakouh N, Benjelloun F, Hulin P, et al. NH3 is involved in the NH4+ transport induced by the functional expression of the human Rh C glycoprotein. J Biol Chem. 2004; 279(16):15975-15983. doi:10.1074/jbc.M308528200

[59] Handlogten ME, Hong S-P, Zhang L, Vander AW, Steinbaum ML, Campbell-Thompson M, Weiner ID. Expression of the ammonia transporter proteins, Rh B Glycoprotein and Rh C Glycoprotein, in the intestinal tract. Am. J. Physiol. Gastrointest. Liver Physiol. 2005; 288: G1036–G1047:

[60] Bosoi CR, Rose CF. Identifying the direct effects of ammonia on the brain. Metab Brain Dis. 2009; 24(1):95-102

[61] Španěl P, Smith D. What is the real utility of breath ammonia concentration measurements in medicine and physiology? J. Breath Res. 2018; 12: 027102.

[62] Spacek LA, Mudalel M, Tittel F, Risby TH, Solga SF. Clinical utility of breath ammonia for evaluation of ammonia physiology in healthy and cirrhotic adults. J. Breath Res. 2015; 9: 047109. doi:10.1088/1752-7155/9/4/047109.

[63] Hibbard T, Killard AJ. Breath Ammonia Analysis: Clinical Application and Measurement. Crit. Rev. Anal. Chem. 2011; 41: 21-35, doi:10.1080/10408347.2011.521729.

[64] Solga SF, Mudalel ML, Spacek LA, Risby TH. Fast and Accurate Exhaled Breath Ammonia Measurement. J. Vis. Exp. 2014; 88: e51658. doi:10.3791/51658.

[65] Lewicki R, Kosterev AA, Bakhirkin YA, Thomazy DM, Doty J, Dong L, Tittel FK. Real Time Ammonia Detection in Exhaled Human Breath with a Quantum Cascade Laser Based Sensor. In: Proceedings of the Conference on Lasers and Electro-Optics and Conference on Quantum electronics and Laser Science Conference; 2-4 June 2009; Baltimore, MD, USA; 2009; p. 1-2.

[66] Petrus M, Bratu AM, Popa C. The response of human body at oxidative stress in subjects with type 2 diabetes: ammonia breath analysis by laser photoacoustic spectroscopy. Rev. Roum. Chim.2016; 61(2): 89-95.

[67] Cristescu SM, Kiss R, Hekkert ST, Dalby M, Harren FJM, Risby TH, Marczin N, Harefield BSI. Real-time monitoring of endogenous lipid peroxidation by exhaled ethylene in patients undergoing cardiac surgery. Am. J. Physiol. Lung Cell. Mol. Physiol. 2014; 307: L509–L515.

[68] Giubileo G, Puiu AP, Dumitras DC. Detection of ethylene in smokers breath by laser photoacoustic spectroscopy. Proc. Spie Int. Soc. Opt. Eng. 200;, 5486: 280-286. doi:10.1117/12.572042.

[69] Borza C, Muntean D, Dehelean C, Săvoiu G, Serban C, Simu G, Andoni M, Butur M, Drăgan S. Chapter 2: Oxidative Stress and Lipid Peroxidation –A Lipid Metabolism Dysfunction. IntechOpen. 2013; p.23-38. http://dx.doi.org/10.5772/51627

[70] Cheesman KH, Slater TF. An introduction to free radical biochemistry. Free radicals Medicine: British Medical Bulletin. 1993; 49(3): 481-494.

[71] Halliwel B, Gutteridge C, Cross C.Free radicals, antioxidants and human disease. Where are you now? J Lab Clin Med. 1993; 119(6): 606-610.

[72] Halliwell B. Free radicals and antioxidants: updating a personal view. Nutr Rev. 2012; 70(5): 257-265.

[73] Devasagayam TP, Tilak JC, Boloor KK, Sane KS, Ghaskadbi SS, Lele RD. Free radicals and antioxidants in human health: current status and future prospects," J. Assoc. Physicians India. 2004; 52: 794-804.

[74] Knight JA. Review: free radicals, antioxidants and the immune system. Ann. Clin. Lab. Sci. 2000; 30(2): 145-158.

[75] Petrus M, Bratu AM, Popa C. Spectroscopic analysis of breath ethylene and oxidativestress relation with glycaemic status in type 2 diabetes. Opt Quant Electron (2017) 49:2. DOI 10.1007/s11082-016-0837-y.

[76] Dumitras DC, Dutu DC, Matei C, Magureanu AM, Petrus M, Popa C. Laser photoacoustic spectroscopy: Principles, instrumentation, and characterization. J. Optoelectron. Adv. Mater. 2007; 9: 3655-3701.

[77] Rattray NJ, Hamrang Z, Trivedi DK, Goodacre R, Fowler SJ. Taking your breath away: metabolomics breathes life in to personalized medicine. Trends in Biotechnology. 2014; 32:538-548.

[78] Lawal O, AhmedWM, Nijsen TME, Goodacre R, Fowler SJ. Exhaled breath analysis: a review of 'breath-taking' methods for off-line analysis. Metabolomics. 2017; 13:110. DOI 10.1007/s11306-017-1241-8.

[79] Quinn M, St Lucia K, Rizzo A. Anatomy, Anatomic Dead Space. [Updated 2020 May 15]. In: StatPearls [Internet]. Treasure Island (FL): StatPearls Publishing; 2020 Jan-. Available from: https://www.ncbi.nlm.nih.gov/books/NBK442016/

[80] Lourenco C, Turner C. Breath analysis in disease diagnosis: methodological considerations and applications. Metabolites. 2014; 4: 465-498.

[81] Harren FJM, Cotti G, Oomens J, te Lintel Hekkert S. Environment: Trace Gas Monitoring. In: Encyclopedia of Analytical Chemistry. Sigrist MW, Meyers RA. Eds.Wiley: Chichester; 2000; Volume 3. p. 2203-2226.

[82] Sigrist MW. Trace gas monitoring by laser photoacoustic spectroscopy and related techniques. Rev. Sci. Instrum. 2003; 74: 486-490.

[83] Bell AG. On the production and reproduction of sound by light. Am. J. Sci. 1880; 20: 305-324.

[84] Bell AG. Upon the production of sound by radiant energy. Phil. Mag. J. Sci. 1881; 11: 510-528.

[85] Tyndall J. Action of an intermittent beam of radiant heat upon gaseous matter. Proc. R. Soc. 1881; 31: 307-317.

[86] Röntgen WC. Über Töne, welche durch intermittierende Bestralung eines Gases entstehen. Ann. Phys. Chem. 1881; 1: 155-159.

[87] Preece WH. On the conversion of radiant energy into sonorous vibrations. Proc. R. Soc. 1881; 31: 506 520.

[88] Tam AC. Applications of photoacoustic sensing techniques. Rev. Mod. Phys. 1986; 58: 381-431.

[89] Sigrist MW. Laser generation of acoustic waves in liquids and gases. J. Appl. Phys. 1986; 60: R83–R121.

[90] Meyer PL,Sigrist MW. Atmospheric pollution monitoring using CO2-laser photoacoustic spectroscopy and other techniques. Rev. Sci. Instrum. 1990; 61: 1779-1807.

[91] Harren FJM, Reuss J. Spectroscopy, photoacoustic. In: Encyclopedia of Applied Physics. Trigg GL Ed. VCH Publishers: New York USA. 1997; Volume 19, p. 413-435.

[92] Miklos A, Hess P, Bozoki Z. Application of acoustic resonators in photoacoustic trace gas analysis and metrology. Rev. Sci. Instrum. 2001; 72: 1937-1955.

[93] Schmid T. Photoacoustic spectroscopy for process analysis. Anal. Bioanal. Chem. 2006; 384: 1071-1086.

[94] Bratu AM, Popa C, Matei C, Banita S, Dutu DCA, Dumitras DC. Removal of interfering gases in breath biomarker measurements. J. Optoelectron. Adv. Mater. 2011; 13: 1045-1050.

[95] Fatani SH, Babakr AT, NourEldin EM, Almarzouki AA. Lipid peroxidation is associated with poor control of type-2 diabetes mellitus. Diabetes Metab. Syndr. Clin. Res. Rev. 2016. doi:10.1016/j.dsx.2016.01.08

[96] Kumavat M, Sharma TK, Singh N, Ghalaut VS, Vardey SK, Shankar V. Antioxidant enzymes and lipid peroxidation in type 2 diabetes mellitus patients with and without nephropathy. N. Am. J. Med. Sci. 2013; 5: 213-219.

[97] Erejuwa OO. Oxidative stress in diabetes mellitus: is there a role for hypoglycemic drugs and/or antioxidants. Oxid. Stress Dis. 2012; 217-246.

[98] Ayala A. Munoz MF, Arguelles S. Lipid peroxidation: production, metabolism, and signaling mechanism of malondialdehyle and 4-hydroxy-2-nonenal. Oxid. Med. Cell. Longev. 2014. doi:10.1155/2014/360438

[99] de Badeira SM, da Guedes GS, da Fonseca LJS, Pires AS, Gelain DP, Moreira JCF. Rabelo LA, Vasconcelos SML, Goulart MOF. Characterization of blood oxidative stress in type 2 diabetes mellitus aptients: increased in lipid peroxidation and SOD activity. Oxid. Med. Cell. Longev. 2012; ID 819310.

[100] Hotamisligil GS. Inflammation and metabolic disorders. Nature. 2006; 444:860-867.

[101] Yu PH, Wang M, Deng YL, Fan H, Shira-Bock L. Involvement of semicarbazide-sensitive amine oxidase-mediated deamination in atherogenesis in KKAy diabetic mice fed with high cholesterol diet.Diabetologia. 2002; 45:1255-1262.

[102] Braatvedt GD, Cundy T, Crooke M, Florkowski C, Mann JI, Lunt H, Jackson R, Orr-Walber B, Kenealy T, Drury PL. Understanding the new HbA1c units for the diagnosis of type 2 diabetes. N. Z. Med. J. 2012, 125: 70-80.

[103] Nasir MN, Thevarajah M, Yean CY. Hemoglobin variants detected by hemoglobin A1c (HbA1c) analysis and the effects on HbA1c measurements. Int. J. Diabetes Dev. Ctries. 2010; 30: 86-90.

[104] Sacks DB.:Hemoglobin variants and hemoglobin A1c analysis: problems solved? Clin Chem. 2003; 49:1245-1247.

[105] Shaw JE, Zimmet PZ, McCarty D, de Courten M. Type 2 diabetes worldwide according to the new classification and criteria. Diabetes Care. 2000; 23: B5–B10.

[106] Rytter E, Vessby B, Asgard R, Johansson C, Sjodin A, Abbramsson-Zetterberg L, Moller L, Basu S. Glycaemic status in relation to oxidative stress and inflammation in well-controlled type 2 diabetes. Br. J. Nutr. 2009; 101: 1423-1426.

[107] Adly AAM. Oxidative stress and disease: an updated review. Res. J. Immunol. 2010; 3: 129-145.

Section 3

# Diabetes Complications

Chapter 7

# Diabetes Microvascular Complications: An Overview of Epigenetic Modifications

*Neerja Aggarwal and Pawan Kumar Kare*

## Abstract

Diabetic nephropathy (DN) and diabetic retinopathy (DR) are two serious and long-standing microvascular complications of type 2 diabetes mellitus (T2DM) whose burden is increasing worldwide due to increasing burden of T2DM. Several factors which may predispose to the development of DN and DR are persistent hyperglycemia and its consequences such as formation of advanced glycation end products (AGEs), activation of hexosamine pathway, polyol pathway, uncontrolled blood pressure, increased oxidative stress, age, family history of kidney disease or hypertension, ethnic background etc. However, the pathophysiological mechanisms of these complications are complicated and not completely understood yet. Hence it is the demand to discover newer approaches to treat these devastating complications completely. Recently, various epigenetic modifications, which are the transmissible alterations in the expressions of a gene, are being studied to understand the pathophysiology of diabetic vascular complications. Metabolic and environmental factors may lead to dysregulated epigenetic mechanisms which might further affect the chromatin structure and related expressions of a gene, which may lead to diabetes-associated complications. Therefore, it is the need to explore its role in vascular complications in the current scenario. In this chapter, various epigenetic studies with regard to DN and DR, epigenome-wide association studies (EWAS) approach, and starting clinical material for such studies have been discussed. We have also summarized the better understanding of epigenetic alterations and their role in microvascular complications of diabetes through this chapter. The better understanding of epigenetic mechanisms and their role in diabetic microvascular complications could be used in clinical management of DN as well as DR or could be helpful to improve the available therapies for these complications.

**Keywords:** diabetes, epigenetics, methylation, histone modification

## 1. Introduction

Diabetes is a chronic metabolic disorder in which blood glucose levels upsurge more than normal. Type 2 diabetes mellitus (T2DM) contributes to the majority of diabetes cases accounting for more than 90% of them. An imbalance of insulin supply and demand results in type 2 diabetes [1]. Decrease in insulin sensitivity accompanied by deficiency of insulin are the two primary pathogenetic defects underlying type 2 diabetes and together explain 85–90% of diabetes [2]. Long term diabetes instigates vascular diseases affecting almost all blood vessels of the body, which further results in increased morbidity and mortality in diabetic populations. Among well-known risk factors of diabetes, non-changeable factors include genetics, age and ethnicity while others are changeable, for example physical activity, adiposity, environmental exposures and diet, via combination of treatment at both individual as well as population level [3]. Type 2 diabetes is frequently seen in older adults, but now-a-days, may be, as a result of increasing physical inactivity, obesity and/or the absence of healthy diet it is also being seen increasingly among children, teenagers and younger adults. Diabetes is globally affecting 425 million people or 8.8% of adult population. By 2045, diabetes is projected to affect about 629 million of adult population in the world [3].

India, now-a-days, is becoming the diabetes capital of the world with estimated prevalence of diabetes as 7.3% and that of pre-diabetes as 10.3% [4]. In the current report (2017), 72.9 million Indians were suffering from diabetes and this is expected to rise to 134.3 million by the year 2045 [3]. Prolonged hyperglycemia is the foremost cause of kidney disease, cardiovascular disorders, retinopathy and neuropathy [5], which are the main vascular complications of diabetes.

## 2. Diabetes mellitus-associated vascular complications

Hyperglycemia triggers damage to the vasculature and thus, leads to the failure of various organs including kidney, heart, retina of eyes and nerves; usually develop after many years of diabetes. This gives rise to the development of vascular complications which are categorized into micro- and macrovascular complications. Microvascular disease or microangiopathy is actually the thickening of walls of small blood vessels so that they bleed and leakage of protein occurs. This narrowing of blood vessels results in decreased blood flow and impairment of oxygen flow throughout the body which leads to the damage of tissues or organs that are extremely sensitive to oxygen levels i.e., kidney cells, nerve cells and retina. On the other hand, macrovascular disease or macroangiopathy is the disease of large blood vessels due to clot formations that further results in the decreased blood flow all through the body. This may cause heart diseases, peripheral vascular diseases or stroke. Both micro- and macrovascular complications are the result of hyperglycemia and it seems that they both may be interconnected but who precedes whom or whether they progress together, it is not clear. Complications of T2DM keep on increasing due to increasing burden of diabetes, thus deteriorating the quality of human life. Smoking, age factor, increased weight, lack of physical activity and high-fat diet are the common risk factors to diabetes complications. Now-a-days diabetic kidney disease (DKD) or DN and diabetic retinopathy (DR) are among the most frequent complications of diabetes. Improved and maintained glycemic control may reduce risk of some of the diabetic complications, but it is not the only factor which, if under control, may reduce the progression of all vascular complications. In this segment, we have elaborated two major microvascular complications of diabetes, i.e., DN and DR.

### 2.1 Diabetic nephropathy

Diabetic nephropathy is the major microvascular complication of diabetes affecting 20–30% of patients with type 2 diabetes mellitus [6], which weaken the quality of life leading to increased morbidity and mortality. Symptoms of DN are less evident in the early years of diabetes, usually develops after many years of diabetes. In India approximately 48% cases of CKD are caused by diabetes [7].

DN is defined as a clinical syndrome characterized by persistent proteinuria, a moderate deterioration of eGFR and an increasing arterial blood pressure [8]. Being the foremost cause of end-stage renal disease (ESRD), it results in considerable morbidity and mortality and incurs massive burden of cost on patient and the society as well. Pathways, specifically renin-angiotensin-aldosterone system (RAAS), have been known to play a central role in the development and progression of nephropathy which eventually triggers numerous inflammatory factors directing to the development of fibrosis in the kidney, hypertension/hyperfilteration in the glomerulus and increased permeability to macromolecules leading to proteinuria [9]. It has been seen that some patients with good glycemic control may develop DN at later stages and patients with poor glycemic control may not always develop DN. This may partly be due to genetic predisposition among various ethnic populations. Presence of diabetic nephropathy within families and the large differences in its incidence among diabetic populations with different ethnicity suggests the contribution of several genetic and epigenetic factors in the development and progression of DN. Till date several candidate genes, that are susceptible to DN, have been recognized with the advancements of molecular techniques via linkage studies, GWAS or candidate gene studies. The important candidate genes includes ADIPOQ [10] and ACACβ [11] from lipid metabolism, GCKR [12] and TCF7L2 [13] from glucose metabolism, transforming growth factor-β1 (TGF-β1) involved in inflammation [14], genes associated with angiogenesis i.e., VEGF-A [15] and RAAS genes i.e., ACE [16] and AGTR1 [17], and recently SLC12A3 [18] whose various polymorphisms are reported to be associated with DN. Genes involved in RAAS have been most extensively investigated in the context of DN. Among RAAS genes, angiotensin converting enzyme (ACE) gene is found to be strongly correlated with DN. For this reason, ACE inhibitors and angiotensin receptor blockers (ARBs) are the first line of drugs for the treatment of diabetic nephropathy that aims to reduce proteinuria. Though these drugs have shown to reverse the progression of albuminuria from macroalbuminuria or microalbuminuria to normoalbuminuria [19], thereby slows down the progression of disease, but are not able to provide a stable renoprotective effect. The response of DN patients to ACE inhibitors or ARBs alone or in combination is also not uniform despite several studies. Moreover, there are some limitations regarding their usage based on particular patient to be treated. Hence, these drugs along with strict glycemic control contribute to some degree of renoprotection, but not complete. Therefore, it is the urge to discover new pathways leading to the development of more specific therapies/treatments to help DN patients and improving their life.

### 2.2 Diabetic retinopathy

Diabetic retinopathy is a medical condition where damage to retina, as a result of high glucose, occurs. It is the most frequent cause of blindness in patients with diabetes. Patients with DR usually does not develop any major symptoms at an early stage but during later stages physiological and metabolic abnormalities can appear leading to blindness, if left untreated. The risk factors associated with DR includes high blood glucose [20], duration and type of diabetes [21], high B.P. [22] and, lipids [23]. Presently it is being diagnosed with the identification of microvascular lesions in the retina. It has been differentiated clinically in 2 categories on the basis of ophthalmic observation: proliferative DR (PDR), the advance stage and; non-proliferative DR (NPDR), the early stage. NPDR can be identified by fundus where hard exudates, microaneurysms or hemorrhages are seen. NPDR is further categorized into mild, moderate and severe NPDR. On the other hand, detection of retinal neovascularization confirms PDR. The risk of progression of DR can be reduced by early detection, but it is difficult to achieve as there is little or no symptoms at early stages. Several molecular mechanisms are thought to involve in the development and progression of DR including polyol pathway, enhanced expression of vascular endothelial growth factor (VEGF), production of advance glycation end products (AGEs), activation of RAAS, hemodynamic alterations, etc. Current treatment involves conventional laser therapy and anti-VEGF or other anti-angiogenic, anti-inflammatory, non-steroidal anti-inflammatory drugs (NSAIDs) treatment. Despite this, reading is also difficult in patients with severe retina loss. Some treatments are precise but they are associated with high cost or side effects. Hence, the discovery of fundamental molecular mechanisms involved is required for the development of more specific interventions. Among genetic predisposition to the disease, several candidate genes have been identified in the past few decades with contradictory findings, although few genes have been found to be associated with DR in mostly studies. Among them, aldose reductase (AKR1B1) is important enzyme in polyol pathway. Activation of this pathway and AKR1B1 polymorphisms are incriminated in the pathogenesis of DR [24]. VEGF is another the most important growth factor activated by hyperglycemia and implicated in the development and progression of DR [25]. Various polymorphisms of VEGF were found to be associated with DR with conflicting results [24]. ACE I/D polymorphism was found to be associated with PDR in a meta-analysis [26]. Receptor for advance glycation end products (RAGE) gene polymorphisms is also reported to be associated with DR in Indian population [27].

The pathophysiology of complications of diabetes is very complex as depicted in **Figure 1**.

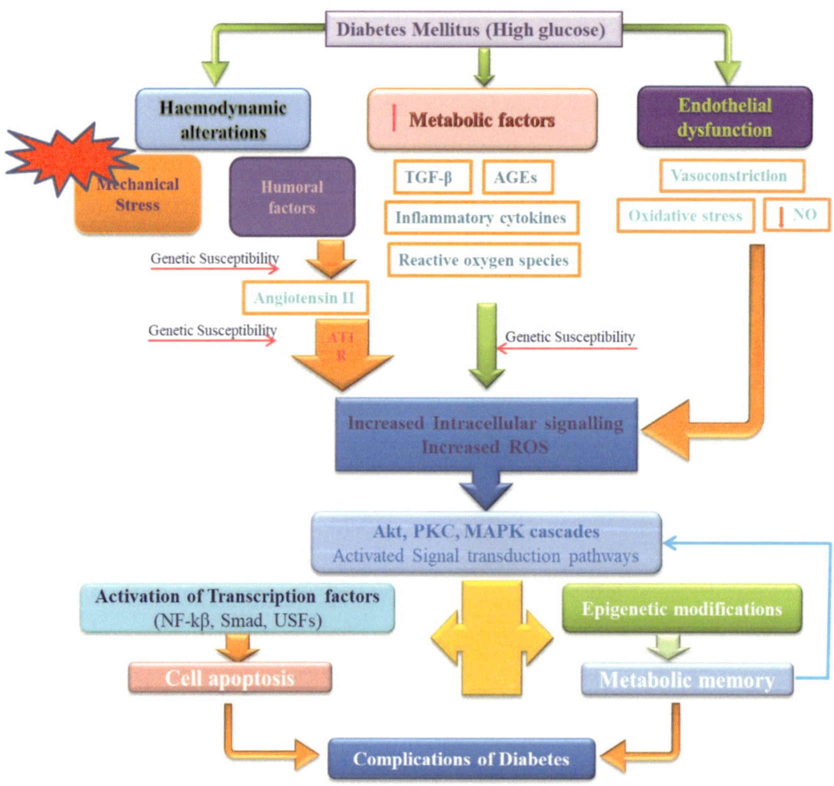


**Figure 1.**
*Signaling pathways facilitating the pathogenesis of microvascular complications of diabetes mellitus.*

*Diabetes-induced hyperglycemia promotes various growth factors which play influential roles in the progression of diabetic complications. These factors act by binding to their specific receptors to initiate multiple downstream signaling cascades involved. Subsequently, these signaling pathways trigger transcription factors and promote their crosstalk with epigenetic mechanisms that lead to diabetic microvascular complications. Transcription factors also interact with epigenetic factors that further participate in metabolic memory. AT1R, Angiotensin II type 1 receptor; AGEs, Advance glycation end products; TGF-β, Transforming growth factor-β1; ROS, Reactive oxygen species; NO, Nitric oxide; Akt, Serine/threonine-specific protein kinase; PKC, Protein kinase C; MAPK, Mitogen-activated protein kinase; NF-κB, Nuclear factor-κB; USFs, Upstream stimulatory factors.*

Several genetic factors and gene polymorphisms have been extensively discovered, studied and implicated in DN as well as DR, but no report is able to provide strong evidence regarding uneven response to available treatment. No drug or treatment is able to provide a stable and long-term protective effect against these complications.

In past few years, a lot of interest has been generated in gene–environment interactions as they seem to be involved in the pathophysiology of diabetes mellitus. Recently, epigenetic mechanisms have been linked to various complications of diabetes, as altered gene expressions are the results of several post-transcriptional modifications (PTMs) of chromatin. Accomplishing complete control of blood glucose is also not sufficient to stop or retard the development and progression of diabetes complications; this proposes the involvement of initial glycemic 'metabolic memory' in various complications of diabetes. So, how epigenetic modifications play the role in diabetic vascular complications is still not completely understood, therefore, we have described the understanding about epigenetic mechanisms and their role in the pathophysiology of diabetic microvascular complications.

## 3. Epigenetics-an addition to current treatment strategy

In mammalian cells, expression of a gene is known to be controlled by genetic as well as epigenetic mechanisms. In the recent times, epigenetic mechanisms have been shown to play substantial roles in the development and progression of diabetes and its microvascular complications. In this section, epigenetic mechanisms have been elaborated in the complications of diabetes.

Epigenetic mechanisms are deprived of any modification in the principal DNA structure which involves vibrant switching within 'active' (euchromatin) and 'inactive' (heterochromatin) positions of chromatin; that determined 'gene activation' and 'gene repression' states and thus biological outcomes [28]. Fundamentally, any change, in the expression of a gene without variation in its nucleotide (DNA) sequence, unlike genetic variations, is known as epigenetic variation. Subsequently, epigenetic studies in diabetic complications may help us to understand the role of epigenetic mechanisms in the alteration of expressions of genes involved in various complications. Hypermethylation at CpG Island in promoter region of a gene is likely to silence its expressions. In contrast, when CpG turns out to be hypomethylated, reverse can takes place [29]. At first, 'epigenetics' term was described by Waddington as 'the casual interaction between genes and their products which bring the phenotype into being' [30]. Epigenetic mechanisms maintains the structure of chromatin to confer transcription memory important for the faithful transmission of gene expression pattern across multiple cell divisions even in the absence of signals that initiated them [31]. Such a control of gene expression by the epigenetic modifications elucidates the mechanisms which triggers our cells with the same DNA to differentiate into numerous cell types with various phenotypes [32, 33]. That's why phenotype of a person is not only decided by its genome but by its epigenome too.

### 3.1 Factors associated with epigenetic mechanisms

The suggested mechanism behind altered expression of a gene was the activation of an intracellular signal by environmental factors, which sequentially specifies the accurate chromatin position for epigenetic alterations [34, 35]. Certain environmental aspects takes place during the course of formation and development of embryo (such as maternal diet and intrauterine nutrition) and such an initial development could influence health and disease conditions even at later stages [36]. Additionally, several other environmental exposures accelerate alterations in epigenetic mechanisms, such as heavy metal exposure, smoking, revelation of pesticides, even insufficiencies of nutrients (such as folate and methionine) [37]. Moreover these mechanisms are also appeared to be altered by age and obesity which may possibly cause type 2 DM [38].

### 3.2 Epigenetic mechanisms in diabetes mellitus and its complications

In past few years, environment has shown a significant role in activating diabetes, although diabetes has a trend to run in family due to intense genetic component. Obesity, older age and sluggish routine with absence of physical doings are the pronounced risk factors for getting hyperglycemia. Diabetes may cause altered epigenetic mechanisms which can direct diabetes-associated complications such as diabetic nephropathy, by altered expression of genes in target cells as depicted in **Figure 2** [39].

*Diabetes mellitus results in the activation of several signaling pathways following activation of alterations in DNA and histone proteins and transcription factors including NF-κB. These mechanisms via chromatin remodeling resulted in regulated target genes expression in targeted tissues along with activation of several ncRNAs including miRNAs, lncRNAs and circRNAs. Such post transcriptional alterations in target tissues resulted in specific key pathological changes in specific tissues and promote the development of specific vascular complication of diabetes. Even after blood glucose control, synchronized crosstalk between various transcription factors and altered epigenetic mechanisms contribute to the metabolic memory and increased expression of ncRNAs that is embroiled in risk of development of microvascular complication of diabetes.*

High glucose can also stimulate abnormalities in DNA at key genes which are well-known to be involved in endothelial dysfunction as evident by sequencing studies in endothelial cells [40]. Augmented DNA methylation at the promoter region of peroxisome proliferator activated receptor gamma coactivator-1 alpha (PPARGC1A) was reported to be associated with decreased expression of PPARGC1A in pancreatic islets [41]. Tewari et al. [42] have demonstrated the decreased transcriptional activity owing to decreased binding of mitochondrial DNA (mtDNA) to DNA polymerase as a result of hypermethylation at regulatory region of DNA polymerase. Global DNA hypomethylation and thereby, anomalous gene expression due to hyperglycemia was observed in the animal model of diabetes, which was further correlated with inadequate wound healing process [43]. Glucose-induced insulin secretion was shown to be influenced by hyper-acetylation of H4 (histone) at promoter region of insulin gene [38]. Hyperglycemic environment exposure to endothelial cells showed the increased expression of p65 subunit of NF-κB along with other inflammatory genes that correspond with increased H3K4me1 alterations on promoter region of p65 subunit [44].

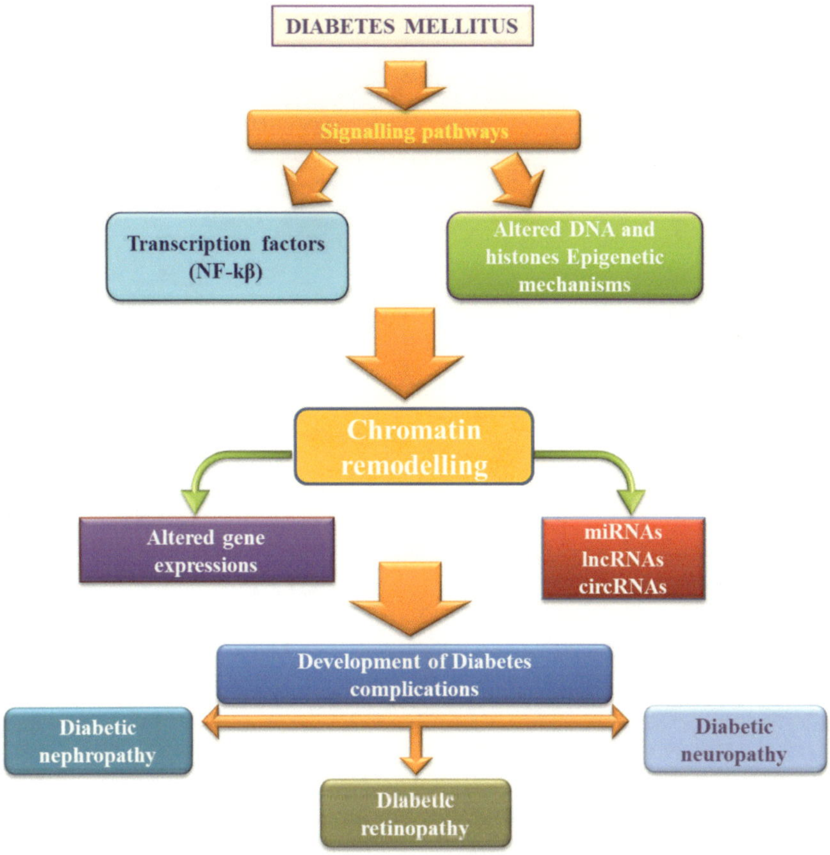


**Figure 2.**
*Pathways preceding the development of microvascular complications of diabetes.*

Hyperglycemia has also shown to alter micro RNA (miRNA), a mechanism of epigenetic modifications, which is also implicated in complications of diabetes. The alteration in miRNA-133a has been reported in cardiomyocyte hypertrophy in diabetes patients [45]. miRNA-320 upregulation was also observed in myocardial microvascular endothelial cells in rat model with type 2 diabetes [46]. The elementary epigenetic modifications viz., (a) methylation of promoter sites in DNA, (b) modifications in histone proteins and, (c) non-coding RNAs facilitated pathways, as illustrated in **Figure 3**, known to modify the expressions of a gene are described as below:

*DNA in chromosomes is packed round the histones to form nucleosomes. Unwrapping and accessibility of nucleosomes is regulated by alterations in histone proteins. DNA methylation involves addition or removal of methyl groups to cytosine residues in CpG islands via DNA methylating enzymes (DNMT) or DNA demethylases, thus, preventing the binding of transcription factors and suppressing respective gene expression. Histone modifications include acetylation, methylation and phosphorylation. HATs/HDACs regulates the acetylation and deacetylation of histone tails, whereas histone methylation is regulated by HMTs/HDMs. Alterations in histone tail coupled with DNA methylation and control the chromatin accessibility or inaccessibility, hence, regulating the expression of various genes. ncRNAs can be act as housekeeping molecules or regulatory molecules. miRNAs act as regulatory molecules among epigenetic mechanisms and are most widely studied mechanism regulating gene expressions at post-transcriptional level. This dynamic condition of chromatin is exposed to modifications by external*

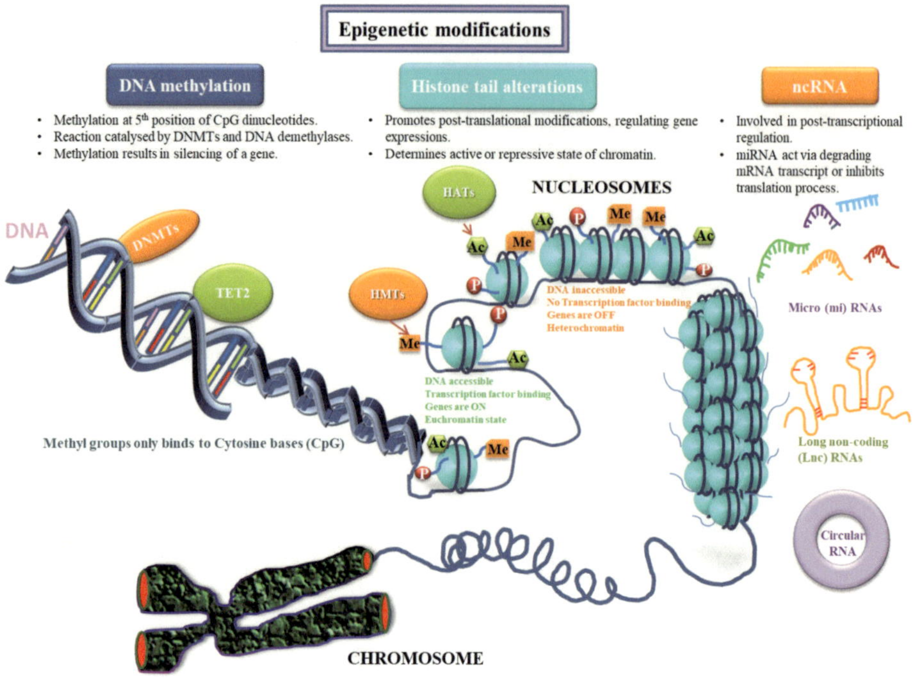


**Figure 3.**
*Framework of inheritable epigenetic modifications.*

*stimuli via regulation of miRNAs, thus directing several pathophysiological outcomes. DNMTs, DNA methyl transferases; HATs, Histone acetyl transferases; HDACs, Histone deacetylases; HMTs, Histone methyl transferases; HDMs, Histone demethylases; ncRNAs, non-coding RNAs, miRNAs, micro RNAs.*

### a. Methylation of DNA

It is the renowned epigenetic modification that is well studied in cancer, and lot of interest has been generated in DNA methylation in the framework of diabetes and its related complications. In detail, DNA undergoes methylation at 5th position of CpG dinucleotides and form 5-methylcytosine, which is a post-replicative mechanism. DNA methylation is extremely dynamic process in the progress of a disease, which tends to alter related gene expressions. These alterations can be reversed by external stimuli. Commonly repression of a gene takes place due to addition of methyl groups at promoter region on DNA, while methylation at gene bodies may regulate their transcription during elongation and also during alternative splicing [31].

DNA methyl transferases (DNMTs) are known to catalyze DNA methylation reaction which, in freshly synthesized DNA, methylates CpG dinucleotides. Hence, to sustain DNA methylation in proliferating cells, DNMTs are vital. Throughout the embryonic development, for *de novo* methylation, presence of DNMT-3a and -3b enzymes is obligatory [47]. The molecular effects of DNA methylation were interceded by a group of methyl binding domain (MBD) proteins. Out of these, merely MBD2 alone is identifiable for methyl-CpG positions, which guides the interaction of methylated DNA to a multifaceted complex encompassing nucleosome remodeling and histone deacetylases (HDACs) bustles, thereby conducting silencing of a gene [48]. DNA methylation is commonly studied by various methods including methylation specific PCR (MS-PCR), methylation sensitive high resolution melt curve (MS-HRM), immunoprecipitation or sequencing approaches. Advantage of MS-HRM is that it offers a low-cost and rapid method for the detection of even low levels of methylation at gene promoters.

Earlier exposure of target cells to high glucose can result in a 'metabolic memory' which results in persistence of its detrimental effects long after glucose stabilization. Diabetes-induced altered epigenetic mechanisms, resulting in modified gene expression in target cells can lead to diabetes-associated complications, such as diabetic nephropathy [39]. In the pathogenesis of DN and ESRD, DNAme (DNA methylation) has been explored by several studies via studying differentially methylated genes related to DN [31, 49, 50]. In a genome-wide methylation analysis (GWAS), significant alterations in DNA methylation in DN patients as compared to control were reported at 19 CpG sites that were found to be associated with the risk of DN. They also correlated the degree of methylation with time to development of DN [50]. In DNA isolated from the saliva of type 2 diabetic patients with end-stage kidney disease (ESRD), differentially site-specific methylation of DNA was recorded at 187 gene targets in comparison to those without ESRD [49]. DN patients have altered DNA methylation at important key gene promoters in comparison to those without DN [50]. However, studies in DN animal models or in renal cells under hyperglycemic conditions were not competent to show any significant changes in DNA methylation patterns [51]. In patients having type 2 diabetes with diabetic nephropathy, global DNA methylation variations were also observed to be associated with albuminuria in a recent study [52]. Noteworthy alterations in histone and DNA methylation patterns were observed to be present in peripheral blood mononuclear cells (PBMCs) of patients with membranous nephropathy [53]. Genome-wide DNA methylation study also depicted modifications in differential DNA methylation profiles among type 1 diabetes patients with or without nephropathy, where degree of methylation is linked with time towards the progression of DN [50].

It has been demonstrated that the promoter of human ACE gene, the most important and widely studied gene in pathophysiology of DN, harbor CpG islands. ACE transcription and expression levels were also observed to be influenced by methylation in its promoter region both in vivo and in vitro [54]. The magnitude of epigenetic alterations, particularly DNA methylation, has been shown to correlate with ACE activity levels [54, 55]. These studies demonstrated an increase in ACE activity with hypomethylation of ACE gene promoter. Also, a relation between epigenetics of ACE gene and I/D polymorphism has been suggested, where decreased DNA methylation in 3 CpG sites of ACE gene was observed in low birth weight (LBW) children with DD genotype although this has not been reported directly in DN patients [55]. Global DNA methylation variations were also observed to be associated with albuminuria in a recent study [52]. Additionally alterations in DNA methylation of ACE promoter are suggested to be a fundamental cause of major depression (MD) and a shared pathogenic factor for bi-directional connection between MD and cardiovascular disorders [56].

Apart from the importance of DNA methylation in DN, their role in DR is not clear, however, DNA methylation has been shown to control the expressions of many genes associated with retinal homeostasis. Previous studies have shown the link of DR development and DNA methylation, which indicates that DR may be associated with epigenetic alterations. In this connection, a GWAS between PDR and healthy controls was conducted in PBMC'S sample and out of 349 identified methylated sites, only 17 genes were observed to be hypermethylated [57]. They assumed that PBMCs could be used as a predictor for diabetic retinopathy. Another study evaluated global DNA methylation levels in blood leukocytes in persons with and without retinopathy [58]. They found a significantly higher global methylation levels in patients with DR than those without DR. These changes were seen to be progressive from non-DR stage to NPDR and eventually to PDR and were independent of hyperglycemia, dyslipidemia, diabetes duration and person's blood pressure. Binding of polymerase gamma 1 (POLG1) to mtDNA (mitochondrial DNA) also results in compromised transcriptional activity as a result of hypermethylation at promoter region of DNA polymerase gamma 1 (POLG1) in the hyperglycemic environment [42]. This study was conducted in rat model of diabetes which showed that the mitochondrial damage in retina of diabetic rats could be diminished/controlled by maintaining stable glycemic control for longer time periods or therapy that targets directly DNA methylation. However, it does not benefit DNA methylation machinery by the reversal of hyper-glycemic environment for shorter duration [59]. In people with diabetes mellitus, it has been seen that activity of Dnmt1 enzyme was elevated in retinal and its capillary cells. However, this was not observed with Dnmt-3a or Dnmt-3b [60, 61]. Similar differential DNA methylation patterns were also observed in persons with PDR [57].

b. **Histone modifications:**

It is the interesting and emerging mechanism that exhibits the addition of methyl groups at histones related to a gene. As DNA is structured into chromosomes in eukaryotic cells, it is tightly wrapped onto series of nucleosomes (the basic unit of chromatin), which are the octamer complexes of small core (a H3-H4 tetramer and two H2A-H2B dimers) linked by linker histone proteins (H1) [62]. These histones are involved in post-translational modifications (PTMs) which may regulate gene expressions. The gene activation and repression are determined by dynamic chromatin structure that directly depends upon these PTMs, as they will allow transformation of inactive or repressive chromatin to euchromatin, the active condition of chromatin. These modifications, like DNA methylation, are able to regulate the gene expression without any change in its DNA sequence. Hence, histone tails can be acetylated, methylated, or phosphorylated. Histones with methylated (Kme) or acetylated (Kac) lysine residues, mostly at amino terminal tails, have been identified. Generally, these modifications are correlated with either gene activation or repression. Like, on one hand, histone lysine acetylation (H3K9ac, H3K14ac and H4K5ac) is generally associated with gene activation that opens the chromatin for the binding of transcription machinery [63]. Histone acetylation is tightly controlled by the equilibrium between acetylation (HATs) and deacetylation (HDACs) enzymes that add or deletes acetyl group. On the other hand, methylation on lysine or arginine residues can be correlated with both, gene activation or gene repression, depending on the residue to be modified. For example, mono- or tri-methylation of Histone 3 at lysine 4 residue (H3K4me, H3K4me3), H3K79me2 [64] and at lysine 36 residue (H3K36me) facilitated by lysine methyl transferases (KMTs) such as SET1/7/9 are associated with gene activation [63]. Although, mono-methylation of histone 3 at lysine residue 9 (H3K9me) mediated by suppressor of variegation 3–9 homolog 1 (SUV39H1) is correlated with gene activation whilst, its trimethylation (H3K9me3) is linked with gene repression [65]. Additionally, H3K27me3 and H4K20 were associated with gene repression. Afterwards, lysine demethylases (LSD1) are there to reverse such steady modifications at H3K4 and H3K9 [66, 67] as a co-repressor or co-activator respectively. Their nomenclature has already been changed from LSD1 to lysine demethylases (KDMs) [68]. In a study in lymphocytes from type 1 diabetic patients, as compared to controls increased H3K9me2 levels were reported to be correlated with immune and inflammatory pathways associated with diabetes and its complications including DN [69]. Such histone modifications at N-terminal are two key mechanisms that may alter development and progression of diabetes and its related complications; they are noteworthy as discussed below.

In DN pathogenesis, expressions of a gene that are associated with DN are regulated by post-translational modifications of histone proteins, apart from DNA methylation. Smad2/3/4 (transcription factors) are activated by TGF-β and also team up with HATs and other chromatin remodeling factors. Alterations in DNA methylation and H3K9Ac at gene promoters were found to be associated with endothelial dysfunction in endothelial cells cultured in hyperglycemic conditions. Among various epigenetic mechanisms, methylation among core histone tails is considered to be the highly stable PTM that could be a key factor in the pathogenesis of various complications of diabetes. Previous studies have studied the role of histone modifications in cultured cells as well as animal model in the presence of TGF-β and high glucose environment, the two key factors in diabetes [70]. They reported an increased H3K9/14Ac at PAI-1 and p21 promoters near Smad/SP1 binding sites. Cultured rat mesangial cells (RMCs), obstructed by TGF-β antibodies, displayed increased levels of p21 and PAI-1 under hyperglycemic conditions. Also in glomeruli of diabetic animal model, increased expressions of PAI-1 and p21 were found to be linked with increased promoter H3K9/14Ac. In the model of DN, TGF-β stimulated expressions of key fibrotic genes were found to be associated with enrichment of histone active chromatin marks (H3K4me1/2/3) and reduced repressive chromatin marks (H3K9me2/3) at their promoters [71]. Collectively, TGF-β plays as an intermediator in hyperglycemia induced histone modifications of promoters of key genes in mesangial cells leading to kidney damage. In glomeruli of diabetic mice, increased chromatin active marks along with decreased repressive marks were observed at PAI-1 and receptor for AGE (RAGE) gene promoters as compared to control, which showed the regulation of histone modifications in kidney in the presence of hyperglycemia [72]. In addition, AT1R inhibitor decreased key indicators of DN and also reversed some of the epigenetic changes in diabetic mice including reduced H3K9/14Ac at PAI-1, RAGE and MCP-1 promoters in diabetic mesangial cells. In the animal models of DN, increased histone active marks (H3K4me2) and decreased repressive marks (H3K27me3) were observed to be associated with the expression of genes related to DN [73]. In the kidney of uninephrectomized db/db mice model, H3K4me2 levels were increased in association with albuminuria, glomerular filtration rate and glomerular cell proliferation, which can be reversed by MCP-1/CCL2 antagonist [74]. In diabetic kidneys, HDAC inhibitor (Trichostatin A) has been observed to block the induction of TGF-β at essential fibrotic genes, both *in vitro* and *in vivo*. This implies major role of HDACs in TGF-β facilitated kidney fibrosis and ECM accumulation [75]. In another study, treatment of renal epithelial cells with Trichostatin A (TSA) resulted in downregulated TGF-β mediated epithelial-to-mesenchymal transition (EMT) [75, 76]. Taken as a whole, these studies demonstrate the involvement of HDACs in renal injury via TGF-β.

Histone post-translational modifications have also been studied extensively in the context of DR. Increased oxidative stress and simultaneous decreased levels of retinal superoxide dismutase (SOD2) are the key features of DR. Increased histone repressive mark (H4K20me3) along with increased NF-κB p65 in association with decreased SOD2 mRNA levels and decreased activation marks (H3K4me1/2) at SOD2 promoters were observed in retinal endothelial cells cultured in high glucose. Acetylation of core histone protein on lysine residues is thought to opens up the DNA, thereby, increased availability for binding of transcription factors. Afterwards, activated proinflammatory transcription factors, for instance NF-κB, binds to particular sequence in DNA and activates and bind coactivators (like p300) having intrinsic HAT activity to the target promoters of target gene. These coactivator molecules then, regulate the expressions of target gene owing to their HAT activity [77]. Contrary to this, recruitment of HDACs results in compact chromatin, coiled DNA and less accessibility for binding of transcription factors to DNA, thereby decreased expression of target gene. Hence, the balance between acetylation and deacetylation of histones regulates the transcription of the gene. Increased HDACs and decreased HATs along with decreased global histone acetylation activities were also found in diabetic retinal cells in the models of diabetic retinopathy [78]. However, reversal of hyperglycemic conditions did not able to restore changes in histone activities. This is in contrast to a study in diabetes where activation of histone acetylation was observed in retinal cells [79]. Pro-apoptotic enzyme, MMP-9, is also observed to be associated with epigenetic alterations in DR [80, 81]. Lysine of histone 3 was reported to be methylated by SUV39H1 resulted in H3k9me3 [82]. Another methyl transferase gene i.e., SUV39H2 is involved in the onset of disease, when methylates histone H3K9 results in the inception of DR [83]. Moreover under hyperglycemic conditions, recruitment of Set7 (HMT) at promoter region of NF-KB p65 unit was linked with its enhanced transcription [44]. Western blotting and mass spectrometry studies in diabetic rat model also confirmed the acetylation of several lysine residues on histones due to hyperglycemia leading to increased expressions of proinflammatory proteins in retina and associated with DR [79].

Oxidative stress also plays a central role in diabetic complications and has been shown to control histone acetylation or deacetylation in diabetic conditions. High blood glucose is known to increase ROS production, which further activates important pathways that are required for the development of DR [84]. ROS is observed to inhibit acetylation of histones by increasing HDAC activity and decreasing HAT activity [85]. Hence, it was believed that there is involvement of ROS in regulating acetylation and deacetylation. Usually, oxidative stress was found to be increased in retina and capillary cells [86]. Thus, it is possible that diabetes via increased ROS production may regulates histone acetylation and deacetylation in retina. Ischemia and hypoxia are also known to promote the process of histone deacetylation [87] and hypoxia in diabetes is the leading cause for neovascularization in retina [88] which indicates the role of retinal hypoxia in diabetic retinopathy via stimulating retinal histone deacetylases. Thus, in hyperglycemia, epigenetic alterations may be involved at a larger level in modulating the expressions of various important genes in pathogenesis of DR.

Various researches on histone protein alterations may suggests that chromatin state is likely to be affected by multiple histone code modifications and hence, screening of various histone alterations at key genes promoters and/or bodies related to DN is crucial. The role of DNA methylation, histone code modifications and changes in epigenetic marks in response to various therapies is not well studied and would be of great concern to see whether these modifications could be altered in response to therapy. In future, more epigenome studies are required to elucidate the mechanisms of pathogenesis of DN that could help in developing better treatment strategies for people suffering from this devastating complication.

c. **Micro RNAs (miRNA):**

Whole transcriptome studies (RNA-sequencing) have uncovered that majority of the transcribed genome (into RNA) is non-coding part, apart from the coding mRNA [89]. Non-coding RNA refers to the RNA that does not code for any protein. These non-coding RNAs are also a part of epigenetic mechanisms that are of immense interest in the context of diabetic complications as they are observed to repress the expressions of target genes via regulating transcription and post-transcription mechanisms. Non-coding RNAs includes small non-coding RNAs (miRNAs approx. 20-22 bp long), circular RNAs (circRNAs) as well as long non-coding RNAs (lncRNAs approx. 200 bp long). They are reported to control the expressions of important genes associated with diabetic complications. In contrast to miRNAs, few studies have observed the role of lncRNAs in DN [90, 91]. miRNAs are usually single stranded RNA of approximately 20–25 nucleotides long. They are well-known non-coding RNAs that involved in post-transcriptional regulation by means of either suppression of translation or degradation of mRNA transcript by binding 3' UTR of target sequences [92, 93]. LncRNAs, instead, are usually longer (>200 bp) than miRNAs (20-22 bp). They function as scaffolds [94] and may regulate miRNA due to their antisense activity [95] and have tissue specific expressions [96]. Similar to mRNA, lncRNAs are formed due to transcription in the presence of RNA polymerase II and undergo splicing, although they are slightly polyadenylated [96]. LncRNAs also participate in modifications of epigenetic marks as they harbor histone methylation marks at H3k4 and H3K36 [97]. They are also reported to be involved in the development and progression of diabetic microvascular complications [98–101]. Recently circular RNAs, the next level of epigenetic regulation, are holding our interest in addition to lncRNAs as they are generated from mRNA via its back-splicing and later on both 5′ and 3′ spliced ends ligated together to form a circular structure. They regulate miRNAs, thereby regulating the expressions of miRNAs targetted genes. They also act as sponge for various miRNAs. Several circRNAs are observed to stimulate the pathogenesis of diabetes-related microvascular complications [102, 103].

On the other hand miRNAs, at first, were portrayed in *C. elegans*, a nematode, during early 1990s. Over 1000 miRNAs in human genome have been identified; lin-4 was the first described miRNA [104]. Various miRNAs are found in humans, algae, plants, animals and viruses [105]. miRNAs, unlike other small RNAs, are derived from the transcripts that themselves can rapidly fold back to form a hairpin-like structure. RNA polymerase II transcribed miRNA as primary transcript (pri-miRNA) in nucleus, where they are later spliced into precursor miRNAs (pre-miRNA) [106, 107] by the action of endonuclease complex. Exportin-5, a protein transport pre-miRNA into the cytoplasm from nucleus where they are further processed to mature miRNA duplex (~ 22 nucleotides) by the action of ribonucleases [107]. One strand of mature miRNAs is selected and loaded on RNA induced silencing complex (RISC) and other stand undergoes the process of degradation [106, 108]. This complex binds to their complementary sequence on mRNA for post-transcriptional suppression. Initially, lin-4 RNA was observed to have complementarity with conserved sites in mRNA of lin-14 [109] within untranslated (3'-UTR) site. But how to find their targets was the primary question in initial times. Algorithm tool, at first, identifies the perfect Watson-Crick pairing to 2–8 nucleotides of miRNAs starting from 5'region [110]. This 7 seven nucleotide sequence (at 5′-end) was termed as 'miRNA seed'. This finding was clearly in agreement with the earlier study which showed that 5′ end is the most conserved region in metazoan miRNAs [111]. Afterwards extending seed match with adding more base pairs to the miRNA continues in both directions, but stopping at discrepancies [110]. Therefore, the silencing effect of target gene by miRNA is via binding of seed sequence at miRNA with the complementary sequence at mRNA in 3'-UTR. miRNAs based therapies would have a better lead in that they can target multiple genes of a particular pathway or process [112]. Because, one miRNA can supress expression of many genes and subsequently one gene can also be targetted by more than one miRNAs. Another advantage is that these miRNAs can cross blood-retina barrier so as to get into the target tissue, which is the foremost obligation with this therapy. In past years, several studies have linked miRNAs with diabetic complications. Henceforth we have, now described the role of miRNAs in the pathogenesis of diabetes complications.

Several miRNAs including miR-29, miR-192, miR-194, miR-200b/c, miR-204, miR-215, miR-216a, miR-217, miR-377 etc. have been found to be associated with DN. Characteristics of DN includes fibrosis, accumulation of extracellular matrix (ECM), podocyte dysfunction and proteinuria [113, 114]. TGF-β has been implicated in the pathogenesis of DN and is found to be upregulated during the progression of DN, which in turn, induce fibrotic events, kidney deterioration and dysfunction [114]. TGF-β has shown to upregulate several miRNAs including miR-192, miR-216a, miR-217 in mesangial cells as well as in kidneys of diabetic mouse models as compared to control group [115–117]. ZEB2, a translation repressor that supress fibrotic gene collagen type 1 Alpha 2 (*Col1a2*), was observed to get suppressed by miR-192, thus, resulted in an increased expression of *Col1a2* gene and contribute to matrix accumulation and kidney fibrosis in DN model [115]. In diabetic mice, increased expressions of p53, TGF-β and miR-192 was reported in renal cortex and was found to be associated with augmented fibrosis and glomerular expansion as compared to control. Moreover, knockout of miR-192 gene resulted in decreased markers of DN. However, conflicting reports to these results are also described. One of such reports observed that TGF-β decreased the expression of miR-192 in cultured proximal tubule cells and concluded that decreased miR-192 levels are associated with increased fibrogenesis in PTCs [118]. Another study also showed that kidney fibrosis was associated with the loss of miR-192 [119]. These contradictory studies showed that the interconnection between DN and miR-192 is much more complicated than it seems. Also, a decreased expression of miR-21 was found in DN and albuminuria was decreased in diabetic mice due to ectopic expression of miR-21 [120]. miR-377 expression was found to be upregulated in DN [121]. It actually alters the levels of MnSOD and PAK1, which in turn, resulted in augmented fibronectin expression in mesangial cells in streptozotocin (STZ)-induced diabetic model, thus contributing to DN progression indirectly. TGF-β induced miR-216a expression has been shown to increased collagen (*Col1a2*) expression [116] and subsequently participates in the fibrogenesis in proximal tubular cells (PTCs) [122]. Another important contributor to DN is VEGF and treatment with anti-VEGF showed to improve kidney functions in diabetic animal model [123]. Earlier miRNA-93 was considered as 'signature miRNA' in both *in vivo* as well as *in vitro* hyperglycemic environment [124]. Long et al. also demonstrated that increased expression of miR-93 resulted in reduced high glucose-stimulated VEGF-A levels via downregulation of the host *MCM7* gene promoter.

Earlier studies have also reported the role of miRNAs in diabetic retinopathy. Neovascularization is the hallmark of DR and several studies have confirmed the importance of miRNAs in neovascularization regulation in retina [125]. Microarray studies recognized increased (miR-146, miR-106a, miR-181, miR-199a, miR-214, miR-424 and miR-451) as well as decreased expressions of various miRNAs (miR-31, miR-150, miR-184) in model of ischemic retinopathy [126]. In retina and retinal endothelial cells (RECs), increased miRNAs corresponding to NF-κB, p53 and VEGF were identified reflecting pathological changes of early DR by means of functional analysis, thus, revealing the role of miRNA in pathogenesis of DR [127]. In diabetes, downregulated miR-200b was detected in retina of diabetic rat model with simultaneous elevated levels of VEGF mRNA and protein. In addition, *in vitro* miR-200b antagonist transfection resulted in elevated VEGF expression [128]. This demonstrates VEGF to be the direct target of miR-200b. During early stage of diabetes, miR-29 shown to be anti-apoptotic for retinal ganglion cells (RGCs) and inner nuclear layer (INL) cells through pro-apoptotic RNA dependent (PKR) signaling pathway [129].

Therefore, this chapter has enlightened the role and contribution of epigenetic mechanisms in the pathogenesis of two major diabetic vascular complications i.e.,

DN and DR. Together all, it indicates the important connection of miRNAs with microvascular complications of diabetes; hence, it would be worth to explore the role of these alterations in the pathophysiology of DN as well as DR. As reviewed in this chapter, methylation in DNA, histone tail alterations and variable expressions of miRNAs are found to be altered in hyperglycemic environment either upregulated or downregulated affecting directly or indirectly. Current treatment for DN and DR is not able to stop the progression of these devastating complications, henceforth, focusing treatment approaches via targeting epigenetic alterations alone or in combination with conventional therapy could provide a new approach to combat or retard the progression of these diabetic complications. However, the fact that a particular miRNA can have multiple targets made it difficult and challenging with few limitations, still it will increase our understanding about the disease pathophysiology.

## 4. Targeting diabetic complications via targeting epigenetic marks

Heritable epigenetic alterations are the results of interactions between environmental (momentary) and genetic (long-standing) components and thus, may play a decisive role in the pathophysiology of diabetic complications. They are able to alter the gene expression, thereby, gene function, the underline mechanism in the pathogenesis of vascular complications of diabetes. Reversible attribute of epigenetic marks provides immense opportunity of developing restorative interventions for treating patients with these complications. Till date, some of the drugs targeting epigenetic marks are already being clinically used for cancer therapy including HDAC inhibitors [130] and DNA methylation inhibitors [131, 132]. However, preclinical studies targeting histone as well as DNA methylation are still in progress [133–135]. Metformin, the current line of drug for treating hyperglycemia, upregulates sirtuin 1 (SIRT1) expression along with downregulating NF-κB expression [136], SIRT1 has been shown to possess $NAD^+$-dependent protein deacetylase activity [137]. In glomerular mesangial cells, SIRT 1 induces antioxidant genes and simultaneously downregulates TGF-β1 and the expression of AGEs-induced fibronectin [138]. In diabetic mice glomeruli, BF175, a SIRT1 agonist, ameliorates hyperglycemia-induced podocyte loss, proving the protective role of SIRT1 against diabetes-induced kidney damage [139]. Recently, angiotensin II (Ang II) of RAAS has been reported to induce the expressions of few non-coding RNAs including miRNAs [140] and lncRNAs [141] as well. Enhancers, the elements that affect transcription of genes and are associated with specific histone modifications [142], when blocked by JQ1, a Bromodomain (an epigenetic reader) inhibitor, also obstructs enhancer functions along with attenuation of Ang II-mediated hypertension and inflammation *in vivo* in vascular smooth muscle cells (VSMCs) [143], hence, strongly supporting the importance of targeting enhancers in Ang II-mediated actions for treating vascular complications. This, in turn, could reveal evidence directing new therapeutic interventions for treatment of diabetic vascular complications. In addition, the modified inhibitor of miR-192 i.e., Locked nucleic acid (LNA) not only downregulates key fibrotic markers of kidney damage but also shown to reduce proteinuria in diabetic mice [144], favoring miRNAs based therapeutic interventions for DN. Several studies have also reported the amelioration of kidney-injury parameters via targeting miR-21 [145–147] implying that its inhibition could be a promising therapeutic intervention in DN. Recently with the use of latest and advanced approach of genome editing i.e., CRISPR-Cas9, locus-specific changes in epigenetic alterations could be generated owing to the fusion of Cas9 proteins with various DNMTs or TETs or histone modification proteins [148–150], thus, reversing the epigenetic marks of important genes involved in the pathogenesis of s disease. Despite extensive ongoing research, more detailed epigenetics-targeted approach is required to combat diabetic microvascular complications.

## 5. Conclusion

In conclusion, discovering specific role and targeting pathways related to epigenetic alterations for the development of therapeutic interventions in T2DM patients with microvascular complications could be promising. Moreover, this will certainly be helpful in increasing our knowledge and developing tools for better and early diagnosis and subsequent more effective treatment of these distressing complications in clinical practice.

## Author details

Neerja Aggarwal[1] and Pawan Kumar Kare[2*]

1 Department of Medicine, University College of Medical Sciences and Guru Teg Bahadur Hospital, Delhi, India

2 Department of Medical Biochemistry, Gandhi Medical College, Bhopal, India

*Address all correspondence to: pawankare4@gmail.com

## References

[1] Tuomilehto J, Lindström J, Eriksson JG, Valle TT, Hämäläinen H, Ilanne-Parikka P, et al. Prevention of type 2 diabetes mellitus by changes in lifestyle among subjects with impaired glucose tolerance. New England Journal of Medicine. 2001;**344**(18):1343-1350

[2] Association AD. 2. Classification and diagnosis of diabetes. Diabetes care. 2015;38(Supplement 1):S8-S16.

[3] Atlas D. International, Federation D. IDF Diabetes Atlas. 7th ed. International Diabetes Federation: Brussels, Belgium; 2015

[4] Anjana RM, Deepa M, Pradeepa R, Mahanta J, Narain K, Das HK, et al. Prevalence of diabetes and prediabetes in 15 states of India: Results from the ICMR–INDIAB population-based cross-sectional study. The Lancet Diabetes & Endocrinology. 2017;**5**(8):585-596

[5] Zhao Y, Ye W, Boye KS, Holcombe JH, Hall JA, Swindle R. Prevalence of other diabetes-associated complications and comorbidities and its impact on health care charges among patients with diabetic neuropathy. Journal of Diabetes and its Complications. 2010;**24**(1):9-19

[6] Shahbazian H, Rezaii I. Diabetic kidney disease; review of the current knowledge. Journal of renal injury prevention. 2013;**2**(2):73

[7] Rajput R, Kumar K, Seshadri K, Agarwal P, Talwalkar P, Kotak B, et al. Prevalence of chronic kidney disease (CKD) in type 2 diabetes mellitus patients: START-India study. JOURNAL OF DIABETES & METABOLISM. 2017;8(2).

[8] Jensen T, Borch-Johnsen K, Kofoed-Enevoldsen A, Deckert T. Coronary heart disease in young type 1 (insulin-dependent) diabetic patients with and without diabetic nephropathy: Incidence and risk factors. Diabetologia. 1987;**30**(3):144-148

[9] Seidegård J, Vorachek WR, Pero RW, Pearson WR. Hereditary differences in the expression of the human glutathione transferase active on trans-stilbene oxide are due to a gene deletion. Proceedings of the National Academy of Sciences. 1988;**85**(19):7293-7297

[10] Amal S, Zidan HE, Rashad NM. Adiponectin gene polymorphisms in Egyptian type 2 diabetes mellitus patients with and without diabetic nephropathy. Molecular biology reports. 2014;**41**(4):2287-2298

[11] Shah VN, Cheema BS, Sharma R, Khullar M, Kohli HS, Ahluwalia TS, et al. ACACβ gene (rs2268388) and AGTR1 gene (rs5186) polymorphism and the risk of nephropathy in Asian Indian patients with type 2 diabetes. Molecular and Cellular Biochemistry. 2013;**372**(1-2):191-198

[12] Deshmukh H, Palmer C, Morris A, Colhoun H. Investigation of known estimated glomerular filtration rate loci in patients with type 2 diabetes. Diabetic medicine. 2013;**30**(10):1230-1235

[13] Hussain H, Ramachandran V, Ravi S, Sajan T, Ehambaram K, Gurramkonda VB, et al. TCF7L2 rs7903146 polymorphism and diabetic nephropathy association is not independent of type 2 diabetes—A study in a south Indian population and meta-analysis. Endokrynologia Polska. 2014;**65**(4):298-305

[14] Jia H, Yu L, Gao B, Ji Q. Association between the T869C polymorphism of transforming growth factor-beta 1 and diabetic nephropathy: A meta-analysis. Endocrine. 2011;**40**(3):372-378

[15] Nazir N, Siddiqui K, Al-Qasim S, Al-Naqeb D. Meta-analysis of diabetic

nephropathy associated genetic variants in inflammation and angiogenesis involved in different biochemical pathways. BMC Medical Genetics. 2014;**15**(1):103

[16] Lu M, Zhang J, Li M, Ge X, Dai X, Zhao J, et al. The angiotensin-I converting enzyme gene I/D variation contributes to end-stage renal disease risk in Chinese patients with type 2 diabetes receiving hemodialysis. Molecular and Cellular Biochemistry. 2016;**422**(1-2):181-188

[17] Currie D, McKnight A, Patterson C, Sadlier D, Maxwell A, Group UWGS. Investigation of ACE, ACE2 and AGTR1 genes for association with nephropathy in type 1 diabetes mellitus. Diabetic medicine. 2010;**27**(10):1188-1194

[18] Seman NA, He B, Ojala JR, Mohamud WNW, Östenson C-G, Brismar K, et al. Genetic and biological effects of sodium-chloride cotransporter (SLC12A3) in diabetic nephropathy. American journal of nephrology. 2014;**40**(5):408-416

[19] Aggarwal N, Kare PK, Varshney P, Kalra OP, Madhu SV, Banerjee BD, et al. Role of angiotensin converting enzyme and angiotensinogen gene polymorphisms in angiotensin converting enzyme inhibitor-mediated antiproteinuric action in type 2 diabetic nephropathy patients. World Journal of Diabetes. 2017;**8**(3):112

[20] Group ER. Retinopathy and nephropathy in type 1 diabetes patients four years after trial of intensive therapy. The New England Journal of Medicine. 2000;**342**:381-389

[21] Klein R, Klein BE, Moss SE, Davis MD, DeMets DL. The Wisconsin epidemiologic study of diabetic retinopathy: II. Prevalence and risk of diabetic retinopathy when age at diagnosis is less than 30 years. Archives of Ophthalmology. 1984;**102**(4):520-526

[22] Matthews DR, Stratton IM, Aldington SJ, Holman RR, Kohner EM, Group UPDS. Risks of progression of retinopathy and vision loss related to tight blood pressure control in type 2 diabetes mellitus: UKPDS 69. Archives of ophthalmology (Chicago, Ill: 1960). 2004;122(11):1631.

[23] Ferris FL, Chew EY, Hoogwerf BJ, Group ETDRSR. Serum lipids and diabetic retinopathy. Diabetes Care. 1996;**19**(11):1291-1293

[24] Abhary S, Hewitt AW, Burdon KP, Craig JE. A systematic meta-analysis of genetic association studies for diabetic retinopathy. Diabetes. 2009;**58**(9):2137-2147

[25] Simó-Servat O, Hernández C, Simó R. Genetics in diabetic retinopathy: Current concepts and new insights. Current Genomics. 2013;**14**(5):289-299

[26] Zhou J-B, Yang J-K. Angiotensin-converting enzyme gene polymorphism is associated with proliferative diabetic retinopathy: A meta-analysis. Acta diabetologica. 2010;**47**(1):187-193

[27] Kumaramanickavel G, Ramprasad VL, Sripriya S, Upadyay NK, Paul PG, Sharma T. Association of Gly82Ser polymorphism in the RAGE gene with diabetic retinopathy in type II diabetic Asian Indian patients. Journal of Diabetes and its Complications. 2002;**16**(6):391-394

[28] Kundu TK. Epigenetics : Development and Disease. 2013.

[29] Aguilera O, Fernández AF, Muñoz A, Fraga MF. Epigenetics and environment: A complex relationship. Journal of Applied Physiology. 2010;**109**(1):243-251

[30] Waddington CH. The epigenotype. International journal of epidemiology. 2011;**41**(1):10-13

[31] Reddy MA, Park JT, Natarajan R, editors. Epigenetic modifications in the pathogenesis of diabetic nephropathy. Seminars in nephrology; 2013: Elsevier.

[32] Probst AV, Dunleavy E, Almouzni G. Epigenetic inheritance during the cell cycle. Nature reviews Molecular cell biology. 2009;**10**(3):192

[33] Feinberg AP. Phenotypic plasticity and the epigenetics of human disease. Nature. 2007;**447**(7143):433

[34] Bramswig NC, Kaestner KH. Epigenetics and diabetes treatment: An unrealized promise? Trends in Endocrinology & Metabolism. 2012;**23**(6):286-291

[35] Berger SL, Kouzarides T, Shiekhattar R, Shilatifard A. An operational definition of epigenetics. Genes & development. 2009;**23**(7):781-783

[36] Roseboom TJ, Van Der Meulen JH, Ravelli AC, Osmond C, Barker DJ, Bleker OP. Effects of prenatal exposure to the Dutch famine on adult disease in later life: An overview. Molecular and cellular endocrinology. 2001;**185**(1-2):93-98

[37] KHAN O. GROVER D. Effect of Methylation on Gene Expression.

[38] Ling C, Groop L. Epigenetics: A molecular link between environmental factors and type 2 diabetes. Diabetes. 2009;**58**(12):2718-2725

[39] Khullar M. Cheema BS. Raut SK. emerging evidence of epigenetic Modifications in vascular Complication of Diabetes. Frontiers in endocrinology. 2017;**8**:237

[40] Pirola L, Balcerczyk A, Tothill RW, Haviv I, Kaspi A, Lunke S, et al. Genome-wide analysis distinguishes hyperglycemia regulated epigenetic signatures of primary vascular cells. Genome Research. 2011;**21**(10):1601-1615

[41] Ling C, Del Guerra S, Lupi R, Rönn T, Granhall C, Luthman H, et al. Epigenetic regulation of PPARGC1A in human type 2 diabetic islets and effect on insulin secretion. Diabetologia. 2008;**51**(4):615-622

[42] Tewari S, Zhong Q, Santos JM, Kowluru RA. Mitochondria DNA replication and DNA methylation in the metabolic memory associated with continued progression of diabetic retinopathy. Investigative ophthalmology & visual science. 2012;53(8):4881-8.

[43] Olsen AS, Sarras MP, Leontovich A, Intine RV. Heritable transmission of diabetic metabolic memory in zebrafish correlates with DNA hypomethylation and aberrant gene expression. Diabetes. 2012;**61**(2):485-491

[44] El-Osta A, Brasacchio D, Yao D, Pocai A, Jones PL, Roeder RG, et al. Transient high glucose causes persistent epigenetic changes and altered gene expression during subsequent normoglycemia. The Journal of experimental medicine. 2008;**205**(10):2409-2417

[45] Feng B, Chen S, George B, Feng Q, Chakrabarti S. miR133a regulates cardiomyocyte hypertrophy in diabetes. Diabetes/metabolism research and reviews. 2010;**26**(1):40-49

[46] Wang X, Qian R, Zhang W, Chen S, Jin H, Hu R. MicroRNA-320 expression in myocardial microvascular endothelial cells and its relationship with insulin-like growth factor-1 in type 2 diabetic rats. Clinical and Experimental Pharmacology and Physiology. 2009;**36**(2):181-188

[47] Patra SK, Deb M, Patra A. Molecular marks for epigenetic identification of developmental and cancer stem cells. Clinical Epigenetics. 2011;**2**(1):27

[48] Klose RJ, Bird AP. Genomic DNA methylation: The mark and its mediators. Trends in biochemical sciences. 2006;**31**(2):89-97

[49] Sapienza C, Lee J, Powell J, Erinle O, Yafai F, Reichert J, et al. DNA methylation profiling identifies epigenetic differences between diabetes patients with ESRD and diabetes patients without nephropathy. Epigenetics. 2011;**6**(1):20-28

[50] Bell CG, Teschendorff AE, Rakyan VK, Maxwell AP, Beck S, Savage DA. Genome-wide DNA methylation analysis for diabetic nephropathy in type 1 diabetes mellitus. BMC Medical Genomics. 2010;**3**(1):33

[51] Reddy MA, Natarajan R. Epigenetics in diabetic kidney disease. Journal of the American Society of Nephrology. 2011;**22**(12):2182-2185

[52] Maghbooli Z, Larijani B, Emamgholipour S, Amini M, Keshtkar A, Pasalar P. Aberrant DNA methylation patterns in diabetic nephropathy. Journal of Diabetes & Metabolic Disorders. 2014;**13**(1):69

[53] Sui WG, He HY, Yan Q, Chen JJ, Zhang RH, Dai Y. ChIP-seq analysis of histone H3K9 trimethylation in peripheral blood mononuclear cells of membranous nephropathy patients. Brazilian Journal of Medical and Biological Research. 2014;**47**(1):42-49

[54] Rivière G, Lienhard D, Andrieu T, Vieau D, Frey BM, Frey FJ. Epigenetic regulation of somatic angiotensin-converting enzyme by DNA methylation and histone acetylation. Epigenetics. 2011;**6**(4):478-489

[55] Rangel M, dos Santos JC, Ortiz PHL, Hirata M, Jasiulionis MG, Araujo RC, et al. Modification of epigenetic patterns in low birth weight children: Importance of hypomethylation of the ACE gene promoter. PLoS One. 2014;**9**(8):e106138

[56] Zill P. DNA Methylation Analysis of the Angiotensin Converting Enzyme (ACE) Gene in Major Depression. 2012;7(7).

[57] Agardh E, Lundstig A, Perfilyev A, Volkov P, Freiburghaus T, Lindholm E, et al. Genome-wide analysis of DNA methylation in subjects with type 1 diabetes identifies epigenetic modifications associated with proliferative diabetic retinopathy. BMC medicine. 2015;**13**(1):182

[58] Maghbooli Z, Hossein-nezhad A, Larijani B, Amini M, Keshtkar A. Global DNA methylation as a possible biomarker for diabetic retinopathy. Diabetes/metabolism research and reviews. 2015;**31**(2):183-189

[59] Mishra M, Kowluru RA. The role of DNA methylation in the metabolic memory phenomenon associated with the continued progression of diabetic retinopathy. Investigative ophthalmology & visual science. 2016;**57**(13):5748-5757

[60] Tewari S, Santos JM, Kowluru RA. Damaged mitochondrial DNA replication system and the development of diabetic retinopathy. Antioxidants & redox signaling. 2012;**17**(3):492-504

[61] Mishra M, Kowluru RA. Epigenetic modification of mitochondrial DNA in the development of diabetic retinopathy. Investigative ophthalmology & visual science. 2015;**56**(9):5133-5142

[62] Luger K, Mäder AW, Richmond RK, Sargent DF, Richmond TJ. Crystal structure of the nucleosome core particle at 2.8 Å resolution. Nature. 1997;**389**(6648):251-260

[63] Glozak M, Seto E. Histone deacetylases and cancer. Oncogene. 2007;**26**(37):5420-5432

[64] Wang Z, Zang C, Rosenfeld JA, Schones DE, Barski A, Cuddapah S,

et al. Combinatorial patterns of histone acetylations and methylations in the human genome. Nature genetics. 2008;**40**(7):897-903

[65] Nightingale KP, O'Neill LP, Turner BM. Histone modifications: Signalling receptors and potential elements of a heritable epigenetic code. Current opinion in genetics & development. 2006;**16**(2):125-136

[66] Cai C, He HH, Gao S, Chen S, Yu Z, Gao Y, et al. Lysine-specific demethylase 1 has dual functions as a major regulator of androgen receptor transcriptional activity. Cell Reports. 2014;**9**(5):1618-1627

[67] Carnesecchi J, Forcet C, Zhang L, Tribollet V, Barenton B, Boudra R, et al. ERRα induces H3K9 demethylation by LSD1 to promote cell invasion. Proceedings of the National Academy of Sciences. 2017;**114**(15):3909-3914

[68] Allis CD, Berger SL, Cote J, Dent S, Jenuwien T, Kouzarides T, et al. New nomenclature for chromatin-modifying enzymes. Cell. 2007;**131**(4):633-636

[69] Miao F, Wu X, Zhang L, Riggs AD, Natarajan R. Histone methylation patterns are cell-type specific in human monocytes and lymphocytes and well maintained at core genes. The Journal of Immunology. 2008;**180**(4):2264-2269

[70] Yuan H, Reddy MA, Sun G, Lanting L, Wang M, Kato M, et al. Involvement of p300/CBP and epigenetic histone acetylation in TGF-β1-mediated gene transcription in mesangial cells. American Journal of Physiology-Renal Physiology. 2013;**304**(5):F601-FF13

[71] Sun G, Reddy MA, Yuan H, Lanting L, Kato M, Natarajan R. Epigenetic histone methylation modulates fibrotic gene expression. Journal of the American Society of Nephrology. 2010;**21**(12):2069-2080

[72] Reddy MA, Sumanth P, Lanting L, Yuan H, Wang M, Mar D, et al. Losartan reverses permissive epigenetic changes in renal glomeruli of diabetic db/db mice. Kidney international. 2014;**85**(2):362-373

[73] Komers R, Mar D, Denisenko O, Xu B, Oyama TT, Bomsztyk K. Epigenetic changes in renal genes dysregulated in mouse and rat models of type 1 diabetes. Laboratory investigation. 2013;**93**(5):543-552

[74] Sayyed SG, Gaikwad AB, Lichtnekert J, Kulkarni O, Eulberg D, Klussmann S, et al. Progressive glomerulosclerosis in type 2 diabetes is associated with renal histone H3K9 and H3K23 acetylation, H3K4 dimethylation and phosphorylation at serine 10. Nephrology dialysis transplantation. 2010;**25**(6):1811-1817

[75] Noh H, Oh EY, Seo JY, Yu MR, Kim YO, Ha H, et al. Histone deacetylase-2 is a key regulator of diabetes-and transforming growth factor-β1-induced renal injury. American Journal of Physiology-Renal Physiology. 2009;**297**(3):F729-FF39

[76] Yoshikawa M, Hishikawa K, Marumo T, Fujita T. Inhibition of histone deacetylase activity suppresses epithelial-to-mesenchymal transition induced by TGF-β1 in human renal epithelial cells. Journal of the American Society of Nephrology. 2007;**18**(1):58-65

[77] Ogryzko VV, Schiltz RL, Russanova V, Howard BH, Nakatani Y. The transcriptional coactivators p300 and CBP are histone acetyltransferases. Cell. 1996;**87**(5):953-959

[78] Zhong Q, Kowluru RA. Role of histone acetylation in the development of diabetic retinopathy and the metabolic memory phenomenon. Journal of Cellular Biochemistry. 2010;**110**(6):1306-1313

[79] Kadiyala CSR, Zheng L, Du Y, Yohannes E, Kao H-Y, Miyagi M, et al. Acetylation of retinal histones in diabetes increases inflammatory proteins effects of minocycline and manipulation of histone acetyltransferase (HAT) and histone deacetylase (HDAC). Journal of Biological Chemistry. 2012;**287**(31):25869-25880

[80] Zhong Q, Kowluru RA. Regulation of matrix metalloproteinase-9 by epigenetic modifications and the development of diabetic retinopathy. Diabetes. 2013;**62**(7):2559-2568

[81] Kowluru RA, Shan Y, Mishra M. Dynamic DNA methylation of matrix metalloproteinase-9 in the development of diabetic retinopathy. Laboratory investigation. 2016;**96**(10):1040-1049

[82] Muramatsu D, Kimura H, Kotoshiba K, Tachibana M, Shinkai Y. Pericentric H3K9me3 formation by HP1 interaction-defective histone methyltransferase Suv39h1. Cell Structure and Function. 2016;**16013**

[83] Joglekar MV, Januszewski AS, Jenkins AJ, Hardikar AA. Circulating microRNA biomarkers of diabetic retinopathy. Diabetes. 2016;**65**(1):22-24

[84] Kanwar M, Kowluru RA. Role of glyceraldehyde 3-phosphate dehydrogenase in the development and progression of diabetic retinopathy. Diabetes. 2009;**58**(1):227-234

[85] Berthiaume M, Boufaied N, Moisan A, Gaudreau L. High levels of oxidative stress globally inhibit gene transcription and histone acetylation. DNA and cell biology. 2006;**25**(2):124-134

[86] Kowluru RA. Diabetic retinopathy: Mitochondrial dysfunction and retinal capillary cell death. Antioxidants & redox signaling. 2005;**7**(11-12):1581

[87] Ellis L, Hammers H, Pili R. Targeting tumor angiogenesis with histone deacetylase inhibitors. Cancer letters. 2009;**280**(2):145-153

[88] Frank R. Retinopathy D. Diabetic retinopathy N Engl J Med. 2004;**350**:48-58

[89] Reddy MA, Natarajan R. Epigenetic mechanisms in diabetic vascular complications. Cardiovascular Research. 2011;**90**(3):421-429

[90] Puthanveetil P, Chen S, Feng B, Gautam A, Chakrabarti S. Long non-coding RNA MALAT 1 regulates hyperglycaemia induced inflammatory process in the endothelial cells. Journal of cellular and molecular medicine. 2015;**19**(6):1418-1425

[91] Long J, Badal SS, Ye Z, Wang Y, Ayanga BA, Galvan DL, et al. Long noncoding RNA Tug1 regulates mitochondrial bioenergetics in diabetic nephropathy. The Journal of clinical investigation. 2016;**126**(11):4205-4218

[92] He L, Hannon GJ. MicroRNAs: Small RNAs with a big role in gene regulation. Nature Reviews Genetics. 2004;**5**(7):522-531

[93] Bartel DP. MicroRNAs: target recognition and regulatory functions. cell. 2009;136(2):215-33.

[94] Spitale RC, Tsai M-C, Chang HY. RNA templating the epigenome. Epigenetics. 2011;**6**(5):539-543

[95] Faghihi MA, Zhang M, Huang J, Modarresi F, Van der Brug MP, Nalls MA, et al. Evidence for natural antisense transcript-mediated inhibition of microRNA function. Genome Biology. 2010;**11**(5):R56

[96] Cabili MN, Trapnell C, Goff L, Koziol M, Tazon-Vega B, Regev A, et al. Integrative annotation of human large intergenic noncoding RNAs

reveals global properties and specific subclasses. Genes & Development. 2011;**25**(18):1915-1927

[97] Guttman M, Amit I, Garber M, French C, Lin MF, Feldser D, et al. Chromatin signature reveals over a thousand highly conserved large non-coding RNAs in mammals. Nature. 2009;**458**(7235):223-227

[98] Yi H, Peng R, Zhang L-y, Sun Y, Peng H-m, Liu H-d, et al. LincRNA-Gm4419 knockdown ameliorates NF-κ B/NLRP3 inflammasome-mediated inflammation in diabetic nephropathy. Cell death & disease. 2017;8(2):e2583-e.

[99] Duan L-J, Ding M, Hou L-J, Cui Y-T, Li C-J, Yu D-M. Long noncoding RNA TUG1 alleviates extracellular matrix accumulation via mediating microRNA-377 targeting of PPARγ in diabetic nephropathy. Biochemical and biophysical research communications. 2017;**484**(3):598-604

[100] Li Y, Xu F, Xiao H, Han F. Long noncoding RNA BDNF-AS inversely regulated BDNF and modulated high-glucose induced apoptosis in human retinal pigment epithelial cells. Journal of Cellular Biochemistry. 2018;**119**(1):817-823

[101] Thomas AA, Feng B, Chakrabarti S. ANRIL: A regulator of VEGF in diabetic retinopathy. Investigative ophthalmology & visual science. 2017;**58**(1):470-480

[102] Hu W, Han Q, Zhao L, Wang L. Circular RNA circRNA_15698 aggravates the extracellular matrix of diabetic nephropathy mesangial cells via miR-185/TGF-β1. Journal of Cellular Physiology. 2019;**234**(2):1469-1476

[103] Zhang S-J, Chen X, Li C-P, Li X-M, Liu C, Liu B-H, et al. Identification and characterization of circular RNAs as a new class of putative biomarkers in diabetes retinopathy. Investigative ophthalmology & visual science. 2017;**58**(14):6500-6509

[104] Lee RC, Feinbaum RL, Ambros V. The C. *elegans* heterochronic gene lin-4 encodes small RNAs with antisense complementarity to lin-14. cell. 1993;75(5):843-54.

[105] Griffiths-Jones S, Saini HK, Van Dongen S, Enright AJ. miRBase: tools for microRNA genomics. Nucleic acids research. 2007;36(suppl_1):D154-D8.

[106] Filipowicz W, Bhattacharyya SN, Sonenberg N. Mechanisms of post-transcriptional regulation by microRNAs: Are the answers in sight? Nature reviews genetics. 2008;**9**(2):102-114

[107] Kim VN. MicroRNA biogenesis: Coordinated cropping and dicing. Nature reviews Molecular cell biology. 2005;**6**(5):376-385

[108] Hutvágner G, Zamore PD. A microRNA in a multiple-turnover RNAi enzyme complex. Science. 2002;**297**(5589):2056-2060

[109] Wightman B, Ha I, Ruvkun G. Posttranscriptional regulation of the heterochronic gene lin-14 by lin-4 mediates temporal pattern formation in C. elegans. Cell. 1993;**75**(5):855-862

[110] Lewis BP, Shih IH, Jones-Rhoades MW, Bartel DP, Burge CB. Prediction of mammalian microRNA targets. Cell. 2003;**115**(7):787-798

[111] Lim LP, Lau NC, Weinstein EG, Abdelhakim A, Yekta S, Rhoades MW, et al. The microRNAs of Caenorhabditis elegans. Genes & development. 2003;**17**(8):991-1008

[112] Caroli A, Cardillo MT, Galea R, Biasucci LM. Potential therapeutic role of microRNAs in ischemic heart disease. Journal of Cardiology. 2013;**61**(5):315-320

[113] Kato M, Park JT, Natarajan R. MicroRNAs and the glomerulus. Experimental Cell Research. 2012;**318**(9):993-1000

[114] Ziyadeh FN, Sharma K. <strong>overview:</strong> combating diabetic nephropathy. Journal of the American Society of Nephrology. 2003;**14**(5):1355-1357

[115] Kato M, Zhang J, Wang M, Lanting L, Yuan H, Rossi JJ, et al. MicroRNA-192 in diabetic kidney glomeruli and its function in TGF-beta-induced collagen expression via inhibition of E-box repressors. Proceedings of the National Academy of Sciences of the United States of America. 2007;**104**(9):3432-3437

[116] Kato M, Wang L, Putta S, Wang M, Yuan H, Sun G, et al. Post-transcriptional up-regulation of Tsc-22 by Ybx1, a target of miR-216a, mediates TGF-{beta}-induced collagen expression in kidney cells. The Journal of biological chemistry. 2010;**285**(44):34004-34015

[117] Kato M, Arce L, Wang M, Putta S, Lanting L, Natarajan R. A microRNA circuit mediates transforming growth factor-β1 autoregulation in renal glomerular mesangial cells. Kidney international. 2011;**80**(4):358-368

[118] Krupa A, Jenkins R, Luo DD, Lewis A, Phillips A, Fraser D. Loss of MicroRNA-192 promotes fibrogenesis in diabetic nephropathy. Journal of the American Society of Nephrology : JASN. 2010;**21**(3):438-447

[119] Wang B, Herman-Edelstein M, Koh P, Burns W, Jandeleit-Dahm K, Watson A, et al. E-cadherin expression is regulated by miR-192/215 by a mechanism that is independent of the profibrotic effects of transforming growth factor-beta. Diabetes. 2010;**59**(7):1794-1802

[120] Zhang Z, Peng H, Chen J, Chen X, Han F, Xu X, et al. MicroRNA-21 protects from mesangial cell proliferation induced by diabetic nephropathy in db/db mice. FEBS letters. 2009;**583**(12):2009-2014

[121] Wang Q, Wang Y, Minto AW, Wang J, Shi Q, Li X, et al. MicroRNA-377 is up-regulated and can lead to increased fibronectin production in diabetic nephropathy. The FASEB Journal. 2008;**22**(12):4126-4135

[122] Fraser DJ, Phillips AO, Zhang X, van Roeyen CR, Muehlenberg P, En-Nia A, et al. Y-box protein-1 controls transforming growth factor-beta1 translation in proximal tubular cells. Kidney International. 2008;**73**(6):724-732

[123] Flyvbjerg A, Dagnæs-Hansen F, De Vriese AS, Schrijvers BF, Tilton RG, Rasch R. Amelioration of long-term renal changes in obese type 2 diabetic mice by a neutralizing vascular endothelial growth factor antibody. Diabetes. 2002;**51**(10):3090-3094

[124] Long J, Wang Y, Wang W, Chang BH, Danesh FR. Identification of microRNA-93 as a novel regulator of vascular endothelial growth factor in hyperglycemic conditions. Journal of biological chemistry. 2010;**285**(30):23457-23465

[125] Lagos-Quintana M, Rauhut R, Meyer J, Borkhardt A, Tuschl T. New microRNAs from mouse and human. RNA (New York, NY). 2003;9(2):175-9.

[126] Shen J, Yang X, Xie B, Chen Y, Swaim M, Hackett SF, et al. MicroRNAs regulate ocular neovascularization. Molecular therapy : the journal of the American Society of Gene Therapy. 2008;**16**(7):1208-1216

[127] Kovacs B, Lumayag S, Cowan C, Xu S. MicroRNAs in early diabetic

retinopathy in streptozotocin-induced diabetic rats. Investigative ophthalmology & visual science. 2011;**52**(7):4402-4409

[128] McArthur K, Feng B, Wu Y, Chen S, Chakrabarti S. MicroRNA-200b regulates vascular endothelial growth factor–mediated alterations in diabetic retinopathy. Diabetes. 2011;**60**(4):1314-1323

[129] Silva VAO, Polesskaya A, Sousa TA, Corrêa VMA, André ND, Reis RI, et al. Expression and cellular localization of microRNA-29b and RAX, an activator of the RNA-dependent protein kinase (PKR), in the retina of streptozotocin-induced diabetic rats. Molecular Vision. 2011;**17**:2228-2240

[130] San-Miguel JF, Hungria VT, Yoon SS, Beksac M, Dimopoulos MA, Elghandour A, et al. Panobinostat plus bortezomib and dexamethasone versus placebo plus bortezomib and dexamethasone in patients with relapsed or relapsed and refractory multiple myeloma: A multicentre, randomised, double-blind phase 3 trial. The Lancet Oncology. 2014;**15**(11):1195-1206

[131] Lübbert M, Suciu S, Baila L, Rüter BH, Platzbecker U, Giagounidis A, et al. Low-dose decitabine versus best supportive care in elderly patients with intermediate-or high-risk myelodysplastic syndrome (MDS) ineligible for intensive chemotherapy: Final results of the randomized phase III study of the European Organisation for Research and Treatment of Cancer leukemia group and the German MDS study group. Journal of clinical oncology. 2011;**29**(15):1987-1996

[132] Almasri J, Alkhateeb HB, Firwana B, Sonbol MB, Damlaj M, Wang Z, et al. A systematic review and network meta-analysis comparing azacitidine and decitabine for the treatment of myelodysplastic syndrome. Systematic reviews. 2018;**7**(1):144

[133] Daigle SR, Olhava EJ, Therkelsen CA, Majer CR, Sneeringer CJ, Song J, et al. Selective killing of mixed lineage leukemia cells by a potent small-molecule DOT1L inhibitor. Cancer Cell. 2011;**20**(1):53-65

[134] Mohammad HP, Smitheman KN, Kamat CD, Soong D, Federowicz KE, Van Aller GS, et al. A DNA hypomethylation signature predicts antitumor activity of LSD1 inhibitors in SCLC. Cancer Cell. 2015;**28**(1):57-69

[135] Issa J-PJ, Roboz G, Rizzieri D, Jabbour E, Stock W, O'Connell C, et al. Safety and tolerability of guadecitabine (SGI-110) in patients with myelodysplastic syndrome and acute myeloid leukaemia: A multicentre, randomised, dose-escalation phase 1 study. The lancet oncology. 2015;**16**(9):1099-1110

[136] Zheng Z, Chen H, Li J, Li T, Zheng B, Zheng Y, et al. Sirtuin 1–mediated cellular metabolic memory of high glucose via the LKB1/AMPK/ROS pathway and therapeutic effects of metformin. Diabetes. 2012;**61**(1):217-228

[137] Sauve AA. Sirtuin chemical mechanisms. Biochimica et Biophysica Acta (BBA)-proteins and. Proteomics. 2010;**1804**(8):1591-1603

[138] Huang K, Huang J, Xie X, Wang S, Chen C, Shen X, et al. Sirt1 resists advanced glycation end products-induced expressions of fibronectin and TGF-β1 by activating the Nrf2/ARE pathway in glomerular mesangial cells. Free Radical Biology and Medicine. 2013;**65**:528-540

[139] Hong Q, Zhang L, Das B, Li Z, Liu B, Cai G, et al. Increased podocyte

Sirtuin-1 function attenuates diabetic kidney injury. Kidney International. 2018;**93**(6):1330-1343

[140] Jin W, Reddy MA, Chen Z, Putta S, Lanting L, Kato M, et al. Small RNA sequencing reveals microRNAs that modulate angiotensin II effects in vascular smooth muscle cells. Journal of Biological Chemistry. 2012;**287**(19):15672-15683

[141] Leung A, Trac C, Jin W, Lanting L, Akbany A, Sætrom P, et al. Novel long noncoding RNAs are regulated by angiotensin II in vascular smooth muscle cells. Circulation research. 2013;**113**(3):266-278

[142] Pott S, Lieb JD. What are super-enhancers? Nature genetics. 2015;**47**(1):8-12

[143] Das S, Senapati P, Chen Z, Reddy MA, Ganguly R, Lanting L, et al. Regulation of angiotensin II actions by enhancers and super-enhancers in vascular smooth muscle cells. Nature Communications. 2017;**8**(1):1467

[144] Putta S, Lanting L, Sun G, Lawson G, Kato M, Natarajan R. Inhibiting microRNA-192 ameliorates renal fibrosis in diabetic nephropathy. Journal of the American Society of Nephrology. 2012;**23**(3):458-469

[145] Zhong X, Chung ACK, Chen H-Y, Dong Y, Meng X, Li R, et al. miR-21 is a key therapeutic target for renal injury in a mouse model of type 2 diabetes. Diabetologia. 2013;**56**(3):663-674

[146] Kölling M, Kaucsar T, Schauerte C, Hübner A, Dettling A, Park J-K, et al. Therapeutic miR-21 silencing ameliorates diabetic kidney disease in mice. Molecular Therapy. 2017;**25**(1):165-180

[147] Chau BN, Xin C, Hartner J, Ren S, Castano AP, Linn G, et al. MicroRNA-21 promotes fibrosis of the kidney by silencing metabolic pathways. Science translational medicine. 2012;4(121):121ra18-ra18.

[148] Hilton IB, D'ippolito AM, Vockley CM, Thakore PI, Crawford GE, Reddy TE, et al. Epigenome editing by a CRISPR-Cas9-based acetyltransferase activates genes from promoters and enhancers. Nature biotechnology. 2015;**33**(5):510-517

[149] Morita S, Noguchi H, Horii T, Nakabayashi K, Kimura M, Okamura K, et al. Targeted DNA demethylation in vivo using dCas9–peptide repeat and scFv–TET1 catalytic domain fusions. Nature biotechnology. 2016;**34**(10):1060-1065

[150] WareJoncas Z, Campbell JM, Martínez-Gálvez G, Gendron WA, Barry MA, Harris PC, et al. Precision gene editing technology and applications in nephrology. Nature Reviews Nephrology. 2018;**14**(11):663-677

Chapter 8

# Predicting Type 2 Diabetes Complications and Personalising Patient Using Artificial Intelligence Methodology

*Leila Yousefi and Allan Tucker*


## Abstract

The prediction of the onset of different complications of disease, in general, is challenging due to the existence of unmeasured risk factors, imbalanced data, time-varying data due to dynamics, and various interventions to the disease over time. Scholars share a common argument that many Artificial Intelligence techniques that successfully model disease are often in the form of a "black box" where the internal workings and complexities are extremely difficult to understand, both from practitioners' and patients' perspective. There is a need for appropriate Artificial Intelligence techniques to build predictive models that not only capture unmeasured effects to improve prediction, but are also transparent in how they model data so that knowledge about disease processes can be extracted and trust in the model can be maintained by clinicians. The proposed strategy builds probabilistic graphical models for prediction with the inclusion of informative hidden variables. These are added in a stepwise manner to improve predictive performance whilst maintaining as simple a model as possible, which is regarded as crucial for the interpretation of the prediction results. This chapter explores this key issue with a specific focus on diabetes data. According to the literature on disease modelling, especially on major diseases such as diabetes, a patient's mortality often occurs due to the associated complications caused by the disease over time and not the disease itself. This is often patient-specific and will depend on what type of cohort a patient belongs to. Another main focus of this study is patient personalisation via precision medicine by discovering meaningful subgroups of patients which are characterised as phenotypes. These phenotypes are explained further using Bayesian network analysis methods and temporal association rules. Overall, this chapter discussed the earlier research of the chapter's author. It explores Artificial Intelligence (IDA) techniques for modelling the progression of disease whilst simultaneously stratifying patients and doing so in a transparent manner as possible. To this end, it reviews the current literature on some of the most common Artificial Intelligent (AI) methodologies, including probabilistic modelling, association rule mining, phenotype discovery and latent variable discovery by using diabetes as a case study.


**Keywords:** diabetes, complex disease progression, artificial intelligence in medicine, patient model, Bayesian statistics, causal networks, data mining, hidden risk factors

## 1. Introduction

Intelligent systems, whether biological or artificial, require the ability to make decisions under uncertainty using the available evidence. Several computational models exhibit some of the required functionality to handle uncertainty. These computational models in Artificial Intelligent (AI) and Machine Learning are judged by two main criteria: ease of creation and effectiveness in decision making. For example, Neural Networks (NNs) which represent complex input/output relations using combinations of simple nonlinear processing elements, are a familiar tool in AI and computational neuroscience. Alternatively, probabilistic networks (also called Bayesian Networks) are a more explicit representation of a domain through modelling the joint probability distribution (the probability of all possible outcomes in a domain). This paper provides a short summary of the previous methods in Intelligent Data Analysis (IDA) in disease progression, decision making and probabilistic modelling of patients. It then describes some existing key methods that can be updated or combined to model multiple diabetes complications in the presence of unmeasured factors. There is considerable research on predicting diabetes, especially Type 2 Diabetes Mellitus (T2DM), complications. Nevertheless, the previous research of the author is discussed in order to address these issues. In particular, these previously proposed methods have contributed to the diabetes literature by explaining unknown risk factors and identifying temporal phenotypes employing hybrid methods (including descriptive and predictive). These suggested methodology includes rule-based methods for an explanation of patient subgroups and a probabilistic framework for modelling data explicitly.

## 2. Literature review: intelligent data analysis in complex disease progression modelling

This article reviews the current literature on some of the most common AI methodologies, including probabilistic modelling, association rule mining, and latent variable discovery. Intelligent Data Analysis (IDA) is a subcategory of AI that is focused on data analysis and modelling. These methods are known to be highly successful in combining advantages of modern data analytics, classical statistics and the expertise of scientists and experts [1–3]. IDA techniques have already proved successful in clinical modelling [4]. A large and growing body of literature has investigated IDA approaches that have shown excellent results modelling cross-sectional clinical data for classification. There has also been substantial modelling on longitudinal data using IDA techniques. However, there is still an urgent need to improve these models to take account of the variability of disease progression from person to person, and explicitly model the time-varying nature of the disease. Many studies have attempted to find automated ways of helping clinicians predict disease progression [5].

For many clinical problems, the underlying structure of unmeasured variables may play an essential role in the progress of the disease. However, it is still a relatively unexplored area. Identifying these unmeasured variables as hidden or latent variables is key. What is more, understanding the semantics behind these unmeasured risk factors can improve the understanding of the disease mechanisms and thus better improve clinical decision making. Interpreting these latent variables is complicated; however, as they may represent different many types of unmeasured information such as social deprivation, missing clinical data, environmental factors, time-based information or some combination of these. To gain trust in any AI model, it is mandatory to understand/explain influencing factors of disease that guide predictions or decisions. This is because clinicians expect to understand AI diagnoses to be able to make decisions. There is a great deal of debate over the importance of explanation in AI models inferred from health data. In particular, there is a balance that needs to be made between the accuracy of complex deep models such as convolutional neural networks (in predictive strategy) and the transparency of models (in descriptive strategy) that aims to model data in a more human way such as expert systems.

A combination of explainable and deep strategies rather than either one of them alone would have a better prognostic value. Furthermore, in order to obtain a more accurate and explainable prediction of progression, the predictive models need to be personalised based on how an individual patient matches historical data by identifying patient subgroups.

## 3. Probabilistic model for time-series analysis

Understanding the pattern of complications associated with the disease has been used significantly in the clinical domain [6]. It provides an insight into the prediction and relative prevention of the associated complications which are expected to occur in a patient follow-up [7]. It generally can lead to less suffering time for patients while saving time and cost to healthcare. However, that is highly dependent on the stage of disease along with the prior occurring complications, which is associated with time-series analysis. In time-series analysis, every disease risk factor and complication is determined by various features in previous patient visits (time interval). At every medical visit, all diabetic patients have a unique profile of symptoms and complications that change over time, regardless of the phase of the disease. This non-stationary characteristic of clinical data collected as part of the monitoring of T2DM creates a difficult context for effective forecasting [8]. Clinical data needs to be considered as time-series data in order to provide a description of the progression of a disease over time. Nevertheless, dealing with time-series patient records is known to be a major issue in the prognosis of comorbidities [9], particularly when time-series data is imbalanced and contains few examples of patients without comorbidities that are common to all patients. In Type 2 Diabetes, for example, once patients are diagnosed with T2DM, half of them show signs of complications [10]. Unfortunately, these life-threatening complications remain undiagnosed for a long time because of the hidden patterns of their associated risk factors [11]. If T2DM is not appropriately managed, the development of serious complications, such as neuropathy, retinopathy, and hypertension lead to disability, premature mortality and financial cost [12]. The prediction process is complex due to the interactions between these complications and other features, as well as between complications themselves. More importantly, each patient has a unique profile of complication occurrence and the status of T2DM risk factors during a patients time-series is subject to change, as their levels may rise and fall over time. Early diagnosis and prevention techniques are needed to reduce the associated mortality and morbidity caused by T2DM complications [13]. Although there are various methodologies for T2DM prediction, for example, risk-prediction equation and Markov models [14], studies that enable early predictions of diabetes using predictive models are limited [15]. The risk-prediction equations suffer from uncertainty as well as performing only one-step-ahead predictions, while Markov models are limited to a small number of discrete risk factors. Other existing literature on investigating the prognosis of T2DM complications [16, 17] focuses particularly on logistic regression and Naive Bayes. Such studies are unsatisfactory for modelling the complex T2DM complications/risk factors. Logistic regression does

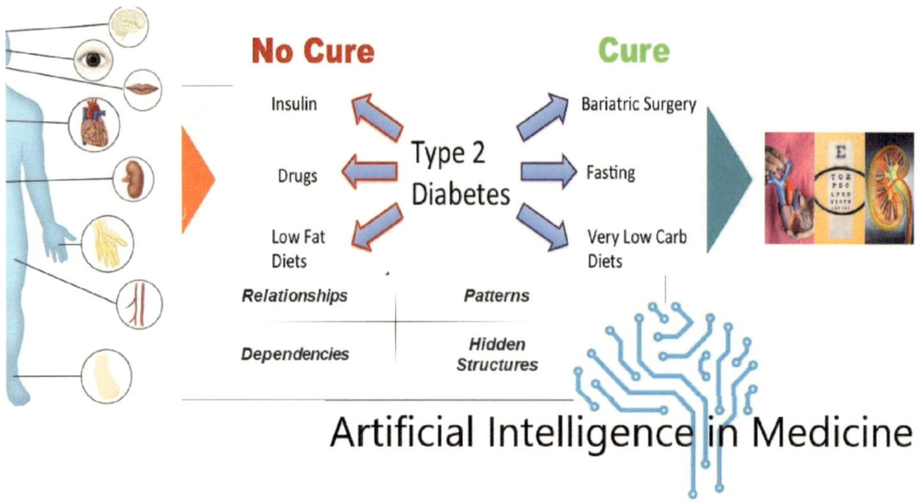


**Figure 1.**
*The organs/muscles affected by the common complications associated with type 2 Diabetes.*

not perform well when there are multiple or non-linear decision limitations. In Naive Bayes, there is an assumption of independence among the risk factors whereas all features are independent of one another.

The major limitation of the previous work in T2DM literature derives from time discretisation in temporal time slices per year. Therefore, in this study, we consider all T2DM patient's follow-up visits regardless of year basis while precisely monitoring the location of change within the unequal number of visits. This chapter suggests that AI in Medicine can provide useful techniques to analyse patient data to be able to find cure for the disease or reduce patient's suffering time (see **Figure 1**).

### 3.1 Dynamic Bayesian networks

In the field of medical informatics, probabilistic IDA techniques are exploited to obtain different clinical solutions. To improve patients' quality of life, there is an urgent need to extend and explore probabilistic IDA methods to investigate the disease complications from a clinical point of view. Thus, a Bayesian Network (BN) decision model was exploited in [18] for supporting the diagnosis of dementia, Alzheimer disease and mild cognitive impairment. Bayesian Network models appear to be well suited T2DM progression modelling, because of their flexibility in modelling spatial and temporal relationships as well as their ease of interpretation [19]. It has been reported that Dynamic Bayesian Networks (DBNs) are simple BNs for modelling time-series data and popular for modelling uncertain noisy time-series clinical data [20]. More importantly, DBNs are probabilistic graphical models that can handle missing data and hidden variables.

Previous work on learning DBNs have inferred both network structures and parameters from (sometimes incomplete) clinical datasets [20]. For example, a recent study presented a DBN method but to analyse fisheries data [21]. Authors in [22] proposed a Bayes Network to predict diabetes on the Pima Indian Diabetes dataset. However, the study failed to consider the time-series analysis. Similarly, authors in another study [23] simulated the health state and complications of type 1 diabetes patients by using partially and entirely learned Bayesian models. Apart from using a different type of Diabetes, this chapter is utilising a different approach from the above studies for the representation of the relationship between T2DM risk factors. Many diseases involved structural changes based upon key stages in the progression, but many models did not appear to take this into account. There has been some work in extending DBNs to model underlying processes that are non-stationary [24]. In [24], clinical features were modelled using a second-order time-series model while time-invariant temporal dependencies were assumed. Among this, some studies, for example, Marini and co-authors conducted research [23] that variables were connected within two-time-series and within the same time slice assumed that the temporal dependencies were time-invariant. In addition, in Marinis paper for learning the network structures, a Tabu search was used based on the Hill climbing algorithm for Bayesian Networks but with no use of latent variables. However, the approach was useful for stratifying patients according to the probability of developing complications, the major limitation of the Marinis work derived from time discretisation in time slices of one year.

Another work in [25] retained the stationary nature of the structure in favour of parameter flexibility, arguing that structure changes lead almost certainly to over-flexibility of the model in short time-series. Alternatively, a paper [26] formalised non-stationary DBN models and suggested MCMC sampling algorithm for learning the structure of the model from time-series biological data. Similarly, authors in [27] estimated the variance in the data structure parameter with an MCMC approach, but the search space was limited to a fixed number of segments and indirect edges only, which is not suitable for T2DM data. Such studies remained narrow and limited by constraints on one or more degrees of freedom: the segmentation points of the time-series, the parameters of the variables, the dependencies between the variables and the number of segments and the ignorance of the incomplete data and latent variable.

### 3.2 Dealing with time-series imbalanced data

Another common problem with classifying complications in longitudinal data is that there may be many more cases where the complication does not manifest compared to those where it does. Early prediction of T2DM complications while discovering the behaviour of associated aggressive risk factors can help to improve a patients quality of life [28]. This study suggests that while there is an association between the latent variable and joint complications in the prognosis of T2DM patients, this relationship is complex. In T2DM data analysis, another challenge can be to classify/group patients in imbalanced clinical data with several binary complications. Models of the time-series data are needed to manage diabetic complications and deal with their imbalanced and complex interactions. In particular, mining time-series is one of the challenging problems in the prognosis of disease. In addition, it has received considerable critical attention in data mining especially when there are rare positive results [29]. It has been reported that a class imbalance in the training data caused by one class (here positive cases) massively outnumbers the examples in another class (negative class) [30]. This situation may occur where the number of positive clinical test results for a complication is not equal or even close to the number of negatives. That can be solved by applying an appropriate balancing strategy in a multi-class classification problem. Different learning techniques deal with imbalanced data, such as oversampling, undersampling, boosting, bagging, bootstrapping, and repeated random sub-sampling [31]. Therefore, this chapter in order to prepare T2DM data for the prediction has utilised these strategies and customised them based on dataset nature (time-series patients records with the unequal number of visits). As a result, various balancing strategies such as pair-sampling, bootstrapping undersampling and over-sampling have been proposed in [32, 33].

The bootstrap approach can be used to identify the significant statistics from classifiers learnt from such data. For example, in a study [34], Li and co-authors provide an extension to the temporal bootstrap approach while applied on cross-sectional data. Similarly, a study conducted in [21], the bootstrap strategy is extended to longitudinal data by sampling pairs of time points, thus enabling the (first-order) temporal nature of the data to be inferred. However, these solutions only can be applicable when the imbalance ratio for all binary complications is similar. Otherwise, it can be more difficult if we need to over-sample one class value and under- sample others in order to reduce bias from data. Overall, the observed balancing strategies from the prior studies have not been sufficient for analysing more than one complication at a time, whereas it was almost impossible to obtain a satisfactory prediction performance enhancement for all complications. As well as modelling unmeasured factors, hidden variables can also be used to model non-stationary processes. This chapter attempts to address this issue by using hidden variables discovery approaches based upon T2DM risk factors/complications dependencies. Before explaining these strategies, it is necessary to understand unmeasured variables and analyse their dependencies that are generated by causal structures.

### 3.3 Causal structure learning and latent variable discovery

Various studies on longitudinal data sets have suggested an association between complications and risk factors of the disease. To discover probabilistic dependencies given clinical data, it is necessary to search the space of belief networks or casual models, which is called casual discovery of BNs [35]. These patterns of dependency with no model based solely upon the observed variables can be explained by using a latent variable. The casual discovery indicates dependencies that are generated by casual structures with unmeasured factors, i.e., hidden variables. Hidden variable modelling, introduced in [36], has a long tradition in casual discovery. One of the research gap in the previous literature of disease prediction is the existence of the unmeasured or latent variables. This is because clinicians cannot measure all risk factors and carry out all kinds of tests, so there are some unmeasured factors that clinicians fail to measure, which need to be discovered at the early stage of diabetes.

Furthermore, Factor Learning (FL) was introduced in [37], which has been known as one method for learning a probabilistic model from data. It can also be helpful to understand latent variables and measure their hypothetical impacts. FL contrasts with most other BN learning methods in that it learns a factor structure. As Martin and co-authors in [37] stated that FL for hidden variables could identify the most probable structures of factors have given the data and suitable priors. However, with a large number of variables, FL methods might be prohibitively expensive. Again in the same research these authors provided a factor structure for learning methods that efficiently utilised hidden variables. Factor structure indicates the joint probability distribution among discrete observed variables. It also contributes an explanation across a small number of variables. Although factor structures are suitable for polynomial time inference, they can cause a reduction in the prediction accuracy and precision; they contribute an explanation across a small number of variables. Nevertheless, these techniques failed to consider prior belief in the factor structure, and therefore, it could be hard to rely on the final structure.

Factor structure indicates the joint probability distribution among discrete observed variables. Interestingly, each factor in a factor structure corresponds to a completely connected dependency graph. Although they are suitable for polynomial time inference, caused reducing accuracy and precision. By contrast, they are not able to decide precisely whether or not latent variables are present, and in consequence there has been some controversy about that status of exploratory versus confirmatory factor analysis. In this regard, casual discovery methods in AI have the advantages as they can discover the actual dependencies and independencies in the data.

The causal discovery of BNs is a critical research territory, which depends on looking through the space of causal models for those which can best clarify a pattern of probabilistic conditions appeared in the data [35]. As a result, [38] showed the integration of structure-search algorithm with a latent variable in a DBNs model. However, the method did not consider the discovery of the long-range dependencies with an equal number of time slices. Similarly, in [39], Bayesian belief networks was used to find the most probable structure, using the K2 algorithm, while adding a hidden variable. Nevertheless, Cooper in [39] applied the K2 method that needs an ordering on the nodes. Witting focused on using hidden variables in a known structure [40]. Cooper in [39] used Bayesian techniques to find the most probable structure and can use this technique to add hidden variables. In principle, exact Bayesian methods for hidden variables could identify the most probable structures of factors given the data and suitable priors. However, with a large number of variables, exact methods are prohibitively expensive. Furthermore, in [41] Silva highlighted the weakness of DAG (Directed Acyclic Graph) models in the marginalisation of Hidden factors and representing the independencies over a subset of features in a DAG with more links. They suggested that Directed mixed graphs (DMGs) are a solution to this drawback. Therefore, they represented how to perform Bayesian inference on two DMGs, such as Gaussian and Probit, which is not the focus of this chapter. Nevertheless, such studies remained narrow and limited by constraints on one or more degrees of freedom: the segmentation points of the time-series, the parameters of the variables, the dependencies between the variables and the number of hidden factors. As a result, Chicharro in [42] analysed causal influences to find the relationship among different brain regions in several disorders. Similar to this chapter, Chicharros research made use of Inductive Causation (IC*) algorithm in the latent process to analyse Granger causality and Dynamic Causal Modelling. However, Chicharros study did not consider DBNs to understand causal influences.

Difficulties arise, however, when an attempt is made to implement a Bayesian Network structure as authors in [43] have argued that the number of potential DAGs over the disease risk factors is super-exponential. Additionally, the real cause-effect relationship DAG is not distinguishable while from equivalent structures when learning only using from observational data. This issue will be worse, especially when each expert has a unique probability of correctly labelling the inclusion or exclusion of edges in the disease structure. As noted by Amirkhani [43], some scoring functions are provided with that score each suitable graph based on the data and experts knowledge. Another research in [44] shows that networks with the fixed structure containing hidden variables can be learned automatically from data using a gradient-descent mechanism similar to that used in neural networks. A few algorithms have been created to understand the structure for Bayesian Networks from both fully observed models and those with hidden variables. Structure Expectation–Maximisation (SEM) has been produced for learning Probabilistic system structure from information with latent factors and missing data. A structure learning algorithm has been created for non-stationary dynamic probabilistic models. For example, REVEAL (REVerse Engineering ALgorithm) has been utilised as a structure learning algorithm, that learns the optimal set of parents for each node of a network independently, based on the information-theoretic concepts of mutual information analysis. However, the two-stage temporal Bayes network (2TBN) cannot be well recovered by the application of REVEAL. A normally utilised structure learning algorithm depends on REVEAL which takes in the ideal arrangement of guardians for every hub of a system autonomously, in light of the theoretical data ideas of common data examination. Be that as it may, the two-arrange fleeting Bayes organise as the 2TBN which cannot be all around recuperated by use of REVEAL. Rijmen in [45] exploited an HMM to study the temporal pattern of symptoms burden in brain tumour patients. He showed that the discovery of symptom experience over time is necessary for treatment and follow-up of patients with symptom-specific intervention. In general, Bayesian learning methods could determine network structure and how the networks variables should be represented along with the causal links among them. Moreover, it addressed the difficulty of qualifying causal relationships in terms of Conditional Probability Tables (CPTs). Witting focused on using hidden variables in a known structure [40] as the knowledge of the latent variable in predictive modelling is important for an understanding of the complex AI models. Discovering latent variables can potentially capture unmeasured effects from clinical data, simplifying complex networks of interactions and giving us a better understanding of disease processes. In addition, it can improve classification accuracy and boost user confidence in the classification models [46]. Elidan and co-authors in [47] emphasised the importance of the presence of hidden variables. In addition, they determined a hidden variable that interacted with observed variables and located them within the Bayesian Network structure. They also showed that networks without hidden variables are clearly less useful because of the increased number of edges needed to model all interactions, which caused overfitting. Despite the productivity of exploring trees of hidden variables to render all observable variables independently [48], these hidden variables were non-optimal with independencies among observable variables. Overall, previous works on learning DBNs have presented both network structures and parameters from clinical data sets and learning parameters for a fixed network of incomplete data, in the presence of missing data and latent variables [20]. Much of the current literature on disease prediction have argued that a complex AI model, with many unexplainable hidden variables, also has several serious drawbacks. Therefore, this chapter has chosen AI DBNs model to learn parameters and latent variables to predict complications. The next section intends to emphasise the explainability of the proposed methodology in order to uncover the meaning behind the latent AI model.

## 4. Black box models and AI in medicine

Investigating unmeasured risk factors can improve the modelling of disease progression and thus enable clinicians to focus on early diagnosis and treatment of unexpected conditions. However, the overuse of hidden variables and lack of explainability can lead to complex models, which are not well understood (being black box in nature). Models need to be understood by clinicians to facilitate transparency and trust.

### 4.1 Explainability in deep learning

This stage outlines and discusses the limitations of Deep Learning approaches that have been proposed, so far, to gain deeper insights into the understanding of black box AI models. AI medical machine such as Deep Learning has become ubiquitous to provide a high-performance prediction. Nevertheless, understanding their mechanisms has become a significant concern worldwide whereby the goal is to gain clinicians and patients trust. The reason behind this is due to several obstacles that arise to interpret the findings, such as the scale of big data, complex interactions, and high-dimensional internal state.

#### *4.1.1 Google's novel approach*

Most medical algorithms proposed by [49], such as AI Doctor designed to reproduce current problem-solving methods (e.g., the detection of cancers). In addition, the concept assignment can help people to strengthen their skills and talents for a computer system that showcased superhuman effectiveness and efficiency.

Google's AI Doctor can be demonstrated how they could be used to provide an explanation further into predictions generated by local classifiers, first from conventional image classification networks to a focused clinical application. The concept attribution approach in AI Doctor offers several promising avenues for future work. In addition to this, the concept assignment can help people to strengthen their skills and talents for a computer system that showcases superhuman effectiveness and efficiency. The concepts of explanatory power are outlined by Google under three principle assumptions/limitations: firstly, comprehension for whatever hidden layer and artificial neurons would offer. This is based on most of the information in a deep neural network consists of hidden layers. Secondly, it recommends that acknowledging the numerous hidden layers and understanding their design on a meta-level would lead to more in-depth modelling. Finally, to comprise how nodes become active, it considers groups of interconnected neurons that trigger at the same time and space. These principles are defined instead of explaining the structural nature of each neuron in each network. This is because the stratification of a network for the categories of interconnected neurons would enable its configurations even more abstractable. This is the main weakness of the black box models.

One of the most highlighted ones is Google's approach to resolve the explainability issues while enabling human-like description of the internal state of a deep network by employing Concept Activation Vectors (CAVs). While medical systems are mostly designed to reproduce current decision-making methods such as the classifier used in the detection of cancers, Google has claimed that its novel strategy can interpret existing clinical data. Although Google has made a claim that the CAVs can directly relate to one's anticipated theories, to draw conclusions about the decision-making process, it needs to consider the human needs of a higher level of understandability.

Nevertheless, cardiac specialists have been critical of the conclusions derived by Google in the clinical domain. With the proper information, AI is optimistic that innovative, unique healthcare insights might be created without human intervention. Unfortunately, this new approach is only established based on extensive and adequate datasets. This is presumably part of the explanation of why Google has established projects as its benchmark research proposal is capturing detailed patients' history of 100,000 population across four years. However, the investigation conducted out by Google did not necessarily indicate that the suggestion was entirely distant. Such as image classifiers that could be applied to low-level structures. The central concept and assumption are to consider a neural network as additional assistance that can cause issues related to the internal representation. As a result, the clinicians commented on the deep explanatory networks. They questioned the hypotheses, by stating that although the AI algorithms and Deep Learning could improve current prediction methods of clinical domain, the research would not be trustworthy unless it had been assessed with caution while a broader range of disease had been explored. Difficulties arose, when an attempt was made in order to implement the principles and these assumptions. It seemed to be evident that their approach was overconfident and yet to be trusted.

### *4.1.2 Prototyping examples in Artificial Neural Networks*

In order to introduce a different perspective on Deep Learning models' interpretability, Zintgra and co-authors [50] conducted a study to simplify the black box structure of Artificial Neural Networks (ANNs). They made use of prototypic examples method that indicate tools in order to diagnose trained ANNs. In general, ANNs analyse discrete decision-making processes and obtain high-performance prediction results.

The prototype examples may be computationally intractable, including a pre-determined normal distribution to prevent the proliferation of unreasonable prototype cases. They provided an explanation of tools to train ANNs based on two datasets. Moreover, it can often be like such a losing battle to describe precisely how ANNs operate mathematically. Therefore, a much more comprehensive pre-processing methodology could also be used in a related development (e.g., generative adversarial network proposed by Goodfellow et al. in [49]). Furthermore, experimental results and hypotheses in ANNs were portrayed and tested only on two datasets. Alternatively, a more detailed analysis is required to rely on the empirical results, which might be achieved by including rich data containing imbalance issue, different types of features. Selection bias was another potential concern because it could involve possible measurement errors. It could be extended through more set of data with various features. Finally, conclusions and interpretations of data were drawn from an inevitably subjective mechanism on the investigator's basis. This was because to examine whether the produced case studies should satisfy the investigator's standards about the phenomena of been modelled (e.g., decisions could be only made by the time it came). This was established based on approaches or standards for collecting and analysing concepts that might be more unbiased. As a result, this could also enable investigators/analysers to understand the implications and weaknesses of the use of ANNs for the discrete decision-making process, which might enhance the strictness of the approach. However, many healthcare methods are required to reconstruct conventional prediction methods (e.g., the identification of cancers), but so far, different ideas to interpret previous clinical records have been discovered.

### *4.1.3 Visualisation in deep learning*

For the time being, the possibility of an AI physician planning to roll new prognosis without direct human intervention is a significant distance in which the more presumably in decades rather than a few years later. Recent developments in several technologies in the Deep Learning area have been powered by the steadily declining expense of computing and storage. That being said, realistic apps, including certain integrated smartphone and electronic devices, have intensified explainability issues for Deep Learning in the black box resource-limited environments. Liu et al. in [51] introduced the leading solution to address these issues where a deteriorated image of Binary Convolutionary Networks caused by binarising Filtres. They offered a range of Circulant Filtres (CiFs) and a Circulant Binary Convolution (CBConv) to strengthen efficiency and to tackle those limitations for Binary Convolutionary functionalities through their proposed Circulant Backpropagation (CBP). Then, CiFs effortlessly was integrated into the current deep neural networks (DCNNs). Enormous research has indicated that perhaps the output difference among one-bit and total-precision DCNNs could be reduced by extending the variety and distributing the filtres. Zintgraf et al. in [52] identified numerous tools to test the model and understand how DCNNs could provide a reliable outcome by using the visualisation method.

Overall, the existing explanatory Deep Learning approaches would need to be adapted for further sophisticated longitudinal modelling strategy (rather than with a multivariate distribution). This would result in better outcomes, for example, in pixel values which could be estimated reliably by everyone's environment while it skewed down much more. By providing the black box models with sufficient data, machine learning seemed to be overconfident that completely different health knowledge could then be generated without user intervention. The black box models of Deep Learning can be simplified in several aspects. For example, if an object is detected, an image detection machine can breakdown back and towards specific attributes including shape, colour and texture of the image, and then reduce the predictions to a mathematical method by checking the classification error and then background diffusion to improve the practises. In particular, in the world that it is possible to fully allocate decision making to computer systems, confidence in AI systems will be hard to achieve. In the future work, one approach that can be applied to the small-sized T2DM dataset can be the use of Bayesian Neural Networks, which will deal with uncertainties in data and model structure by exploiting the advantages of both Neural Networks and Bayesian modelling. To conclude, AI can improve current methods of medical diagnosis in terms of interpretability but cautioned that the technology would need to be more evaluated to be trusted by both patients and practitioners.

In black box models, it can be challenging to determine what is coordinating the visible patterns. Such models are problematic not only for lack of transparency but also for possible biases inherited by the algorithms from clinicians mistakes [53]. This issue is caused based on the human errors and biased sampling of training data as well as the underestimation of the impact of the risk factors underlying behaviour/ pattern. In general, as observed from prior studies, it is difficult to obtain performance enhancement while simultaneously trying to explain hidden factors. Lakkaraju in [54] suggested that there is a trade-off between patient personalisation (in a descriptive analysis) and prediction performance (in predictive analysis). Generally speaking, an improvement in explainability is often possible through a less accurate model or at a higher cost of the predictive accuracy (in a Black box model) [6]. There are quite few research studies on predicting T2DM complications and T2DM black box models. However, studies on explaining an unknown risk factor/ latent phenotype by using a hybrid data mining methodology (including descriptive and predictive) are rare to find in literature. Therefore, this study attempts to open the AI, black box model by using both predictive and descriptive strategies.

## 5. Patient personalisation and explanation

Most of the previously published studies in diabetes prediction have tended to focus on all patients as one integrated database rather than separating patients [16]. It can be challenging to stratify patients based on their longitudinal data in order to determine what is triggering the visible patterns that may be specific to one cohort of patients. There is some research, such as [55] that assesses the disease prediction performance based upon different IDA techniques. For example, the onset of the disease is modelled in [56] while other studies focus on patient modelling [57]. The approach described in this chapter aims to personalise patients by using unsupervised methodologies to group time-series patient data.

The proposed descriptive strategy in this chapter has been regarded as a useful tool known as association rules to detect interesting relationships among T2DM complications.

### 5.1 Time-series clustering

Time-series clustering is often problematic [58], especially when we need to analyse risk factors from matching patterns across time. The literature on time-series clustering and pattern discovery has highlighted several studies [59]. There have been some qualitative measures for clustering time-series data, which captured similar risk factor patterns in dynamic temporal data, regardless of whether the correlation between them was linear or not [60]. However, they did not seem to be very suitable for a long and an unequal number of time-series data (e.g., T2DM data). For instance, authors in [59] proposed an algorithm to cluster patients based on clinical data whilst utilising the clustering information for identifying distinct patterns. Altiparmak in [59] provided a slope-wise comparison method (SWC) to find the correlation between local distance vectors of patients visits, and group clinical test results into different sub-groups, based upon the related risk factors, by using feature selection. In their method each cluster of patients was considered as a transaction data that included a pattern indicating which cluster belonged to each patient. Authors in [61] used a similar method [59] in clustering, but they clustered fixed length time-series. Ceccon and coauthors [62] exploited a variation of the naive Bayes classifier with a hidden variable for segmenting patients into disease sub-types. Ceccon's study intended to enhance the classification performance of Glaucoma patients based upon visual field data. Nevertheless, they only focused on standard/static BNs (instead of DBNs) to infer the parameter in a cross-sectional dataset. Moreover, they failed to analyse the influences of multiple hidden variables on the prediction results.

### 5.2 Pattern discovery and association rules mining

It has previously been observed that patients with T2DM are also at an increased risk of microvascular comorbidities, including nephropathy, neuropathy, and retinopathy [63]. The underlying pattern of T2DM complications and how their co-occurrence is followed/caused/related by other complications associated with the disease, known as the major source of mortality and morbidity in T2DM [64]. That is because predicting a target complication can be challenging without the consideration of the effects of its associated complications. Similar to Diabetic type 1 patients, although genetic factors impact on developing T2DM, it is believed ignorance of developing complications harms patients' life. What is more, T2DM patients develop a different profile of complications and features, which changes over time per follow-up visit. One of the most important factors in the high number of dependencies among T2DM features and complications is the appearance of unmeasured risk factors. Surprisingly, the effect of understanding unmeasured variables, which play an important role in disease prediction, does not seems that closely examined.

Understanding these associated patterns has a remarkable actual value and can significantly being used in the clinical domain [6]. It provides an insight into the prediction and relative prevention of the associated complications which are expected to occur in patient followups [7]. It also leads to less suffering time for patients while saves time and cost to healthcare. However, that is highly dependent on the stage of disease along with the prior occurring complications, which is associated with time-series analysis. In time-series analysis, every disease risk factor and complication is determined by various features in previous patient visits (time interval). To better understand the complications of the disease and their effects, this chapter clusters patient the associated rules among the complications. It attempts to address this issue and present an informative rules/ordering pattern of patient behaviour, with an aim to capture the complexities of the associated complications' over time. The proposed descriptive strategy has been regarded as a useful tool known as association rules (ARs) to detect interesting relationships among T2DM complications.

Temporal Association Rules (TARs) [65] is an extension to association rules [66] to analyse basket data that includes a temporal dimension to order related items. Many algorithms with temporal rules work by dividing the temporal transitions database into different partitions based on the time granularity obliged. For example, different mining algorithms were reformulated and presented to reflect the new general temporal association rules. These include Progressive Partition Minder (PPM), Segmented Progressive Filter (SPF), and TAR algorithm [65–67]. Various algorithms have been proposed for the incremental mining of temporal association rules, especially for numerical attributes [68]. Allen's rules [69] generalised abstracted time-series data into a relation (PRECEDES) to find TARs in [70]. Various ways were proposed to explore the problem of temporal association rules discovery [71]. Nevertheless, previous studies performed discovering association rules on a given subset specified by the time [72], whilst not considering the specific exhibition period of the elements.

Association Rule Mining (ARM) finds frequent patterns by mining ARs with the use of two basic parameters of support and confidence [73]. The majority of the previous ARM algorithms worked by dividing the temporal transitions database into different partitions based on the time granularity obliged.

Difficulties arise with TARs when there are some rare rules of particular interest [74]. Many studies have employed the most common filtering metrics rather than support and confidence in order to detect interesting rules [75]. There is a controversy to this, as a study in the literature argued that a conservative ARM methodology only based on a fixed and rigid threshold for the filtering metrics could be problematic. A few studies attempted to mine frequent underlying patterns of diabetic complications [76]. The frequent pattern mining research significantly affects data mining techniques in longitudinal data. A post-processing approach in [77] attempted to extract interesting subsets of temporal rules within T2DM data. However, it only considered characteristic patterns of administrative data without the appearance of latent variables. Other researchers have undertaken association rule mining of clinical data [78, 79]. Lee et al. attempted to address the issue in [67] and have led to the proposal of the concept of general TARs, where the items were allowed to have varying exhibition periods, and their support was made based on that accordingly. Another research conducted by Plasse et al. in [80] looked at finding homogeneous groups of variables. They suggested that a variable clustering method could be applied to the data in order to achieve a better result in pattern discovering methodology. However, their strategy to mine ARs differed from this chapter in which the number of rules was reduced only based on hierarchical clustering applied to items, not to multiple identical binary attributes. Among these, some methods uncovered temporal patterns and relationships among clinical variables, including causal information [81], numeric time-series analysis [82]. Nevertheless, considering all of this evidence, none of the above studies has clustered uneven time-series clinical data based on a hidden variable for extracting temporal phenotype and behaviours of patients.

## 6. The suggested methodology

This chapter, so far, has described the research gap in the modelling and explaining of complex disease processes and thus given the motivation behind the suggested methodology. The previously discussed methods suffer from some limitations in addressing imbalance issues, complex and temporal relationships between (sometimes unmeasured) factors, and the identification of different underlying characteristics of disease for different subgroups of the population. There is considerable research on predicting T2DM complications. Among these, studies on explaining unknown risk factors and identifying temporal phenotypes by using

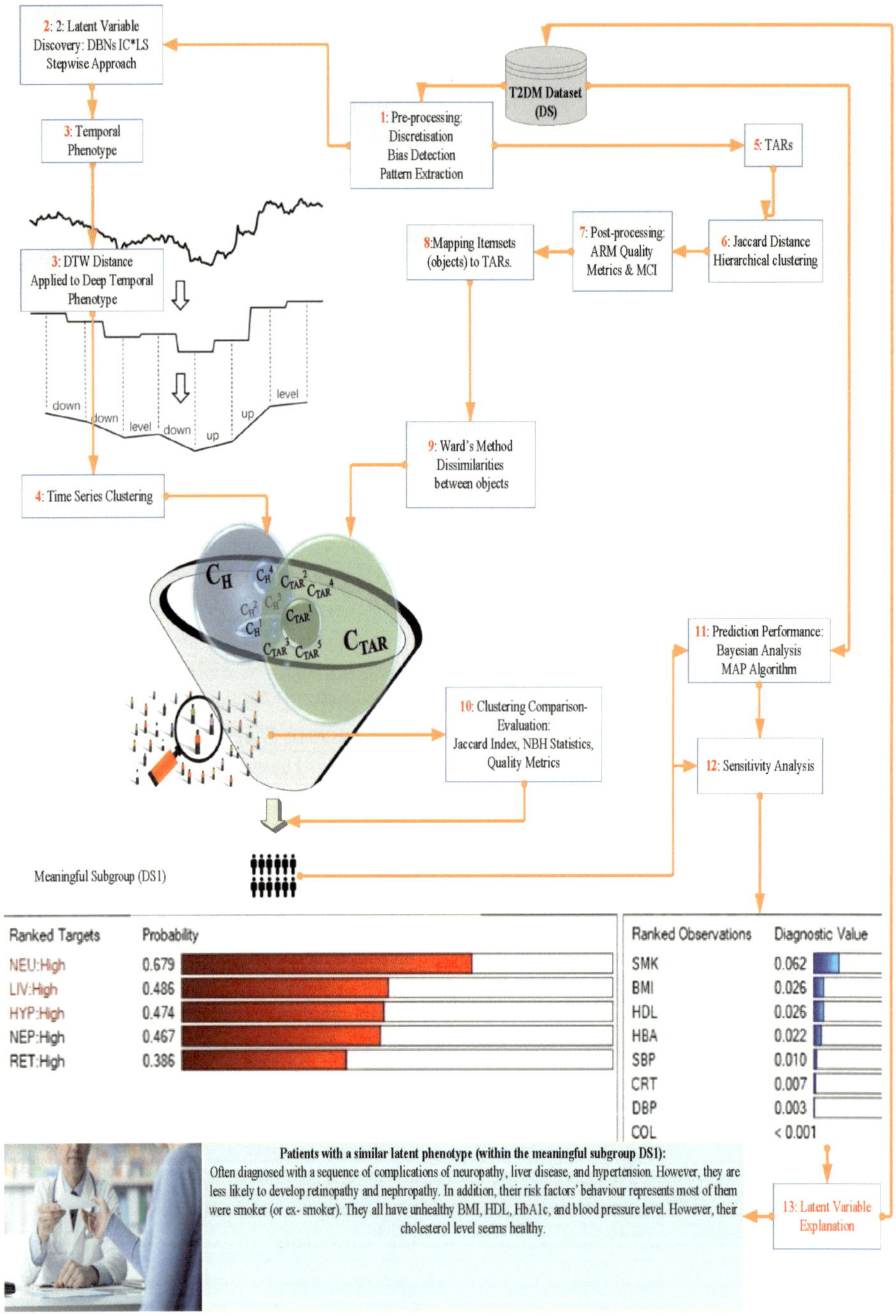


**Figure 2.**
*The proposed hybrid methodology to find explainable subgroup of patients by personalising diabetic patients in precision medicine. This figure is an abstract methodology explained in Figures 1–4 in the previous work in [83].*

hybrid methods (including descriptive and predictive) are rare to find in literature. It represented the reason of the earlier research conducted by the author in [32, 33, 83–85]. The current work of this chapter's author has attempted to address these issues in the previous research in [32, 33, 84], after describing the case study data as a starting point, the suggested methodology is explored as a framework for modelling real time-series clinical data. In the recent work conducted in [83, 85], the identification of informative hidden factors is investigated followed by methods to cluster patients into meaningful subgroups along with the identification of a latent temporal phenotype and the characterisation of these groups using temporal association rules (as illustrated in **Figure 2**).

## 7. Type 2 Diabetes as a case study

The World Health Organisation (WHO) reported that Type 2 Diabetes Mellitus (T2DM) accounts for at least 90% of all diabetes types. Another study in WHO revealed that T2DM patients are at increased risk of long-term vascular comorbidities, which is known as "underlying cause of death" and severe phenotype of the disease [86]. It has previously been observed that patients with T2DM are also at an increased risk of microvascular comorbidities, including nephropathy, neuropathy, and retinopathy [86]. Similar to Diabetic type 1 patients, although genetic factors impact on developing T2DM, it is believed ignorance of developing complications harms patient life because it may develop a different profile of complications and features, which changes over time per follow-up visit. However, these life-threatening complications remain undiagnosed for a long time because of the hidden patterns of their associated risk factors [11]. The underlying pattern of the complications is known as the major source of mortality and morbidity in T2DM and how their co-occurrence is followed/caused by other complications associated with the disease [64]. That is because predicting a target complication can be challenging without the consideration of the effects of its associated complications.

### 7.1 Data description

The observed dataset in this chapter is similar to the data utilised in the previous study of Diabetes patients in [83] of pre-diagnosed T2DM patients aged twenty five to sixty five years (inclusive) that were recruited from clinical followups at the "IRCCS Instituti Clinic Scientifici" (ICS) Maugeri of Pavia, Italy. The MOSAIC project funds the information based on the seventh Framework Program of the European Commission, Theme ICT201152 Virtual Physiological Human (600914) from 2009 to 2013. These consists of physical examinations and laboratory data for complications and risk factors (predictors) in T2DM which were selected supported existing literature on T2DM [76, 87–90] as well as the recommendations from the clinicians at ICS. These are Retinopathy (RET), Hypertension (HYP), Nephropathy (NEP), Neuropathy (NEU) and LIVer disease (LIV) (see **Table 1**). Here, the predictors are known and selected from the dataset: Body Mass Index (BMI), Systolic Blood Pressure (SBP), High-density Lipoprotein (HDL), Glycated Haemoglobin (HbA1c or HBA), Diastolic Blood pressure (DBP), ChOLesterol (COL), Smoking habit (SMK) and Creatinine (CRT). Control Values for T2DM risk factors are classified in **Table 2** illustrates three clinical level of risk, particularly low (zero), medium (one) and high (two). In T2DM data, the worsening level of the microvascular diseases and HYP is known as a significant cause of death [91]. Even though micro-vascular complications such as RET, NEP, NEU are less frequent comparing to HYP, an inadequate estimation of them causes long-term suffering

| Node ID | Target complication | Diagnosis outcome[a] | Clinical risk class[b] |
|---|---|---|---|
| 2 | Retinopathy (RET) | {Negative,Positive} | {low,high} |
| 3 | Neuropathy (NEU) | {Negative,Positive} | {low,high} |
| 4 | Nephropathy (NEP) | {Negative,Positive} | {low,high} |
| 5 | Liver Disease (LIV) | {Negative,Positive} | {low,high} |
| 6 | Hypertension (HYP) | {Negative,Positive} | {low,high} |

[a]*Negative test result, Positive test result.*
[b]*Low clinical risk, High clinical risk.*

**Table 1.**
*The description of T2DM target complication, clinical node control values, and discretised states [83].*

| Node ID | T2DM risk factors | Control value[a] | Discretised value[b] |
|---|---|---|---|
| 1 | HbA1c (HBA) | $6.6 \pm 1.2$ (%) | {low,medium,high} |
| 7 | Body Mass Index (BMI) | $26.4 \pm 2.4$ (kg/m$^2$) | {low,medium,high} |
| 8 | Creatinine (CRT) | $0.9 \pm 0.2$ (mg/dL) | {low,medium,high} |
| 9 | Cholesterol (COL) | $0.9 \pm 0.2$ (mg/dL) | {low,medium,high} |
| 10 | High-Density Lipoprotein (HDL) | $1.1 \pm 0.3$ (mmol/l) | {low,medium,high} |
| 11 | Diastolic Blood Pressure (DBP) | $91 \pm 12$ (mmHg) | {low,medium,high} |
| 12 | Systolic Blood Pressure (SBP) | $148 \pm 19$(mmHg) | {low,medium,high} |
| 13 | Smoking Habit (SMK) | {0,1,2} | {low,medium,high} |

[a]*(Mean ± SD).*
[b]*low, medium, high.*

**Table 2.**
*The description of the T2DM clinical features, risk factors, control values, and the discretised states [83].*

and life-threatening comorbidities [64]. Fowler and co-authors in [7] researched type 2 Diabetic American patients. This research utilised T2DM key risk factors such as HbA1c, SBP, and DBP to investigate relationships among complications such as HYP, NEP, RET, and NEU. In addition, LIV is a severe phenotype of diabetes and associated with T2DM complications, especially NEU [92]. Litwak analysed Russian diabetic patients in [93] which referred to the influence of macro-vascular and micro-vascular disease on one anther. For example, important features in T2DM dataset such as blood pressure, HDL, lipid, BMI, and HbA1c influence diabetic patients' complications. They also revealed that HDL has a negative effect on HYP, NEP, NEU, and RET, whereas HbA1c negatively associated with HYP. Again, a study conducted by Ramachandran [94] referred to the high prevalence of NEU and RET in Type 2 diabetes in India. Similarly, research in [76] suggested that most of the diabetic patients have objective evidence for some variety of NEU, but only a few of them have identified by symptoms. This research also showed that there is a strong association among NEP, NEU, and RET. This study only concentrates on five binary complications as the predictive target classes in a binary classification problem (with two categories of classes: "high" or "low" risk). Furthermore, a complication class value of low risk (zero) represents a patient visit in which the complication is not present; otherwise, it is at high risk (one). For instance, a complication class value of zero represents a patient visit in which the complication is not present; otherwise, it is one. Alternatively, other risk factors associated with a patient (symptoms/clinical tests) are abstracted in the multi-class classification problems with more than two targets including high, medium, and low risk patient, according to a diabetes experts definitions [95, 96]. For each patient in T2DM dataset, time-series analysis is described in Appendix A with definition of the related notations.

## 8. Experimental results and conclusions

This section summarises the clinical implications and shows how the obtained experimental findings in the previous works [83, 84, 97] and their significance have led to developing explanatory AI models. For example **Table 3** illustrated the promising results obtained by the proposed Stepwise approach discussed in [33, 84].

In **Table 4**, the prediction performance of the underlying patterns of complications for these patients within the discovered subgroup dataset (was introduced in [83] as DS1 and discovered using the descriptive strategy) was analysed and compared to all patients belonged to DS (the raw T2DM dataset). It also suggested that DS1 (by personalising patients) could be considered as a dataset with less uncertainty than DS. In order to describe the inference problem in this chapter, the causal relationships seemed to be a reliable option to represent static and dynamic correlations between T2DM risk factors. The causal inference has a greater focus on distinguishing causes from other associations than on uncovering detailed temporal relationships. Therefore, in this work ([83]), several predictive strategies in order to

| Percentage (%) | Accuracy | Sensitivity | Specificity | Precision |
|---|---|---|---|---|
| No Hidden variable in [32] | 48 | 53 | 48 | 53 |
| Stepwise IC* in [33] (Step1) | 60 | 40 | 80 | 70 |
| Enhanced stepwise in [97] (Step1) | 80 | 51 | 98 | 97 |
| Stepwise IC* in [33] (Step2) | 78 | 98 | 58 | 68 |
| Enhanced stepwise in [97] (Step2) | 95 | 80 | 96 | 86 |
| Stepwise IC* in [33] (Step3) | 78 | 98 | 58 | 68 |
| Enhanced stepwise in [97] (Step3) | 95 | 81 | 96 | 82 |
| Enhanced stepwise in [97] (Step4) | 96 | 81 | 97 | 092 |
| Enhanced stepwise in [97] (Step5) | 95 | 82 | 97 | 85 |

**Table 3.**
*Comparison of our new and enhanced stepwise IC*LS approach in [97] with its previous version (stepwise IC*) in [33] and without latent variable in [32].*

| Complication | Accuracy | |
|---|---|---|
| | DS | DS1 |
| NEP | 0.81 | 0.93 |
| LIV | 0.77 | 0.88 |
| HYP | 0.91 | 0.99 |
| NEU | 0.76 | 0.81 |
| RET | 0.81 | 0.79 |
| All | 0.81 | 0.88 |

**Table 4.**
*The overall prediction accuracy of T2DM complications for patients in DS is compared to DS1.*

test whether the descriptive approaches have contributed to improving the prediction performance of the ordering patterns of complications.

## 8.1 Clinical implications

This study offered several valuable insights into the prediction challenges in diabetes and similar diseases and explained how they could be tackled. First, throughout this chapter, appropriate machine learning techniques were conducted to model complex interactions among the complications, risk factors and unmeasured factors. For instance, the use of probabilistic graphical models provided a significant improvement in the accuracy of predictive models while reducing uncertainty in disease management. Having adopted DBNs to learn hidden risk factors and effectively understand the AI black box model was the key contribution of this research. The temporal phenotype was identified to represent the overall patterns of disease risk factors for each patient based on the discovered hidden variables over time. The descriptive analytics, in [97], provided valuable insights into the hidden variable effects on stratifying patients into different sub-groups, whether or not they developed the same complications. These findings also explained the influence of the latent variable on the bootstrapped data. Phenotype discovery was utilised to categorise and investigate meaningful subgroups of patients based on how an individual matches historical data. The hybrid type methods in discovering meaningful subgroups and explaining temporal phenotype also led to a better understanding of clinical data as well as aiding to interpret the unmeasured factors while demonstrating their risks.

## 8.2 Future works

The generalisability of the results presented in this study is subject to certain limitations as follows: This research was conducted to explain and discover the unmeasured factors with a few patients and relatively few features. Thus, this study focused on time-series complex clinical dataset like T2DM, which was a small-sized dataset with an unequal number of patient's follow-up visits (which is common in clinical data). This study was specific to T2DM concept and Bayesian modelling; hence, one fundamental criticism could be the bias towards this dataset and whether the method could be developed in other fields of clinical data in the future. In order to help overcome the limitations discussed in the previous section, the following recommendations are suggested: The originality of the proposed study consisted in its innovative, analytical, and methodological strategies to predict and explain complex clinical data to improve patients' quality of life. A natural progression of this work for a better generalisability should involve extending the latent DBNs model with more hidden variables to capture a greater variety of unmeasured factors to characterise critical changes and produce interesting findings that account more for better explainability and predictability. In addition, to address the limitation related to the small-sized dataset, this work could be extended to further investigation and experimentation into clinical impacts and environmental factors, such as family history, pollution, and glucose. More research also might be conducted to monitor disease progression effectively and detect the underlying patterns of complications, which could provide clinicians with a better understanding of the obtained findings. For example, a greater focus on phenotype discovery could enable assessment of the long-term effects of the temporal phenotype on the patient, which might be done by following qualitative approaches to support the obtained findings from the biomedical literature. The generalisability of the findings obtained in this study might be tested on other data with potentially non-stationary, complex, and incomplete data. For instance, the pre-processing approaches, statistical analysis, temporal phenotype, MCI algorithm and the DBNs model could be applied to another complex data (e.g., COVID-19). Therefore, in a new project, a similar patient model to this research was mainly employed, which primarily concentrated on helping healthcare staff in their understanding of how COVID-19 spread and how they could be better prepared.

In the current work as a Post-Doctorate research fellow at Brunel University and University City London (UCL) associated with the BHF Alan Turing Institute jointly funded research project with the collaborators of the project in UCL and GSK. This project aims to develop a computational tool to investigate the action of drug compounds for the treatment of cardiovascular disease and type 2 diabetes which involves: firstly, the construction of a cardiovascular disease (CVD) and Type-II diabetes (T2D) relevant metabolic measures networks, using repeated measures. Secondly, the combination of different causal networks on the same set of metabolic measures. Lastly, the integration to the system of available drug targets and disease information for testing CVD and T2D drugs.

## Acknowledgements

I thank the following individuals for their expertise and assistance throughout all aspects of this study and for their insightful suggestions and careful reading of the manuscript. Dr. Stephen Swift, Dr. Mahir Arzoky and clinicians/scientist at Pavia hospital; especially Lucia Saachi and Luca Chiovato for providing the dataset and their professional advice.

## Author details

Leila Yousefi* and Allan Tucker
Life Science Department, College of Health, Medicine and Life Sciences, Brunel University London, United Kingdom

*Address all correspondence to: leila.yousefi@brunel.ac.uk

## References

[1] R. Bellazzi. Big data and biomedical informatics: a challenging opportunity. *Yearbook of medical informatics*, 9(1):8, 2014.

[2] M. R. Berthold, C. Borgelt, F. Höppner, and F. Klawonn. *Guide to intelligent data analysis: how to intelligently make sense of real data*. Springer Science & Business Media, 2010.

[3] D. J. Hand. Intelligent data analysis: Issues and opportunities. In *International Symposium on Intelligent Data Analysis*, pages 1–14. Springer, 1997.

[4] R. Bellazzi, F. Ferrazzi, and L. Sacchi. Predictive data mining in clinical medicine: a focus on selected methods and applications. *Wiley Interdisciplinary Reviews: Data Mining and Knowledge Discovery*, 1(5):416–430, 2011.

[5] M. B. Sesen, T. Kadir, R.-B. Alcantara, J. Fox, and M. Brady. Survival prediction and treatment recommendation with bayesian techniques in lung cancer. In *AMIA Annual Symposium Proceedings*, volume 2012, page 838. American Medical Informatics Association, 2012.

[6] T. Wang and Q. Lin. Hybrid predictive model: When an interpretable model collaborates with a black-box model. *arXiv preprint arXiv: 1905.04241*, 2019.

[7] M. J. Fowler. Microvascular and macrovascular complications of diabetes. *Clinical diabetes*, 26(2):77–82, 2008.

[8] M. A. Van Gerven, B. G. Taal, and P. J. Lucas. Dynamic bayesian networks as prognostic models for clinical patient management. *Journal of biomedical informatics*, 41(4):515–529, 2008.

[9] M. Van der Heijden, M. Velikova, and P. J. Lucas. Learning bayesian networks for clinical time series analysis. *Journal of biomedical informatics*, 48:94–105, 2014.

[10] R. Turner, R. Holman, D. Matthews, S. Oakes, P. Bassett, I. Stratton, C. Cull, S. Manley, and V. Frighi. Uk prospective diabetes study (ukpds). viii. study design, progress and performance. *Diabetologia*, 34(12):877–890, 1991.

[11] K.-H. Yoon, J.-H. Lee, J.-W. Kim, J. H. Cho, Y.-H. Choi, S.-H. Ko, P. Zimmet, and H.-Y. Son. Epidemic obesity and type 2 diabetes in asia. *The Lancet*, 368(9548):1681–1688, 2006.

[12] U. Diabetes. Diabetes: facts and stats. *Diabetes UK*, 3:1–21, 2014.

[13] S. Mani, Y. Chen, T. Elasy, W. Clayton, and J. Denny. Type 2 diabetes risk forecasting from emr data using machine learning. In *AMIA annual symposium proceedings*, volume 2012, page 606. American Medical Informatics Association, 2012.

[14] E. Mueller, S. Maxion-Bergemann, D. Gultyaev, S. Walzer, N. Freemantle, C. Mathieu, B. Bolinder, R. Gerber, M. Kvasz, and R. Bergemann. Development and validation of the economic assessment of glycemic control and long-term effects of diabetes (eagle) model. *Diabetes technology and therapeutics*, 8(2):219–236, 2006.

[15] S. E. Inzucchi and R. S. Sherwin. The prevention of type 2 diabetes mellitus. *Endocrinology and Metabolism Clinics*, 34 (1):199–219, 2005.

[16] A. Dagliati, A. Malovini, P. Decata, G. Cogni, M. Teliti, L. Sacchi, C. Cerra, L. Chiovato, and R. Bellazzi. Hierarchical bayesian logistic regression to forecast metabolic control in type 2 dm patients. In *AMIA Annual*

*Symposium Proceedings*, volume 2016, page 470. American Medical Informatics Association, 2016.

[17] A. Dagliati, A. Marinoni, C. Cerra, P. Decata, L. Chiovato, P. Gamba, and R. Bellazzi. Integration of administrative, clinical, and environmental data to support the management of type 2 diabetes mellitus: From satellites to clinical care. *Journal of diabetes science and technology*, 10(1):19–26, 2016.

[18] F. L. Seixas, B. Zadrozny, J. Laks, A. Conci, and D. C. M. Saade. A bayesian network decision model for supporting the diagnosis of dementia, alzheimer s disease and mild cognitive impairment. Computers in biology and medicine, 51: 140–158, 2014.

[19] J. Pearl. Probabilistic reasoning in intelligent systems. 1988. *San Mateo, CA: Kaufmann*, 23:33–34.

[20] K. P. Murphy and S. Russell. Dynamic bayesian networks: representation, inference and learning. 2002.

[21] N. Trifonova, A. Kenny, D. Maxwell, D. Duplisea, J. Fernandes, and A. Tucker. Spatio-temporal bayesian network models with latent variables for revealing trophic dynamics and functional networks in fisheries ecology. *Ecological Informatics*, 30:142–158, 2015.

[22] Y. Guo, G. Bai, and Y. Hu. Using bayes network for prediction of type-2 diabetes. In *2012 International Conference for Internet Technology and Secured Transactions*, pages 471–472. IEEE, 2012.

[23] S. Marini, E. Trifoglio, N. Barbarini, F. Sambo, B. Di Camillo, A. Malovini, M. Manfrini, C. Cobelli, and R. Bellazzi. A dynamic bayesian network model for long-term simulation of clinical complications in type 1 diabetes. *Journal of biomedical informatics*, 57:369–376, 2015.

[24] A. Tucker, X. Liu, and D. Garway-Heath. Spatial operators for evolving dynamic bayesian networks from spatio-temporal data. In *Genetic and Evolutionary ComputationGECCO 2003*, pages 205–205. Springer, 2003.

[25] M. Grzegorczyk and D. Husmeier. Non-stationary continuous dynamic bayesian networks. In *Advances in Neural Information Processing Systems*, pages 682–690, 2009.

[26] J. W. Robinson and A. J. Hartemink. Learning non-stationary dynamic bayesian networks. *Journal of Machine Learning Research*, 11(Dec):3647–3680, 2010.

[27] M. Talih and N. Hengartner. Structural learning with time-varying components: tracking the cross-section of financial time series. *Journal of the Royal Statistical Society: Series B (Statistical Methodology)*, 67(3):321–341, 2005.

[28] A. Lloyd, W. Sawyer, and P. Hopkinson. Impact of long-term complications on quality of life in patients with type 2 diabetes not using insulin. *Value in Health*, 4(5):392–400, 2001.

[29] Q. Yang and X. Wu. 10 challenging problems in data mining research. *International Journal of Information Technology & Decision Making*, 5(04): 597–604, 2006.

[30] L. Litwak, S.-Y. Goh, Z. Hussein, R. Malek, V. Prusty, and M. E. Khamseh. Prevalence of diabetes complications in people with type 2 diabetes mellitus and its association with baseline characteristics in the multinational a 1 chieve study. *Diabetology and metabolic syndrome*, 5(1):57, 2013.

[31] N. Japkowicz and S. Stephen. The class imbalance problem: A systematic study. *Intelligent data analysis*, 6(5):429–449, 2002.

[32] L. Yousefi, L. Saachi, R. Bellazzi, L. Chiovato, and A. Tucker. Predicting comorbidities using resampling and dynamic bayesian networks with latent variables. In *Computer-Based Medical Systems (CBMS), 2017 IEEE 30th International Symposium on*, pages 205–206. IEEE, 2017.

[33] L. Yousefi, A. Tucker, M. Al-luhaybi, L. Saachi, R. Bellazzi, and L. Chiovato. Predicting disease complications using a stepwise hidden variable approach for learning dynamic bayesian networks. In *2018 IEEE 31st International Symposium on Computer-Based Medical Systems (CBMS)*, pages 106–111. IEEE, 2018.

[34] G. Liang. An effective method for imbalanced time series classification: Hybrid sampling. In *Australasian Joint Conference on Artificial Intelligence*, pages 374–385. Springer, 2013.

[35] X. Zhang, K. B. Korb, A. E. Nicholson, and S. Mascaro. Latent variable discovery using dependency patterns. *arXiv preprint arXiv: 1607.06617*, 2016.

[36] C. SPEARMAN. " general intelligence," objectively determined and measured. *American Journal of Psychology*, 15:201–293, 1904.

[37] J. Martin and K. VanLehn. Discrete factor analysis: Learning hidden variables in bayesian networks. Technical report, Technical report, Department of Computer Science, University of Pittsburgh, 1995.

[38] X. Boyen, N. Friedman, and D. Koller. Discovering the hidden structure of complex dynamic systems. In *Proceedings of the Fifteenth conference on Uncertainty in artificial intelligence*, pages 91–100. Morgan Kaufmann Publishers Inc., 1999.

[39] L. co Todorovski, B. Cestnik, and M. Kline. Qualitative clustering of short time-series: A case study of firms reputation data. *IDDM-2002*, 141, 2002.

[40] F. Wittig. Learning bayesian networks with hidden variables for user modeling. In *UM99 User Modeling*, pages 343–344. Springer, 1999.

[41] R. Silva and Z. Ghahramani. The hidden life of latent variables: Bayesian learning with mixed graph models. *Journal of Machine Learning Research*, 10 (Jun):1187–1238, 2009.

[42] D. Chicharro and S. Panzeri. Algorithms of causal inference for the analysis of effective connectivity among brain regions. *Frontiers in neuroinformatics*, 8:64, 2014.

[43] H. Amirkhani, M. Rahmati, P. J. Lucas, and A. Hommersom. Exploiting experts knowledge for structure learning of bayesian networks. *IEEE transactions on pattern analysis and machine intelligence*, 39(11):2154–2170, 2017.

[44] S. Russell, J. Binder, D. Koller, and K. Kanazawa. Local learning in probabilistic networks with hidden variables. In *IJCAI*, volume 95, pages 1146–1152, 1995.

[45] F. Rijmen, E. H. Ip, S. Rapp, and E. G. Shaw. Qualitative longitudinal analysis of symptoms in patients with primary and metastatic brain tumours. *Journal of the Royal Statistical Society: Series A (Statistics in Society)*, 171(3): 739–753, 2008.

[46] N. Friedman, K. Murphy, and S. Russell. Learning the structure of dynamic probabilistic networks. In *Proceedings of the Fourteenth conference on Uncertainty in artificial intelligence*, pages 139–147. Morgan Kaufmann Publishers Inc., 1998.

[47] G. Elidan, N. Lotner, N. Friedman, and D. Koller. Discovering hidden variables: A structure-based approach.

In *Advances in Neural Information Processing Systems*, pages 479–485, 2001.

[48] J. Pearl. *Probabilistic reasoning in intelligent systems: networks of plausible inference*. Elsevier, 2014.

[49] E. Choi, M. T. Bahadori, A. Schuetz, W. F. Stewart, and J. Sun. Doctor ai: Predicting clinical events via recurrent neural networks. In *Machine Learning for Healthcare Conference*, pages 301–318, 2016.

[50] M. Khashei, M. Bijari, and G. A. R. Ardali. Improvement of auto-regressive integrated moving average models using fuzzy logic and artificial neural networks (anns). *Neurocomputing*, 72(4–6):956–967, 2009.

[51] Y. Li, S. Swift, and A. Tucker. Modelling and analysing the dynamics of disease progression from cross-sectional studies. *Journal of biomedical informatics*, 46(2):266–274, 2013.

[52] L. M. Zintgraf, T. S. Cohen, and M. Welling. A new method to visualize deep neural networks. *arXiv preprint arXiv:1603.02518*, 2016.

[53] D. Pedreschi, F. Giannotti, R. Guidotti, A. Monreale, S. Ruggieri, and F. Turini. Meaningful explanations of black box ai decision systems. In *Proceedings of the AAAI Conference on Artificial Intelligence*, volume 33, pages 9780–9784, 2019.

[54] H. Lakkaraju, E. Kamar, R. Caruana, and J. Leskovec. Faithful and customizable explanations of black box models. In *Proceedings of the 2019 AAAI/ACM Conference on AI, Ethics, and Society*, pages 131–138, 2019.

[55] S. Ceccon, D. F. Garway-Heath, D. P. Crabb, and A. Tucker. Exploring early glaucoma and the visual field test: Classification and clustering using bayesian networks. *IEEE journal of biomedical and health informatics*, 18(3): 1008–1014, 2014.

[56] P. J. Lucas, L. C. Van der Gaag, and A. Abu-Hanna. Bayesian networks in biomedicine and health-care, 2004.

[57] L. Peelen, N. F. de Keizer, E. de Jonge, R.-J. Bosman, A. Abu-Hanna, and N. Peek. Using hierarchical dynamic bayesian networks to investigate dynamics of organ failure in patients in the intensive care unit. *Journal of biomedical informatics*, 43(2):273–286, 2010.

[58] S. Aghabozorgi, A. S. Shirkhorshidi, and T. Y. Wah. Time-series clustering–a decade review. *Information Systems*, 53: 16–38, 2015.

[59] F. Altiparmak, H. Ferhatosmanoglu, S. Erdal, and D. C. Trost. Information mining over heterogeneous and high-dimensional time-series data in clinical trials databases. *IEEE Transactions on Information Technology in Biomedicine*, 10(2):254–263, 2006.

[60] S. Colagiuri. Glycated haemoglobin (hba1c) for the diagnosis of diabetes mellitus–practical implications. *Diabetes research and clinical practice*, 93(3):312, 2011.

[61] G. Das, K.-I. Lin, H. Mannila, G. Renganathan, and P. Smyth. Rule discovery from time series. In *KDD*, volume 98, pages 16–22, 1998.

[62] S. Ceccon, D. Garway-Heath, D. Crabb, and A. Tucker. The dynamic stage bayesian network: identifying and modelling key stages in a temporal process. *Advances in Intelligent Data Analysis X*, pages 101–112, 2011.

[63] R. Raman, A. Gupta, S. Krishna, V. Kulothungan, and T. Sharma. Prevalence and risk factors for diabetic microvascular complications in newly diagnosed type ii diabetes mellitus. sankara nethralaya diabetic retinopathy

epidemiology and molecular genetic study (sn-dreams, report 27). *Journal of Diabetes and its Complications*, 26(2): 123–128, 2012.

[64] K. R. Munana. Long-term complications of diabetes mellitus, part i: Retinopathy, nephropathy, neuropathy. *Veterinary Clinics: Small Animal Practice*, 25(3):715–730, 1995.

[65] W. Wang, J. Yang, and R. Muntz. Tar: Temporal association rules on evolving numerical attributes. In *Data Engineering, 2001. Proceedings. 17th International Conference on*, pages 283–292. IEEE, 2001.

[66] R. Agrawal, T. Imieliński, and A. Swami. Mining association rules between sets of items in large databases. In *Acm sigmod record*, volume 22, pages 207–216. ACM, 1993.

[67] C.-H. Lee, M.-S. Chen, and C.-R. Lin. Progressive partition miner: an efficient algorithm for mining general temporal association rules. *IEEE Transactions on Knowledge and Data Engineering*, (4):1004–1017, 2003.

[68] T. F. Gharib, H. Nassar, M. Taha, and A. Abraham. An efficient algorithm for incremental mining of temporal association rules. *Data & Knowledge Engineering*, 69(8):800–815, 2010.

[69] J. F. Allen et al. Towards a general theory of action and time. *Artificial intelligence*, 23(2):123–154, 1984.

[70] L. Sacchi, C. Larizza, C. Combi, and R. Bellazzi. Data mining with temporal abstractions: learning rules from time series. *Data Mining and Knowledge Discovery*, 15(2):217–247, 2007.

[71] J. M. Ale and G. H. Rossi. An approach to discovering temporal association rules. In *Proceedings of the 2000 ACM symposium on Applied computing-Volume 1*, pages 294–300, 2000.

[72] H. Jen-Wei and C. M. S. Dai Bi-Ru. Twain: Two-end association miner with precise frequent exhibition periods. *ACM Transactions on Knowledge Discovery from Data*, 8(2):800–815, 2007.

[73] Q. Zhao and S. S. Bhowmick. Association rule mining: A survey. *Nanyang Technological University, Singapore*, page 135, 2003.

[74] J. Mennis and J. W. Liu. Mining association rules in spatio-temporal data: An analysis of urban socioeconomic and land cover change. *Transactions in GIS*, 9(1):5–17, 2005.

[75] P.-N. Tan, V. Kumar, and J. Srivastava. Selecting the right objective measure for association analysis. *Information Systems*, 29(4):293–313, 2004.

[76] P. J. Dyck, K. Kratz, J. Karnes, W. J. Litchy, R. Klein, J. Pach, D. Wilson, P. O'brien, and L. Melton. The prevalence by staged severity of various types of diabetic neuropathy, retinopathy, and nephropathy in a population-based cohort: the rochester diabetic neuropathy study. *Neurology*, 43(4):817–817, 1993.

[77] G. F. Cooper and E. Herskovits. A bayesian method for the induction of probabilistic networks from data. *Machine learning*, 9(4):309–347, 1992.

[78] A. Doddi, S. Marathe, D. C. Ravi, and S. Torney. Discovery of association rules in medical data. *Medical informatics and the Internet in medicine*, 26(1):25–33, 2001.

[79] C. Ordonez, C. A. Santana, and L. De Braal. Discovering interesting association rules in medical data. In *ACM SIGMOD workshop on research issues in data mining and knowledge discovery*, pages 78–85. Citeseer, 2000.

[80] M. Plasse, N. Niang, G. Saporta, A. Villeminot, and L. Leblond. Combined

use of association rules mining and clustering methods to find relevant links between binary rare attributes in a large data set. *Computational Statistics and Data Analysis*, 52(1): 596–613, 2007.

[81] S. Mani and G. F. Cooper. Causal discovery using a bayesian local causal discovery algorithm. In *Medinfo*, pages 731–735, 2004.

[82] G. Sparacino, A. Facchinetti, A. Maran, and C. Cobelli. Continuous glucose monitoring time series and hypo/hyperglycemia prevention: requirements, methods, open problems. *Current diabetes reviews*, 4(3):181–192, 2008.

[83] L. Yousefi, S. Swift, M. Arzoky, L. Saachi, L. Chiovato, and A. Tucker. Opening the black box: Personalizing type 2 diabetes patients based on their latent phenotype and temporal associated complication rules. *Computational Intelligence*, 2020.

[84] L. Yousefi, S. Swift, M. Arzoky, L. Saachi, L. Chiovato, and A. Tucker. Opening the black box: Discovering and explaining hidden variables in type 2 diabetic patient modelling. In *2018 IEEE International Conference on Bioinformatics and Biomedicine (BIBM)*, pages 1040–1044. IEEE, 2018.

[85] L. Yousefi, S. Swift, M. Arzoky, L. Sacchi, L. Chiovato, and A. Tucker. Opening the black box: Exploring temporal pattern of type 2 diabetes complications in patient clustering using association rules and hidden variable discovery. In *2019 IEEE 32nd International Symposium on Computer-Based Medical Systems (CBMS)*, pages 198–203. IEEE, 2019.

[86] U. P. D. S. Group et al. Uk prospective diabetes study 16: overview of 6 years' therapy of type ii diabetes: a progressive disease. *Diabetes*, 44(11): 1249–1258, 1995.

[87] A. Z. Ali, M. Hossain, R. Pugh, et al. Diabetes, obesity and hypertension in urban and rural people of bedouin origin in the united arab emirates. *The Journal of tropical medicine and hygiene*, 98(6): 407–415, 1995.

[88] S. Concaro, L. Sacchi, C. Cerra, P. Fratino, and R. Bellazzi. Mining health care administrative data with temporal association rules on hybrid events. *Methods of information in medicine*, 50 (02):166–179, 2011.

[89] K. G. Tolman, V. Fonseca, A. Dalpiaz, and M. H. Tan. Spectrum of liver disease in type 2 diabetes and management of patients with diabetes and liver disease. *Diabetes care*, 30(3): 734–743, 2007.

[90] R. Turner, H. Millns, H. Neil, I. Stratton, S. Manley, D. Matthews, and R. Holman. Risk factors for coronary artery disease in non-insulin dependent diabetes mellitus: United kingdom prospective diabetes study (ukpds: 23). *Bmj*, 316(7134):823–828, 1998.

[91] M. Cusick, A. D. Meleth, E. Agron, M. R. Fisher, G. F. Reed, G. L. Knatterud, F. B. Barton, M. D. Davis, F. L. Ferris, E. Y. Chew, et al. Associations of mortality and diabetes complications in patients with type 1 and type 2 diabetes: early treatment diabetic retinopathy study report no. 27. *Diabetes Care*, 28(3):617–625, 2005.

[92] P. Thuluvath and D. Triger. Autonomic neuropathy and chronic liver disease. *QJM: An International Journal of Medicine*, 72(2):737–747, 1989.

[93] C. Liu, W. Ding, Y. Hu, X. Xia, B. Zhang, J. Liu, and D. Doermann. Circulant binary convolutional networks for object recognition. *IEEE Journal of Selected Topics in Signal Processing*, 2020.

[94] A. Ramachandran, C. Snehalatha, K. Satyavani, E. Latha, R. Sasikala, and

V. Vijay. Prevalence of vascular complications and their risk factors in type 2 diabetes. *The Journal of the Association of Physicians of India*, 47(12): 1152–1156, 1999.

[95] R. Bellazzi, L. Sacchi, and S. Concaro. Methods and tools for mining multivariate temporal data in clinical and biomedical applications. In *2009 Annual International Conference of the IEEE Engineering in Medicine and Biology Society*, pages 5629–5632. IEEE, 2009.

[96] R. Bellazzi and B. Zupan. Predictive data mining in clinical medicine: current issues and guidelines. *International journal of medical informatics*, 77(2): 81–97, 2008.

[97] L. Yousefi, M. Al-Luhaybi, L. Sacchi, L. Chiovato, and A. Tucker. Identifying latent variables in dynamic bayesian networks with bootstrapping applied to type 2 diabetes complication prediction. 2020.

Chapter 9

# The Role of Gender in the Onset, Development and Impact of Type 2 Diabetes Mellitus and Its Co-Morbidities

*Féaron C. Cassidy, Sinead Lafferty and Cynthia M. Coleman*

## Abstract

Almost half a billion people worldwide are living with diabetes mellitus (DM). Complications associated with DM are common and approximately half of those people with DM suffer from at least one comorbidity. There is high mortality, morbidity and cost associated with these comorbidities which include cardiovascular disease, retinopathy, nephropathy, neuropathy and osteopathy. Gender influences the relative risk of developing complications from DM via differing mechanisms – both directly and indirectly. Generally, an increased relative risk of cardiovascular disease and kidney disease is noticed in women with DM compared to the non-DM context, where rates of both are much higher in men. Men appear to be at greater risk of diabetic retinopathy and also of insensate diabetic neuropathy, whereas women suffer from an increased rate of painful diabetic neuropathy compared to men. These differences are not clear cut and vary regionally and temporally, indicating that the field would benefit from further research on both the epidemiology and physiological mechanism of the observed patterns. These differences should be taken into account in treatment programmes for DM and its comorbidities.

**Keywords:** gender, diabetes, diabetic complications, diabetic comorbidities

## 1. Introduction

Diabetes mellitus (DM) is a metabolic disease characterised by elevated blood glucose levels resultant of insufficient production or action of insulin, resulting in Type 1 (T1DM) and Type 2 (T2DM) respectively. Chronic hyperglycaemia is responsible for an array of severe macro- and micro-vascular complications resulting in numerous health complications. These include cardiovascular disease, retinopathy, nephropathy, neuropathy and osteopathy. Globally, more than 450 million adults are living with DM, while the annual death toll of DM is over 4 million people [1]. 70% of recorded deaths where T2DM is a contributing factor are due to T2DM comorbidities rather than T2DM itself, indicating insufficient or ineffective treatment of comorbidities [1, 2]. This statistic emphasises the importance of treating not only T2DM but also the complications associated with it, which are often present despite seemingly effective T2DM management.

The cost of treating T2DM includes the direct management of the disease with medication and medical visits as well as that of treating the associated complications and comorbidities which account for 53% of the total cost of T2DM patient care [3]. This puts the annual global healthcare expenditure on complications alone at $324 billion as of 2014 [4]. The continued increase in the healthcare budget spending on DM complications tracks the overall increased prevalence of the disease, but is also dependent on the likelihood of those complications within the DM population. Age is positively correlated with both onset of T2DM and its complications [5, 6]. In some middle income countries T2DM per capita is approaching 30% and increasing, these extraordinarily high rates of disease are intersecting with increasing life expectancy, which is also increasing fastest in middle-income countries [7, 8]. This will further compound the prevalence of T2DM complications and the associated morbidity, mortality and financial costs as the duration of disease and the average age of people living with it increases [9].

Despite a slightly increased prevalence of DM in men than women, more women than men die from DM and its associated complications [1]. Here we discuss the contribution of gender as a variable in the development of T2DM, its associated comorbidities and resulting mortality rates.

## 2. Gender differences in DM prevalence and mortality

The global prevalence of DM in adults aged 20–79 years is 9.3%, with slightly fewer women (9%) than men (9.6%) estimated to be living with the disease [1]. Prevalence of DM is increasing globally and though there is some evidence in high-income countries that incidence level is stabilising, the incidence in low- and middle-income countries continues to increase [1, 10]. The overall global prevalence of DM continues to increase both due to this increased incidence and due to the reduced mortality associated with DM as diagnosis and treatment continue to improve.

The major risk factors for the development of T2DM are obesity and poor diet. The higher prevalence of DM among men is despite generally higher rates of obesity in women globally - 15% of women and 11% of men were estimated to be in the obese category in 2016 [11, 12]. This epidemiological finding has been supported by studies at the individual level, which demonstrate that men have increased insulin resistance and develop T2DM at a younger age and lower BMI than women. This is primarily due to their overall propensity for visceral and hepatic deposition of lipid [11, 13–16]. In contrast, women tend to experience preferential subcutaneous deposition of lipid. These female and male pattern adipose distributions, commonly referred to as pear- and apple-shaped obesity respectively, are regulated by sex hormones and apple/central adiposity is independently correlated with T2DM status irrespective of BMI or gender [16, 17]. Though this bias exists currently and on a global level, there is high geographical and temporal variability [1, 18]. Despite men's physiologically higher propensity toward the development of T2DM, up until recently higher prevalence was recorded in women than men globally, and still is in many regions [1, 18]. This statistic correlates with what is known about obesity, a robust predictor of T2DM [19].

Although obesity has been recognised since ancient times, it effected a very low proportion of the population even up until the 1960s (1–2% in England at the time) and has only been described as posing a serious threat to public health in the last 50 years [20]. This rapid onset of obesity at the population level has correlated with the change in lifestyle and diet associated with development and westernisation, and, has disproportionately affected women [19]. In all countries assessed, the prevalence of obesity is higher in women during the growth phase of increasing obesity prevalence within that country [19, 21–26]. Only as obesity levels stabilise does the prevalence of obesity in men reach that of women [27, 28]. As would be expected, this generally tracks with what is known regarding the prevalence of T2DM in women and men over time. 100 years ago, rates of T2DM were higher in women in all regions assessed [18, 29]. Now in 2020, Europe, North America, South-East Asia and the Western pacific IDF regions have recorded either higher rates in men or no difference between genders, while the Africa, Middle East and Central America regions record higher rates of T2DM in women [1].

This may in part explain why despite their metabolically preferential adipose expansion, and lower propensity to T2DM itself, women have higher DM-associated mortality, with 2.3 million women and 1.9 million men dying from DM or DM-associated complications in 2019 alone [1, 7, 30, 31]. However, considering the majority of T2DM-associated mortality is due to associated complications rather than T2DM itself, this also indicates a higher risk of either developing complications or to enhanced severity of those complications in women. The IDF also record increased spending on women with T2DM than men, which may reflect higher rates of comorbidity in this group [1]. Whether gender impacts comorbidity outcomes in response to T2DM has been assessed in studies investigating individual complications, these are discussed below.

### 2.1 Cardiovascular disease

Cardiovascular disease (CVD), including cardiomyopathy, congestive heart failure, stroke and peripheral arterial disease, is the most prevalent cause of both morbidity and mortality in patients with DM [32–35]. The increased risk of death from CVD compared to the general population has been estimated at being between 1.6 and 2.6 times greater in individuals with T2DM depending on the form of CVD [1, 36–38].

The T2DM milieu increases CVD risk via a number of pathways. Atherosclerosis build-up is accelerated by the combination of hyperglycaemia, insulin resistance and increased free fatty acid release. In tandem, blood pressure is increased; hyperglycaemia impedes the production of nitric oxide (NO), while free fatty acid release resultant from insulin resistance reduces the bioavailability of NO (reviewed in [39]). NO has a vasoprotective role through increasing vasodilation, and therefore reducing blood pressure, as well as inhibiting inflammation and platelet activation [40]. The upregulation of inflammatory signalling pathways, including AGEs (advanced glycation end-products) and their receptor; RAGE, further promotes plaque deposition (reviewed in [39, 41]). The culmination of these processes is a patient at high risk of cardiovascular insult. While rates of CVD have decreased in patients with and without T2DM over the past few decades, risk of an event and risk of mortality from CVD remain higher in patients with T2DM [42, 43]. This is at least in part due to high rates of inability to achieve glycaemic control, but even in cases of robust glucose control, there is an increased level of risk that remains, indicating a metabolic memory of the hyperglycaemia present prior to control of T2DM [44]. This is exacerbated the longer the person has been diagnosed with T2DM. The mode of modulation of this metabolic memory is discussed in Cooper et al. [45], where both epigenetic mechanisms and immune memory are put forward. The treatment of patients with T2DM with standard CVD treatment regimens largely ameliorates this risk [46].

In women there is a 44% greater T2DM-associated risk of coronary heart disease (CHD) than in men [47]. The vastly increased risk of CVD in T2DM-diagnosed women is so great that it has been proposed as the primary attribute accounting for high diabetes-associated mortality in this population [30], see **Table 1**. In the general population men are at greater risk for CVD which is explained by the protective functions of oestrogens [54]. Primarily estradiol, for which there is receptors on cardiomyocytes, acts in a cardioprotective manner with numerous mechanisms for its action described in the literature (by improving mitochondrial function and reducing reactive oxygen species (ROS), via anti-fibrotic action in extracellular matrix remodelling, by stimulation of angiogenesis, via eNOS-dependent vasodilation, or possibly via aromatase action) as reviewed in Iorga et al., 2017 [55]. It is hypothesised that T2DM reverses the protective functions of oestrogens via immune-modulation [48]. As well as this increased disease burden, women with CHD and T2DM are at a nearly three times higher risk of death from CHD than men with CHD and T2DM [52]. A statistic that is likely related to the fact that women are less likely to be prescribed appropriate blood pressure and lipid lowering drugs [56–60].

Androgens, hormones which promote the development of male characteristics in vertebrates, have been shown to up-regulate the expression of known atherosclerosis associated genes in monocyte-derived macrophages from male donors but not from female donors [47]. However, men with hypogonadotropic hypogonadism (decreased androgen levels) have worse cardiovascular health and outcomes and are at increased risk of T2DM [61, 62]. Additionally, testosterone therapy has been shown to increase lean mass and insulin sensitivity in a small study of men with this condition [63].

As is the case with CHD, T2DM has been identified as an independent risk factor for stroke with a relative risk of 2.1 compared to the general population [64]. In the non-diabetic population, women have a higher lifetime risk of stroke despite lower risk in the majority of age categories [65]. Their risk increases over the age of 85 and the higher life time risk is a likely a factor of this combined with women's longer life expectancy [65]. Additionally, that female gender is associated with poorer outcome and increased risk of post-stroke disability is due to both differences in the types of strokes experienced by women and men and the significantly older age at which women experience stroke [65]. Women diagnosed with T2DM are at a 27% greater risk of stroke compared to men with T2DM, an effect which correlates with HbA1c levels [66]. Women are also less likely to achieve target levels for HbA1c [67]. Additionally, each 1% increase from baseline HbA1c is associated with a 5% increase in risk of stroke for women whereas the same increase from baseline in men is only associated with a 1% increase in risk of stroke [66]. This association is stronger in women over 55 years of age than those under 55, supporting a protective role of oestrogens, which are lost following menopause [68].

| Study location | Measure | Hazard ratio | | Reference |
|---|---|---|---|---|
| | | Women | Men | |
| Finland | Myocardial infarction | **14.40** | 2.90 | Juutilainen et al. 2004 [48] |
| USA | CHD mortality | **3.30** | 1.90 | Barrett-Connor et al. 1991 [49] |
| Italy | Stroke | **2.56** | 1.89 | Policardo et al. 2015 (varied by age) [50] |
| Asia Pacific | CHD mortality | **2.54** | 2.03 | Woodward et al. 2003 [51] |
| Taiwan | CHD mortality | **2.46** | 1.83 | Lin et al. 2013 [52] |
| USA | PAD | 1.72 | **2.12** | Palumbo & Joseph Melton III 1995 [53] |

**Table 1.**
*T2DM hazard ratio for CVD events by gender.*

While a number of studies have found women with DM at higher risk of stroke, Dhamoon et al. found that this increased risk disappeared when other factors including medication were accounted for [69]. This highlights a trend in the treatment of women in general for CVD, whereby a focus by doctors and the public on men's cardiovascular health has resulted in a greater risk to women who have not received a similar increase in attention to symptoms and biomarkers [70].

### 2.2 Diabetic retinopathy

Diabetic retinopathy is a leading cause of preventable visual impairment, effecting many in the working age demographic with significant personal and socioeconomic consequences [1]. It presents in approximately one third of patients with DM [71]. There are two main forms of diabetic retinopathy: nonproliferative and proliferative diabetic retinopathy. Nonproliferative retinopathy, also known as background diabetic retinopathy, is the early stages of the disorder in which hyperglycaemia leads to vascular cell apoptosis and neural damage within the retina but without major symptoms or an effect on vision. Proliferative diabetic retinopathy is the advanced form of diabetic retinopathy which is brought on by progressive retinal ischemia and results in vision loss through complications such as retinal detachment, neovascular glaucoma and vitreous haemorrhage [72].

Men appear to be at greater risk than women of developing diabetic retinopathy as well as progressing to proliferative retinopathy [73], see **Table 2**. Interestingly this pattern was not found in a large study in China [78], where there was found to be no effect of gender on the prevalence of diabetic retinopathy in people with DM [78].

While, in general, improvement in diabetic retinopathy status appears to be associated with improved glycaemic control and blood pressure, these factors cannot be attributed to the greater chance of improvement observed in women compared to men. Women in the UKPDS study were found to have a higher incidence of risk factors than the men in that study, including older age, more obesity, higher blood pressure, higher fasting plasma glucose levels, higher glycosylated haemoglobin levels, higher plasma cholesterol levels, higher insulin levels and increased insulin resistance [77].

| Study | DR type | Women (%) | Men (%) | P value | Reference |
|---|---|---|---|---|---|
| CURES | DR | 15 | **21** | <0.0001 | Rema et al. 2005 [74] |
| GADPVD | DR | 22 | **24** | <0.0001 | Hammes et al. 2015 [75] |
| NHANES | DR | 26 | **32** | <0.05 | Zhang et al. 2010 [76] |
| | V-DR | 4 | 6 | >0.05 | |
| UKPDS | DR | 35 | 39 | None | Kohner et al. 1998 [77] |
| | V-DR | 5 | **8** | <0.001 | |
| CCSS | DR | 31 | 30 | ns | Liu et al. 2017 [78] |
| | V-DR | 14 | 14 | ns | |
| WESDR | DR | Hazard ratio men = 1.3 | | 0.002 | Klein et al. 2008 [79] |

*NHANES = The National Health and Nutrition Examination Survey, USA; UKPDS = The United Kingdom Prospective Diabetes Study; WESDR = Wisconsin Epidemiological Study of Diabetic Retinopathy, Wisconsin, USA; GADPVD = German/Austrian Diabetes-Patienten-Verlaufsdokumentation Database, Germany and Austria; CURES = Chennai Urban Rural Epidemiology Study, Chennai City, India; v-DR = vision-threatening DR. Statistically significant values bolded. ns = not significant; none = no statistical analysis performed.*

**Table 2.**
*Prevalence of diabetic retinopathy in women and men with DM.*

It has been hypothesised alterations to sex hormone levels may be in part responsible for the increased chance of retinopathy progression in males. Sex hormone-binding globulin (SHBG) levels were found to be reduced in men who progressed to proliferative retinopathy as compared to those whose retinopathy did not progress over a 6 year period [80]. SHBG binds sex hormones, and lower levels allow for increased sex hormone activity, in men this would be associated with increased androgenicity.

### 2.3 Diabetic kidney disease

Diabetic kidney disease (DKD) is characterised by increased urinary albumin excretion in individuals living with DM who have not been diagnosed with any other renal disease [81]. It affects 20–40% of patients with T2DM and is the primary cause of kidney disease in patients who require renal replacement therapy [82]. Chronic Kidney Disease (CKD) in the absence of DM is more prevalent and more severe in men, but this gender disparity is not as striking in the case of DM-induced CKD (i.e. DKD) [83–85]. While some studies have found that men retain a significantly greater chance of developing DKD with DM [86, 87], others have found a similar prevalence of DKD women and men [88], see **Table 3**.

| Study | Measure | Women (%) | Men (%) | P value | Reference |
|---|---|---|---|---|---|
| Saudi Arabia | Prevalence | 41 | **59** | $p < 0.001$ | Al-Rubeaan et al. 2014 [86] |
| Denmark | Cumulative Incidence | 18 | **35** | 0.02 | Gall et al. 1997 [87] |
| NHANES | Prevalence | 39 | 40 | None | Wu et al. 2016 [88] |
| Korea | Odds ratio (OR) | OR for men = 1.31 | | 0.0024 | Yang et al. 2011 [89] |

*Statistically significant values bolded. None = no statistical analysis performed.*

**Table 3.**
*Prevalence of diabetic kidney disease in women and men with DM.*

This increased relative risk in women mirrors the loss of protection from oestrogens seen in CVD rates in women with DM, and as per CVD, protection from CKD in women has also been recorded to be lost after menopause [90]. This, along with evidence from animal models supports a role for oestrogens and/or androgens in CKD progression that is blunted or lost in a DM setting [91, 92]. Mouse models of both menopause (ovariectomy) and DM demonstrate worsened nephropathy [93, 94]. The mechanism by which estradiol or other sex hormones may impact CKD risk is unknown but both direct action on the kidney (eg. podocyte viability) or indirect action (eg. due to increased blood pressure or via transforming growth factor-β (TGF-β)-induced collagen synthesis) have been posited [84, 95, 96].

### 2.4 Diabetic neuropathy

Diabetic neuropathy (DN) is one of the most frequently observed complications in diabetic populations, averaging at about 20% of people with T2DM globally – though much higher estimates are observed in older populations and in communities with suboptimal therapeutic adherence (eg. up to 66% in older women in rural South Carolina, USA) [97, 98]. DN is characterised by nerve damage resultant from hyperglycaemia, with a correlation between risk of development and the duration and severity of hyperglycaemia [99, 100]. Symptoms of diabetic neuropathy include pain, idiopathic sensations (paraesthesia), excessive sensitivity to stimulus, loss of sensitivity, loss of coordination and altered sense of position [101]. These symptoms are associated with considerable morbidity, impacting quality of life [102]. The mechanism for nerve damage is through loss of protection and nutrient-provision from Schwann cells, leading eventually to axonal loss, most likely due to both high blood glucose levels and the absence of insulin, for which there are high affinity receptors throughout the nervous system [103, 104].

DN is the most significant contributor to diabetic foot syndrome (DFS) and results in a high risk of lower extremity amputation (LEA) among individuals living with DM [105]. DFS is characterised by the presence of foot ulcers and is causative of over 130,000 LEAs annually in the USA alone, this is approximately 0.6% of people with DM in the USA [10, 106]. The percentage of people with DM who experience DFS and the percentage of those who go on to have an amputation vary between countries, with higher rates of amputation in Sub-Saharan Africa, the Caribbean and parts of Latin America [107, 108]. The USA also has a high rate when compared to other developed countries [109].

Generally, men have a younger onset of DN and more severe symptoms, including higher rates of foot ulceration [100, 102, 110, 111]. Therefore, men are more likely to undergo a lower-extremity amputation (LEA) than women and at younger ages [102, 112–116], see **Table 4**. Globally, the number of people in 2016 who had amputations which were attributed to DM is 6.8 million people, with 4.1 million (60%) of those being men [107].

Although it has been hypothesised that lower rates of ulceration and/or LEA in women are due to indirect effects such as less physical work, superior preventative foot care and following care instructions [123–127], women and men have the same rate of ulceration when severity of DN is taken into account and equal rates of LEA within a population who have ulcers [111, 128]. Furthermore, though it has been reported that women heal ulcers more effectively than men [126], this study was in

| **Prevalence of DN in diabetic populations by gender** | | | | |
|---|---|---|---|---|
| **Study location** | **Women (%)** | **Men (%)** | **Significance** | **Reference** |
| Qatar | 22 | 24 | ns | Ponirakis et al. 2020 [117] |
| India | 8 | 10 | P = 0.001 | Sharath Kote et al. 2013 [118] |
| UK | 19 | 23 | P < 0.0001 | Abbott et al. 2011 [97] |
| Bangladesh | 19 | 21 | None | Mørkrid, Ali and Hussain 2010 [119] |
| UK | 29 | 29 | None | Young et al. 1993 [120] |
| Sri Lanka | 26 | 20 | p < 0.01 | Katulanda et al. 2012 [121] |
| **Incidence of LEA in diabetic populations by gender** | | | | |
| **Study Location** | **Women (per 100,000)** | **Men (per 100,000)** | **Significance** | **Reference** |
| USA | 28 | **55** | p < 0.05 | Correa-de-Araujo et al. 2006 [122] |
| Sweden | 192 | 197 | None | Johannesson et al. 2008 [113] |
| Spain | 145 | 583 | None | Almaraz et al. 2012 [116] |
| USA | 300 | 600 | None | Margolis et al. 2011 [112] |

*Statistically significant values bolded. ns = not significant; none = no statistical analysis performed.*

**Table 4.**
*Prevalence of DN and incidence of LEA in women and men.*

the context of a therapeutic bioengineered human dermal substitute, while studies of ulcer healing generally demonstrate no effect of gender on ulcer healing [129].

Therefore, the physiological link between DN and gender remains unclear and interestingly height alone, with men being on average taller than women, may be the greatest predictor of the incidence of DN [130]. This may explain the regional variation in DN prevalence differences by gender, as average height also varies geographically. For example average adult male height in the USA (where men experience higher rates of DN) is 175 cm compared to men in Sri Lanka, (where lower rates of DN are recorded in men compared to women) and the average height of men is 166 cm. The absence of a direct effect of gender on DN is corroborated by studies in mice which demonstrate similar nerve tissue dysfunction in female and male mice [131].

DN can be classified as painful or insensate and interestingly, painful DN is more prevalent in women and does not correlate with height [97, 118, 130, 132, 133]. This specific form of DN has independent risk factors from overall DN and seriously impacts on quality of life due to persistent sensation of pain in effected individuals [134, 135]. Why painful DN associates with the female gender is unknown but there is evidence of a genetic predisposition to the disorder based on high heritability [135]. This difference in painful DN between women and men may be attributable to the differences in pain processing, for which many hypotheses have been proposed to explain the differences present between genders, rather than differences related to DM or even DN specifically [136, 137].

### 2.5 Diabetic osteopathy

Bone health can be measured in a number of ways, including dual-energy x-ray absorptiometry (DXA) scan or measurement of bone turnover markers in the blood, however, the clinical importance of the disease lies in the elevated rate of fracture [138, 139]. In the non-diabetic population, the lifetime prevalence of hip fracture is significantly greater in women than in men [140]. This is driven by the higher rate of bone-turnover in postmenopausal women which results in decreased bone mineral density (BMD) culminating in osteoporosis [141–144]. As diagnosis and treatment for osteoporosis have increased, in conjunction with lower smoking rates and higher average BMI, the rate of hip fracture is decreasing. However, with an ageing population the absolute number of hip fractures is predicted to increase [139, 140]. Compounding this challenge in managing orthopaedic health is the increased fracture risk in people living with T2DM [145–149]. Contrary to the osteoporotic context, this increase in fracture risk is despite generally increased BMD in the T2DM population [148, 150, 151].

T2DM is associated with a relative risk of hip fracture of 1.3 with greater durations of T2DM increasing this risk [152, 153]. The presence of T2DM also increases the odds ratio of poor fracture healing, resulting in a malunion or non-union [154]. Hospital stay length and mortality following orthopaedic procedures are also increased in people with T2DM [149, 155]. The increased risk of fracture is present in both women and men, with contradicting evidence regarding whether women or men are preferentially impacted in terms of fracture risk by T2DM, while worse outcomes post-operatively seem to be more prevalent in men [149, 152, 153, 155, 156], see **Table 5**. Regardless, it is important that the increased risk of osteopathy in men with T2DM leads to appropriate intervention, where currently the emphasis of bone health is on women, in the T2DM context both women and men need to be considered.

Although DM-associated complications such as neuropathy and retinopathy increase the risk of falls which may result in fracture, the increased relative risk in

*DOI: http://dx.doi.org/10.5772/intechopen.94271*

| Study | Measure | Women | Men | Significance | Reference |
|---|---|---|---|---|---|
| Korea | HR | 1.7 | 1.8 | None | Kim et al. 2017 [156] |
| USA | HR | 1.5 | 1.5 | ns | Melton et al. 2008 [143] |
| Scotland | IRR | 1- | 1- | ns | Hothersall et al. 2014 [157] |
| Meta-Analysis | **RR** | **1.3** | 1.1 | $p < 0.001$ | Vilaca et al. 2020 [153] |
| | RR | 2.1 | 2.8 | ns | Janghorbani et al. 2007 [158] |
| | RR | 1.1 | Baseline | ns | Fan et al.2016 [152] |

*Statistically significant values bolded.HR = hazard ratio; IRR = incidence risk ratio; RR = relative risk; ns = not significant; none = no statistical analysis performed.*

**Table 5.**
*Summary of hip fracture risk in women and men living with T2DM.*

fracture remains when these variables are taken into account [159]. The reason for the increase in fracture risk in individuals with T2DM is not well characterised, but several hypotheses exist. DM induces systemic changes including inflammation and the generation of ROS which can negatively impact bone remodelling and changes in bone structure and mineral distribution [160–162], reviewed by [163]. People with T2DM have also been recorded as having lower density specifically of cortical bone and a more heterogeneous distribution of mineral, indicating compromising structural alterations that would yield impaired mechanical strength and increase the risk of fracture [160, 162]. Additionally, alterations to the mesenchymal stem cells (MSCs) responsible for maintaining bone homeostasis and for stimulating repair following an injury have also been reported [164–167]. Finally, pharmaceutical choice has also been reported to impact on the future risk of fracture in the DM population - thiazolidinediones have been associated with bone fragility while DPP4i and Metformin may reduce relative fracture risk [168–175].

In order to understand the gender aspect of the role of DM in bone health, recent publications investigated the aetiology of this increased fracture risk in men living with T2DM, identifying correlations with high levels of follicle-stimulating hormone and reduced estradiol with fracture risk [176]. There is also a discrepancy in the prescription of pharmaceuticals aimed at treating DM between women and men. For example, men are prescribed thiazolidinediones more often than women [177]. The disparity within the literature regarding the impact of gender in T2DM-induced fracture risk indicates the complexity of the question, with confounding variables such as the impact of pharmaceuticals, age, BMI, duration of diabetes and the presence of other diabetes-associated comorbidities.

## 3. Conclusions

DM is a growing global pandemic. DM is associated with several severe complications which have a major impact on patient outcomes and quality of life, and which make up a considerable component of healthcare budgets worldwide. Diabetic complications include cardiovascular disease, retinopathy, nephropathy, neuropathy (including diabetic foot syndrome) and osteopathy. Gender has been proposed across numerous studies as an important variable in the risk of development of these complications. However, teasing apart the role of gender is complex. Both the physiological impact of sex and the psychosocial impact of gender on behaviour and treatment are confounded by numerous factors. These include direct and indirect biological traits that associate with each gender, from hormone levels (which are vastly different for women post-menopause) to average height, life span and access to appropriate treatment. Many of these biological traits, and also psychosocial and socioeconomic traits that impact risk vary widely geographically. Understanding the epidemiology and physiological mechanisms of DM-associated complications, including the role of gender, allows for the implementation of appropriate treatment and research programmes that ultimately reduce morbidity and mortality.

In the non-DM population, oestrogens such as estradiol are protective against some of these comorbidities but the protective effects are often diminished in a DM context. This pattern is evident in both CVD and CKD where women with DM undergo a much larger relative increase in risk compared to men. Numerous studies have also shown that women are less often prescribed ACE inhibitors and lipid lowering drugs, including statins [56–60]. This prescription bias compounds the higher rates of CVD and CKD in women with T2DM, leading to increased mortality rates, a major factor in the high T2DM-assocaited mortality in women [30]. Therefore, particular awareness needs to be paid to the gender discrepancy in patient care in the context of T2DM in order to address this inequality and improve outcomes for women living with T2DM.

The onset of diabetic retinopathy is also linked to sex hormones - with levels of androgens correlating to likelihood of diagnosis. There is therefore increased incidence of diabetic retinopathy in men compared to women. Contrasting to this, neuropathy incidence, though higher in men, does not correlate directly with gender but instead with height which is a predictor of neuropathy development in both diabetic and non-diabetic populations [111, 118]. Therefore the higher rates in men in many regions are likely due to the greater average height of men with the causality possibly being longer nerve fibres which are more susceptible to injury and take longer to heal [111, 118].

Diabetic osteopathy is one of the less-reported complications of DM. People living with T2DM experience higher fracture rates both due to increased rates of falling and due to poorer bone health, which is present despite increased BMD [159]. In terms of the role of gender in diabetic osteopathy, the disorder follows an opposite pattern to that seen in CVD and DKD. Poor bone health experienced primarily by women in the non-DM population as they age is largely absent in men, but in the context of DM there is an increased relative risk for men to experience, for example, hip fracture [149, 156]. Fractures such as these are associated with high morbidity, especially functional limitations that results in loss of independence – physically and economically [178].

Interestingly, the overall mortality rates and cost of treatment associated with DM are higher in women than in men despite the general preponderance of comorbidity in men. A number of factors may explain this discrepancy. Firstly, women with DM are older, and epidemiologically there is increased cost of treatment and higher mortality with age. Secondly, regions with high DM-associated mortality (low- and middle-income countries) also report higher rates of DM in women [1]. Finally, men are reported to develop DM with a reduced risk-factor burden (eg. lower BMI). Though this indicates a greater risk of DM development for men, it also signifies that women, once they do develop DM, are diagnosed with such along with a greater set of risk factors for DM complications. These risk factors include inadequate blood glucose control, high blood pressure, high BMI and reportedly less frequent exercise [179]. Though not all women will experience pregnancy, for those that do, their glycaemic control during this time is a strong predictor of future development of T2DM [180]. Targeting those women who experience gestational diabetes for education or treatment options for T2DM would be an effective way of reducing diabetic burden in women and therefore reducing associated morbidity and mortality of T2DM globally [181, 182].

With such a large proportion of society effected by DM and the fact that the major risk factors for T2DM comprise a generally unhealthy lifestyle, the lines between complications of the disease itself and disorders that are simply comorbid, but potentially highly important and relevant to the DM population, become blurred. For example, T2DM is a risk factor for vascular dementia, more so in women compared to men [183]. Women with T2DM also have increased depressive symptoms compared to men with T2DM and these symptoms correlate with worsening T2DM biological profiles [179]. Studying the role of gender in this wider range of comorbidities will be important for a greater understanding of the interplay between common modifiable risk factors and those non-communicable diseases that are increasing in prevalence worldwide. This will ultimately benefit the future wellbeing of those that live with DM.

Gender also plays a role in response to and adherence to medication. While it has been demonstrated that there is no overall difference in medication adherence between women and men, Walker et al. demonstrated a significantly reduced adherence to Metformin in women and this was specifically related to women reporting worse adverse effects from the drug [179, 184]. Although advancements in therapies for DM include expensive pharmaceutical agents which are likely to increase the cost of treatment of DM per patient, significant reduction to overall spend may be achieved through effective reduction of complications [185]. Fewer complications and reduced severity of complications are not only beneficial for the overall costs of DM but also due to the obvious significant reduction in morbidity and mortality that would be associated. It is important that current and future medications are assessed for differential effects between women and men. A more recently explored treatment option, which has potential to rescue many of the disorders associated with T2DM is cell therapy. For many DM comorbidities, MSCs, for example, have been proposed as having a mechanistic role in both pathology and/or recovery [165, 186, 187]. There are fewer MSCs in the bone marrow of people with T2DM and considering the role of MSCs in repair and in reduction of inflammation, they are well poised as an effective treatment option [165]. Furthermore, there does not appear to be an impact of gender on the functioning of MSCs in tissue repair indicating they could benefit both women and men with T2DM comorbidity [165].

In conclusion, there are important implications of gender in terms of the risk of DM itself and subsequently the disorders caused by and associated with it. These differences need to be taken into account in research into T2DM and its complications as well as in the treatment of those individuals diagnosed with the disease. The observed interplay between T2DM and gender warrants further epidemiological and molecular analyses in order to achieve a more complete understanding of the role of gender in the onset and prognosis of diabetic complications. This review also demonstrates that in terms of biomedical research it is of crucial importance for studies to include both genders in their research, and for gender to be recorded as a variable. This supports recommendations made by the SAGER (Sex and Gender Equity in Research) guidelines [188]. It will also be important to further study the mechanism by which gender exerts the described effects, which will be different for different comorbidities of DM, and will likely vary by region.

## Acknowledgements

Research Alliance under the MRCG-HRB Joint Funding Scheme, grant number HRB-MRCG-2016-2.

## Conflict of interest

The authors declare no conflict of interest with regard to the content of this chapter.

## Note

In writing about the effect of gender on the development of diabetic complications in this review, it should be noted that only two genders are referred to due to the lack of data in the current literature on people who identify otherwise. We have chosen to use the term gender rather than sex, as it encompasses the combined physiological and psychosocial impacts on health discussed.


## Author details

Féaron C. Cassidy[1*], Sinead Lafferty[2] and Cynthia M. Coleman[2]

1 Department of Biology, Kathleen Lonsdale Human Health Institute, Maynooth University, Maynooth, Ireland

2 College of Medicine, Nursing and Health Science, School of Medicine, Regenerative Medicine Institute (REMEDI), National University of Ireland Galway (NUI Galway), Galway, Ireland

*Address all correspondence to: fearon.cassidy@mu.ie

## References

[1] International Diabetes Federation. IDF Diabetes Atlas Ninth Edition 2019. 2019.

[2] Park J, Peters PA. Mortality from diabetes mellitus, 2004 to 2008: A multiple-causeof-death analysis. Heal Reports 2014;25:12-6.

[3] Zhuo X, Zhang P, Hoerger TJ. Lifetime Direct Medical Costs of Treating Type 2 Diabetes and Diabetic Complications. Am J Prev Med 2013;45:253-61. https://doi.org/10.1016/J.AMEPRE.2013.04.017.

[4] Da J, Fernandes R, Ogurtsova K, Linnenkamp U, Guariguata L, Seuring T, et al. IDF Diabetes Atlas estimates of 2014 global health expenditures on diabetes 2016. https://doi.org/10.1016/j.diabres.2016.04.016.

[5] Morgan CL, Currie CJ, Stott NCH, Smithers M, Butler CC, Peters JR. The prevalence of multiple diabetes-related complications. Diabet Med 2000;17:146-51. https://doi.org/10.1046/j.1464-5491.2000.00222.x.

[6] Suastika K, Dwipayana P, Siswadi M, Tuty RA. Age is an Important Risk Factor for Type 2 Diabetes Mellitus and Cardiovascular Diseases. Glucose Toler., InTech; 2012. https://doi.org/10.5772/52397.

[7] IDF. IDF Diabetes Atlas Eighth edition 2017. 2017.

[8] ROSER M. Life Expectancy. OurWorldInDataOrg 2018. https://ourworldindata.org/life-expectancy.

[9] Harding JL, Pavkov ME, Magliano DJ, Shaw JE, Gregg EW. Global trends in diabetes complications: a review of current evidence. Diabetologia 2019;62:3-16. https://doi.org/10.1007/s00125-018-4711-2.

[10] U.S. Department of Health and Human Services, Centers for Disease Control and Prevention. National Diabetes Statistics Report 2020 Estimates of Diabetes and Its Burden in the United States. 2020.

[11] Kautzky-Willer A, Harreiter J, Pacini G. Sex and Gender Differences in Risk, Pathophysiology and Complications of Type 2 Diabetes Mellitus. Endocr Rev 2016;37:278-316. https://doi.org/10.1210/er.2015-1137.

[12] World Health Organisation. Obesity and overweight 2020. https://www.who.int/news-room/fact-sheets/detail/obesity-and-overweight (accessed August 18, 2020).

[13] Geer EB, Shen W. Gender differences in insulin resistance, body composition, and energy balance. Gend Med 2009;6:60-75. https://doi.org/10.1016/J.GENM.2009.02.002.

[14] Berry DC, Stenesen D, Zeve D, Graff JM. The developmental origins of adipose tissue. Development 2013;140:3939-49. https://doi.org/10.1242/dev.080549.

[15] Jeffery E, Wing A, Holtrup B, Sebo Z, Kaplan JL, Saavedra-Peña R, et al. The Adipose Tissue Microenvironment Regulates Depot-Specific Adipogenesis in Obesity. Cell Metab 2016;24:142-50. https://doi.org/10.1016/j.cmet.2016.05.012.

[16] Nordström A, Hadrévi J, Olsson T, Franks PW, Nordström P. Higher Prevalence of Type 2 Diabetes in Men Than in Women Is Associated With Differences in Visceral Fat Mass. J Clin Endocrinol Metab 2016;101:3740-6. https://doi.org/10.1210/jc.2016-1915.

[17] Snijder MB, Dekker JM, Visser M, Bouter LM, Stehouwer C DA, Kostense PJ, et al. Associations of hip

and thigh circumferences independent of waist circumference with the incidence of type 2 diabetes: the Hoorn Study. Am J Clin Nutr 2003;77:1192-7. https://doi.org/10.1093/ajcn/77.5.1192.

[18] Gan D, International Diabetes Federation. Diabetes atlas 2000. 2000.

[19] Kumanyika S, Jeffery RW, Morabia A, Ritenbaugh C, Antipatis VJ. Obesity prevention: The case for action. Int J Obes 2002;26:425-36. https://doi.org/10.1038/sj.ijo.0801938.

[20] Kirby M. Too Much of a Good Thing? Society, Affluence and Obesity in Britain, 1940-1970. ESharp 2012:44-63.

[21] Chen Y, Peng Q, Yang Y, Zheng S, Wang Y, Lu W. The prevalence and increasing trends of overweight, general obesity, and abdominal obesity among Chinese adults: A repeated cross-sectional study. BMC Public Health 2019;19:1293. https://doi.org/10.1186/s12889-019-7633-0.

[22] Lemamsha H, Randhawa G, Papadopoulos C. Prevalence of overweight and obesity among Libyan men and women. Biomed Res Int 2019;2019. https://doi.org/10.1155/2019/8531360.

[23] Australian Institute of Health and Welfare. The health of Australia's males, Overweight and obesity - Australian Institute of Health and Welfare n.d. https://www.aihw.gov.au/reports/men-women/male-health/contents/lifestyle-and-risk-factors/overweight-and-obesity (accessed August 28, 2020).

[24] Australian Institute of Health and Welfare. The health of Australia's females, Mothers - Australian Institute of Health and Welfare n.d. https://www.aihw.gov.au/reports/men-women/female-health/contents/lifestyle-risk-factors/overweight-and-obesity (accessed August 28, 2020).

[25] Craig M. Hales, M.D., Margaret D. Carroll, M.S.P.H., Cheryl D. Fryar, M.S.P.H., and Cynthia L. Ogden PD. Prevalence of Obesity and Severe Obesity Among Adults: United States, 2017-2018. 2020.

[26] Von Hippel PT, Nahhas RW. Extending the history of child obesity in the United States: The fels longitudinal study, birth years 1930-1993. Obesity 2013;21:2153-6. https://doi.org/10.1002/oby.20395.

[27] Kanter R, Caballero B. Global gender disparities in obesity: A review. Adv Nutr 2012;3:491-8. https://doi.org/10.3945/an.112.002063.

[28] Ameye H, Swinnen J. Obesity, income and gender: The changing global relationship. Glob Food Sec 2019;23:267-81. https://doi.org/10.1016/j.gfs.2019.09.003.

[29] Gale EAM, Gillespie KM. Diabetes and gender. Diabetologia 2001;44:3-15. https://doi.org/10.1007/s001250051573.

[30] Roche MM, Wang PP. Sex differences in all-cause and cardiovascular mortality, hospitalization for individuals with and without diabetes, and patients with diabetes diagnosed early and late. Diabetes Care 2013;36:2582-90. https://doi.org/10.2337/dc12-1272.

[31] Saeedi P, Salpea P, Karuranga S, Petersohn I, Malanda B, Gregg EW, et al. Mortality attributable to diabetes in 20-79 years old adults, 2019 estimates: Results from the International Diabetes Federation Diabetes Atlas, 9th edition. Diabetes Res Clin Pract 2020;162:108086. https://doi.org/10.1016/j.diabres.2020.108086.

[32] Baena-Díez JM, Peñafiel J, Subirana I, Ramos R, Elosua R, Marín-Ibañez A, et al. Risk of Cause-Specific Death in Individuals With Diabetes: A Competing Risks Analysis. Diabetes

Care 2016;39:1987-95. https://doi.org/10.2337/dc16-0614.

[33] Bertoni AG, Krop JS, Anderson GF, Brancati FL. Diabetes-Related Morbidity and Mortality in a National Sample of U.S. Elders. Diabetes Care 2002;25:471-5. https://doi.org/10.2337/DIACARE.25.3.471.

[34] Deshpande AD, Harris-Hayes M, Schootman M. Epidemiology of diabetes and diabetes-related complications. Phys Ther 2008;88:1254-64. https://doi.org/10.2522/ptj.20080020.

[35] Pantalone KM, Hobbs TM, Wells BJ, Kong SX, Kattan MW, Bouchard J, et al. Clinical characteristics, complications, comorbidities and treatment patterns among patients with type 2 diabetes mellitus in a large integrated health system. BMJ Open Diabetes Res Care 2015;3:e000093. https://doi.org/10.1136/bmjdrc-2015-000093.

[36] The Emerging Risk Factors Collaboration. Diabetes mellitus, fasting blood glucose concentration, and risk of vascular disease: a collaborative meta-analysis of 102 prospective studies. Lancet 2010;375:2215-22. https://doi.org/10.1016/S0140-6736(10)60484-9.

[37] Sarwar N, Gao P, Kondapally Seshasai SR, Gobin R, Kaptoge S, Di Angelantonio E, et al. Diabetes mellitus, fasting blood glucose concentration, and risk of vascular disease: A collaborative meta-analysis of 102 prospective studies. Lancet 2010;375:2215-22. https://doi.org/10.1016/S0140-6736(10)60484-9.

[38] Woodward M. The effects of diabetes on the risks of major cardiovascular diseases and death in the Asia-Pacific region. Diabetes Care 2003;26:360-6. https://doi.org/10.2337/diacare.26.2.360.

[39] Beckman JA, Creager MA, Libby P. Diabetes and Atherosclerosis. JAMA 2002;287:2570. https://doi.org/10.1001/jama.287.19.2570.

[40] Moncada S, Palmer RMJ, Higgs EA. The Discovery of Nitric Oxide as the Endogenous Nitrovasodilator. 1988.

[41] Koulis C, Kanellakis P, Pickering RJ, Tsorotes D, Murphy AJ, Gray SP, et al. Role of bone-marrow- and non-bone-marrow-derived receptor for advanced glycation end-products (RAGE) in a mouse model of diabetes-associated atherosclerosis. Clin Sci (Lond) 2014;127:485-97. https://doi.org/10.1042/CS20140045.

[42] Matheus AS de M, Tannus LRM, Cobas RA, Palma CCS, Negrato CA, Gomes M de B. Impact of diabetes on cardiovascular disease: an update. Int J Hypertens 2013;2013:653789. https://doi.org/10.1155/2013/653789.

[43] Wang CCL, Hess CN, Hiatt WR, Goldfine AB. Atherosclerotic Cardiovascular Disease and Heart Failure in Type 2Diabetes – Mechanisms, Management, and ClinicalConsiderations. Circulation 2016;133:2459. https://doi.org/10.1161/CIRCULATIONAHA.116.022194.

[44] Riddle MC, Ambrosius WT, Brillon DJ, Buse JB, Byington RP, Cohen RM, et al. Epidemiologic relationships between A1C and all-cause mortality during a median 3.4-year follow-up of glycemic treatment in the ACCORD trial. Diabetes Care 2010;33:983-90. https://doi.org/10.2337/dc09-1278.

[45] Cooper ME, El-Osta A, Allen TJ, Watson AMD, Thomas MC, Jandeleit-Dahm KAM. Metabolic Karma-The Atherogenic Legacy of Diabetes: The 2017 Edwin Bierman Award Lecture. Diabetes 2018;67:785-90. https://doi.org/10.2337/dbi18-0010.

[46] Gæde P, Vedel P, Larsen N, Jensen GVH, Parving H-H, Pedersen O.

Multifactorial Intervention and Cardiovascular Disease in Patients with Type 2 Diabetes. N Engl J Med 2003;348:383-93. https://doi.org/10.1056/NEJMoa021778.

[47] Ng MKC, Quinn CM, McCrohon JA, Nakhla S, Jessup W, Handelsman DJ, et al. Androgens up-regulate atherosclerosis-related genes in macrophages from males but not females: molecular insights into gender differences in atherosclerosis. J Am Coll Cardiol 2003;42:1306-13.

[48] Juutilainen A, Kortelainen S, Lehto S, Rönnemaa T, Pyörälä K, Laakso M. Gender difference in the impact of type 2 diabetes on coronary heart disease risk. Diabetes Care 2004;27:2898-904.

[49] Barrett-Connor EL, Cohn BA, Wingard DL, Edelstein SL. Why Is Diabetes Mellitus a Stronger Risk Factor for Fatal Ischemic Heart Disease in Women Than in Men? JAMA 1991;265:627. https://doi.org/10.1001/jama.1991.03460050081025.

[50] Policardo L, Seghieri G, Francesconi P, Anichini R, Franconi F, Seghieri C, et al. Gender difference in diabetes-associated risk of first-ever and recurrent ischemic stroke. J Diabetes Complications 2015;29:713-7. https://doi.org/10.1016/J.JDIACOMP.2014.12.008.

[51] Woodward M, Zhang X, Barzi F, Pan W, Ueshima H, Rodgers A, et al. The effects of diabetes on the risks of major cardiovascular diseases and death in the Asia-Pacific region. Diabetes Care 2003;26:360-6. https://doi.org/10.2337/diacare.26.2.360.

[52] Lin G-M, Li Y-H, Lin C-L, Wang J-H, Han C-L. Gender differences in the impact of diabetes on mortality in patients with established coronary artery disease: A report from the Eastern Taiwan integrated health care delivery system of Coronary Heart Disease (ET-CHD) registry, 1997-2006. J Cardiol 2013;61:393-8. https://doi.org/10.1016/J.JJCC.2013.02.007.

[53] Palumbo PJ, Joseph Melton III L. Peripheral Vascular Disease and Diabetes. In: National Diabetes Data Group, National Institute of Diabetes and Digestive and Kidney Diseases NI of H, editor. Diabetes Am. - Ronald Aubert. 2nd ed., National Diabetes Data Group, National Institute of Diabetes and Digestive and Kidney Diseases, National Institutes of Health; 1995, p. 401-8.

[54] Roeters van Lennep JE, Westerveld HT, Erkelens DW, van der Wall EE. Risk factors for coronary heart disease: implications of gender. Cardiovasc Res 2002;53:538-49.

[55] Iorga A, Cunningham CM, Moazeni S, Ruffenach G, Umar S, Eghbali M. The protective role of estrogen and estrogen receptors in cardiovascular disease and the controversial use of estrogen therapy. Biol Sex Differ 2017;8:33. https://doi.org/10.1186/s13293-017-0152-8.

[56] Lenzen MJ, Rosengren A, Scholte op Reimer WJM, Follath F, Boersma E, Simoons ML, et al. Management of patients with heart failure in clinical practice: differences between men and women. Heart 2008;94:e10. https://doi.org/10.1136/hrt.2006.099523.

[57] Baumhäkel M, Müller U, Böhm M. Influence of gender of physicians and patients on guideline-recommended treatment of chronic heart failure in a cross-sectional study. Eur J Heart Fail 2009;11:299-303. https://doi.org/10.1093/eurjhf/hfn041.

[58] Nilsson PM, Theobald H, Journath G, Fritz T. Gender differences in risk factor control and treatment profile in diabetes: a study in 229 Swedish primary health care centres. Scand J Prim Health

Care 2004;22:27-31. https://doi.org/10.1080/02813430310003264.

[59] Graversen L, Christensen B, Borch-Johnsen K, Lauritzen T, Sandbaek A. General practitioners' adherence to guidelines on management of dyslipidaemia: ADDITION-Denmark. Scand J Prim Health Care 2010;28:47-54. https://doi.org/10.3109/02813430903335216.

[60] Fu AZ, Zhang Q, Davies MJ, Pentakota S-R, Radican L, Seck T. Underutilization of statins in patients with type 2 diabetes in US clinical practice: a retrospective cohort study. Curr Med Res Opin 2011;27:1035-40. https://doi.org/10.1185/03007995.2011.567257.

[61] Hackett G. Type 2 diabetes and testosterone therapy. World J Men?S Heal 2019;37:31-44. https://doi.org/10.5534/wjmh.180027.

[62] Stoian AP, Andronache LF, Ginghina O. Testosterone therapy, new opportunities in diabetes mellitus. 2018.

[63] Dhindsa S, Ghanim H, Batra M, Kuhadiya ND, Abuaysheh S, Sandhu S, et al. Insulin Resistance and Inflammation in Hypogonadotropic Hypogonadism and Their Reduction after Testosterone Replacement in Men with Type 2 Diabetes. Diabetes Care 2016;39:82-91. https://doi.org/10.2337/dc15-1518.

[64] Ergul A, Kelly-Cobbs A, Abdalla M, Fagan SC. Cerebrovascular complications of diabetes: focus on stroke. Endocr Metab Immune Disord Drug Targets 2012;12:148-58.

[65] Petrea RE, Beiser AS, Seshadri S, Kelly-Hayes M, Kase CS, Wolf PA. Gender Differences in Stroke Incidence and Poststroke Disability in the Framingham Heart Study. Stroke 2009;40:1032-7. https://doi.org/10.1161/STROKEAHA.108.542894.

[66] Peters SAE, Huxley RR, Sattar N, Woodward M. Sex Differences in the Excess Risk of Cardiovascular Diseases Associated with Type 2 Diabetes: Potential Explanations and Clinical Implications. Curr Cardiovasc Risk Rep 2015;9:36. https://doi.org/10.1007/s12170-015-0462-5.

[67] Choe S-A, Kim JY, Ro YS, Cho S-I. Women are less likely than men to achieve optimal glycemic control after 1 year of treatment: A multi-level analysis of a Korean primary care cohort. PLoS One 2018;13:e0196719. https://doi.org/10.1371/journal.pone.0196719.

[68] Chen Y, Huang Y-C, Yan CH, Chiu KY, Wei Q, Zhao J, et al. Abnormal subchondral bone remodeling and its association with articular cartilage degradation in knees of type 2 diabetes patients. Bone Res 2017;5:17034. https://doi.org/10.1038/boneres.2017.34.

[69] Dhamoon MS, Liang JW, Zhou L, Stamplecoski M, Kapral MK, Shah BR. Sex Differences in Outcomes after Stroke in Patients with Diabetes in Ontario, Canada. J Stroke Cerebrovasc Dis 2018;27:210-20. https://doi.org/10.1016/J.JSTROKECEREBROVASDIS.2017.08.028.

[70] Wexler DJ, Grant RW, Meigs JB, Nathan DM, Cagliero E. Sex disparities in treatment of cardiac risk factors in patients with type 2 diabetes. Diabetes Care 2005;28:514-20. https://doi.org/10.2337/DIACARE.28.3.514.

[71] Lee R, Wong TY, Sabanayagam C. Epidemiology of diabetic retinopathy, diabetic macular edema and related vision loss. Eye Vis 2015;2:17. https://doi.org/10.1186/s40662-015-0026-2.

[72] Danis RP, Davis MD. Proliferative Diabetic Retinopathy. Diabet. Retin., Totowa, NJ: Humana Press; 2008, p. 29-65. https://doi.org/10.1007/978-1-59745-563-3_2.

[73] Ozawa GY, Bearse MA, Adams AJ. Male-female differences in diabetic retinopathy? Curr Eye Res 2015;40:234-46. https://doi.org/10.3109/02713683.2014.958500.

[74] Rema M, Premkumar S, Anitha B, Deepa R, Pradeepa R, Mohan V. Prevalence of Diabetic Retinopathy in Urban India: The Chennai Urban Rural Epidemiology Study (CURES) Eye Study, I. Investig Opthalmology Vis Sci 2005;46:2328. https://doi.org/10.1167/iovs.05-0019.

[75] Hammes H-P, Welp R, Kempe H-P, Wagner C, Siegel E, Holl RW, et al. Risk Factors for Retinopathy and DME in Type 2 Diabetes—Results from the German/Austrian DPV Database. PLoS One 2015;10:e0132492. https://doi.org/10.1371/journal.pone.0132492.

[76] Zhang X, Saaddine JB, Chou C-F, Cotch MF, Cheng YJ, Geiss LS, et al. Prevalence of Diabetic Retinopathy in the United States, 2005-2008. JAMA 2010;304:649. https://doi.org/10.1001/jama.2010.1111.

[77] Kohner EM, Aldington SJ, Stratton IM, Manley SE, Holman RR, Matthews DR, et al. United Kingdom Prospective Diabetes Study, 30. Arch Ophthalmol 1998;116:297. https://doi.org/10.1001/archopht.116.3.297.

[78] Liu Y, Song Y, Tao L, Qiu W, Lv H, Jiang X, et al. Prevalence of diabetic retinopathy among 13473 patients with diabetes mellitus in China: a cross-sectional epidemiological survey in six provinces. BMJ Open 2017;7:e013199. https://doi.org/10.1136/bmjopen-2016-013199.

[79] Klein R, Knudtson MD, Lee KE, Gangnon R, Klein BEK. The Wisconsin Epidemiologic Study of Diabetic Retinopathy: XXII the twenty-five-year progression of retinopathy in persons with type 1 diabetes. Ophthalmology 2008;115:1859-68. https://doi.org/10.1016/j.ophtha.2008.08.023.

[80] Haffner SM, Klein R, Moss SE, Klein BE. Sex hormones and the incidence of severe retinopathy in male subjects with type I diabetes. Ophthalmology 1993;100:1782-6. https://doi.org/10.1016/S0161-6420(93)31398-9.

[81] Gross JL, de Azevedo MJ, Silveiro SP, Canani LH, Caramori ML, Zelmanovitz T. Diabetic nephropathy: diagnosis, prevention, and treatment. Diabetes Care 2005;28:164-76. https://doi.org/10.2337/diacare.28.1.164.

[82] Gheith O, Farouk N, Nampoory N, Halim MA, Al-Otaibi T. Diabetic kidney disease: world wide difference of prevalence and risk factors. J Nephropharmacology 2016;5:49-56.

[83] Goldberg I, Krause I. THE ROLE OF GENDER IN CHRONIC KIDNEY DISEASE. 2016.

[84] Silbiger SR. Raging hormones: Gender and renal disease. Kidney Int 2011;79:382-4. https://doi.org/10.1038/ki.2010.474.

[85] NEUGARTEN J, ACHARYA A, SILBIGER SR. Effect of Gender on the Progression of Nondiabetic Renal Disease. J Am Soc Nephrol 2000;11.

[86] Al-Rubeaan K, Youssef AM, Subhani SN, Ahmad NA, Al-Sharqawi AH, Al-Mutlaq HM, et al. Diabetic nephropathy and its risk factors in a society with a type 2 diabetes epidemic: a Saudi National Diabetes Registry-based study. PLoS One 2014;9:e88956. https://doi.org/10.1371/journal.pone.0088956.

[87] Gall MA, Hougaard P, Borch-Johnsen K, Parving HH. Risk factors for development of incipient and overt diabetic nephropathy in patients with non-insulin dependent diabetes mellitus: prospective, observational study. BMJ 1997;314:783-8. https://doi.org/10.1136/BMJ.314.7083.783.

[88] Wu B, Bell K, Stanford A, Kern DM, Tunceli O, Vupputuri S, et al. Understanding CKD among patients with T2DM: prevalence, temporal trends, and treatment patterns—NHANES 2007-2012. BMJ Open Diabetes Res Care 2016;4:e000154. https://doi.org/10.1136/bmjdrc-2015-000154.

[89] Yang C-W, Park JT, Kim YS, Kim YL, Lee Y-S, Oh Y-S, et al. Prevalence of diabetic nephropathy in primary care type 2 diabetic patients with hypertension: data from the Korean Epidemiology Study on Hypertension III (KEY III study). Nephrol Dial Transplant 2011;26:3249-55. https://doi.org/10.1093/ndt/gfr011.

[90] Coggins CH, Lewis JB, Caggiula AW, Castaldo LS, Klahr S, Wang SR, et al. Differences between women and men with chronic renal disease. Nephrol Dial Transplant 1998;13:1430-7. https://doi.org/10.1093/ndt/13.6.1430.

[91] Kang DH, Yu ES, Yoon K Il, Johnson R. The Impact of Gender on Progression of Renal Disease: Potential Role of Estrogen-Mediated Vascular Endothelial Growth Factor Regulation and Vascular Protection. Am J Pathol 2004;164:679-88. https://doi.org/10.1016/S0002-9440(10)63155-0.

[92] Gluhovschi A, Petrica L, Gluhovschi C. Chronic kidney disease and the involvement of estrogen hormones in its pathogenesis and progression Article in Romanian journal of internal medicine = Revue roumaine de médecine interne ·. 2012.

[93] Keck M, Romero-Aleshire MJ, Cai Q, Hoyer PB, Brooks HL. Hormonal status affects the progression of STZ-induced diabetes and diabetic renal damage in the VCD mouse model of menopause. Am J Physiol Physiol 2007;293:F193-9. https://doi.org/10.1152/ajprenal.00022.2007.

[94] Silbiger S, Neugarten J. Gender and human chronic renal disease. Gend Med 2008;5. https://doi.org/10.1016/j.genm.2008.03.002.

[95] Suzuki H, Kondo K. Chronic kidney disease in postmenopausal women. Hypertens Res 2012;35:142-7. https://doi.org/10.1038/hr.2011.155.

[96] Doublier S, Lupia E, Catanuto P, Periera-Simon S, Xia X, Korach K, et al. Testosterone and 17B-estradiol have opposite effects on podocyte apoptosis that precedes glomerulosclerosis in female estrogen receptor knockout mice. Kidney Int 2011;79:404-13. https://doi.org/10.1038/ki.2010.398.

[97] Abbott CA, Malik RA, van Ross ERE, Kulkarni J, Boulton AJM. Prevalence and Characteristics of Painful Diabetic Neuropathy in a Large Community-Based Diabetic Population in the U.K. Diabetes Care 2011;34:2220-4. https://doi.org/10.2337/dc11-1108.

[98] Pruitt J, Moracho-Vilrriales C, Threatt T, Wagner S, Wu J, Romero-Sandoval EA, et al. Identification, prevalence, and treatment of painful diabetic neuropathy in patients from a rural area in South Carolina. J Pain Res 2017;10:833-43. https://doi.org/10.2147/JPR.S129139.

[99] Groener JB, Jende JME, Kurz FT, Kender Z, Treede RD, Schuh-Hofer S, et al. Understanding diabetic neuropathy—from subclinical nerve lesions to severe nerve fiber deficits: A cross-sectional study in patients with type 2 diabetes and healthy control subjects. Diabetes 2020;69:436-47. https://doi.org/10.2337/db19-0197.

[100] Booya F, Bandarian F, Larijani B, Pajouhi M, Nooraei M, Lotfi J. Potential risk factors for diabetic neuropathy: a case control study. BMC Neurol 2005;5:24. https://doi.org/10.1186/1471-2377-5-24.

[101] Lechleitner M, Abrahamian H, Francesconi C, Kofler M. Diabetische Neuropathie. Wien Klin Wochenschr 2016;128:73-9. https://doi.org/10.1007/s00508-015-0930-4.

[102] Aaberg ML, Burch DM, Hud ZR, Zacharias MP. Gender differences in the onset of diabetic neuropathy. J Diabetes Complications 2008;22:83-7.

[103] Mizisin AP. Mechanisms of diabetic neuropathy: Schwann cells. Handb. Clin. Neurol., vol. 126, Elsevier B.V.; 2014, p. 401-28. https://doi.org/10.1016/B978-0-444-53480-4.00029-1.

[104] Feldman EL, Nave K-A, Jensen TS, Bennett DLH. New Horizons in Diabetic Neuropathy: Mechanisms, Bioenergetics, and Pain. Neuron 2017;93:1296-313. https://doi.org/10.1016/J.NEURON.2017.02.005.

[105] Tuttolomondo A, Maida C, Pinto A. Diabetic foot syndrome: Immune-inflammatory features as possible cardiovascular markers in diabetes. World J Orthop 2015;6:62-76. https://doi.org/10.5312/wjo.v6.i1.62.

[106] Pecoraro RE, Reiber GE, Burgess EM. Pathways to Diabetic Limb Amputation: Basis for Prevention. Diabetes Care 1990;13:513-21. https://doi.org/10.2337/diacare.13.5.513.

[107] Zhang Y, Lazzarini PA, McPhail SM, van Netten JJ, Armstrong DG, Pacella RE. Global Disability Burdens of Diabetes-Related Lower-Extremity Complications in 1990 and 2016. Diabetes Care 2020;43:964-74. https://doi.org/10.2337/dc19-1614.

[108] Boulton AJM. The diabetic foot: grand overview, epidemiology and pathogenesis. Diabetes Metab Res Rev 2008;24:S3-6. https://doi.org/10.1002/dmrr.833.

[109] Renzi R, Unwin N, Jubelirer R, Haag L. An international comparison of lower extremity amputation rates. Ann Vasc Surg 2006;20:346-50. https://doi.org/10.1007/s10016-006-9044-9.

[110] Zhang P, Lu J, Jing Y, Tang S, Zhu D, Bi Y. Global epidemiology of diabetic foot ulceration: a systematic review and meta-analysis†. Ann Med 2017;49:106-16. https://doi.org/10.1080/07853890.2016.1231932.

[111] Dinh T, Veves A. The influence of gender as a risk factor in diabetic foot ulceration. Wounds 2008.

[112] Margolis DJ, Malay DS, Hoffstad OJ, Leonard CE, MaCurdy T, de Nava KL, et al. Incidence of diabetic foot ulcer and lower extremity amputation among Medicare beneficiaries, 2006 to 2008: Data Points #2. Agency for Healthcare Research and Quality (US); 2011.

[113] Johannesson A, Larsson GU, Ramstrand N, Turkiewicz A, Wiréhn AB, Atroshi I. Incidence of lower-limb amputation in the diabetic and nondiabetic general population: A 10-year population-based cohort study of initial unilateral and contralateral amputations and reamputations. Diabetes Care 2009;32:275-80. https://doi.org/10.2337/dc08-1639.

[114] Alvarsson A, Sandgren B, Wendel C, Alvarsson M, Brismar K. A retrospective analysis of amputation rates in diabetic patients: Can lower extremity amputations be further prevented? Cardiovasc Diabetol 2012;11. https://doi.org/10.1186/1475-2840-11-18.

[115] Al-Rubeaan K, Al Derwish M, Ouizi S, Youssef AM, Subhani SN, Ibrahim HM, et al. Diabetic foot complications and their risk factors from a large retrospective cohort study. PLoS One 2015;10. https://doi.org/10.1371/journal.pone.0124446.

[116] Almaraz MC, González-Romero S, Bravo M, Caballero FF, Palomo MJ,

Vallejo R, et al. Incidence of lower limb amputations in individuals with and without diabetes mellitus in Andalusia (Spain) from 1998 to 2006. Diabetes Res Clin Pract 2012;95:399-405. https://doi.org/10.1016/j.diabres.2011.10.035.

[117] Ponirakis G, Elhadd T, Chinnaiyan S, Dabbous Z, Siddiqui M, Al-muhannadi H, et al. Prevalence and management of diabetic neuropathy in secondary care in Qatar. Diabetes Metab Res Rev 2020;36. https://doi.org/10.1002/dmrr.3286.

[118] Sharath Kote GS, Bhat AN, Thajuddeen K, Ismail MH, Gupta A. Peripheral insensate neuropathy-is height a risk factor? J Clin Diagnostic Res 2013;7:296-301. https://doi.org/10.7860/JCDR/2013/5140.2751.

[119] Mørkrid K, Ali L, Hussain A. Risk factors and prevalence of diabetic peripheral neuropathy: A study of type 2 diabetic outpatients in Bangladesh. Int J Diabetes Dev Ctries 2010;30:11-7. https://doi.org/10.4103/0973-3930.60004.

[120] Young MJ, Boulton AJM, Macleod AF, Williams DRR, Onksen PHS. A multicentre study of the prevalence of diabetic peripheral neuropathy in the United Kingdom hospital clinic population. vol. 36. 1993.

[121] Katulanda P, Ranasinghe P, Jayawardena R, Constantine GR, Sheriff MHR, Matthews DR. The prevalence, patterns and predictors of diabetic peripheral neuropathy in a developing country. Diabetol Metab Syndr 2012;4:21. https://doi.org/10.1186/1758-5996-4-21.

[122] Correa-de-Araujo R, McDermott K, Moy E. Gender differences across racial and ethnic groups in the quality of care for diabetes. Women's Heal Issues 2006;16:56-65. https://doi.org/10.1016/j.whi.2005.08.003.

[123] Moura Neto A, Zantut-Wittmann DE, Fernandes TD, Nery M, Parisi MCR. Risk factors for ulceration and amputation in diabetic foot: Study in a cohort of 496 patients. Endocrine 2013;44:119-24. https://doi.org/10.1007/s12020-012-9829-2.

[124] Rossaneis MA, Haddad M do CFL, Mathias TA de F, Marcon SS. Diferenças entre mulheres e homens diabéticos no autocuidado com os pés e estilo de vida. Rev Lat Am Enfermagem 2016;24. https://doi.org/10.1590/1518-8345.1203.2761.

[125] Hjelm K, Nyberg P, Apelqvist J. Gender influences beliefs about health and illness in diabetic subjects with severe foot lesions. J Adv Nurs 2002;40:673-84. https://doi.org/10.1046/j.1365-2648.2002.02427.x.

[126] Marston WA. Risk factors associated with healing chronic diabetic foot ulcers: The importance of hyperglycemia. Ostomy Wound Manag 2006;52:26-39.

[127] Vedhara K, Beattie A, Metcalfe C, Roche S, Weinman J, Cullum N, et al. Development and preliminary evaluation of a psychosocial intervention for modifying psychosocial risk factors associated with foot re-ulceration in diabetes. Behav Res Ther 2012;50:323-32. https://doi.org/10.1016/j.brat.2012.02.013.

[128] Ugwu E, Adeleye O, Gezawa I, Okpe I, Enamino M, Ezeani I. Predictors of lower extremity amputation in patients with diabetic foot ulcer: Findings from MEDFUN, a multi-center observational study. J Foot Ankle Res 2019;12:34. https://doi.org/10.1186/s13047-019-0345-y.

[129] Gubara Musa H, E. Ahmed M. Associated risk factors and management of chronic diabetic foot ulcers exceeding 6 months' duration. Diabet Foot Ankle

2012;3:18980. https://doi.org/10.3402/dfa.v3i0.18980.

[130] Sorensen L, Molyneaux L, Yue DK. Insensate versus painful diabetic neuropathy: the effects of height, gender, ethnicity and glycaemic control. Diabetes Res Clin Pract 2002;57:45-51. https://doi.org/10.1016/S0168-8227(02)00010-4.

[131] O'Brien PD, Hur J, Robell NJ, Hayes JM, Sakowski SA, Feldman EL. Gender-specific differences in diabetic neuropathy in BTBR ob/ob mice. J Diabetes Complications 2016;30:30-7. https://doi.org/10.1016/j.jdiacomp.2015.09.018.

[132] Alkhatatbeh M, Abdul-Razzak KK. Neuropathic pain is not associated with serum vitamin D but is associated with female gender in patients with type 2 diabetes mellitus. BMJ Open Diabetes Res Care 2019;7:690. https://doi.org/10.1136/bmjdrc-2019-000690.

[133] Kim SS, Won JC, Kwon HS, Kim CH, Lee JH, Park TS, et al. Prevalence and clinical implications of painful diabetic peripheral neuropathy in type 2 diabetes: Results from a nationwide hospital-based study of diabetic neuropathy in Korea. Diabetes Res Clin Pract 2014;103:522-9. https://doi.org/10.1016/j.diabres.2013.12.003.

[134] Davies M, Brophy S, Williams R, Taylor A. The prevalence, severity, and impact of painful diabetic peripheral neuropathy in type 2 diabetes. Diabetes Care 2006;29:1518-22. https://doi.org/10.2337/dc05-2228.

[135] Galer BS, Gianas A, Jensen MP. Painful diabetic polyneuropathy: Epidemiology, pain description, and quality of life. Diabetes Res Clin Pract 2000;47:123-8. https://doi.org/10.1016/S0168-8227(99)00112-6.

[136] Boerner KE, Chambers CT, Gahagan J, Keogh E, Fillingim RB, Mogil JS. Conceptual complexity of gender and its relevance to pain. Pain 2018;159:2137-41. https://doi.org/10.1097/j.pain.0000000000001275.

[137] Fillingim RB. Sex, Gender, and Pain. Princ. Gender-Specific Med. Gend. Genomic Era Third Ed., Elsevier; 2017, p. 481-96. https://doi.org/10.1016/B978-0-12-803506-1.00038-3.

[138] Eastell R, Szulc P. Use of bone turnover markers in postmenopausal osteoporosis. Lancet Diabetes Endocrinol 2017;5:908-23. https://doi.org/10.1016/S2213-8587(17)30184-5.

[139] Ström O, Borgström F, Kanis JA, Compston J, Cooper C, McCloskey E V., et al. Osteoporosis: Burden, health care provision and opportunities in the EU. Arch Osteoporos 2011;6:59-155. https://doi.org/10.1007/s11657-011-0060-1.

[140] Hopkins RB, Pullenayegum E, Goeree R, Adachi JD, Papaioannou A, Leslie WD, et al. Estimation of the lifetime risk of hip fracture for women and men in Canada. Osteoporos Int 2012;23:921-7. https://doi.org/10.1007/s00198-011-1652-8.

[141] ALBRIGHT F, SMITH PH, RICHARDSON AM. POSTMENOPAUSAL OSTEOPOROSIS. J Am Med Assoc 1941;116:2465. https://doi.org/10.1001/jama.1941.02820220007002.

[142] Garnero P, Sornay-Rendu E, Chapuy M-C, Delmas PD. Increased bone turnover in late postmenopausal women is a major determinant of osteoporosis. J Bone Miner Res 2009;11:337-49. https://doi.org/10.1002/jbmr.5650110307.

[143] Melton LJ, Atkinson EJ, O'Fallon WM, Wahner HW, Riggs BL. Long-term fracture prediction by bone mineral assessed at different skeletal sites. J Bone Miner Res

1993;8:1227-33. https://doi.org/10.1002/jbmr.5650081010.

[144] Black DM, Cummings SR, Genant HK, Nevitt MC, Palermo L, Browner W. Axial and appendicular bone density predict fractures in older women. J Bone Miner Res 1992;7:633-8. https://doi.org/10.1002/jbmr.5650070607.

[145] Napoli N, Chandran M, Pierroz DD, Abrahamsen B, Schwartz A V., Ferrari SL, et al. Mechanisms of diabetes mellitus-induced bone fragility. Nat Rev Endocrinol 2017;13:208-19. https://doi.org/10.1038/nrendo.2016.153.

[146] Moayeri A, Mohamadpour M, Mousavi S, Shirzadpour E, Mohamadpour S, Amraei M. Fracture risk in patients with type 2 diabetes mellitus and possible risk factors: a systematic review and meta-analysis. Ther Clin Risk Manag 2017;Volume 13:455-68. https://doi.org/10.2147/TCRM.S131945.

[147] Liao CC, Lin CS, Shih CC, Yeh CC, Chang YC, Lee YW, et al. Increased risk of fracture and postfracture adverse events in patients with diabetes: Two nationwide population-based retrospective cohort studies. Diabetes Care 2014;37:2246-52. https://doi.org/10.2337/dc13-2957.

[148] De Liefde II, Van Der Klift M, De Laet CEDH, Van Daele PLA, Hofman A, Pols HAP. Bone mineral density and fracture risk in type-2 diabetes mellitus: The Rotterdam Study. Osteoporos Int 2005;16:1713-20. https://doi.org/10.1007/s00198-005-1909-1.

[149] Galbraith AS, Sanz-Nogués C, Glynn S, Coleman CM, Murphy C. Diabetes Mellitus and Gender Have a Negative Impact on the Outcome of Hip Fracture Surgery—A Pilot Study. J Orthop Res 2020;38:834-42. https://doi.org/10.1002/jor.24517.

[150] Napoli N, Schwartz A V, Schafer AL, Vittinghoff E, Cawthon PM, Parimi N, et al. Vertebral Fracture Risk in Diabetic Elderly Men: The MrOS Study. J Bone Miner Res 2018;33:63-9. https://doi.org/10.1002/jbmr.3287.

[151] Lunt M, Masaryk P, Scheidt-Nave C, Nijs J, Poor G, Pols H, et al. The effects of lifestyle, dietary dairy intake and diabetes on bone density and vertebral deformity prevalence: The EVOS study. Osteoporos Int 2001;12:688-98. https://doi.org/10.1007/s001980170069.

[152] Fan Y, Wei F, Lang Y, Liu Y. Diabetes mellitus and risk of hip fractures: a meta-analysis. Osteoporos Int 2016;27:219-28. https://doi.org/10.1007/s00198-015-3279-7.

[153] Vilaca T, Schini M, Harnan S, Sutton A, Poku E, Allen IE, et al. The risk of hip and non-vertebral fractures in type 1 and type 2 diabetes: A systematic review and meta-analysis update. Bone 2020;137. https://doi.org/10.1016/j.bone.2020.115457.

[154] Zura R, Xiong Z, Einhorn T, Watson JT, Ostrum RF, Prayson MJ, et al. Epidemiology of fracture nonunion in 18 human bones. JAMA Surg 2016;151. https://doi.org/10.1001/jamasurg.2016.2775.

[155] Kannegaard PN, van der Mark S, Eiken P, Abrahamsen B. Excess mortality in men compared with women following a hip fracture. National analysis of comedications, comorbidity and survival. Age Ageing 2010;39:203-9. https://doi.org/10.1093/ageing/afp221.

[156] Kim SH, Kim YM, Yoo JS, Choe EY, Kim TH, Won YJ. Increased risk of hip fractures in Korean patients with type 2 diabetes: a 6-year nationwide population-based study. J Bone Miner Metab 2017;35:623-9. https://doi.org/10.1007/s00774-016-0798-z.

[157] Hothersall EJ, Livingstone SJ, Looker HC, Ahmed SF, Cleland S, Leese GP, et al. Contemporary risk of hip fracture in type 1 and type 2 diabetes: A national registry study from Scotland. J Bone Miner Res 2014;29:1054-60. https://doi.org/10.1002/jbmr.2118.

[158] Janghorbani M, Van Dam RM, Willett WC, Hu FB. Systematic review of type 1 and type 2 diabetes mellitus and risk of fracture. Am J Epidemiol 2007;166:495-505. https://doi.org/10.1093/aje/kwm106.

[159] Schwartz A V. Diabetes Mellitus: Does it Affect Bone? Calcif Tissue Int 2003;73:515-9. https://doi.org/10.1007/s00223-003-0023-7.

[160] Burghardt AJ, Issever AS, Schwartz A V., Davis KA, Masharani U, Majumdar S, et al. High-Resolution Peripheral Quantitative Computed Tomographic Imaging of Cortical and Trabecular Bone Microarchitecture in Patients with Type 2 Diabetes Mellitus. J Clin Endocrinol Metab 2010;95:5045-55. https://doi.org/10.1210/jc.2010-0226.

[161] Moseley KF, Doyle ME, Jan De Beur SM. Diabetic serum from older women increases adipogenic differentiation in mesenchymal stem cells. Endocr Res 2018:1-11. https://doi.org/10.1080/07435800.2018.1441868.

[162] Parle E, Tio S, Behre A, Carey JJ, Murphy CG, O'Brien TF, et al. Bone Mineral Is More Heterogeneously Distributed in the Femoral Heads of Osteoporotic and Diabetic Patients: A Pilot Study. JBMR Plus 2020;4. https://doi.org/10.1002/jbm4.10253.

[163] Murray CE, Coleman CM. Impact of Diabetes Mellitus on Bone Health. Int J Mol Sci 2019;20:4873. https://doi.org/10.3390/ijms20194873.

[164] Ferland-mccollough D, Maselli D, Spinetti G, Sambataro M, Sullivan N, Blom A, et al. MCP-1 Feedback Loop Between Adipocytes and Mesenchymal Stromal Cells Causes Fat Accumulation and Contributes to Hematopoietic Stem Cell Rarefaction in the Bone Marrow of Patients With Diabetes. Diabetes 2018;67:1380-94. https://doi.org/10.2337/db18-0044.

[165] Cassidy FC, Shortiss C, Murphy CG, Kearns SR, Curtin W, De Buitléir C, et al. Impact of Type 2 Diabetes Mellitus on Human Bone Marrow Stromal Cell Number and Phenotypic Characteristics. Int J Mol Sci 2020;21:2476. https://doi.org/10.3390/ijms21072476.

[166] Phadnis SM, Ghaskadbi SM, Hardikar AA, Bhonde RR. Mesenchymal stem cells derived from bone marrow of diabetic patients portrait unique markers influenced by the diabetic microenvironment. Rev Diabet Stud 2009;6:260-70. https://doi.org/10.1900/RDS.2009.6.260.

[167] Park D, Spencer JA, Koh BI, Kobayashi T, Fujisaki J, Clemens TL, et al. Endogenous bone marrow MSCs are dynamic, fate-restricted participants in bone maintenance and regeneration. Cell Stem Cell 2012;10:259-72. https://doi.org/10.1016/j.stem.2012.02.003.

[168] Dombrowski S, Kostev K, Jacob L. Use of dipeptidyl peptidase-4 inhibitors and risk of bone fracture in patients with type 2 diabetes in Germany—A retrospective analysis of real-world data. Osteoporos Int 2017;28:2421-8. https://doi.org/10.1007/s00198-017-4051-y.

[169] Monami M, Dicembrini I, Antenore A, Mannucci E. Dipeptidyl peptidase-4 inhibitors and bone fractures: A meta-analysis of randomized clinical trials. Diabetes Care 2011;34:2474-6. https://doi.org/10.2337/dc11-1099.

[170] Zhu ZN, Jiang YF, Ding T. Risk of fracture with thiazolidinediones: An updated meta-analysis of randomized clinical trials. Bone 2014;68:115-23. https://doi.org/10.1016/j.bone.2014.08.010.

[171] Aubert RE, Herrera V, Chen W, Haffner SM, Pendergrass M. Rosiglitazone and pioglitazone increase fracture risk inwomen andmen with type 2 diabetes. Diabetes, Obes Metab 2010;12:716-21. https://doi.org/10.1111/j.1463-1326.2010.01225.x.

[172] Bilik D, McEwen LN, Brown MB, Pomeroy NE, Kim C, Asao K, et al. Thiazolidinediones and fractures: Evidence from translating research into action for diabetes. J Clin Endocrinol Metab 2010;95:4560-5. https://doi.org/10.1210/jc.2009-2638.

[173] Kahn SE, Zinman B, Lachin JM, Haffner SM, Herman WH, Holman RR, et al. Rosiglitazone-associated fractures in type 2 diabetes. Diabetes Care 2008;31:845-51. https://doi.org/10.2337/dc07-2270.

[174] Habib ZA, Havstad SL, Wells K, Divine G, Pladevall M, Williams LK. Thiazolidinedione use and the longitudinal risk of fractures in patients with type 2 diabetes mellitus. J Clin Endocrinol Metab 2010;95:592-600. https://doi.org/10.1210/jc.2009-1385.

[175] Xu H, Wang Z, Li X, Fan M, Bao C, Yang R, et al. Osteoporosis and Osteopenia Among Patients With Type 2 Diabetes Aged ≥50: Role of Sex and Clinical Characteristics. J Clin Densitom 2020;23:29-36. https://doi.org/10.1016/j.jocd.2019.04.004.

[176] Jing Y, Wang X, Yu J, Wang X, Zhou Y, Tao B, et al. Follicle-stimulating hormone and estradiol are associated with bone mineral density and risk of fractures in men with type 2 diabetes mellitus. J Diabetes 2020;12:426-37. https://doi.org/10.1111/1753-0407.13011.

[177] Krämer HU, Raum E, Rüter G, Schöttker B, Rothenbacher D, Rosemann T, et al. Gender disparities in diabetes and coronary heart disease medication among patients with type 2 diabetes: results from the DIANA study. Cardiovasc Diabetol 2012;11:88. https://doi.org/10.1186/1475-2840-11-88.

[178] Youm T, Koval KJ, Zuckerman JD. The economic impact of geriatric hip fractures. Am J Orthop (Belle Mead NJ) 1999;28:423-8.

[179] Chiu C-J, Wray LA. Gender Differences in Functional Limitations in Adults Living with Type 2 Diabetes: Biobehavioral and Psychosocial Mediators. Ann Behav Med 2011;41:71-82. https://doi.org/10.1007/s12160-010-9226-0.

[180] Noctor E, Dunne FP. Type 2 diabetes after gestational diabetes: The influence of changing diagnostic criteria. World J Diabetes 2015;6:234-44. https://doi.org/10.4239/wjd.v6.i2.234.

[181] Ratner RE. Prevention of type 2 diabetes in women with previous gestational diabetes. Diabetes Care 2007;30:S242-5. https://doi.org/10.2337/dc07-s223.

[182] England LJ, Dietz PM, Njoroge T, Callaghan WM, Bruce C, Buus RM, et al. Preventing type 2 diabetes: public health implications for women with a history of gestational diabetes mellitus. Am J Obstet Gynecol 2009;200:365.e1-365.e8. https://doi.org/10.1016/j.ajog.2008.06.031.

[183] Chatterjee S, Peters SAE, Woodward M, Arango SM, Batty GD, Beckett N, et al. Type 2diabetes as a risk factor for dementia in women compared with men: A pooled analysis of 2.3 million people comprising more than 100,000 cases of dementia. Diabetes Care 2016;39:300-7. https://doi.org/10.2337/dc15-1588.

[184] Walker EA, Molitch M, Kramer MK, Kahn S, Ma Y, Edelstein S, et al. Adherence to preventive medications: predictors and outcomes in the Diabetes Prevention Program. Diabetes Care 2006;29:1997-2002. https://doi.org/10.2337/dc06-0454.

[185] McEwen LN, Casagrande SS, Kuo S, Herman WH. Why Are Diabetes Medications So Expensive and What Can Be Done to Control Their Cost? Curr Diab Rep 2017;17. https://doi.org/10.1007/s11892-017-0893-0.

[186] Alvino VV, Fernández-Jiménez R, Rodriguez-Arabaolaza I, Slater S, Mangialardi G, Avolio E, et al. Transplantation of Allogeneic Pericytes Improves Myocardial Vascularization and Reduces Interstitial Fibrosis in a Swine Model of Reperfused Acute Myocardial Infarction. J Am Heart Assoc 2018;7. https://doi.org/10.1161/JAHA.117.006727.

[187] Shin L, Peterson DA. Impaired Therapeutic Capacity of Autologous Stem Cells in a Model of Type 2 Diabetes. Stem Cells Transl Med 2012;1:125-35. https://doi.org/10.5966/sctm.2012-0031.

[188] Heidari S, Babor TF, De Castro P, Tort S, Curno M. Sex and Gender Equity in Research: rationale for the SAGER guidelines and recommended use. Res Integr Peer Rev 2016;1:2. https://doi.org/10.1186/s41073-016-0007-6.

Chapter 10

# Microvascular Complications of Diabetes Mellitus: Focus on Diabetic Retinopathy (DR) and Diabetic Foot Ulcer (DFU)

*Ana Maria Dascalu, Dragos Serban, Nikolaos Papanas, Peter Kempler, Manfredi Rizzo, Daniela Stana, Gabriela Roman and Anca Pantea Stoian*

## Abstract

Diabetic retinopathy and diabetic foot ulcer are the most frequent, but also the most disabling complications of diabetes mellitus, with a sinister impact on patients' quality of life. Microvascular changes related to the deleterious effect of chronic hyperglycemia play an important role in the pathophysiology of both clinical entities by multiple molecular pathways. Vision-threating diabetic retinopathy may be treated by laser photocoagulation, anti-vascular endothelial growth factor (VEGF) agents and vitreoretinal surgery. Diabetic foot lesions are best treated by revascularization if needed, off-loading, infection control and therapeutic adjuncts (e.g. special dressings). Treatment should ideally be offered by a multidisciplinary expert team. Prevention and early detection, along with adequate control of glucose, lipids and arterial hypertension are of paramount importance to avoid and mitigate these fearful complications.

**Keywords:** microvascular complications, diabetic retinopathy, risk factors, ophthalmoscopy, angiography, laser photocoagulation, diabetic foot, diabetic neuropathy, treatment

## 1. Introduction

In diabetes (DM), chronic complications related to the direct or indirect effects of prolonged hyperglycemia on the vasculature have been classified into macrovascular and microvascular complications, depending on the size of affected vessels and the pathophysiological mechanisms involved. Microvascular disease includes retinopathy, nephropathy and neuropathy.

Diabetic retinopathy, one of the first manifestations of microvascular disease, remains today, despite improvements in monitoring and treatment, one of the leading causes of blindness worldwide. Epidemiological studies estimate that approximately 40% of subjects with DM type I over 40 years of age have retinal microvascular changes, of which 8.2% exhibit impaired visual acuity [1, 2]. Both DM types are associated with impaired retinal microcirculation. After 20 years from the onset of DM, almost all patients with type 1 DM (T1DM) and over 60% of those with type 2 DM (T2DM) will be affected [3]. Furthermore, decreased vision as a result of diabetic retinopathy has a negative impact on the quality of life of patients and their ability to successfully manage DM [4].

Diabetic foot results from diabetic neuropathy and/or peripheral arterial disease and affects annually between 9.1 to 26.1 million [5]. It is a chronic disabling and progressive complication, with potential deformities, chronic ulcerations and infections. Diabetic foot ulcers (DFUs) are encountered in 15% of DM patients, of whom 15-20% reach amputations. The latter lead to increased morbidity and decreased quality of life, but also an important burden on national healthcare systems, with increased health costs and hospitalization [6, 7].

## 2. Diabetic retinopathy

### 2.1 Risk factors

#### *2.1.1 DM duration and poor glycemic control*

Diabetic retinopathy (DR) is a chronic complication associated with long DM duration and poor glycemic control, the overall incidence of DR and of vision-threatening forms of DR (VTDR) being higher in T1DM than in T2DM [8].
The United Kingdom Prospective Diabetes Study (UKPDS) showed that both the incidence and progression of DR correlate with elevated $HbA_{1c}$, emphasizing the importance of good glycemic control to prevent visual impairment [9]. Every 1% decrease in $HbA_{1c}$ leads to a 40% reduction in the risk of developing retinopathy, a 25% reduction in the risk of progression to vision-threatening retinopathy, and a 15% reduction in the risk of blindness [10].

#### *2.1.2 Arterial hypertension*

The correlations between cardiovascular risk factors and the occurrence and evolution of DR are still a subject of study. However, there is clear evidence that the processes of arteriolosclerosis and the mechanical trauma to the vascular endothelium caused by elevated systolic and diastolic blood pressure are both cofactors in worsening DR. Some but not all studies have shown a negative impact of high blood pressure on DR [9, 11, 12]. The UKPDS has demonstrated a significant correlation between systolic arterial hypertension and DR incidence in T2DM. Thus, patients with blood pressure (BP) > 140 mmHg have a 2.8 times higher risk of developing DR than those with BP <125 mmHg. In the study of Lurbe et al. [13], in a cumulative exposure model, $HbA_{1c}$ and elevated diastolic BP values are predictive factors for the occurrence and progression of RD. In the Wisconsin Epidemiologic Study of Diabetic Retinopathy (WESDR), diastolic BP emerged as a significant risk factor for DR progression in T1DM, but no correlations were found for systolic BP or T2DM [14, 15]. Therapeutic lowering BP was found to have a protective role on retinal lesions in several studies supporting the recommendations for tight blood pressure control to further prevent visual loss n T2DM [9, 14, 16].

#### *2.1.3 Lipidic disorders and serum LDL*

Unlike glycemic control, the role of serum lipids in DR pathogenesis is less clear. There is no parameter in the lipid profile that is strictly associated with the incidence or progression of DR. However, elevated total cholesterol, LDL-cholesterol, Apo B and Apo B/Apo A ratio are correlated with the appearance of hard exudates, these being lipoprotein extravasations in the retinal capillaries. Hadjadj et al. showed that serum triglyceride levels are correlated with the occurrence of nephropathy and retinopathy in patients with T1DM [17]. Several randomized trials confirmed that the treatment of dyslipidemia can prevent the development of DR [14, 15, 18–21].

#### *2.1.4 Genetic predisposition*

Several studies have revealed that in young adults with T1DM, genetic predisposition for the development of DR is connected with the presence of HLA DR3/DR4 antigens. Furthermore, different alleles for codification of cytokines and chemokines, as well as vascular endothelial growth factor (VEGF) and transforming growth factor (TGF)beta1 were characterized, explaining different predisposition for DR in diabetic patients. VEGF plays a key role in increased microvascular permeability and neovascularization in proliferative diabetic retinopathy. The VEGF gene is located on chromosome 6 (6p21.3) and is highly polymorphic in the promoter region, correlated with VEGF expression and activity. In a study by Buranczynska et al., the presence of the D allele at −2549 in the promoter region of the VEGF gene enhanced gene expression [22]. The DD genotype was associated with DR but not with nephropathy, suggesting a cell-specific target of the VEGF isoform. In a study of Jalal and Kalia, regarding the polymorphism of VEGF genes in India, allele A and AA genotype of rs2146323 were significantly correlated both with incidence and with severity of DR [23]. Awata et al. described C (−634) G polymorphism of VEGF gene to be related to macular edema as well as diabetic retinopathy [24]. Ray et al. identified VEGF −460 C genotype to increase VEGF basal promoter activity by 71%, leading to a 2.5 increased risk of proliferative DR [25]. TGF beta signaling is considered to have an immunosuppressive role in the retina. Disorders affecting this pathway lead, at least in experimental animal models, to loss of pericytes, microaneurysms and leakage, finding resembling diabetic retinopathy [26]. Beránek et al. found a more frequent incidence of 915G/C (R25P) polymorphism of TGF beta gene in patients with DR compared to control subjects [27].

#### *2.1.5 Pregnancy*

Hormonal alterations during pregnancy were found to be an independent risk factor both for onset and for progression of DR, especially PDR, posing many challenges regarding the management of these patients [28–30]. Another mechanism is pregnancy-induced hypertension and pre-eclampsia [31].

#### *2.1.6 Ocular and systemic inflammation*

Recent studies focus on the significance of inflammation in the developments of DR [32–36]. There is strong evidence that ischemia and retinal hypoxia induce release of VEGF and inflammatory molecules at the level of endothelial and glial cells. Furthermore, several studies support the idea that ocular inflammatory disorders, such as prolonged post cataract surgery healing, uveitis, keratitis, are related to DR progression [32–36].

There are increased evidences that chronic systemic inflammation is also related to increased risk of DR onset and progression. In an experimental animal model, recurrent exposure to systemic LPS leads to injury of capillary endothelium and in vivo thinning of the retina in hyperglycemic mice, but not in healthy controls [37]. There are clinical evidences of increased incidence of DR and PDR in long standing non-healing foot ulcer, that could be explained due to the associated chronic low-grade systemic inflammation [38–42].

#### *2.1.7 Antidiabetic treatment and macular edema*

The correlations between antidiabetic mellitus medication and the risk of macular edema is still a subject of research. In a comprehensive systematic review and meta-analyses, Zhu and col. found that insulin use, as well as thiazolinedione (TZD) and meglitinide might increase the risk of macular edema, metformin has no statistically significant effect, while the use of sulfonylureas seems to have a protective role [43]. The physiopathological mechanisms are not completely understood, but experimental studies indicate that insulin and TZD may induce changes in retinal flow and increased expression of VEGF and breakdown of retinal-vascular barrier [43–46].

### 2.2 Pathophysiology

The pathological changes that lead to diabetic retinopathy are attributable to 3 main factors:

- small vessel wall damage:
- changes in blood flow
- alterations in platelet function

#### *2.2.1 Lesions in small vessel wall*

Microvascular changes in the retinal capillaries are due to chronic hyperglycemia by different mechanisms, such as:

##### *2.2.1.1 Aldose-reductase and intracellular polyol pathway*

Aldose reductase is an enzyme that converts glucose to sorbitol, which induces osmotic stress by intracellular accumulation. In animal models, this phenomenon leads to microaneurysmal dilatations of the vascular wall, basal membrane thickening and loss of the pericytes [47]. However, experimental studies of treatment with aldose reductase inhibitors have not obtained satisfactory clinical results.

##### *2.2.1.2 Advanced glycosylated end products (AGEs)*

Chronic hyperglycemia leads to non-enzymatic glycation or glycoxidation of proteins, resulting in accumulation of AGEs. This process affects both intra- and extracellular proteins, resulting in functional impairment. Deposits of AGEs in the extracellular matrix and subendothelial space lead to permanent alterations of intercellular junctions, monocyte migration and activation of nuclear factor (NF)-$\kappa$B along with activation of pro-inflammatory pathways [48, 49]. In experimental models, increased AGEs accumulation is associated with loss of pericytes and microaneurysm formation in retinal capillaries [50].

##### *2.2.1.3 Oxidative stress and ROS*

Hyperglycemia induces mitochondrial dysfunction and endoplasmic reticulum stress, with increased production of free radicals and reactive oxygen species (ROS) accumulation [49]. These degrade lipids, proteins and ribonucleic acid (RNA) chains.

Furthermore, experimental studies have proved a "hyperglycemic memory": in subjects with long periods of poor glycemic control, reversal of hyperglycemia fails to normalize increased oxidative activity in the retina [51]. Treatment with antioxidants and vitamin E alleviates endothelial dysfunction, but does not prevent the onset and progression of DR and other microvascular complications. Isolated experimental blockade of each of these pathways does not stop retinal microvascular damage, suggesting that the effects of hyperglycemia are manifested at the cellular and extracellular levels. Recently, experimental and clinical studies have demonstrated that inflammation biomarkers and pathways play a significant role in the aggravation of lesions and the evolution towards retinal neovascularization. A large array of cytokines and chemokines were found in increased concentrations in patients with DM, both in ocular samples and in serum: interleukin (Il)1beta, Il 2, 4, 6, 8, TNFalfa and (monocyte chemoattractant protein) MCP-1 [38, 42, 52–54]. Recent works have revealed that the TXNIP/NLRP3 Inflammasome activation pathways may contribute to pathologic neovascularization encountered in advanced stages of PDR [50, 54, 55].

#### *2.2.1.4 Nitric oxide (NO) deficiency*

Hyperglycemia induces decreased synthesis and increased consumption of NO by multiple pathways: activation of protein kinase C (PKC) in endothelial cells, oxidation of the reduced form of nicotinamide adenine dinucleotide phosphate (NADPH) via aldose reductase pathway, and non-enzymatic production of superoxide by AGEs. NO plays key roles in microcirculation, by regulation of arteriolar tone, platelet stabilization and preventing leukocyte adherence at the vascular wall. Decreased local levels of NO promotes vasoconstriction, microvascular occlusions and secondary retinal ischemia.

### *2.2.2 Changes in blood flow and platelet function*

General changes in blood favor small vessel obstructions with secondary retinal ischemia:

- increased hematocrit and blood viscosity related to high liver synthesis of fibrinogen and alfa2 globulins
- more rigid erythrocytes, with increased tendency to thrombosis
- increased platelet adhesion and aggregation
- activation of peripheral leukocytes, increased adherence to endothelial cells via beta-2 integrin expression and synthesis of mediators of inflammation

#### *2.2.2.1 Pigmented Epitelium Derived Factor (PEDF) decrease and retinal neurodegeneration*

PEDF is a trophic factor expressed by a multitude of retinal cells, an antagonist of VEGF. It decreases vascular permeability and plays an antioxidant role, protecting retinal cells from ROS. In the experimental setting, PEDF is decreased in aqueous and vitreous humor, early in preclinical stages of DR. The pathogenic mechanisms are supposed to be related with decreased insulin, as well as increased toxic mediators, such as glutamate. These early changes may induce mild changes in color vision, contrast sensitivity, visual field and electroretinogram oscillatory potentials [56–60].

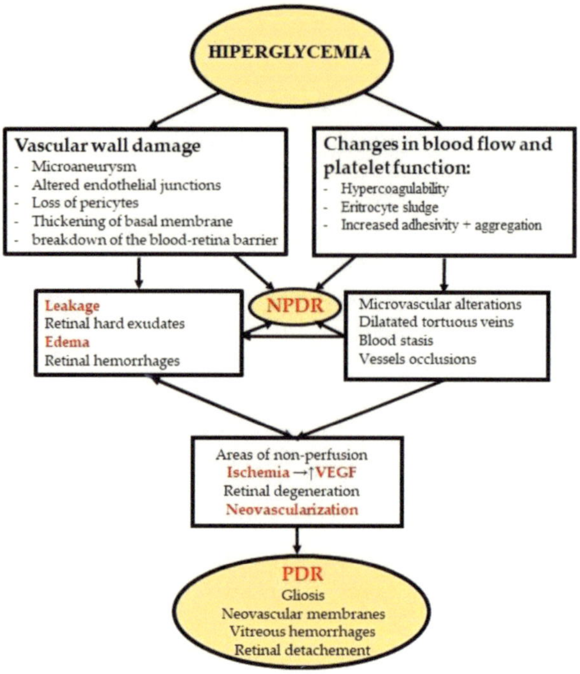


**Figure 1.**
*Pathogenesis of diabetic retinopathy.*

All these molecular mechanisms may lead to:

- alteration of tight junctions in endothelial cells, compromising the blood-retinal barrier, increasing extravasation of fluid in the retinal space and the formation of lipoprotein exudates and retinal edema

- loss of pericytes, with the appearance of focal vascular dilations and microaneurysms

- thickening, hyalinization of the basement membranes, with loss of elasticity of the vascular wall and autoregulatory capacity. This, together with the alterations of blood flow and platelets, favors microvascular occlusions, with the appearance of ischemic, hypoxic retinal areas.

The first areas affected by thrombosis and ischemia are in the middle retinal periphery, and the answer is to release a range of mediators, of which the key role is played by VEGF, which promotes retinal neovascularization and interruption of blood flow in many areas (optical disc, macula, iridocorneal angle and iris). The response to retinal hypoperfusion, a maladaptive protective mechanism, leads to the appearance of fragile new vessels, prone to repeated bleeding and leakage, ultimately destroying normal retinal architecture (**Figure 1**).

### 2.3 Clinical manifestations of DR

Fundus examination documents the presence and severity of retinal lesions. Clinical signs include:

- **Microaneurysms:** tiny round red dots, typically located initially temporal to the fovea; sometimes hard to be differentiated from dot hemorrhages in ophthalmoscopy; they are best shown by fluorescein angiography

- **Retinal hemorrhages**: a) "dot-blot" hemorrhages result from the venous end of the capillaries and are located in the middle layer of the retina; b) "flame-shaped" hemorrhages arise from pre-capillary arterioles and are located more superficially in the retinal nerve fiber layer

- **Retinal edema:** elevated, white-greyish appearance of the involved area; may be a consequence of leakage and fluid accumulation or of retinal ischemia (intracellular retinal edema). When foveal region is involved, it may assume a cystoid appearance and fluorescein angiography reveal a flower-petal pattern

- **Hard exudates:** these are well delineated, small, bright yellowish retinal lesions, formed by extravasated lipoproteins and lipid-filled macrophages and are mainly located in the outer plexiform layer. They are considered a sign of current or previous macular edema. When located in the macular region, they tend to organize in a circinate manner. They could resorb spontaneously months after the leakage is stopped, otherwise, chronic leakage leads to enlargement of the exudates and cholesterol accumulation.

- **"Cotton wool" spots**: these are small, whitish, fluffy superficial lesions, that cover the underlying retinal vessels and bear the significance of focal retinal ischemia and infarction. They are composed by neuronal debris and can disappear in time by autolysis and phagocytosis.

- **Venous loops and venous beading (VB):** these frequently occur adjacent to areas of nonperfusion and bear the significance of increasing retinal ischemia

- **Intraretinal microvascular abnormalities (IRMA):** these are arteriolo-venous shunts, bypassing the capillary bed, and are considered an indicator of capillary occlusion and retinal ischemia. Together with VB, they are considered the most significant predictor of progression to PDR [58].

- **Neovessels:** these are thin, with a single cell layer wall, extremely fragile, with a lace-like appearance and may be situated at the surface of the optic disk or elsewhere, in general at the periphery of the areas of non-perfusion. They can be best evidenced by fluorescein angiography and optical coherence tomography (OCT).

### 2.4 Staging of DR

Dr is classically referred as: non-proliferative (NPDR) and proliferative (PDR). The classification is determined by the presence of retinal neovascularization. Recent Guidelines of International Council of Ophthalmology for Diabetic Eye Care recommends the following staging system, based on findings encountered in ophthalmoscopy, to be used in clinical practice (**Table 1**).

The ICO guidelines also refer to the location, extension of the diabetic macular edema (DME), as it is an important cause of decreased vision in DR, even in the absence of neovessels. Central involved DME is considered to be an area of retinal thickening in the macula that does involve the central subfield zone (of 1 mm in diameter).

| DR | Findings on Dilated Ophthalmoscopy |
|---|---|
| No apparent DR | No abnormalities |
| Mild NPDR* | Microaneurysms only |
| Moderate NPDR | Microaneurysms + other signs:<br>• dot and blot hemorrhages<br>• hard exudates<br>cotton wool spots |
| Severe NPDR | Moderate NPDR with any of the following:<br>• Intraretinal hemorrhages ≥20 in each quadrant;<br>• Definite venous beading (VB) in 2 quadrants;<br>• Intraretinal microvascular abnormalities (IRMA) in 1 quadrant;<br>and no signs of proliferative retinopathy |
| PDR* | Severe non-proliferative DR + one of the followings:<br>Neovascularization<br>Vitreous/preretinal hemorrhage |

**NPDR: non proliferative diabetic retinopathy; *PDR: proliferative diabetic retinopathy*

**Table 1.**
*International Classification of Diabetic Retinopathy [57].*

## 2.5 Clinical forms of DR associated with high risk of vision loss

Diabetic maculopathy is the most frequent cause of decreased vision encountered in patients with T2DM. It can be manifest in every stage of the DR and represents the involvement of the fovea by hard exudates, macular edema due to fluid extravasation or by macular ischemia. In early stages, the loss of vision is mild; however, if untreated, it can may to permanent photoreceptor damage.

DME is considered clinically significant if [61–63]:

- located at or within 500 μm of the center of the macula
- hard exudates at or within 500 μm of the center if associated with thickening of adjacent retina
- the area of retinal thickening is larger than one optic disc area and is located within 1 disc diameter of the center of macula

### *2.5.1 Advanced diabetic ocular disease*

Advanced diabetic disease can remain asymptomatic for a long period of time, due to slow proliferation of the retinal neovessels and their location, usually in mid-periphery. It consists of retinal neovessels that grow into elevated fibrovascular membranes that enter the vitreous body, leading to serious complications: vitreous hemorrhage and retinal detachment [62]. Proliferation of the abnormal vessels at the level of iris and iridocorneal angle led to neovascular glaucoma, with poor clinical outcomes. Ophthalmological periodical screening is extremely important in early identifying and referral to laser therapy. In advanced stages, serious complications appear and the vision loss is irreversible.

Diabetic maculopathy is the most frequent cause of decreased vision encountered in patients with T2DM.

## 2.6 Diagnosis of DR

Early detection of DR depends on educating DM subjects, as well as their families, friends, and health care providers about the importance of regular eye examination. This holds true for asymptomatic subjects as well.

Initial ophthalmological examination in a patient with suspected/confirmed DR should include the following:

- Visual acuity
- Measurement of intraocular pressure (IOP), due to the possible risk of developing neovascular glaucoma
- Slit-lamp exam +/- gonioscopy if iris neovascularization is observed or IOP is elevated
- Fundus examination with dilated pupil

A variety of imaging techniques are useful to detect, classify and monitor DR, as well as efficacy of treatment: fundus photography, fluorescein angiography, optic coherence tomography (OCT) and OCT angiography.

### *2.6.1 Ophthalmoscopy and Fundus Photography*

Currently, the two most sensitive methods are retinal photography and slit-lamp examination through dilated pupils. Direct ophthalmoscopy by ophthalmologists or trained technicians yields 80% sensitivity and >90% specificity [64]. It is cheap and is considered the method of choice. Fundus photography has the advantage of creating a permanent record, and for that reason, it is the preferred method for retinopathy assessment (**Figures 2–4**).

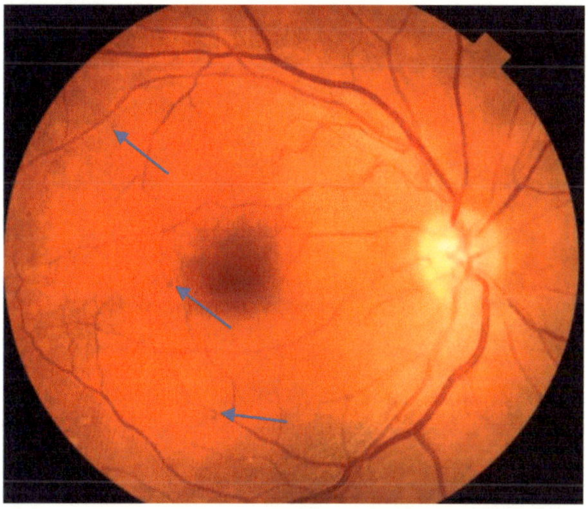

**Figure 2.**
*"Background" diabetic retinopathy: few dot hemorrhages (blue arrows) (Dr. Ana Dascalu's private collection, Emergency University Hospital Bucharest, Ophthalmology Department).*

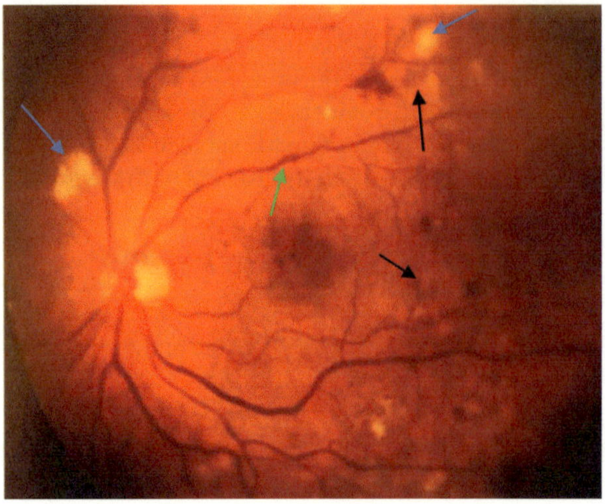

**Figure 3.**
*Retinophotography: Severe NPRD: multiple dot and blot hemorrhages, hard exudates, cotton wool spots (blue arrows), macular edema, VB (green arrow) and IRMA (black arrows) (Dr. Daniela Stana's private collection, Emergency University Hospital Bucharest, Ophthalmology Department, PhD thesis).*

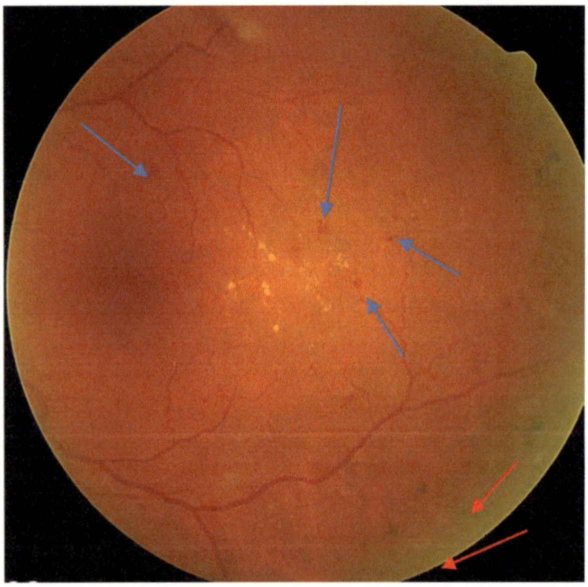

**Figure 4.**
*Incipient PDR: large ischemic area situated temporally to the macular region, with hard exudates, dots hemorrhages, venous loops, IRMA and intraretinal neovessels; in the mid periphery, pigmented lesions post laser photocoagulation (Dr Ana Dascalu's private collection, Emergency University Hospital Bucharest, Ophthalmology Department).*

### 2.6.2 Fluorescein angiography

Fluorescein angiography is an invasive, costly, and time-consuming technique but is a sensitive method to detect vascular changes due to rupture of the inner and outer blood retinal barrier in the course of DR [63, 65, 66]. The retinal vasculature is visualized with great accuracy: the examiner may identify tiny microaneurysms and differentiate between microaneurysms (hyperfluorescent) and punctiform hemorrhage (hypofluorescence by masking effect). It is an indispensable exploration before planning different laser treatment, for example to distinguish retinal edema by leakage (which appears white due to dye accumulation) from ischemic retinal edema (which appears as hypofluorescent). In the latter case, the application of laser impacts is not recommended because it leads to exacerbation of retinal ischemia (**Figure 5**).

#### *2.6.3 Optical coherence tomography (OCT) and OCT-angiography (OCT-A)*

OCT is a completely non-invasive, reproducible and quantifiable. It provides high-resolution images of the retinal layers, choroid, vitreous gel, and the vitreo-retinal interface and has become the gold standard for diagnosis, assessment of treatment response, and follow-up up of patients with diabetic macular edema.

OCT angiography (OCTA) is a new non-invasive imaging technique that employs motion contrast imaging to high-resolution volumetric blood flow information, rapidly generating images similar to angiographic images [63, 65–67]. It provides a highly detailed view of the retinal vasculature, which allows for accurate delineation of the foveal avascular zone (FAZ) and detection of subtle microvascular abnormalities, including FAZ enlargement, areas of capillary non-perfusion, and intraretinal cystic spaces [66]. The possibility of detecting microvascular changes in diabetic eyes before the presence of visible microaneurysms may have important implications in the future. In this sense, OCTA could be able to quickly identify subjects at risk of DM (**Figures 6** and 7).

### 2.7 Treatment

#### *2.7.1 Primary prevention*

Follow-up of patients with DR involves the ophthalmologist and the diabetologist. Extensive studies in large groups of diabetic patients have shown the beneficial role of strict control of blood glucose, hypertension and dyslipidemia in both

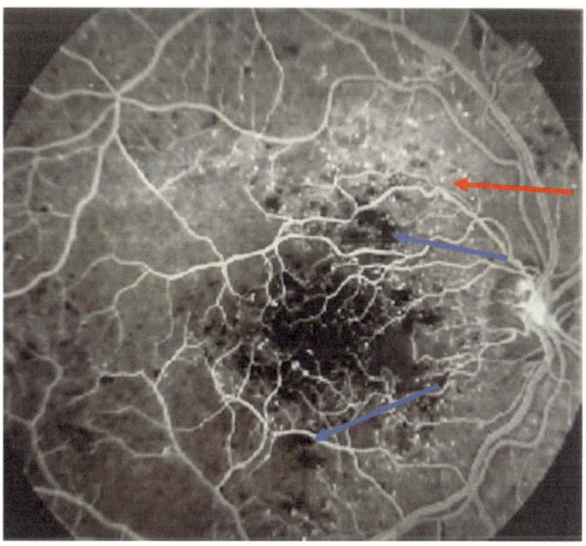

**Figure 5.**
*Fluorescein Angiography: Severe NPRD: numerous microaneurysms (hyperfluorescent dots), areas of non-perfusion (hypofluorescent, blue arrows), venous loops and IRMA, with diffuse leakage (hyperfluorescent, red arrow) (Dr Daniela Stana's private collection, PhD Thesis, Emergency University Hospital Bucharest, Ophthalmology Department).*

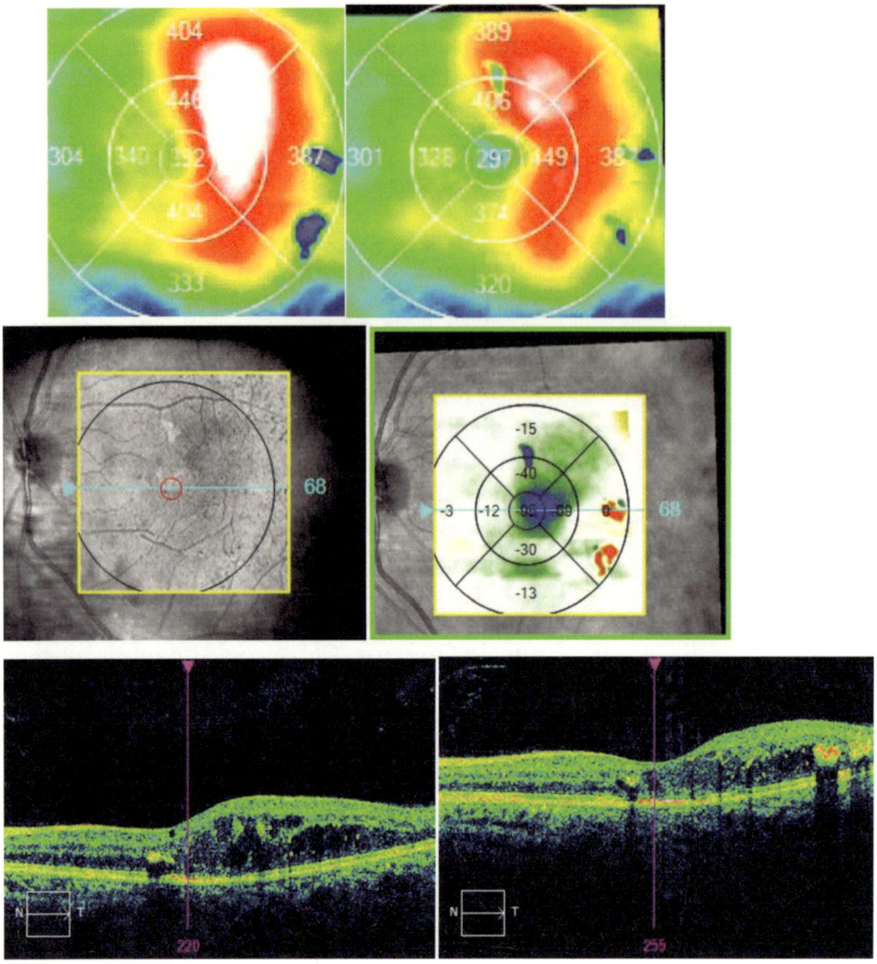

**Figure 6.**
*Optical coherence tomography (OCT) macular change analysis (before and 1 month after intravitreal anti = VEGF): hard exudates intraretinal edema with disorganization of the normal foveal architecture; macular and paramacular temporal edema decreases in area and height (Dr. Ana Dascalu's private collection, Emergency University Hospital Bucharest, Ophthalmology Department).*

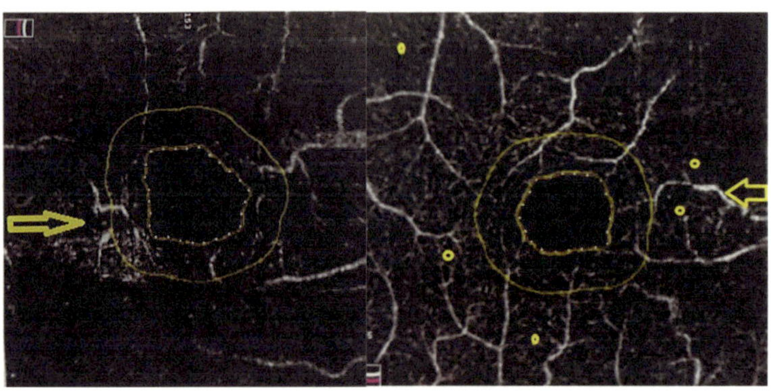

**Figure 7.**
*OCT-A: (a) enlargement of FAZ and perifoveolar area of microvascular abnormalities; (b) mild FAZ enlargement, multiple microaneurysms (Dr. Daniela Stana's private collection, PhD Thesis, Emergency University Hospital Bucharest, Ophthalmological Department).*

preventing and slowing the progression of DR. DCCT and UKPDS showed the importance of a good glycemic control in preventing microvascular damage in diabetes [68, 69]. Furthermore, every decrease with 10 mm Hg of systolic blood pressure is associated with a reduction of 35% in the risk of DR progression and of 50% in the risk of blindness [69]. Maintaining $HbA_{1c}$ below 7.0% (53 mmol/mol) and a systolic blood pressure below 140 mmHg is considered a realistic therapeutic target in clinical practice. Currently, the recommended serum lipid levels in DM are an optimal LDL cholesterol concentration of <100 mg/dl and desirable triglycerides levels of <150 mg/dl [69–72].

#### *2.7.2 Retinopathy screening*

DR remains clinically silent, a long period of time until damages become irreversible. Ophthalmologic monitoring of DM subjects is essential. Frequency of screening depends on the severity of DR and the co-existence of risk factors. The follow-up schedule recommended by the ICO (International Council of Ophthalmology) Guidelines for Diabetic Eye Care is presented in **Table 2** [61].

#### *2.7.3 Laser photocoagulation*

##### *2.7.3.1 Classical laser*

Laser therapy has been used in DR for over 60 years and remains the mainstay of treating the ischemic retina. Applied early in severe NPDR and PDR, laser therapy leads to the prevention/regression of neovascularization and to the remission of retinal edema. Clinical studies confirm the effectiveness of laser photocoagulation by reducing vision loss by approximately 50% in patients with PDR. It is based on application of 1000-2000 laser shots, lasting 100 milliseconds, 200-250 mW of power with a size of 200-500 micrometers at the level of the middle and extreme periphery of the retina, spaced at a distance by a spot diameter, in order to destroy

| **DR staging** | **Follow-up Schedule for ophthalmologists** | **Therapy** |
|---|---|---|
| No apparent DR | 1-2 years | Observation |
| Mild NPDR | 6-12 months | Observation |
| Moderate NPDR | 3-6 month | Observation |
| Severe NPDR | <3 months; | Pan-retinal photocoagulation should be considered |
| Proliferative DR | <1 month; | Pan-retinal photocoagulation |
| Stable (Treated) PDR | 6-12 months | Observation |
| **Diabetic Macular Edema severity** | **Follow-up Schedule for management by ophthalmologists** | |
| Noncentral-involved DME | 3-6 month; | Focal laser photocoagulation should be considered |
| Central-involved DME | 1-3 month; | Focal laser photocoagulation/ anti-VEGF therapy should be considered |
| Stable DME | 3-6 month | Observation |

**Table 2.**
*ICO Guidelines for Diabetic Eye Care: screening and follow-up schedule for diabetic retinopathy.*

the VEGF-secreting ischemic retina. Immediate complications are related to eye discomfort (tingling sensation/low-intensity pain) and mild ocular inflammation (caused by retinal burns). For this reason, it is recommended to space the laser photocoagulation in 3-4 sessions. In the long run, potential complications include hemeralopia, "fan shaped" visual field changes, or even concentric narrowing of the visual field through widening of scars and subretinal fibrosis. Other less frequent side effects are membrane injury, with secondary choroidal neovascularization, damage of ciliary nerves with permanently mydriasis and loss of accommodation, uveal effusion, angle closure glaucoma, serous retinal detachment, and vitreous hemorrhage [73–75].

#### *2.7.3.2 Multispot laser*

This technique allows the delivery of laser shots in a much shorter time and in a semi-automatic manner. These are much finer and at a lower intensity, threshold or subthreshold, causing lesser heat and consequently inflammation in the pigmented retinal epithelium. Clinical studies have shown that the effectiveness of the method is similar to classical laser, but fewer complications are encountered regarding retinal scarring and the impact on the visual field.

#### *2.7.3.3 Laser photocoagulation in diabetic macular edema (DME)*

In the case of exudative non-central DME, laser treatment may be considered as an alternative or in combination with intravitreal injections with anti-VEGF. In this case, the laser spots are finer, with a size of 50-100 μm, and lower energy. Laser treatment is inefficient in the case of ischemic macular edema, and so fluorangiography is necessary before therapeutic planning. In the early treatment diabetic retinopathy study (ETDRS) study, when comparing laser photocoagulation with no treatment, there was a decrease in DME from 24% to 12% after 3 years follow-up, while visual acuity improved in only 3% of patients [76].

### *2.7.4 Intravitreal anti-VEGF*

Clinical and experimental studies have revealed increased VEGF concentration in ocular samples early in the evolution of DR, documenting its role both in increased vascular permeability and in vascular proliferation. Hence, anti-VEGF agents were used first in the treatment of DME and later in PDR management [77] (**Table 3**).

Clinical studies showed that Pegaptanib is the least effective in preventing neovascularization. Comparative studies between bevacizumab, ranibizumab and aflibercept found that they are all effective to decrease DME. However, aflibercept is most powerful in subjects with worse visual acuity [77, 78]. Still, the effect of intravitreal anti- VEGF is temporary and intravitreal therapy should be repeated according to clinical outcome.

### *2.7.5 Intravitreal steroids*

In cases of DME resistant to anti-VEGF therapy after 3 monthly injections, intravitreal triamcinolone injection or fluocinolone are a therapeutic alternative to reduce DME and improve vision [79]. Their main untoward effects are cataract and transient increase of intraocular pressure.

| | Description of the molecule | FDA approval | Dose |
|---|---|---|---|
| **Pegaptanib** (Macugen; Eyetech Inc, Cedar Knolls, NJ, USA) | RNA aptamer that binds to the heparin binding site of the VEGF-A165 isomer | For wet age related macular degeneration only | 0.3 mg /0.09ml |
| **Bevacizumab** (Avastin; Genentech, San Francisco, CA, USA) | Full-length recombinant humanized anti-VEGF monoclonal antibody | No; "off-label" use | 1.25 to 2.5 mg (0.05-0.1ml) |
| **Ranibizumab** (Lucentis; Genentech, San Francisco, CA, USA/ Novartis Ophthalmics, Basel, Switzerland) | Recombinant fragment of the humanized anti-VEGF monoclonal antibody; increased binding affinity for all VEGF isoforms | Yes | 0.3 or 0.5 mg in 0.05 mL |
| **Aflibercept** (Eylea; Regeneron, Tarrytown, NY, USA) | Recombinant fusion protein of the binding domains of human VEGF-R1 and VEGF-R2, fused with the Fc domain of human IgG1 bind VEGF with greater affinity compared to other anti VEGF and prevent activation of VEGF-R | Yes | 2mg/0.05mL |

**Table 3.**
*Anti VEGF agents used in DME treatment.*

### *2.7.6 Surgical management of DR*

Vitreoretinal surgery is crucial in managing advanced DR, in order to mitigate visual loss. Its main indications include vitreous hemorrhage interfering with photocoagulation, tractional and combined tractional and rhegmatogenous retinal detachment, dense premacular hemorrhage and DME with with vitreo-macular traction [80]. The objectives of surgical removal of the vitreous (vitrectomy) include removal of vitreous opacity (usually blood) and/or fibrovascular proliferation, relieving retinal traction, achieving retinal reattachment, and allowing completion of scatter laser photocoagulation. A large case series showed that sight threatening complications are rare and in approximately 90% of cases, vision is improved or stabilized [81]. Vitrectomy may also be beneficial for maculopathy when traction from the vitreous gel contributes to fluid accumulation.

## 3. Diabetic foot ulcers (DFUs)

### 3.1 Risk factors

The main risk factors of DFUs include DM duration and high $HbA_{1c}$ [82–88]. The EURO-Diab group has identified hypertension, smoking and lipid disorders (hypertriglyceridemia, hypercholesterolemia) as additional risk factors [82, 83]. In Western countries, the male sex appears to be more commonly affected, with a risk ratio of 1.6. The co-existence of other microvascular complications (DR, nephropathy) increases the risk of DFUs.

Precipitating trauma is important. However, history of trauma is only identified in 48% of patients with DFUs. By contrast, foot injury without an apparent cause usually results from repeated minor injuries by inappropriate footwear [88–90].

Amin and Doupis have estimated that 45-60% of DFUs are mainly due to neuropathy, while 45% of DFUs are due to both diabetic neuropathy and peripheral arterial disease [87]. Like DR, diabetic neuropathy is also a very frequent DM complication and its prevalence increases with DM duration [90]. The other important driver of DFUs is ischemia from peripheral arterial disease (PAD). Visual impairment, foot deformities and past history of DFU also increase the risk of DFUs [85, 86].

### 3.2 Pathophysiology

The underlying mechanisms of DFUs include diabetic neuropathy, PAD and infection.

Diabetic neuropathy may affect the motor, sensory and autonomic nerves. Thickening of the basement membranes, endothelial hyperplasia in the vasa nervorum lead to thinning of the vascular lumen and secondary ischemia [90, 91]. On the other hand, metabolic disorders caused by chronic hyperglycemia, with the formation of AGEs, polyol pathways, increased oxidative stress levels and enzymatic activation of PKC also have direct toxic effects on nerve fibers.

Autonomic neuropathy causes arteriolo-venular shunts with secondary decreased blood flow in capillaries, but also anhidrosis, resulting in dry skin, thin, prone to cracking and ulceration. Sensory neuropathy leads to sensory (inability to feel warm/cold, pain, pressure), rendering the foot prone to undetected acute or chronic traumas [90, 91]. Motor neuropathy leads to imbalance between plantar flexors and extensors, with characteristic deformities, such as hammer toe, claw toe etc, and leading to high planter pressures in some small foot areas [92–94].

PAD leads to lower-extremity ischemia. In diabetes, it is usually located in the infra-popliteal arteries, less so at the iliofemoral level [89, 95]. Ischemia portends even more ominous outcomes [91, 96].

Pesently, micro and macrocirculatory disorders are considered not as separate entities, but more as a continuum in DM [97], neovascularization of vasa vasorum, with secondary hemorrhages and platelet aggregation facilitating the progression of atherosclerosis and intraluminal obstruction.

DFUs are frequently infected. The most common germs involved are staphylococci and streptococci, but deep infections are usually polymicrobial including gram positive, gram negative and even anaerobic germs [98, 99]. Chronic hyperglycemia and chronic hypoxia predispose to severe infections [99].

#### *3.2.1 Clinical signs-staging systems*

DFU represents any full-thickness ulcer below the ankle in DM. The initial signs and symptoms depend on the pathophysiological mechanism involved (neuropathy and/or PAD). Subjects with diabetic neuropathy are usually initially asymptomatic, but a minority of them may later develop neuropathic symptoms (numbness, paresthesia, lancinating or burning pain) with nocturnal exacerbation. In the event of PAD, intermittent claudication or even ischemic rest pain and gangrene may develop (**Figure 8**).

Usually, DFUs develop in an area exposed to increased pressure, with a nonhealing tendency, often neglected in early stages due to diminished pain sensation. In the vent of infection, signs of local inflammation may be added (redness, swelling, pain, pus secretion etc).

Several staging systems were developed in order to characterize the pathogenic pathway and the severity and extension of ulcer. The International Working Group on the Diabetic Foot Risk Classification System (IWGDF) refers mainly at the severity of neuropathy and coexistence or not of the peripheral ischemia [100], while the Wagner classification describes the extension and depth [101] (**Tables 4** and 5).

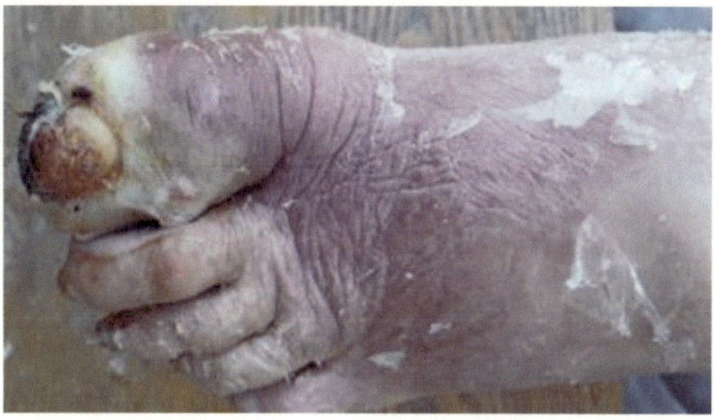

**Figure 8.**
*Distal toe gangrene and extensive infection and inflammation at the level of the forefoot and mid foot (Dr. Dragos Serban's private collection).*

| | |
|---|---|
| Grade 0 | Intact sensation |
| Grade 1 | Diminished sensation |
| Grade 2 | Diminished sensation+ foot deformities (hammertoes, claw toes) +/-peripheral arterial disease |
| Grade 3 | Previous/present ulcer or amputation |

**Table 4.**
*IWGDF risk classification [96].*

| | |
|---|---|
| Grade 0 | No ulcer in high-risk patients |
| Grade 1 | Superficial ulcer |
| Grade 2 | Ulceration involving tendons, ligaments, muscles, joints, not exposed to bone, without cellulitis or abscess |
| Grade 3 | Deeper ulcers, with frequent bone complications of osteomyelitis, abscesses or cellulitis. |
| Grade 4 | Forefoot gangrene. |
| Grade 5 | Gangrene extended to midfoot/hindfoot |

**Table 5.**
*Wagner Classification of DFU [101].*

## 3.3 Diagnosis

### 3.3.1 Clinical examination

Patient history is necessary to provide information on DM duration, glycemic control, associated risk factors and any prior lesions/amputations.

Clinical examination should look for skin disorders, foot deformities, nail lesions, blisters etc. also be documented. It must also include an evaluation of neuropathic deficits, PAD and infection. Signs of limb threatening infection include bullae, ecchymoses, soft tissue crepitus and rapid spread of infection [102, 103].

*Evaluation of sensory neuropathy* is very important to establish whether the patient has lost the protective sensation, making him prone to accidental trauma. Hot/cold discrimination, pain perception, light touch and vibration perception, as well as protective sensation must be tested [95–99]. The latter is best assessed by the 10 g Semmes Weinstein monofilament or the measurement of the vibration perception threshold (VPT) with a neurothesiometer [93–95, 102, 103]. Tendon reflexes and muscular strength are also a part of the examination [95–99]. Finally, sudomotor dysfunction (reduced sweat production) is best examined by the Neuropad indicator test, which is based on a colour change from blue to pink [96, 97]. Indeed, this test has recently been identified as an independent risk factor of DFUs at 5 years [104].

#### *3.3.1.1 Peripheral neuropathy screening*

Evaluation of bilateral sensorial neuropathy in clinical practice requires neurological trained specialist and electrophysiological tests, which an increased burden on the national healthcare systems. In order to better select the patients who are more probably affected by neuropathy, a simpler tool was developed in 1994, namely Michigan Neuropathy Screening Instrument (MNSI) [105, 106]. It comprises a 2-step evaluation: first, a 15-item self-administered questionnaire that is scored by summing abnormal responses, followed by lower extremity examination (deformities, non-healing ulcers), assessment of ankle reflexes and of vibratory sensation. According to Herman and col., a score of more than 4 should raise the suspicion of peripheral sensorial neuropathy [106].

#### *3.3.1.2 Peripheral arterial disease*

Documenting the presence and the severity of ischemia is extremely important. Examination includes: a) palpation of peripheral pulses at the dorsalis pedis and the posterior tibial arteries; b) measurement of the ankle-brachial index (ABI) by a Doppler device [99, 100]. ABI evaluates the ratio of systolic arterial pressure at the brachial over the ankle level [107, 108]. Normal values range between 0.9-1.3, while values exceeding 1.3 point to calcified, uncompressible arteries, in which case the test cannot be used [99]. Similarly, one may measure the toe-brachial index (TBI), given that small digital arteries are rarely calcified: TBI<0.7 confirms the diagnosis of PAD [108]. More sophisticated evaluation (ultrasound, angiography) are used when necessary, especially to guide interventional treatment [95–99].

#### *3.3.1.3 Assessment of the severity of the infection*

If infection is suspected, it is best to use a tissue culture to identifying pathogens [109, 110]. X-rays, computed tomography and magnetic resonance imaging are used to evaluate bone infection or abscess formation, as well as to guide surgical treatment [86, 96, 97].

## 3.4 DFU management

### *3.4.1 Prophylaxis of DFU*

Patients at risk of DFU should be managed by an interdisciplinary approach, including a diabetologist, a vascular surgeon, a podiatrist, a general surgeon, an orthopedic surgeon, a plastic surgeon and other specialists [82, 94, 102]. Stringent glycemic control is essential both in primary prevention of DFU and in ensuring wound healing. Management of high blood pressure and dyslipidemia is also important [86, 96, 97].

High-risk patients need education about the importance of wearing comfortable footwear, rigorous local hygiene, keeping feet dry and avoiding possible causes of local trauma (including barefoot walking) and frequent self-examinations [86, 96, 97]. Callus debridement, off-loading, and correct treatment of nail pathology are simple but extremely efficient measures for the prevention of foot ulcers [86, 96, 97]. LEADER trial suggests that treatment with liraglutide in patients with type 2 diabetes and at high risk of CV events did not increase the risk of DFU events and was associated with a significantly lower risk of DFU-related amputations compared with placebo [109].

#### *3.4.2 Therapeutic management of DFUs: main principles*

Management of DFUs is aimed at correcting the pathogenic triad of neuropathy, PAD and infection. Off-loading with appropriate footwear and/or casts, debridement of callus and/or necrotic tissue, revascularization (by-pass grafting or intraluminal angioplasty) and infection control are the top priorities [86, 96, 97]. These may be aided by special dressings, skin substitutes, growth factors and other modalities [111–116]. Special care must be taken to recognize and promptly deal with emergencies requiring surgery and other urgent interventions [117].

## 4. Conclusions

Diabetic retinopathy and diabetic foot ulcer are both disabling complications, with a significant impact on the patient's quality of life and healthcare systems [118]. Microvascular impairment and local inflammation play a significant role in the both pathological mechanisms. Prevention and early detection, along with optimal control of blood sugar, hyperlipemia and arterial hypertension are the most efficacious measures against these fearful complications.

## Conflict of interest

Peter Kempler has received honoraria from and/or is an advisory member of the following companies: Ely Lilly, Novo Nordisk, Novartis, Miro, Boehringer-Ingelheim, Woerwag-Pharma, Pfizer, Sanofi, Di-Care Zrt., 77 Elektronika Kft., Teva, Astra-Zeneca.

## Author details

Ana Maria Dascalu[1,2], Dragos Serban[1,3*], Nikolaos Papanas[4], Peter Kempler[5], Manfredi Rizzo[6,7], Daniela Stana[2], Gabriela Roman[8,9] and Anca Pantea Stoian[10]

1 Faculty of Medicine, "Carol Davila" University of Medicine and Pharmacy, Bucharest, Romania

2 Ophthalmology Department, Emergency University Hospital Bucharest, Romania

3 IVth General Surgery Department, Emergency University Hospital Bucharest, Romania

4 Diabetes Centre-Diabetic Foot Clinic, Second Department of Internal Medicine, Democritus University of Thrace, University Hospital of Alexandroupolis, Greece

5 Department of Medicine and Oncology, Semmelweis University, Hungary

6 Division of Endocrinology, Diabetes and Metabolism, Department of Medicine, University of South Carolina, Columbia, SC, USA

7 Department of Health Promotion, Mother and Child Care, Internal Medicine and Medical Specialties, University of Palermo, Italy

8 Department of Diabetes and Nutrition Diseases, Iuliu Hatieganu University of Medicine and Pharmacy, Cluj-Napoca, Romania

9 Clinical Center of Diabetes, Emergency Clinical County Hospital Cluj, Cluj-Napoca, Romania

10 Diabetes, Nutrition and Metabolic Diseases Department, "Carol Davila" University of Medicine, Bucharest, Romania

*Address all correspondence to: dragos.serban@umfcd.ro

## References

[1] Ciulla TA, Amador AG, Zinman B. Diabetic retinopathy and diabetic macular edema: pathophysiology, screening, and novel therapies. Diabetes Care. 2003 Sep;26(9):2653-2664. doi: 10.2337/diacare.26.9.2653.

[2] Klein R, Knudtson MD, Lee KE, Gangnon R, Klein BE. The Wisconsin Epidemiologic Study of Diabetic Retinopathy XXII: the twenty-five-year progression of retinopathy in persons with type 1 diabetes. Ophthalmology 2008;115(11):1859-1868.

[3] Fong DS, Aiello L, Gardner TW, King GL, Blankenship G, Cavallerano JD, Ferris FL 3rd, Klein R; American Diabetes Association. Retinopathy in diabetes. Diabetes Care. 2004;27 Suppl 1:S84-S87.

[4] Nathan DM, DER Group. The diabetes control and complications trial/epidemiology of diabetes interventions and complicationsstudy at 30 years: overview. Diabetes Care 2014;37(1): 9-16.

[5] Armstrong DG, Boulton AJM, Bus SA. Diabetic foot ulcers and their recurrence. N Engl J Med. 2017 Jun 15;376(24):2367-2375.

[6] Everett E, Mathioudakis N. Update on management of diabetic foot ulcers. Ann N Y Acad Sci. 2018 Jan;1411(1):153-165.

[7] Moss SE, Klein R, Klein BE. Long-term incidence of lower-extremity amputations in a diabetic population. Arch Fam Med 1996;5:391-398

[8] Yau, J. W., Rogers, S. L., Kawasaki, R., Lamoureux, E. L., Kowalski, J. W., Bek, T., ... & Haffner, S. (2012). Global prevalence and major risk factors of diabetic retinopathy. *Diabetes care*, *35*(3), 556-564.

[9] King P, Peacock I, Donnelly R. The UK prospective diabetes study (UKPDS): clinical and therapeutic implications for type 2 diabetes. Br J Clin Pharmacol. 1999 Nov;48(5):643-648. doi: 10.1046/j.1365-2125.1999.00092.x.

[10] Barsegian A, Kotlyar B, Lee J, Salifu MO, McFarlane SI. Diabetic Retinopathy: Focus on Minority Populations. Int J Clin Endocrinol Metab. 2017;3(1):034-045. doi: 10.17352/ijcem.000027.

[11] UK Prospective Diabetes Study Group. Tight blood pressure control and risk of macrovascular and microvascular complications in type 2 diabetes (UKPDS 38). BMJ 1998;317:703-713.

[12] Liu L, Quang ND, Banu R, Kumar H, Tham YC, Cheng CY, Wong TY, Sabanayagam C. Hypertension, blood pressure control and diabetic retinopathy in a large population-based study. PLoS One. 2020 Mar 5;15(3):e0229 665.

[13] Lurbe, E., Redon, J., Kesani, A., Pascual, J. M., Tacons, J., Alvarez, V., & Batlle, D. (2002). Increase in nocturnal blood pressure and progression to microalbuminuria in type 1 diabetes. *New England Journal of Medicine*, *347*(11), 797-805.

[14] **Klein R**, Klein BEK, Moss SE, *et al.* The Wisconsin Epidemiologic Study of Diabetic Retinopathy. XVII. The 14-year incidence and progression of diabetic retinopathy and associated risk factors in type 1 diabetes. Ophthalmology 1998; 105:1801-1815.

[15] **Klein R**, Klein BEK, Moss SE, *et al.* Is blood pressure a predictor of the incidence or progression of diabetic retinopathy? Arch Intern Med 1989;149:2427-2432.

[16] Donaldson, M., Dodson, P. Medical treatment of diabetic retinopathy. *Eye* **17,** 550-562 (2003).

[17] Hadjadj S, Duly-Bouhanick B, Bekherraz A, BrIdoux F, Gallois Y, Mauco G, Ebran J, Marre M. Serum triglycerides are a predictive factor for the development and the progression of renal and retinal complications in patients with type 1 diabetes. Diabetes Metab. 2004;30(1):43-51.

[18] Klein BE, Moss SE, Klein R, Surawicz TS. The Wisconsin Epidemiologic Study of Diabetic Retinopathy. XIII. Relationship of serum cholesterol to retinopathy and hard exudate. Ophthalmology. 1991;98(8):1261-1265.

[19] Yu JY, Lyons TJ. Modified Lipoproteins in Diabetic Retinopathy: A Local Action in the Retina. J Clin Exp Ophthalmol. 2013 Dec 18;4(6):314. doi: 10.4172/2155-9570.1000314..

[20] Ankit BS, Mathur G, Agrawal RP, Mathur KC. Stronger relationship of serum apolipoprotein A-1 and B with diabetic retinopathy than traditional lipids. Indian J Endocrinol Metab. 2017 Jan-Feb;21(1):102-105.

[21] Chew EY, Klein ML, Ferris FL 3rd, Remaley NA, Murphy RP, Chantry K, Hoogwerf BJ, Miller D. Association of elevated serum lipid levels with retinal hard exudate in diabetic retinopathy. Early Treatment Diabetic Retinopathy Study (ETDRS) Report 22. Arch Ophthalmol. 1996;114(9):1079-1084.

[22] Buraczynska M, Ksiazek P, Baranowicz-Gaszczyk I, Jozwiak L. Association of the VEGF gene polymorphism with diabetic retinopathy in type 2 diabetes patients, *Nephrology Dialysis Transplantation*, 22 (3):827-832, 2007.

[23] Jalal D, Kalia K: Impact of *VEGF* Gene Polymorphisms on Progression of Diabetic Retinopathy in an Indian Population, Biochemistry and Molecular Biology, 31(S1) 780.10-780.10, 2017.

[24] Awata T, Kurihara S, Takata N, Neda T, Iizuka H, Ohkubo T, Osaki M, Watanabe M, Nakashima Y, Inukai K, Inoue I, Kawasaki I, Mori K, Yoneya S, Katayama S. Functional VEGF C-634G polymorphism is associated with development of diabetic macular edema and correlated with macular retinal thickness in type 2 diabetes. Biochem Biophys Res Commun. 2005 Aug 5;333(3):679-685. doi: 10.1016/j.bbrc.2005.05.167. PMID: 15963467.

[25] Ray D, Mishra M, Ralph S, Read I, Davies R, Brenchley P: Association of the VEGF Gene With Proliferative Diabetic Retinopathy But Not Proteinuria in Diabetes, Diabetes Mar 2004, 53 (3) 861-864; **DOI:** 10.2337/diabetes.53.3.861

[26] Braunger BM, Leimbeck SV, Schlecht A, Volz C, Jägle H, Tamm ER. Deletion of ocular transforming growth factor β signaling mimics essential characteristics of diabetic retinopathy. *Am J Pathol*. 2015;185(6):1749-1768.

[27] Beránek M, Kanková K, Benes P et al., "Polymorphism R25P in the gene encoding transforming growth factor-beta (TGF-$\beta$1) is a newly identified risk factor for proliferative diabetic retinopathy," *American Journal of Medical Genetics*, vol. 109, no. 4, pp. 278-283, 2002.

[28] Anjum, A., et al. "Diabetic Retinopathy and Sex Hormones." *OSR Journal of Dental and Medical Sciences (IOSR-JDMS)* 16.1 (2017): 110-5.

[29] Akushichi M, et al. "A Case of Progressive Diabetic Retinopathy Related to Pregnancy Followed on Optical Coherence Tomography Angiography." *Ophthalmic Surgery, Lasers and Imaging Retina* 50.6 (2019): 393-397.

[30] Jesia H, Chew EY. "Retinopathy in diabetic pregnancy." *A Practical Manual of Diabetes in Pregnancy* (2017): 269.

[31] Rosenn, B., Miodovnik, M., Kranias, G., Khoury, J., Combs, C. A., Mimouni, F., ... & Lipman, M. J. (1992). Progression of diabetic retinopathy in pregnancy: association with hypertension in pregnancy. *American journal of obstetrics and gynecology*, *166*(4), 1214-1218.

[32] Knol JA, van Kooij B, de Valk HW, Rothova A. Rapid progression of diabetic retinopathy in eyes with posterior uveitis. Am J Ophthalmol. 2006 Feb;141(2):409-412. doi: 10.1016/j.ajo.2005.09.005. PMID: 16458715.

[33] Denniston, Alastair K., et al. "The UK Diabetic Retinopathy Electronic Medical Record (UK DR EMR) Users Group, Report 2: real-world data for the impact of cataract surgery on diabetic macular oedema." *British Journal of Ophthalmology* 101.12 (2017): 1673-1678.

[34] Chung, Jin, et al. "Effect of cataract surgery on the progression of diabetic retinopathy." *Journal of Cataract & Refractive Surgery* 28.4 (2002): 626-630.

[35] Rübsam A, Parikh S, Fort PE. Role of Inflammation in Diabetic Retinopathy. *Int J Mol Sci*. 2018;19(4):942. Published 2018 Mar 22. doi:10.3390/ijms19040942

[36] Oswal KS, Sivaraj RR, Murray PI, Stavrou P. Clinical course and visual outcome in patients with diabetes mellitus and uveitis. *BMC Res Notes*. 2013;6:167. Published 2013 Apr 29. doi:10.1186/1756-0500-6-167

[37] Vagaja NN, Binz N, McLenachan S, et al: Influence of endotoxin-mediated retinal inflammation on phenotype of diabetic retinopathy in Ins2Akita miceBritish Journal of Ophthalmology 2013;97:1343-1350.

[38] Demircan N., Safran B.G., Soylu M., Ozcan A.A., Sizmaz S. Determination of vitreous interleukin-1 (IL-1) and tumour necrosis factor (TNF) levels in proliferative diabetic retinopathy. Eye (London) 2006;20:1366-1369. doi: 10.1038/sj.eye.6702138.

[39] Yoshida S., Yoshida A., IsHibashi T., Elner S.G., Elner V.M. Role of MCP-1 and MIP-1alpha in retinal neovascularization during postischemic inflammation in a mouse model of retinal neovascularization. J. Leukoc. Biol. 2003;73:137-144. doi: 10.1189/jlb.0302117.

[40] Rusnak S., Vrzalova J., Sobotova M., Hecova L., Ricarova R., Topolcan O. The measurement of intraocular biomarkers in various stages of proliferative diabetic retinopathy using multiplex xmap technology. J. Ophthalmol. 2015;2015:424783. doi: 10.1155/2015/424783

[41] Doganay S., Evereklioglu C., Er H., Turkoz Y., Sevinc A., Mehmet N., Savli H. Comparison of serum no, TNF-alpha, IL-1beta, SIL-2r, IL-6 and il-8 levels with grades of retinopathy in patients with diabetes mellitus. Eye (London) 2002;16:163-170. doi: 10.1038/sj/eye/6700095.

[42] Chalam K.V., Grover S., Sambhav K., Balaiya S., Murthy R.K. Aqueous interleukin-6 levels are superior to vascular endothelial growth factor in predicting therapeutic response to bevacizumab in age-related macular degeneration. J. Ophthalmol. 2014;2014:502174. doi: 10.1155/2014/502174.

[43] Zhu W, Meng Y, Wu Y, Lu J: Anti-diabetic medications and risk of macular edema in patients with type 2 diabetes: a systemic review and meta-analysis, Int J Clin Exp Med 2018;11(12):12889-12901

[44] Poulaki V, Qin W, Joussen AM, Hurlbut P, Wiegand SJ, Rudge J, Yancopoulos GD and Adamis AP. Acute intensive insulin therapy exacerbates

diabetic blood-retinal barrier breakdown via hypoxia-inducible factor-1alpha and VEGF. J Clin Invest 2002; 109: 805-815.

[45] Merante D, Menchini F, Truitt KE and Bandello FM. Diabetic macular edema: correlations with available diabetes therapies--evidence across a qualitative review of published literature from MEDLINE and EMBASE. Drug Saf 2010; 33: 643-652.

[46] Liazos E, Broadbent DM, Beare N and Kumar N. Spontaneous resolution of diabetic macular oedema after discontinuation of thiazolidenediones. Diabet Med 2008; 25: 860-862.

[47] Shin ES, Sorenson CM, Sheibani N. Diabetes and retinal vascular dys-function. J Ophthalmic Vis Res. 2014 Jul-Sep;9(3):362-73. doi: 10.4103/2008-322X.143378. PMID: 25667739; PMCID: PMC4307665.

[48] Rodríguez ML, Pérez S, Mena-Mollá S, Desco MC, Ortega ÁL. Oxidative Stress and Microvascular Alterations in Diabetic Retinopathy: Future Therapies. Oxid Med Cell Longev. 2019 Nov 11;2019:4940825.

[49] Martins, B.; Amorim, M.; Reis, F.; Ambrósio, A.F.; Fernandes, R. Extracellular Vesicles and MicroRNA: Putative Role in Diagnosis and Treatment of Diabetic Retinopathy. *Antioxidants* **2020**, *9*, 705.

[50] Robinson R, Barathi VA, Chaurasia SS, Wong TY, Kern TS. Update on animal models of diabetic retinopathy: from molecular approaches to mice and higher mammals. Dis Model Mech. 2012 Jul;5(4):444-456.

[51] Intine RV, Sarras MP Jr. Metabolic memory and chronic diabetes complications: potential role for epigenetic mechanisms. Curr Diab Rep. 2012 Oct;12(5):551-559. doi: 10.1007/s11892-012-0302-7.

[52] Raczyńska D Zorena K, Urban B, Zalewski D, Skorek A, Malukiewicz G, Sikorski BL. "Current Trends in the Monitoring and Treatment of Diabetic Retinopathy in Young Adults", *Mediators of Inflammation*, vol. 2014, Article ID 492926, 13 pages, 2014. https://doi.org/10.1155/2014/492926

[53] Wu H., Hwang D.K., Song X., Tao Y. Association between aqueous cytokines and diabetic retinopathy stage. J. Ophthalmol. 2017;2017:9402198. doi: 10.1155/2017/9402198.

[54] Chang YC, Wu WC. Dyslipidemia and diabetic retinopathy. *Rev Diabet Stud*. 2013;10(2-3):121-132. doi:10.1900/RDS.2013.10.121

[55] Loukovaara, S., Piippo, N., Kinnunen, K., Hytti, M., Kaarniranta, K. and Kauppinen, A. (2017), NLRP3 inflammasome activation is associated with proliferative diabetic retinopathy. Acta Ophthalmol, 95: 803-808.

[56] Wheeler SE, Lee NY. Emerging Roles of Transforming Growth Factor β Signaling in Diabetic Retinopathy. J Cell Physiol. 2017 Mar;232(3):486-489. doi: 10.1002/jcp.25506. Epub 2016 Sep 21. PMID: 27472503.

[57] Lopes De Jesus CC. Diabetic Retinopathy, Diabetic Retinopathy, Mohammad Shamsul Ola, IntechOpen, 2012. DOI: 10.5772/28955. Available from: https://www.intechopen.com/books/diabetic-retinopathy/diabetic-retinopathy

[58] De La Cruz JP, Gonzalez-Correa JA, Guerrero A, De la Cuesta FS, et al. Pharmacological approach to diabetic retinopathy. Diabetes/metabolism research and reviews 2004;20:91-113.

[59] Siemianowicz K, Gminski J, Telega A, Wójcik A, Posielezna B, Grabowska-Bochenek R,Francuz T. Blood antioxidant parameters in patients with diabetic retinopathy.

International Journal of Molecular Medicine 2004;14:433-437.

[60] Mamputu JC, Renier G. Advanced glycation end-products increase monocyte adhesion to retinal endothelial cells through vascular endothelial growth factor-induced ICAM-1 expression: inhibitory effects of antioxidants. Journal of Leukocyte Biology 2004;75:1062-1069.

[61] http://www.icoph.org/downloads/Diabetic-Retinopathy-Scale.pdf

[62] Kanski J, Bowling B: Kanski's Clinical Ophthalmology 8th Edition, Saunders Ltd, 2015.

[63] Corcóstegui B, Durán S, González-Albarrán MO, Hernández C, Ruiz-Moreno JM, Salvador J, Udaondo P, Simó R. Update on Diagnosis and Treatment of Diabetic Retinopathy: A Consensus Guideline of the Working Group of Ocular Health (Spanish Society of Diabetes and Spanish Vitreous and Retina Society). J Ophthalmol. 2017;2017:8234186. doi: 10.1155/2017/8234186. Epub 2017 Jun 11.

[64] Jiménez-Báez MV, Márquez-González H, Bárcenas-Contreras R, Morales-Montoya C, Espinosa-García LF. (2015). Early diagnosis of diabetic retinopathy in primary care. *Colombia Médica*, *46*(1), 14-18.

[65] Spaide R. F., Klancnik J. M., Jr., Cooney M. J. Retinal vascular layers imaged by fluorescein angiography and optical coherence tomography angiography. *JAMA Ophthalmology*. 2015;133:45-50.

[66] Khadamy J, Abri Aghdam K, Falavarjani KG. An Update on Optical Coherence Tomography Angiography in Diabetic Retinopathy. J Ophthalmic Vis Res. 2018 Oct-Dec;13(4):487-497. doi: 10.4103/jovr.jovr_57_18.

[67] de Barros Garcia JM, Isaac DL, Avila M. Diabetic retinopathy and OCT angiography: clinical findings and future prespectives. *International Journal of Retina and Vitreous*. 2017;3:p. 14. doi: 10.1186/s40942-017-0062-2.

[68] Hsu CR, Chen YT, Sheu WH. Glycemic variability and diabetes retinopathy: a missing link. J Diabetes Complications. 2015 Mar;29(2):302-306. doi: 10.1016/j.jdiacomp.2014.11.013. Epub 2014 Dec 3. PMID: 25534877.

[69] Scanlon PH, Aldington SJ, Stratton IM. Epidemiological issues in diabetic retinopathy. Middle East Afr J Ophthalmol 2014;20:293-300. DOI: 10.4103/0974-9233.120007

[70] Berco E, Rappoport D, Pollack A, Kleinmann G, Greenwald Y: Management of Diabetic Retinopathy and Other Ocular Complications in Type 1 Diabetes, Major Topics in Type 1 Diabetes, Kenia Pedrosa Nunes, 2015, IntechOpen, DOI: 10.5772/61276.

[71] American Diabetes Association, author. Management of Dyslipidemia in Adults in Diabetes. Diabetes Care. 2007;25(1):S74–S77.

[72] Patel JI, Jenkins L, Benjamin L, Webber S. Dilated pupils and loss of accommodation following diode panretinal photocoagulation with sub-tenon local anaesthetic in four cases. Eye Lond Engl. 2002;16(5):628-632. doi: 10.1038/sj.eye.6700004.

[73] Moriarty AP, Spalton DJ, Shilling JS, Ffytche TJ, Bulsara M. Breakdown of the blood-aqueous barrier after argon laser panretinal photocoagulation for proliferative diabetic retinopathy. Ophthalmology. 1996;103(5):833-838. doi: 10.1016/S0161-6420(96)30607-6.

[74] Fong DS, Girach A, Boney A. Visual side effects of successful scatter laser photocoagulation surgery for proliferative diabetic retinopathy: a

literature review. Retina. 2007; 27(7):816-824. doi: 10.1097/IAE.0b013e318042d32c.

[75] Mori, Y., Suzuma, K., Uji, A. *et al.* Restoration of foveal photoreceptors after intravitreal ranibizumab injections for diabetic macular edema. *Sci Rep* **6,** 39161 (2016). https://doi.org/10.1038/srep39161

[76] Romero-Aroca P, Reyes-Torres J, Baget-Bernaldiz M, Blasco-Suñe C. Laser treatment for diabetic macular edema in the 21st century. Curr Diabetes Rev. 2014 Mar;10(2):100-12. doi: 10.2174/1573399810666140402123026. PMID: 24852439; PMCID: PMC4051253.

[77] Zhao Y, Singh RP. The role of anti-vascular endothelial growth factor (anti-VEGF) in the management of proliferative diabetic retinopathy. Drugs Context. 2018 Aug 13;7:212532. doi: 10.7573/dic.212532.

[78] Wells JA, Glassman AR, Ayala AR, Jampol LM, Aiello LP, Antoszyk AN, Arnold-Bush B, Baker CW, Bressler NM, Browning DJ, Elman MJ, Ferris FL, Friedman SM, Melia M, Pieramici DJ, Sun JK, Beck RW: Diabetic Retinopathy Clinical Research Network,. Aflibercept, bevacizumab, or ranibizumab for diabetic macular edema. N Engl J Med. 2015 Mar 26;372(13):1193-1203. doi: 10.1056/NEJMoa1414264.

[79] Busch, C., Zur, D., Fraser-Bell, S. *et al.* Shall we stay, or shall we switch? Continued anti-VEGF therapy versus early switch to dexamethasone implant in refractory diabetic macular edema. *Acta Diabetol* **55,** 789-796 (2018).

[80] Ellis D, Burgess PI, Kayange P. Management of diabetic retinopathy. Malawi Medical Journal : the Journal of Medical Association of Malawi. 2013 Dec;25(4):116-120..

[81] Tesfaye S, Chaturvedi N, Eaton SE, *et al.* Vascular risk factors and diabetic neuropathy. N Engl J Med 2005; 352: 341-350.

[82] Vincent AM, Hinder LM, Pop-Busui R, *et al.* Hyperlipidemia: a new therapeutic target for diabetic neuropathy. J Peripher Nerv Syst 2009; 14: 257-267.

[83] Amin N, Doupis J. Diabetic foot disease: From the evaluation of the "foot at risk" to the novel diabetic ulcer treatment modalities. World J Diabetes. 2016 Apr 10;7(7):153-164. doi: 10.4239/wjd.v7.i7.153.

[84] Edo AE, Edo GO, Ezeani IU. Risk factors, ulcer grade and management outcome of diabetic foot ulcers in a Tropical Tertiary Care Hospital. Niger Med J. 2013 Jan;54(1):59-63. doi: 10.4103/0300-1652.108900

[85] Armstrong DG, Boulton AJM, Bus SA. Diabetic foot ulcers and their recurrence. N Engl J Med 2017;376: 2367-2375

[86] Boulton AJM, Armstrong DG, Kirsner RS, et al. Diagnosis and management of diabetic foot complications. Arlington (VA): American Diabetes Association; January 2020. PMID: 32105420

[87] Shahi SK, Kumar A, Kumar S, Singh SK, Gupta SK, Singh TB. Prevalence of diabetic foot ulcer and associated risk factors in diabetic patients from North India. J Diabetic Foot Complications. 2012;4:83-91.

[88] Moss SE, Klein R, Klein BE. The prevalence and incidence of lower extremity amputation in a diabetic population. Arch Intern Med. 1992;152: 610-616.

[89] Sharma M, Sharma A, Gothwal SR, Dixit S, Lunia AK, Sharma M. Diabetic foot ulcers: A prospective study of 100 patients based on wound based severity score. IOSR J Dent Med Sci. 2014;13:79-89.

[90] Yagihashi S, Mizukami H, Sugimoto K. Mechanism of diabetic

neuropathy: Where are we now and where to go? J Diabetes Investig. 2011 Jan 24;2(1):18-32. doi: 10.1111/j.2040-1124.2010.00070.x.

[91] Boulton AJ, Vinik AI, Arezzo JC, *et al.* Diabetic neuropathies: a statement by the American Diabetes Association. Diabetes Care 2005; 28: 956-962

[92] Strotmeyer ES, de Rekeneire N, Schwartz AV, *et al.* Sensory and motor peripheral nerve function and lower-extremity quadriceps strength: the health, aging and body composition study. J Am Geriatr Soc 2009; 57: 2004-2010.

[93] Vinik AI, Liuzze FJ, Holland MT, *et al.* Diabetic neuropathies. Diabetes Care 1992; 15: 1926-1975

[94] Rogers LC, Frykberg RG, Armstrong DG, Boulton AJ, Edmonds M, Van GH, Hartemann A, Game F, Jeffcoate W, Jirkovska A, Jude E, Morbach S, Morrison WB, Pinzur M, Pitocco D, Sanders L, Wukich DK, Uccioli L. The Charcot foot in diabetes. Diabetes Care. 2011 Sep;34(9):2123-2129.

[95] Pendsey SP. Understanding diabetic foot. Int J Diabetes Dev Ctries. 2010; 30(2):75-79.

[96] Boulton AJM. The diabetic foot: grand overview, epidemiology and pathogenesis. Diabetes Metab Res Rev. 2008;24 Suppl 1:S3-S6.

[97] Papanas N, Maltezos E. The diabetic foot: established and emerging treatments. Acta Clin Bleg 2007; 62(4): 230-238.

[98] Ziegler D, Papanas N, Schnell O, Nguyen BDT, Nguyen KT, Kulkantrakorn K et al. Current concepts in the management of diabetic polyneuropathy. J diabetes Investig 2020;Sep 12 [Online ahead of print].

[99] Papanas N. Diabetic neuropathy collection: progress in diagnosis and screening. Diabetes Ther 2020;11: 761-764.

[100] Papanas N, Paschos P, Papazoglou D, Papatheodorou K, Paletas K, Maltezos E, Tsapas A. Accuracy of the Neuropad test for the diagnosis of distal symmetric polyneuropathy in type 2 diabetes. Diabetes Care. 2011;34(6):1378-1382.

[101] Papanas N, Boulton AJ, Malik RA, Manes C, Schnell O, Spallone V et al. A simple new non-invasive sweat indicator test for the diagnosis of diabetic neuropathy. Diabet Med. 2013;30(5):525-534.

[102] Brownrigg JR, Apelqvist J, Bakker K, Schaper NC, Hinchliffe RJ. Evidence-based management of PAD & the diabetic foot. Eur J Vasc Endovasc Surg. 2013;45(6):673-681. doi:10.1016/j. ejvs.2013.02.014

[103] Vas, PRJ, Edmonds, M, Kavarthapu, V, et al. The diabetic foot attack: "tis too late to retreat!" Int J Low Extrem Wounds. 2018;17:7-13.

[104] Panagoulias GS, Eleftheriadou I, Papanas N, Manes C, Kamenov Z, Tesic D et al. Dryness of foot skin assessed by the visual indicator test and risk of diabetic foot ulceration: a prospective observational study. Front Endocrinol (Lausanne). 2020;11:625.

[105] Feldman EL, Stevens MJ, Thomas PK, Brown MB, Canal N, Greene DA. A practical two-step quantitative clinical and electrophysiological assessment for the diagnosis and staging of diabetic neuropathy. Diabetes Care. 1994 Nov;17(11):1281-1289. doi: 10.2337/ diacare.17.11.1281. PMID: 7821168.

[106] Herman WH, Pop-Busui R, Braffett BH, et al. Use of the Michigan Neuropathy Screening Instrument

as a measure of distal symmetrical peripheral neuropathy in Type 1 diabetes: results from the Diabetes Control and Complications Trial/Epidemiology of Diabetes Interventions and Complications. *Diabet Med*. 2012;29(7):937-944. doi:10.1111/j.1464-5491.2012.03644.x

[107] Høyer C, Sandermann J, Petersen LJ. The toe-brachial index in the diagnosis of peripheral arterial disease. J Vasc Surg. 2013 Jul;58(1):231-238. doi: 10.1016/j.jvs.2013.03.044.

[108] Potier L, Halbron M, Bouilloud F, Dadon M, Le Doeuff J, Ha Van G, Grimaldi A, Hartemann-Heurtier A. Ankle-to-brachial ratio index underestimates the prevalence of peripheral occlusive disease in diabetic patients at high risk for arterial disease. Diabetes Care. 2009;32(4):e44.

[109] Dhatariya K, Bain SC, Buse JB, Simpson R, Tarnow L, Kaltoft MS, Stellfeld M, Tornøe K, Pratley RE; LEADER Publication Committee on behalf of the LEADER Trial Investigators. The Impact of Liraglutide on Diabetes-Related Foot Ulceration and Associated Complications in Patients With Type 2 Diabetes at High Risk for Cardiovascular Events: Results From the LEADER Trial. Diabetes Care. 2018 Oct;41(10):2229-2235. doi: 10.2337/dc18-1094.

[110] Demetriou M, Papanas N, Panopoulou M, Papatheodorou K, Bounovas A, Maltezos E. Tissue and swab culture in diabetic foot infections: neuropathic versus neuroischemic ulcers. Int J Low Extrem Wounds. 2013;12(2): 87-93.

[111] Demetriou M, Papanas N, Panagopoulos P, Panopoulou M, Maltezos E. Antibiotic resistance in diabetic foot soft tissue infections: a series from Greece. Int J Low Extrem Wounds. 2017;16(4):255-259.

[112] Papanas N, Maltezos E. Becaplermin gel in the treatment of diabetic neuropathic foot ulcers. Clin Interv Aging. 2008;3(2):233-240.

[113] Eleftheriadou I, Samakidou G, Tentolouris A, Papanas N, Tentolouris N. Nonpharmacological management of diabetic foot ulcers: an update. Int J Low Extrem Wounds. 2020; Oct 19:1534734620963561. doi: 10.1177/1534734620963561. Online ahead of print.

[114] Papanas N, Demetzos C, Pippa N, Maltezos E, Tentolouris N. Efficacy of a new heparan sulfate mimetic dressing in the healing of foot and lower extremity ulcerations in type 2 diabetes: a case series. Int J Low Extrem Wounds. 2016; 15(1):63-67.

[115] Perren S, Gatt A, Papanas N, Formosa C. Hyperbaric oxygen therapy in ischaemic foot ulcers in type 2 diabetes: a clinical trial. Open Cardiovasc Med J. 2018;12:80-85.

[116] Papanas N, Papachristou S, Kefala C, Kyroglou S. Use of the new Vergenix soft tissue repair matrix to heal a chronic neuropathic diabetic foot ulcer. Int J Low Extrem Wounds. 2020;19(2):205-206.

[117] Vas PRJ, Edmonds M, Kavarthapu V, Rashid H, Ahluwalia R, Pankhurst C, Papanas N. The diabetic foot attack: "'tis too late to retreat!" Int J Low Extrem Wounds. 2018;17(1):7-13.

[118] Papanas N, Papi M, Rerkasem K. A wealth of science. Int J Low Extrem Wounds. 2020;19(1):5-6

Chapter 11

# Cardiovascular Risk/Disease in Type 2 Diabetes Mellitus

*Gabriela Roman and Anca Pantea Stoian*

## Abstract

People with Type 2 diabetes mellitus (T2DM) have a 2–3 times higher cardiovascular risk (CVR) than people without diabetes. Atherosclerotic cardiovascular disease (ASCVD) is the major cause of morbidity and mortality in T2DM. Over 30% of those with T2DM have CVD (cardiovascular disease), and over half die from it, mainly from coronary heart disease. The presence of T2DM reduces life expectancy by 10–14 years. The European Society of Cardiology stratifies the CVR into *moderate* (young patients, with a short duration of diabetes, no risk factors), *high* (duration of diabetes >10 years, no target organ damage, plus any additional risk factor) and *very high* (patients with established CVD, target organ injury three CVD risk factors: age, hypertension, dyslipidemia, obesity, or Type 1 diabetes mellitus (T1DM) over 20 years duration). The American Association of Clinical Endocrinologists (AACE) considers that diabetes per se involves high risk. Heart failure (HF) is the second most common complication after obstructive peripheral arterial disease. T2DM associates a 75% higher risk of CV mortality or hospitalization for HF. A multifactorial approach is required to reduce CV morbidity and mortality.

**Keywords:** cardiovascular risk, cardiovascular disease, type 2 diabetes mellitus

## 1. Introduction

Diabetes mellitus (DM), a very complex and heterogeneous chronic disease, is associated with chronic complications generated by alteration of the endothelium at all arterial vascular territory levels. The micro-and macro-vascular complications affect the entire body; their pathogenic mechanisms are intricate and involve multiple pathways and risk factors. The main risk factors are insulin resistance/hyperinsulinemia, hyperglycemia, dyslipidemia, hypercholesterolemia, hypertension, smoking, obesity/overweight, all of which cause endothelial dysfunction. Consequently, they appear vasoconstriction, oxidative stress, subclinical inflammation, vascular calcification and thrombosis, essential pathogenic elements in the process of atherogenesis/macroangiopathy and microangiopathy [1].

Cardiovascular disease is considered a major cause of morbidity and mortality among people with diabetes, with a significantly increased prevalence compare with people without diabetes. The risk increases with the level of glycaemia, the duration of diabetes and the number of risk factors. People with T2DM have much earlier and more extensive process of accelerated atherosclerosis, more vulnerable and larger volume atherosclerotic plaques and coronary artery lumen with a smaller diameter, compared to people without DM. The pathogenic complex is influenced by genetic factors, age, personal history and a pro-risk lifestyle (unhealthy eating, sedentary lifestyle, smoking, sleep disorders, psychosocial stress and depression) [1].

The macrovascular complications mainly refer to the atherosclerotic cardiovascular disease, represented by coronary artery disease (acute and chronic coronary syndrome) (CAD), chronic peripheral artery disease (PAD) and cerebrovascular disease (CBV). A particular complication is heart failure (HF). The pathogenic mechanisms of micro-and macro-angiopathy are extremely complex, with multiple interactions at the molecular-cellular and vascular-organic level.

Although all complications declined in the last decades, the most significant decreases in diabetes-related complications occurred for heart attack and stroke, especially for people aged 75 years and older. The CVD risk and mortality rate has declined in both the general population [2] and the people with diabetes [3]. However, diabetes, mainly T2DM, continues to be an important generator of cardiovascular disease. As the number of patients with diabetes is predicted to increase, reaching 700 million in 2045 [4], it is expected that the number of people with CVD will also increase. Thus, these major diabetes complications continue to place a heavy burden on health care systems.

## 2. Cardiovascular risk

### 2.1 Cardiovascular risk factors in diabetes

The concept of cardiovascular risk began to be of interest in the 1930s. Studies of cardiovascular disease epidemiology and its causes began in the 1950s, with Framingham Heart Study being one of the first. This extended program has demonstrated the existence of multiple CVR factors over the years, introducing in the literature and medical concept the term "risk factor". Among the study's first results, high blood pressure, hypercholesterolemia, and smoking are considered traditional, classic, risk factors. Subsequently, Framingham study and other epidemiological studies, have identified other risk factors, including obesity, diabetes, dyslipidemia, sedentary lifestyle. Thus diabetes is associated with a 2- to 3-fold increase in the risk of developing CVD and glucose intolerance with a 1.5-fold increase [5–7]. In addition to hyperglycemia, diabetes, mainly T2DM, is accompanied by other cardiovascular risk factors, within the metabolic syndrome: insulin resistance, abdominal obesity, atherogenic dyslipidemia (hypertriglyceridemia, low HDL-C (High-density lipoprotein cholesterol), LDL-C (low density lipoprotein cholesterol particles), remnant lipoproteins, postprandial hyperlipidemia), high blood pressure, prothrombotic, proinflammatory and oxidative stress state, microalbuminuria, non-alcoholic fatty liver disease [8].

High blood pressure increases 2–4 times the risk of CVD, kidney and death, atherogenic dyslipidemia induces a residual CVR, even under statin treatment and LDL-C control and abdominal obesity, as a component of metabolic syndrome, significantly increases the risk of coronary heart disease, stroke and death [9–11].

### 2.2 Cardiovascular risk in T2DM

Overall, people with T2DM have 2 to 4 times increased risk of cardiovascular morbidity and mortality than individuals without diabetes. This risk increases with the increase of fasting glycaemia since the stages of prediabetes. The risk for CAD is rising by 160%, for ischemic heart disease by 127%, for stroke by 56%, for CVD death by 132% [4], and for HF is 2–4 times higher in men and five times higher in women, compared to those without diabetes [5].

Epidemiological studies have revealed that the excess relative risk of vascular events is more significant in women, at younger ages, in long-standing DM and in the presence of microvascular complications, mainly renal disease or proteinuria [12].

Although T2DM was initially considered a "cardiovascular risk equivalent" [12–14], it has since been shown that CVR, mainly CAD risk, is not similar for all persons with diabetes, but is highly heterogeneous. Thus, the CVR should be differentiated based on the presence of other CVR factors or overt CVD.

For T1DM, The Swedish National Diabetes Register has shown actual results in CVD and CV death prevalence. [13] For T1DM, 27,195 patients were stratified by age and sex. Early-onset at 1–10 years of age was correlated with an HR (hazard ratio) of 7.38 for CV mortality, 30.95 for acute myocardial infarction (MI), and 12.9 for heart failure (HF). Progress of T1DM between 1 and 10 years of age resulted in a loss of 17.7 years of life in women and 14.2 years in men. [13] Notwithstanding, T2DM is more common than T1DM.These results confirm the loss of years of life in both populations, which is more severe in the younger patients and in young-onset female individuals with T2DM, highlighting the need for early and intensive risk-factor interventions in these clusters of patients. [12]

The European Society of Cardiology stratifies the CVR into three risk categories, including T1DM, considering that presence of DM overall represents a significant risk factor for CVD:

- **moderate:** young patients (T1DM aged <35 years or T2DM aged <50 years), with DM duration <10 years, without other risk factors,
- **high:** patients with DM duration ≥10 years without target organ damage plus any other additional risk factor, and
- **very high:** patients with DM and established CVD, or further target organ damage (proteinuria, renal impairment defined as eGFR <30 mL/min/1.73 m$^2$, left ventricular hypertrophy, or retinopathy), or three or more major risk factors (age, hypertension, dyslipidemia, smoking, obesity), or early-onset T1DM of >20-year duration [12].

The American Association of Clinical Endocrinologists (AACE) stratifies the CVR into three levels: **high** (DM without other CVR factors), **very high** (DM with at least one CVR factor), and **extreme risk** (overt CVD in those with DM, chronic kidney disease) [15].

T2DM is reputed as an independent risk factor for the development of HF. Higher levels of glycated hemoglobin A1c (HbA1c) in T2DM patients have been associated with significantly more incident HF cases than in patients with T2DM and lower HbA1c levels. The incidence is even higher in patients with established CAD, in which each 1% increase in HbA1c level was associated with a 36% increased risk for HF hospitalization [16].

### 2.3 Cardiovascular risk assessment

A rational and successful approach to reducing the CVR involves stratifying risk and the periodic evaluation of the outcomes. Accurate CVD risk estimation in people with T2DM without established CVD can identify patients at high risk of developing CVD and can thus be used to adapt the intensity and complexity of appropriate treatment. For practice, CVR assessment scores which can be applied in diabetes are beneficial. Several CVR calculation scores in DM have been developed. The first is the result of the United Kingdom Prospective Diabetes Study (UKPDS), in which, in people newly diagnosed with T2DM, the effect of intensive treatment on the evolution of chronic complications compared to conventional treatment was followed. UKPDS Risk Engine estimates the risk of fatal and non-fatal coronary events and fatal and non-fatal stroke at 15 and 30 years, in people with T2DM without CV disease, considering the duration of DM, age, gender, ethnicity, smoking, presence of atrial fibrillation, the level of HbA1c, systolic blood pressure, total cholesterol and HDL-C (https://www.dtu.ox.ac.uk/riskengine/) [17].

Another score (Advance Risk Engine) is based on ADVANCE and ADVANCE-ON studies. It refers to patients with T2DM without CVD, is based on the usual parameters and estimates the risk of major CV events at four years, the risk of renal events at five years and the risk of major vascular disease at ten years (www.advanceriskengine.com) [18].

The American Heart Association (AHA) and American College of Cardiology (ACC), developed a risk score to estimate the ten-year risk for the first ASCVD event (non-fatal myocardial infarction or CHD death, or fatal/non-fatal stroke) (available online at tools.acc.org/ASCVD-Risk-Estimator-Plus) [19].

Based on the ACCORD trial population, the BRAVO risk engine has been recently developed. It contains three separate modules addressed to events (stroke, MI, HF, angina, revascularization surgery, renal events, blindness, hypoglycemia), risk factors and mortality [20].

None of these CVR estimation scores is perfect, so clinical judgment and consideration of CVR factors are important for setting and selecting appropriate therapeutic goals and interventions.

## 3. Cardiovascular disease

The high impact that T2DM has on the CVD has generated numerous studies, and population analyzes in order to determine the prevalence of the cardiovascular pathologies in people with diabetes. Although the description and the diagnostic criteria used to define the different manifestations of CVD were different across the epidemiologic studies, overall, the results show that CVD is a major cause of comorbidity and mortality among patients with T2DM. Thus, the CVD, including myocardial infarction, stroke, angina, heart failure, atherosclerosis and coronary artery disease, is present in 32.2% of people with T2DM. The most frequent type of CVD seems to be the CAD (21.2%), males having higher rates (18.7%) than females (14.3%) [21]. A large cohort of 1,921,260 individuals, 1.8% with T2DM, followed 5.5 years, has been analyzed in terms of the most common initial manifestations of CVD. In T2DM individuals, peripheral artery disease was the most frequent first presentation (16.2%) followed by HF (14.1%), significantly higher compared with those without diabetes [22]. The prevalence of CVD and the incidence of primary adverse outcomes is higher in women with T2DM than their male counterparts ($RR = 9.29$; $P < 0.0001$ for CVD and $RR = 5.25$; $P < 0.0001$ for incident major adverse outcomes [23]. Data from the UK Biobank showed that a cardiovascular event's excess risk was approximately 50% higher in women ($HR = 1.96$) than in men, and more importantly, the incidence of myocardial infarction (MI) [A1] was higher in men than in women(28.8%). This observation was exciting since the sex differences were the same in all age-related groups and were attenuated with increasing age, from 0.27 (0.18 to 0.41), in 45 years age cluster versus 0.45 (0.40 to 0.50) in 65 years age cluster. [24].

Although diabetes-related excess mortality is lower in the contemporary era than previously, T2DM is associated with a two to six times increased risk of CVD mortality than people without diabetes. Cardiovascular disease accounts for 52% of deaths in type 2 DM [25]. MI is considered to be the main cause of death for individuals with diabetes mellitus.

T2DM is a significant predictor of HF, independent of the simultaneous presence of hypertension and coronary heart disease. In diabetes, HF has multiple risk factors: hyperglycemia, insulin resistance, age, ischemic heart disease, high blood pressure, left ventricular hypertrophy, diffuse, accelerated and severe atherosclerosis. Even in the absence of CAD, microvascular complications, arterial thickening and fibrosis, endothelial and vasomotor dysfunction, increase the risk of HF. The risk of HF is 2–4 times higher in men and five times higher in women compared to those without diabetes, according to Framingham Heart Study [5, 16].

The presence of DM in those hospitalized for HF worsens the prognosis, prolongs hospitalization, and increases the number of hospitalizations and the risk of death. In stable forms of HF, T2DM is an independent predictor of hospitalization and mortality, regardless of the ejection fraction [26]. Patients with T2DM have a 2.5-fold increased risk of developing HF and a 75% higher risk of CV mortality or hospitalization for HF than those without DM [27].

HF with preserved ejection fraction (HFpEF) is a frequent phenotype in T2DM and is related to an important risk of morbidity and mortality than those without diabetes, with multiple comorbidities, reduced exercise capacity, increased markers of inflammation, fibrosis, endothelial dysfunction, congestion, increased left ventricular pressure [28].

At similar ejection fraction values, patients with T2DM have a higher NYHA functional class, and more expressed symptoms than those without diabetes. Left ventricular (LV) diastolic dysfunction can be detected in approximately 75% of patients with T2DM, even in the early stages. The degree of hyperglycemia and its duration correlate with LV diastolic dysfunction's severity, with the increased risk of HF and CV mortality [16].

A retrospective cohort study that included 208,792 adults with diabetes has analyzed the impact of varying combinations of heart disease, stroke, moderate chronic kidney disease (CKD) on mortality, over a median follow-up of 8.5 years [29]. The effect of heart diseases, stroke, CKD, and the combination of these conditions on all-cause mortality has been found to be independent and cumulative. The mortality risks were 1.75 times, 2.63 times, and 3.58 times greater for patients with one, two, and all three above mentioned conditions, and life expectancy for a 40-year-old with one, two, and three conditions was reduced with 20, 25, and 30 years for men and 25, 30, and 35 years, respectively, for women, compared with patients without these diseases [29].

Diabetes is the most known cause of CKD, and end-stage renal disease, more than 50% of people with DM are likely to develop CKD. CKD, especially severe CKD, has a significant impact on life expectancy and mortality risk in patients with diabetes. The risk of CV death increases as renal function declines (eGFR <60 ml/min/1.73 $m^2$ and/or ACR (albumin-creatinine ratio) ≥10 mg/g) [30]. Rates of HF are approximately 3-times higher in patients with eGFR <60 ml/min/1.7 $m^2$ [31].

The CardioRenal Metabolic Syndrome (CaReMe) has been introduced as terminology to describe the ongoing relationship between obesity, diabetes, kidney disease and heart failure with preserved systolic function, with significant mortality implications rate and therapeutic interventions [32].

Within CVD, diabetic cardiomyopathy or "cardiac microvascular disease", is a phenotype with distinct manifestations, described as a "structural and functional alteration of the myocardium, in the absence of hypertension, ischemic coronary heart disease, valvulopathies, or other FRCV, in patients with diabetes, especially with long-term diabetes and poor control." Fibrosis, stiffness, and cardiac hypertrophy are basic changes, which are initially associated with diastolic dysfunction, LV hypertrophy and reduced compliance with preserving the ejection fraction, later evolving into systolic dysfunction clinically manifest HF [16, 33]. As risk factors of diabetic cardiomyopathy, hyperglycemia, dyslipidemia, altered energy metabolism, dysregulated insulin signaling, inflammation, endoplasmic reticular stress, mitochondrial dysfunction, oxidative stress and accumulation of advanced glycation end-products (AGEs) and activation of the renin-angiotensin-aldosterone system (RAAS) are described [33].

## 4. Hyperglycemia and CVD relationship

Compared with individuals without diabetes, patients with T2DM are disproportionately affected by CVD morbidity and mortality. Most of this excess risk is associated with an increased prevalence of risk factors such as hypertension, dyslipidemia, and obesity in these patients. However, hyperglycemia, as a distinct characteristic of DM, appears to be an independent risk factor for all-cause and CVD mortality independent of other modifiable CVD risk factors:

- Increased HbA1c is associated with coronary heart disease [34],
- Long-term intraindividual variability of HbA1c or basal blood glucose is associated with micro-and macro-vascular complications and with an increased risk of important adverse CV events [35–37],
- 24-hour glycemic variability, greater than 35.9 mg/dl, is independently associated with an increased risk of left ventricular diastolic dysfunction, even in asymptomatic patients and with a preserved ejection fraction (odds ratio: 3.67; $p < 0.05$) [38],
- Basal glycemia >126 mg/dl was associated with a risk of fatal/non-fatal coronary heart disease, fatal/non-fatal stroke of 39% in women and 48% in men [39],
- Each 1-point increase in HbA1c is associated with an 8% increase in the risk of HF and a 36% increased risk for HF hospitalization [16, 39],
- The onset of diabetes in young people and the long duration of diabetes, are associated with an increased risk of mortality, mainly CV, due to ischemic disease and stroke [40, 41],
- The risk of coronary artery disease increases in diabetic patients by 11% for each 1% increment in HbA1c greater than 6.5%. In adults with diabetes, but without baseline CVD, an HbA1c of 9% is correlated with an increased risk of myocardial infarction or acute coronary syndrome (odds ratio [OR] = 1.18), stroke (OR = 1.29) and heart failure (OR = 1.37) [42],
- Severe hypoglycemia is linked with an increased risk of recurrence (especially in T1DM) and an increased risk of CV events, including death. In the Veteran Affairs Diabetes Trial, severe hypoglycemia was associated in the following 3 months with CV events (HR = 1.9; $p = 0.03$), CV mortality (HR = 3.7; $p = 0.01$) and mortality of any cause (HR = 2.4; $p = 0.02$) [43].

## 5. Therapeutic approach

The major objectives of clinical management in T2DM are preventing or delaying chronic complications, increasing life expectancy, and quality. The basic principle of clinical management is the "patient-centred" approach, respectively, the intervention's individualisation [19]. The significant reduction of cardiovascular morbidity/mortality implies a multifactorial approach, addressed simultaneously to all CV risk factors. The 7.8-year STENO-2 study, which included patients with T2DM with increased CV risk (microalbuminuria), showed that the multifactorial approach significantly reduced mortality from any cause (20% reduction in absolute risk), 13% in CV mortality and 29% in the absolute risk of CV events [44, 45]. The 21-year assessment showed that life expectancy was extended by eight years in the intensive care group, and the relative risk of HF was reduced by 76% [45]. Analysis of data from an extensive registry has shown that in people with T2DM, simultaneous control of major CV risk factors (blood glucose, blood pressure, cholesterol and lifestyle, no smoking), can reduce over 60% of cardiovascular and coronary atherosclerotic events [46]. Patients with diabetes who have five risk-factor variables within the target ranges (HbA1c, LDL-cholesterol, blood pressure, no albuminuria and no smoking) seem to have lower or no excess risk of overall death or myocardial infarction and/or stroke, as similar to the general population, as shown in a study that included 271,174 patients with T2DM registered in the Swedish National Diabetes Register [47].

### 5.1 Specific therapeutic targets

The specific targets of clinical management are presented in **Table 1**.

### 5.2 Lifestyle optimization

Lifestyle interventions addressed to optimize nutrition, increase physical activity, control body weight, stop smoking, are the cornerstone for T2DM therapy, for both glycemic and other CV risk factors [19, 50]. In terms of CV risk control, lifestyle management aims to, and it is proven to achieve [51]:

- Control of body weight and improvements of obesity-related complications,
- Improvement of glycemic control,
- Lowering of blood pressure,
- Improvement of the lipid profile
- Improvement of fitness, well-being and mental health.

Although the Look AHEAD (Action for Health in Diabetes) study did not show. that intensive lifestyle optimization reduces CV events in people with diabetes and obesity, it showed significant control of CV risk factors, with fewer medication requirements and long-term weight loss maintenance (4.7% at eight years) [52].

#### *5.2.1 Medical nutrition therapy*

Medical nutrition therapy is based on healthy eating principles. Its goals are to promote and support healthful eating patterns, with various nutrient-dense foods

| Risk factors | Therapeutic targets |
|---|---|
| HbA1c [19] | < 7% (53 mmol/mol), for most patients<br>< 6,5% (48 mmol/mol), if the target can be achieved without hypoglycemia† (usually younger patients, short duration of diabetes, longer life expectancy, no complications)<br>< 8% (64 mmol/mol), for patients with long-standing diabetes, complex glucose-lowering treatment including insulin, history of severe hypoglycemia, limited life expectancy, advanced microvascular or macrovascular, multiple complications and comorbidities |
| Fasting glycemia, postprandial glycemia, glycemic variability [19] | • Fasting/pre-meal glycemia = 80–130 mg/dl<br>• Postprandial glycemia (1–2 hours) < 180 mg/dl<br>• Reduced glycemic variability (< 36%)<br>• Avoidance of hypoglycemia:<br>> 70% time in range (70–180 mg/dL/3.9–10.0 mmol/L)<br>< 4% glucose range below 70 mg (3.9 mmol/L) |
| Blood pressure [18, 19] | < 130/80 mmHg (≥ 65 years = 130–139/70–79 mmHg) |
| Lipids [12] | • LDL-cholesterol:<br>< 100 mg/dl - moderate CV risk<br>< 70 mg/dl and > 50% reduction - high CV risk<br>< 55 mg/dl and > 50% reduction – very high CV risk<br>• Non-HDL-col <85 mg/dl in patients at very high CVR, and < 100 mg/dl in those at high CVR<br>• HDL-cholesterol >40 mg/dl in men and > 45 mg/dl in women *<br>• Triglycerides <150 mg/dl * |
| Body weight [19] | > 5–10% weight loss and<br>• long term weight loss maintenance |
| Lifestyle [19] | • Physical activity<br>• Healthy nutrition, caloric adjusted<br>• No smoking<br>• No/moderate alcohol intake |

*†Glucose range below 70 mg/dl in less then 4% of the measurements determined by continuous glucose monitoring or ambulatory glycemic profile per day [19, 49].*
**Not a goal but indicates a lower risk.*

**Table 1.**
*Therapeutic targets in T2DM (adapted by [12, 19, 48, 49]).*

in appropriate portion sizes. To ensure adherence and effectiveness, nutritional interventions should be individualized by meeting individual's needs, personal and cultural preferences, access to healthy foods, the pleasure of eating, and providing practical tools to implement the recommendations [50].

Dietary interventions can reduce HbA1c with up to 2% [50]. Caloric intake should be adapted to maintain body weight control. General recommendations are to avoid saturated lipids and foods with a high glycemic index. The Mediterranean diet, the DASH diet (Dietary Approaches to Stop Hypertension), plant-based diets, are recommended for their proven benefits. Carbohydrates should come from foods rich in fibers: vegetables, legumes, whole grains, fruits. Lipids should be mainly mono- and polyunsaturated and omega-3. Supplementation with minerals or vitamins is only recommended in case of deficiency. Hydration is important, with the selection of non-caloric drinks. Consumption of alcohol in moderate amounts is acceptable, but special attention should be paid to the risk of hypoglycemia, hyperglycemia and additional caloric intake. Sodium intake should be <2,300 mg/day [50].

#### *5.2.2 Physical activity*

Most patients' recommended physical activity is at least 150 minutes/week, at least three times/week, moderate/high intensity, aerobic, 2–3 sessions/week of endurance and flexibility exercises. Reducing the time spent in sedentary lifestyle is also an important recommendation [50].

### 5.3 Pharmacotherapy

#### *5.3.1 Pharmacotherapy of hyperglycemia*

The pharmacotherapy of hyperglycemia should be patient-centred, addressed to reduce glycemia and the overall CVR [53]. Metformin remains the first step of the treatment. It is initiated simultaneously with lifestyle optimization, from the diagnosis, and is continued throughout the treatment, associated with the other therapeutic classes. It is stopped in case of intolerance and at an eGFR <30 mL/min/1.73 $m^2$. For patients with established ASCVD or indicators of high ASCVD risk, established kidney disease, or heart failure, the guidelines recommend the medication with demonstrated CVD benefit, independent of the HbA1c value: SGLT-2 inhibitor (sodium-glucose cotransporter 2 inhibitor – empagliflozin, canagliflozin, dapagliflozin) or GLP-1RA (glucagon-like peptide 1 receptor agonist – semaglutide, liraglutide, dulaglutide, long-acting exenatide, lixisenatide) (**Table 2**) [12, 19, 53–59].

For patients without the conditions mentioned above, a second or third agent's choice as an add-on to metformin is based on CV safety, the effect on body weight, and avoidance of hypoglycemia. Sulfonylureas have controversial CV effects. To date, the ADVANCE study (Action in Diabetes and Vascular Disease: Preterax

| **GLP-1 RA/Study** | | | | |
|---|---|---|---|---|
| | **MACE** | **CV mortality** | **hHF** | **Renal effects** |
| Liraglutide (LEADER) [54] | HR = 0.87 (0.78–0.97) | HR = 0.78 (0.66–0.93) | NS | HR = 0.78 (0.67–0.92) |
| Semaglutide (SUSTAIN) [55] | HR = 0.74 (0.58–0.95) * | NS | NS | HR = 0.64 (0.46–0.88) |
| Dulaglutide (REWIND) [56] | HR = 0·88 (0·79–0·99) | NS | NS | HR = 0·85 (0·77–0·93) |
| **SGLT2-inh/Study** | | | | |
| Empagliflozin (EMPAREG-OUTCOME) [57] | HR = 0.86 (0.74–0.99) | HR = 0.62 (0.49–0.77) | HR = 0.65 (0.50–0.85) | HR = 0.61 (0.53–0.70) |
| Canagliflozin (CANVAS) [58] | HR = 0.86 (0.75–0.97) | HR = 0.78 (0.67–0.91) (CV mortality and hHF) | HR = 0.67 (0.52–0.87) | HR = 0.60 (0.47–0.77) |
| Dapagliflozin (DECLARE-TIMI 58) [59] | NS | HR = 0.83 (0.73–0.95) (CV mortality and hHF) | HR = 0.73 (0.61–0.88) | HR = 0.53 (0.43–0.66) |

**Table 2.**
*Antihyperglycemic agents with proven CVD/CKD/hHF benefits [12, 19, 53–59].*

and Diamicron MR Controlled Evaluation) is the only one that has shown that gliclazide is CV neutral and has beneficial effects in reducing kidney disease [60]. The PROactive study (PROspective pioglitAzone Clinical Trial In macroVascular Events) which included patients with T2DM treated with pioglitazone in secondary prevention, demonstrated benefits of reducing events (myocardial infarction, stroke), but also increased risk for heart failure [61]. DPP-IV-inhibitors (dipeptidyl peptidase IV), are CV safe, body weight neutral, and with low risk for hypoglycemia. Insulin therapy is initiated at HbA1c values above 10%, or in the presence of symptoms of hyperglycemia. New generations of basal insulin analogues are recommended, preferably in association with GLP-1 RA [53].

Mention: only the statistically significant results are included in the table; HR-hazard ratio; NS-non statistically significant; MACE-major adverse cardiovascular events: CV mortality, non-fatal myocardial infarction and non-fatal stroke; hHF- hospitalization for heart failure; Renal effects: new or worsening nephropathy (persistent macroalbuminuria, persistent doubling of the serum creatinine level and a creatinine clearance of less than 45 ml per minute per 1.73 m2 of body-surface area, or the need for continuous renal-replacement therapy); LEADER- Liraglutide Effect and Action in Diabetes: Evaluation of Cardiovascular Outcome Results; SUSTAIN-Efficacy and Safety of Semaglutide Once-weekly Versus Placebo in Drug-naïve Subjects With Type 2 Diabetes; EXSCEL- Exenatide Study of Cardiovascular Event Lowering Trial; EMPA-REG-OUTCOME-The Empagliflozin Cardiovascular Outcome Event Trial in Type 2 Diabetes Mellitus Patients–Removing Excess Glucose; CANVAS- Canagliflozin Cardiovascular Assessment Study; DECLARE-TIMI 58-Dapagliflozin Effect on Cardiovascular Events–Thrombolysis in Myocardial Infarction 58.

Unfortunately, the Exenatide Study of Cardiovascular Event Lowering (EXSCEL) was unable to demonstrate that once-weekly exenatide can achieve a statistically significant reduction in the incidence of major adverse cardiovascular events, compare to placebo [62].

DAPA-HF study ("Dapagliflozin and Prevention of Adverse Outcomes in Heart Failure"), which included patients with heart failure (ejection fraction <40% and NYHA class II-IV or symptoms) has demonstrated, after a median of 18.2 months of treatment with dapagliflozin vs. placebo, a significant reduction (HR = 0.74) of the primary composite outcome (worsening heart failure or death from cardiovascular causes) and the secondary outcomes (cardiovascular death or heart-failure hospitalization) (HR = 0.75) [63]. A similar design has been used in EMPEROR-Reduced trial (Empagliflozin Outcome Trial in Patients with Chronic Heart Failure and a Reduced Ejection Fraction). Compare to placebo, empagliflozin has significantly reduced the primary composite outcome of death from cardiovascular causes or hospitalization for HF (HR = 0.75) and the total number of hospitalizations for heart failure (HR = 0.70) [64].

### *5.3.2 Pharmacotherapy of hypertension*

At a systolic blood pressure ≥ 140 mmHg and/or diastolic blood pressure ≥ 90 mmHg, drug therapy is necessary in combination with non-pharmacological treatment [12, 19]. An association of antihypertensive classes is often needed, with a renin-angiotensin-aldosterone system (RAAS) blocker, and a calcium channel blocker or diuretic. A RAAS blocker is recommended particularly in the presence of microalbuminuria, albuminuria, proteinuria, or LV hypertrophy. Dual therapy is recommended as first-line treatment, with a combination of a RAAS blocker with a calcium channel blocker or thiazide/thiazide-like diuretic. It is recommended that at least one antihypertensive drug to be administered in the evening [12]. In the case of resistant hypertension, if therapeutic targets are not met with three classes of antihypertensive drugs (including a diuretic), a mineralocorticoid receptor antagonist (spironolactone) is added. Fixed combinations are preferred to increase adherence [12, 19].

#### 5.3.3 Pharmacotherapy of dyslipidemia

LDL-cholesterol is the first therapeutic target. Depending on the risk class, statins are used in moderate doses (Atorvastatin 10–20 mg, Rosuvastatin 5–10 mg, Simvastatin 20–40 mg) or high doses (Atorvastatin 40–80 mg, Rosuvastatin 20–40 mg) [12, 19, 48]. If LDL-C target is not reached, ezetimibe or PCSK9 inhibitors (evolocumab or alirocumab) are added. In the presence of atherogenic dyslipidemia (persistent triglycerides >200 mg/dl), the fenofibrate can be added to statin. The lipid arm of ACCORD study showed a further 31% reduction in CV events' relative risk in this combination. Omega-3 fatty acids can further reduce the level of triglycerides in a dose of >2 g/day. The "Reduction of Cardiovascular Events with EPA-Intervention Trial (REDUCE-IT) study", showed that 2 grams icosapent ethyl (EPA), administered twice daily, was associated with 25% relative risk reduction ($P < 0.001$) in major adverse CV events (MACE), compared to placebo [65].

#### 5.3.4 Antithrombotic/anticoagulant pharmacotherapy

If there is no contraindication, in individuals with T2DM over the age of 50, at high/very high CV risk, in the presence of the family history of premature atherosclerotic disease, hypertension, dyslipidemia, smoking, chronic kidney disease, aspirin (75–100 mg/day) may be considered in primary prevention. Aspirin (75–162 mg/day), or clopidogrel (75 mg/day) are recommended for secondary prevention. Dual antiplatelet therapy (low-dose aspirin and P2Y12 inhibitors: ticagrelor, clopidogrel, prasugrel) is recommended after an acute coronary syndrome, for a period of one year, possibly with benefits and longer use [12, 19].

Rivaroxaban 2.5 mg administered twice daily in combination with 100 mg aspirin, in T2DM patients with stable atherosclerotic vascular disease, has been shown to significantly reduce the primary outcome of CV death, stroke, myocardial infarction and major adverse limb events including amputation, but with more major bleeding events than those assigned to aspirin alone [66, 67].

#### 5.3.5 Surgical procedures

a. Bariatric surgery is associated with the most important and sustained weight loss, with significant improvements in CV risk factors, including remission of T2DM, cardiac functional parameters and coronary events. The criteria for recommending bariatric surgery in people with T2DM are [68, 69]:

   - BMI $\geq$ 40 kg/m$^2$
   - BMI = 35.0–39.9 kg/m$^2$ if long-term weight loss and improvement of comorbidities by non-surgical methods could not be achieved
   - BMI = 30.0–34.9 kg/m$^2$ in certain situations [69]

b. Myocardial revascularization strategies, either percutaneous coronary intervention (PCI) with drug-eluting stents (DES), preferably the newer-generation everolimus-eluting stents, or coronary artery bypass graft surgery (CABG), are strongly recommended in patients with T2DM. Based on the coronary anatomy complexity, PCI may represent an alternative to CABG for lower complexity, while CABG is recommended for intermediate-to-high anatomical complexity [19].

## 6. Conclusions

T2DM is a major cardiovascular risk factor. CVD is frequent, associated with high mortality.

The clinical management of T2DM must be early, multifactorial, intensive, and patient-centred. Lifestyle intervention and a combination of several classes of drugs should be addressed to all cardiovascular risk factors.

## Author details

Gabriela Roman[1*] and Anca Pantea Stoian[2]

1 Clinical Center of Diabetes, Nutrition and Metabolic Diseases, "Iuliu Hațieganu" University of Medicine and Pharmacy, Cluj-Napoca, Romania

2 Department of Diabetes, Nutrition and Metabolic Diseases, "Carol Davila" University of Medicine and Pharmacy, Bucharest, Romania

*Address all correspondence to: groman@umfcluj.ro

## References

[1] Low Wang CC, Hess CN, Hiatt WR, et al. Clinical Update: Cardiovascular Disease in Diabetes Mellitus Atherosclerotic Cardiovascular Disease and Heart Failure in Type 2 Diabetes Mellitus – Mechanisms, Management, and Clinical Considerations. Circulation. 2016;133:2459. DOI: 10.1161/CIRCULATIONAHA.116.022194

[2] Mensah GA., Wei GS., Sorlie PD, et al. Decline in Cardiovascular Mortality: Possible Causes and Implications. Circ Res. 2017, 120(2): 366-380. DOI: 10.1161/CIRCRESAHA.116.309115

[3] Harding JL, Pavkov ME, Magliano DJ, et al. Global trends in diabetes complications: a review of current evidenceDiabetologia. 2019; 62:3-16. DOI: 10.1007/s00125-018-4711-2

[4] IDF DIABETES ATLAS. Ninth edition, 2019. www. https://www.diabetesatlas.org/upload/resources/2019/IDF_Atlas_9th_Edition_2019.pdf. [Accessed: 2020-09-15]

[5] Kannel WB, McGee DL. Diabetes and cardiovascular disease. The Framingham study. JAMA. 1979;241:2035-2038. DOI: 10.1001/jama.1979.03290450033020

[6] Kannel WB, McGee DL. Diabetes and glucose intolerance as risk factors for cardiovascular disease: the Framingham study. Diabetes Care. 1979;2:120-126. DOI: 10.2337/diacare.2.2.120

[7] O'Donnella CJ, Elosua R. Cardiovascular Risk Factors. Insights From Framingham Heart Study. Rev Esp Cardiol. 2008;61(3):299-310. DOI: 10.1016/S1885-5857(08)60118-8

[8] Alberti K.G.M.M., Eckel RH, Grundy SM., et al. Harmonizing the Metabolic Syndrome. A Joint Interim Statement of the International Diabetes Federation Task Force on Epidemiology and Prevention; National Heart, Lung, and Blood Institute; American Heart Association; World Heart Federation; International Atherosclerosis Society; and International Association for the Study of Obesity. Circulation. 2009;120:1640-1645. DOI:10.1161/CIRCULATIONAHA.109.192644

[9] Ferrannini E, Cushman WC. Diabetes and hypertension: The bad companions. The Lancet, 2012;380: 601-610. DOI: 10.1016/S0140-6736(12)60987-8

[10] Xiao C, Dash S, Morgantini C et al. Pharmacological targeting of the atherogenic dyslipidemia complex: The next frontier in CVD prevention beyond lowering LDL cholesterol. Diabetes 2016;65:1767-1778. DOI: 10.2337/db16-0046

[11] Eeg-Olofsson K., Cederholm J, Nilsson PM, et al. Risk of cardiovascular disease and mortality in overweight and obese patients with type 2 diabetes: an observational study in 13,087 patients. Diabetologia, 2009, 52: 65. DOI: 10.1007/s00125-008-1190-x

[12] Cosentino F, Grant PJ, Aboyans V, et al. 2019 ESC Guidelines on diabetes, pre-diabetes, and cardiovascular diseases developed in collaboration with the EASD: The Task Force for diabetes, pre-diabetes, and cardiovascular diseases of the European Society of Cardiology (ESC) and the European Association for the Study of Diabetes (EASD). European Heart Journal, 2020 (41), 2: 255-323. DOI: 10.1093/eurheartj/ehz486

[13] Rawshani A, Sattar N, Franzen S, Rawshani A, Hattersley AT, Svensson AM, Eliasson B, Gudbjornsdottir S. Excess mortality and

cardiovascular disease in young adults with type 1 diabetes in relation to age at onset: a nationwide, register-based cohort study. Lancet 2018;392:477-486.

[14] Haffner SM, Lehto S, Rönnemaa T, et al. Mortality from Coronary Heart Disease in Subjects with Type 2 Diabetes and in Nondiabetic Subjects with and without Prior Myocardial Infarction. N Engl J Med 1998; 339:229-234. DOI: 10.1056/NEJM199807233390404

[15] Garber AJ, Abrahamson MJ, Barzilay JI, et al. Consensus Statement by the American Association of Clinical Endocrinologists and American College of Endocrinology on the comprehensive type 2 diabetes management algorithm – 2018 Executive summary. Endocrine practice, 2018, 24 (1). DOI: 10.4158/CS-2018-0535

[16] Seferović PM, Petrie MC, Filippatos GS, et al. Type 2 diabetes mellitus and heart failure: a position statement from the Heart Failure Association of the European Society of Cardiology. Eur J Heart Fail, 2018, 20: 853-872. DOI:10.1002/ejhf.1170

[17] Stevens RJ, Kothari V, Adler AI, et al on behalf of the United Kingdom Prospective Diabetes Study (UKPDS) Group. The UKPDS Risk Engine: a model for the risk of coronary heart disease in type 2 diabetes Clinical Science 2001;101:671-679. DOI:10.1042/cs1010671

[18] Kengne AP. The ADVANCE cardiovascular risk model and current strategies for cardiovascular disease risk evaluation in people with diabetes. Cardiovasc J Afr. 2013;24(9-10):376-381. DOI: 10.5830/CVJA-2013-078

[19] American Diabetes Association. Cardiovascular Disease and Risk Management: Standards of Medical Care in Diabetes, 2020. Diabetes Care 2020;43(Suppl. 1):S111–S134. DOI: 10.2337/dc20-s010

[20] Shao H, Fonseca V, Stoecker C, et al. Novel risk engine for diabetes progression and mortality in USA: Building, Relating, Assessing, and Validating Outcomes (BRAVO). Pharmacoeconomics, 2018;36:1125-1134. DOI: 10.1007/s40273-019-00807-3

[21] Einarson TR, Acs A, Ludwig C, Panton UH. Prevalence of cardiovascular disease in type 2 diabetes: a systematic literature review of scientific evidence from across the world in 2007-2017. Cardiovasc Diabetol (2018) 17:83. DOI: 10.1186/s12933-018-0728-6

[22] Shah AD, Langenberg C, Rapsomaniki E, et al. Type 2 diabetes and incidence of cardiovascular diseases:a cohort study in 1·9 million people. Lancet Diabetes Endocrinol. 2015; 3: 105-113. DOI: 10.1016/S2213-8587(14)70219-0

[23] Succurro E, Fiorentino TV, Miceli S, et al. Relative Risk of cardiovascular Disease Is Higher in Women With Type 2 Diabetes, but Not in Those With Prediabetes, as Compared With Men. Diabetes Care, 2020, dc201401; DOI: 10.2337/dc20-1401

[24] Millett ERC, Peters SAE, Woodward M. Sex differences in risk factors for myocardial infarction: cohort study of UK Biobank participants. BMJ, 2018, 363:k4247. DOI:10.1136/bmj.k4247

[25] Morrish NJ, Wang SL, Stevens LK, et al. Mortality and causes of death in the WHO Multinational Study of Vascular Disease in Diabetes. Diabetologia. 2001;44 Suppl 2:S14-S21. DOI: 10.1007/pl00002934

[26] Low Wang CC, Hess CN, Hiatt W.R., et al. Clinical Update: Cardiovascular Disease in Diabetes Mellitus Atherosclerotic Cardiovascular Disease and Heart Failure in Type 2 Diabetes Mellitus – Mechanisms, Management, and Clinical

Considerations. Circulation. 2016;133:2459. DOI: 10.1161/ CIRCULATIONAHA.116.022194

[27] Maack C., Lehrke M., Backs J., et al. Heart failure and diabetes: metabolic alterations and therapeutic interventions: a state-of-the-art review from the Translational Research Committee of the Heart Failure Association–European Society of Cardiology. European Heart Journal, 2018; 39, 4243-4254. DOI: 10.1093/ eurheartj/ehy596

[28] Kelly McHugh, DeVore A.D., Wu J. Heart Failure With Preserved Ejection Fraction and Diabetes. JACC State-of-the-Art Review. J Am Coll Cardiol. 2019;73:602-11. DOI: 10.1016/j. jacc.2018.11.033

[29] Wan EYF, Chin WY, Yu YET, et al. The Impact of Cardiovascular Disease and Chronic Kidney Disease on Life Expectancy and Direct Medical Cost in a 10-year Diabetes Cohort Study. Diabetes Care 2020 May; dc192137. DOI: 10.2337/ figshare.12194913.

[30] Chronic Kidney Disease Prognosis Consortium, Matsushita K, van der Velde M, Astor BC et al. Association of estimated glomerular filtration rate and albuminuria with all-cause and cardiovascular mortality in general population cohorts: a collaborative meta-analysis. Lancet. 2010, 12; 375(9731): 2073-2081. DOI: 10.1016/ S0140-6736(10)60674-5

[31] Kottgen A, Russell SD, Loehr LR, et al. Reduced Kidney Function as a Risk Factor for Incident Heart Failure: The Atherosclerosis Risk in Communities (ARIC) Study. JASN Apr 2007, 18 (4) 1307-1315; DOI: 10.1681/ ASN.2006101159

[32] Connell AW, Sowers JR. The CardioRenal metabolic syndrome. J Am Soc Hypertens. 2014;8(8):604-606. DOI: 10.1016/j.jash.2014.07.003

[33] Thomas MC. Type 2 Diabetes and Heart Failure: Challenges and Solutions. Current Cardiology Reviews, 2016, 12, 249-255. DOI: 10.2174/1573403X1266616060 6120254

[34] Yeung SLA, Luo S, Schooling M. The Impact of Glycated Hemoglobin (HbA1c) on Cardiovascular Disease Risk: A Mendelian Randomization Study Using UK Biobank. Diabetes Care. 2018 Sep;41(9):1991-1997. DOI: 10.2337/ dc18-0289

[35] Takao T, Matsuyama Y, Yanagisawa H, et al. Association between HbA1c variability and mortality in patients with type 2 diabetes. J Diabetes Complications, 2014;28:494-499. DOI: 10.1016/j. jdiacomp.2014.02.006

[36] Sun B., He F., Gao Y, et al. Prognostic impact of visit-to-visit glycemic variability on the risks of major adverse cardiovascular outcomes and hypoglycemia in patients with different glycemic control and type 2 diabetes. Endocrine, 2019, https://doi. org/10.1007/s12020-019-01893-1

[37] Zhou JJ, Schwenke DC, Bahn G, Reaven P. Glycemic Variation and Cardiovascular Risk in the Veteran's Affairs Diabetes Trial. Diabetes Care. 2018 Oct;41(10):2187-2194. DOI:10.2337/dc18-0548

[38] Yokota S, Tanaka H, Mochizuki Y. et al. Association of glycemic variability with left ventricular diastolic function in type 2 diabetes mellitus. JACC, 2019 (73) 9:764. DOI:10.1186/ s12933-019-0971-5

[39] Dunlay SM, Givertz MM, Aguilar D, et al. Type 2 Diabetes Mellitus and Heart Failure: A Scientific Statement From the American Heart Association and the Heart Failure Society of AmericaCirculation. 2019, 140:e294–e324. DOI:10.1161/ CIR.0000000000000691

[40] Huo L, Magliano DJ, Rancière F, et al. Impact of age at diagnosis and duration of type 2 diabetes on mortality in Australia 1997-2011. Diabetologia, 2018, 61:1055-1063. DOI: 10.1007/s00125-018-4544-z

[41] Sattar N., Rawshani A, Franzén S, et al. Age at Diagnosis of Type 2 Diabetes Mellitus and Associations With Cardiovascular and Mortality Risks. Findings From the Swedish National Diabetes Registry. Circulation. 2019; 2019 May 7;139(19):2228-2237. DOI: 10.1161/CIRCULATIONAHA.118.037885

[42] Vazquez-Benitez G, Desai JR, Xu S et al. Preventable major cardiovascular events associated with uncontrolled glucose, blood pressure, and lipids and active smoking in adults with diabetes with and without cardiovascular disease: a contemporary analysis. Diabetes Care, 2015, 38(5): 905-912. DOI: 10.2337/dc14-1877

[43] Davis SN, Duckworth W, Emanuele N, et al. Effects of Severe Hypoglycemia on Cardiovascular Outcomes and Death in the Veterans Affairs Diabetes Trial. Diabetes Care 2019;42:157-163. DOI:10.2337/dc18-1144

[44] Gæde P, Lund-Andersen H, Parving H-H, Pedersen O. Effect of a Multifactorial Intervention on Mortality in Type 2 Diabetes. N Engl J Med. 2008; 358:580-591. DOI: 10.1056/NEJMoa0706245

[45] Gæde, P, Oellgaard J, Carstensen B, et al. Years of life gained by multifactorial intervention in patients with type 2 diabetes mellitus and microalbuminuria: 21 years follow-up on the Steno-2 randomised trial. Diabetologia, 2016, 59: 2298. DOI: 10.1007/s00125-016-4065-6

[46] Fan W, Song Y, Inzucchi SE, et al. Composite cardiovascular risk factor target achievement and its predictors in US adults with diabetes: The Diabetes Collaborative Registry. Diabetes Obes Metab, 2019;21:1121-1112. DOI: 10.1111/dom.13625

[47] Rawshani A, Rawshani A, Franzén S, et al. Risk Factors, Mortality, and Cardiovascular Outcomes in Patients with Type 2 Diabetes. N Engl J Med 2018; 379:633-644. DOI: 10.1056/NEJMoa1800256

[48] Mach F, Baigent C, Catapano AL, et al. 2019 ESC/EAS Guidelines for the management of dyslipidaemias: lipid modification to reduce cardiovascular risk. European Heart Journal (2020) 41, 111188. DOI:10.1093/eurheartj/ehz455

[49] American Diabetes Association. Glycemic Targets: Standards of Medical Care in Diabetes – 2021. Diabetes Care 2021;44(Suppl. 1):S73–S84. DOI: 10.2337/dc21-S006

[50] American Diabetes Association. Facilitating Behavior Change and Well-being to Improve Health Outcomes: Standards of Medical Care in Diabetes—2020. Diabetes Care 2020 Jan; 43(Supplement 1): S48-S65. DOI: 10.2337/dc20-S005

[51] Sun Y, You W, Almeida F, Estabrooks P, Davy B. The Effectiveness and Cost of Lifestyle Interventions Including Nutrition Education for Diabetes Prevention: A Systematic Review and Meta-Analysis. J Acad Nutr Diet. 2017 Mar;117(3):404-421.e36. doi: 10.1016/j.jand.2016.11.016. PMID: 28236962; PMCID: PMC5330213.

[52] Wing RR, Bolin P, Brancati FL, et al.; Look AHEAD Research Group. Cardiovascular effects of intensive lifestyle intervention in type 2 diabetes. N Engl J Med 2013;369:145-154. DOI: 10.1056/NEJMoa1212914

[53] American Diabetes Association. Pharmacologic Approaches to Glycemic Treatment: Standards of Medical Care in Diabetes—2020. Diabetes Care Jan

2020, 43 (Supplement 1) S98-S110; DOI: 10.2337/dc20-S009

[54] Marso SP., Daniels GH., Kirstine Brown-Frandsen, et al. Liraglutide and Cardiovascular Outcomes in Type 2 Diabetes. N Engl J Med. 2016, 28;375(4):311-22. DOI: 10.1056/NEJMoa1603827

[55] Marso SP., Bain SC., Consoli A., et al. Semaglutide and Cardiovascular Outcomes in Patients with Type 2 Diabetes. N Engl J Med, 2016; 375:1834-1844. DOI: 10.1056/NEJMoa1607141

[56] Gerstein H.C., Colhoun HM., Dagenais GR., et al. Dulaglutide and cardiovascular outcomes in type 2 diabetes (REWIND): a double-blind, randomised placebo-controlled Trial. Lancet 2019; 394: 121-130. DOI: 10.1016/S0140-6736(19)31149-3

[57] Zinman B., Wanner C., Lachin JM., et al. Empagliflozin, Cardiovascular Outcomes, and Mortality in Type 2 Diabetes. N Engl J Med 2015; 373:2117-2128. DOI: 10.1056/NEJMoa1504720

[58] Neal B., Perkovic V., Mahaffey KW., et al. Canagliflozin and Cardiovascular and Renal Events in Type 2 Diabetes. N Engl J Med 2017; 377:644-657. DOI: 10.1056/NEJMoa1611925

[59] Wiviott SD., Raz I., Bonaca MP., et al. Dapagliflozin and Cardiovascular Outcomes in Type 2 Diabetes. N Engl J Med 2019; 380:347-357. DOI: 10.1056/NEJMoa1812389

[60] The ADVANCE Collaborative Group. Intensive Blood Glucose Control and Vascular Outcomes in Patients with Type 2 Diabetes. N Engl J Med 2008; 358:2560-2572. DOI: 10.1056/NEJMoa0802987

[61] Erdmann E., Dormandy J., Wilcox R., et al. PROactive 07: pioglitazone in the treatment of type 2 diabetes: results of the PROactive study. Vasc Health Risk Manag. 2007,3(4): 355-370. PMID: 17969365; PMCID: PMC2291341.

[62] Holman RR, Bethel MA, Mentz RJ, et al. Effects of Once-Weekly Exenatide on Cardiovascular Outcomes in Type 2 Diabetes. N Engl J Med. 2017, 28;377(13):1228-1239. DOI: 10.1056/NEJMoa1612917

[63] McMurray J.J.V., Solomon S.D., Inzucchi S.E. et al. Dapagliflozin in Patients with Heart Failure and Reduced Ejection Fraction. N Engl J Med 2019;381:1995-2008. DOI: 10.1056/NEJMoa1911303

[64] Packer M., Anker S.D., Butler J., et al. Cardiovascular and renal outcomes with empagliflozin in heart failure. N Engl J Med. Published online August 29, 2020.DOI: 10.1056/NEJMoa2022190

[65] Bhatt DL, Steg PG, Miller M, et al. Cardiovascular risk reduction with icosapent ethyl for hypertriglyceridemia. N Engl J Med 2019;380:11-22. DOI: doi: 10.1056/NEJMoa1812792

[66] Connolly SJ, Eikelboom JW, Bosch J, et al. Rivaroxaban with or without aspirin in patients with stable coronary artery disease: an international, randomised, double-blind, placebo-controlled trial. Lancet 2018;391: 205-218. DOI: 10.1016/S0140-6736(17)32458-3.

[67] Anand SS, Bosch J, Eikelboom JW, et al. Rivaroxaban with or without aspirin in patients with stable peripheral or carotid artery disease: an international, randomised, double-blind, placebo-controlled trial. Lancet 2018;391:219-229. DOI: 10.1016/S0140-6736(17)32409-1

[68] Fisher DP, Johnson E, Haneuse S, et al. Association Between Bariatric Surgery and Macrovascular Disease Outcomes in Patients With Type 2

Diabetes and Severe Obesity. JAMA. 2018;320(15):1570-1582. DOI: 10.1001/jama.2018.14619

[69] American Diabetes Association. Obesity Management for the Treatment of Type 2 Diabetes: Standards of Medical Care in Diabetes 2020. Diabetes Care 2020;43(Suppl. 1):S89–S97. DOI:10.2337/dc20-S008

Chapter 12

# Type 2 Diabetes Mellitus: Cardiovascular Autonomic Neuropathy and Heart Rate Variability

*Sultana Ferdousi and Phurpa Gyeltshen*

## Abstract

Type 2 Diabetes Mellitus is associated with both macro- and microvascular complications. One among the latter, is cardiovascular autonomic neuropathy (CAN). CAN is attributed to cardiac arrhythmias and sudden death. Underlying pathogenesis of cardiac autonomic neuropathy is chronic hyperglycemia induced oxidative stress causing neuronal necrosis, apoptosis and death, leading to the sympathetic and parasympathetic nerve dysfunction. The balance between sympathetic and parasympathetic nervous system is reflected by heart rate variability (HRV). HRV describes "the variations of both instantaneous heart rate and R-R intervals which in turn reflects the cardiac autonomic nervous control". HRV measured at rest is a marker of autonomic nerve function status. Thus, HRV test is recommended to diagnose diabetic CAN. Time domain parameters predominantly reflect overall autonomic activity and parasympathetic nervous system (PNS) modulations. Frequency domain parameters either reflect, sympathetic nervous system (SNS) activity, PNS activity, or the balance between the two activities. Nonlinear HRV indices marks PNS influences, SNS influences and sympatho-vagal balance. Almost all these HRV parameters are remarkably reduced in T2DM due to cardiac autonomic dysfunction. HRV is an important simple and noninvasive diagnostic tool to detect CAN.

**Keywords:** type 2 diabetes mellitus, oxidative stress, heart rate variability, cardiac autonomic neuropathy, time domain, frequency domain

## 1. Introduction

Diabetes mellitus "is a group of metabolic diseases characterized by hyperglycemia resulting from defects in insulin secretion, insulin action, or both" [1]. World Health Organization (WHO) estimated that about 422 million of global population were suffering from diabetes mellitus in 2014 [2]. This number is estimated to have reached to more than 500 million in 2018 [3]. From the total diabetes mellitus population, 90–95% belongs to T2DM categorey [4].

T2DM is associated with both acute and chronic complications: microvascular and macrovascular complications [5]. Diabetic autonomic neuropathy (DAN) is one of the microvascular complications [6]. DAN causes autonomic dysfunction of many organs and cardiovascular autonomic dysfunction due to diabetic CAN is the most life-threatening condition [7]. Thus, CAN has been found associated with cardiac arrhythmias, silent myocardial infarction and sudden deaths in T2DM patients [8]. CAN progresses through a prolonged subclinical to clinical form [7, 9]. Clinical CAN or late stage CAN occurs due to both parasympathetic and sympathetic denervation of heart and it may be manifested by resting tachycardia, orthostatic hypotension, exercise intolerance and silent myocardial ischemia. But subclinical or early stage CAN is characterized by predominant damage to the vagus nerve innervating the heart with subsequent upper hand in sympathetic drive resulting in resting cardiac autonomic balance characterized by resting tachycardia [9]. However, sub-clinical CAN ensues largely from functional alteration of autonomic nerves and is considered a reversible disorder [10].

Reduced HRV is the earliest sign of subclinical CAN [11]. HRV refers to a variation of RR intervals in time [12, 13]. HRV measured at rest is a marker of autonomic balance as well as cardiac sympathetic and parasympathetic tonic activity [13]. HRV is assessed through time domain, frequency domain and nonlinear metrics of electrocardiogram (ECG) recording [13]. HRV is reduced in type 2 diabetic patients with CAN compared to those without CAN [14].

## 2. Autonomic nervous system regulation of cardiovascular functions

Autonomic nervous system (ANS), a portion of peripheral nervous system, has two subdivisions viz. sympathetic and parasympathetic nervous system. They are responsible for regulating the functions of almost organs of the body via visceral reflexes. Centrally, ANS activities or reflexes are integrated and controlled by hypothalamus, brain stem and spinal cord. Heart and blood vessels are innervated by sympathetic and parasympathetic nerve fibers. Thus, their functions are largely regulated by ANS apart from other regulating factors to adapt to different short-term or long-term physiological/pathological changes of the internal environment of the body.

### 2.1 Regulation of cardiac functions

The main function of the heart is to pump blood into the closed circuit of circulation. The efficiency of this mechanical property of the heart depends on normal electrophysiology of the heart which per se depends on normal structural and functional integrity of sinus atrial node (SA node) and rest of the conducting system of the hear t. Autonomic nervous system plays crucial role in controlling both electrical and mechanical properties of the heart. However, the degree of influence of sympathetic and parasympathetic nerves on heart functions depends on their abundance of innervation in different parts of the heart.

Sympathetic nervous system via right and left cardiac nerves innervate atria and ventricles (including conducting system). Right cardiac nerve predominantly innervates SA node and it has more influence on heart rate (HR) and on the other hand left cardiac nerve predominantly controls myocardial contractility. Thus, the net effect of sympathetic stimulation is to increase HR, conduction velocity and strength of myocardial contractility. Parasympathetic nervous system through right and left vagus nerves innervate predominantly atrial muscle and very sparsely ventricular myocardium. Right vagus nerve primarily innervates the SA node and left vagus nerve innervates mainly atrio-ventricular node (AV node). Thus, the net effect of parasympathetic stimulation is to decrease HR and slightly decrease strength of heart contractility. Dynamic interaction occurs between sympathetic and parasympathetic divisions. However, during rest, parasympathetic tone predominates over sympathetic tone. Therefore, resting HR is mainly controlled by the vagal nerve tone [15]. Hence, resting HR is a marker of vagal nerve function status [15].

### 2.2 Regulation of vascular functions

Arteries and veins are innervated only by sympathetic nerve fibers, whereas, capillaries do not have any autonomic nerve innervation. Thus, vasomotor tone of almost all blood vessels is mainly determined by sympathetic tone. Sympathetic stimulation causes vasoconstriction and vice versa. Parasympathetic nerve fibers do innervate some blood vessels of salivary glands, gastrointestinal glands and genital erectile tissues.

## 3. Diabetic autonomic neuropathy

DAN is quite common, yet remained mostly undiagnosed and micro-vascular complications of T2DM are affecting many organ systems (gastrointestinal, genitourinary, cardiovascular) of the body [7]. However, CAN is clinically the most important form of DAN as it is associated with life-threatening complications (arrhythmias, silent MI) and sudden death [9]. The underlying pathophysiology of DAN is still unclear; however, it has been attributed to chronic hyperglycemia induced oxidative stress and inflammation with subsequent neuronal injury and death [9, 16–19].

### 3.1 Hyperglycemia induced oxidative stress and inflammation

Oxidative stress and inflammation are interlinked, as one causes another and vice versa, and they occur even under normal physiological conditions. However, these two phenomena last for a brief period as they are suppressed by intrinsic negative feedback mechanisms; increased production of antioxidants and anti-inflammatory cytokines [19]. But, in certain chronic diseases like T2DM these altered states of internal environment sustain for a prolonged period as positive feedback mechanisms overrides the negative feedback mechanisms [19]. In addition, reduced parasympathetic nerve function due to autonomic dysfunction in T2DM leads to chains of inflammatory responses [20]. Thus, oxidative stress and inflammation are very prominent features in T2DM linked to both microvascular and macrovascular complications associated with T2DM [19]. Certain cells are particularly susceptible to hyperglycemic induced injury as their intracellular glucose concentration increases in a linear fashion with respect to the extracellular glucose level [16]. This is especially true for endothelial cells and neurons as the transport of glucose through their cell membranes is mediated by insulin-independent GLUTs [16].

Hyperglycemia induces overproduction of mitochondrial superoxide in endothelial cells of large and small blood vessels and neuronal axons [9, 16]. This leads to intracellular accumulation of reactive oxygen species (ROS) with subsequent activation of five major metabolic pathways: polyol pathway flux, increased formation of advanced glycation end-products (AGEs), increased expression of the receptor for AGEs and its activating ligands, activation of protein kinase C (PKC) isoforms, and overactivity of the hexosamine pathway [9, 16]. Over activity of these five metabolic pathways leads to accumulation of toxic metabolic derivatives and pro-inflammatory substances, bringing about following consequences: vascular endothelial damage, vasoconstriction, neuronal hypoxia, neuronal cell necrosis, neuronal apoptosis and axonal degeneration (**Figure 1**) [9, 16, 19, 21, 22].

### 3.2 Cardiovascular autonomic neuropathy

CAN defined as the "impairment of autonomic control of the cardiovascular system in the setting of diabetes after exclusion of other causes" [23]. The prevalence of CAN varies from 31–73% in T2DM patients [17]. The T2DM patients with a higher age, longer duration of diabetes, poor and perhaps unstable glycaemic control, comorbid diabetic polyneuropathy, retinopathy and nephropathy, hypertension (on treatment), and other cardiovascular risk factors (in particular obesity and metabolic dyslipidaemia) are high risk of developing CAN [24].

CAN results from impairment of autonomic regulation on heart and blood vessels with consequent alteration of cardiovascular hemodynamic functions [20]. Underlying pathogenesis of CAN first damages longest autonomic nerve. Thus, CAN initially (subclinical CAN) begins with reduced parasympathetic control, as vagus is the longest autonomic nerve, with the consequent sympathovagal imbalance. Hence, reduced HRV is the earliest marker of CAN [20]. Subclinical CAN be even seen in prediabetes [24]. As subclinical CAN progresses

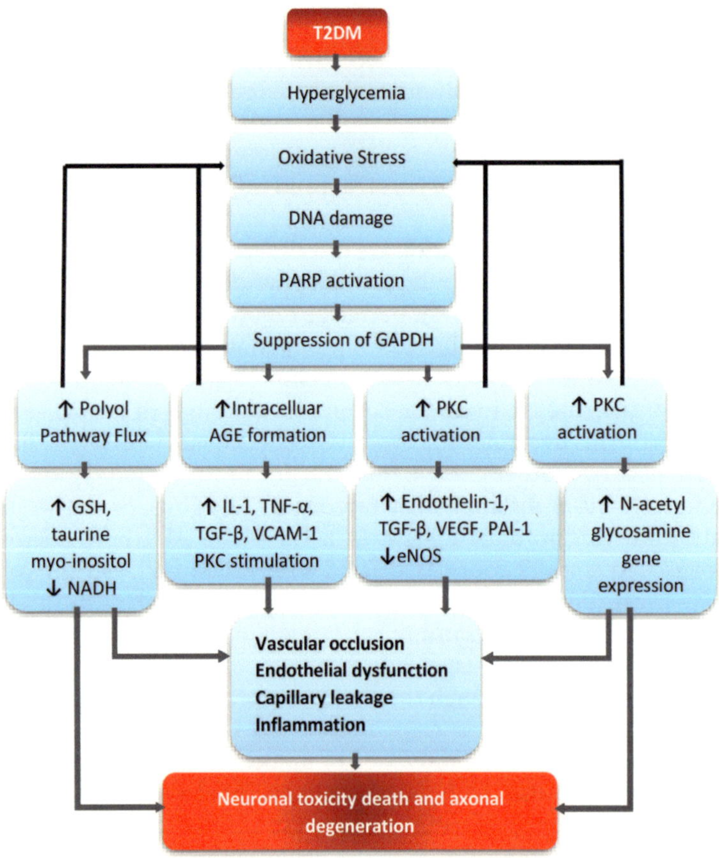


**Figure 1.**
*Summary of the mechanisms that relate hyperglycemia to microvascular complications in patients with diabetes [9, 15, 18, 20, 21]. PKC: Protein kinase C; AGE: Advanced glycation end-products; GAPDH: Glyceraldehyde-3 phosphate dehydrogenase; GSH: Glutathione; NADH: Nicotinamide adenine dinucleotide; TGF-β: Transforming growth factor; VEGF: Vascular endothelial growth factor; PAI-1: Plasminogen activator inhibitor-1; eNOS: Endothelial nitric oxide.*

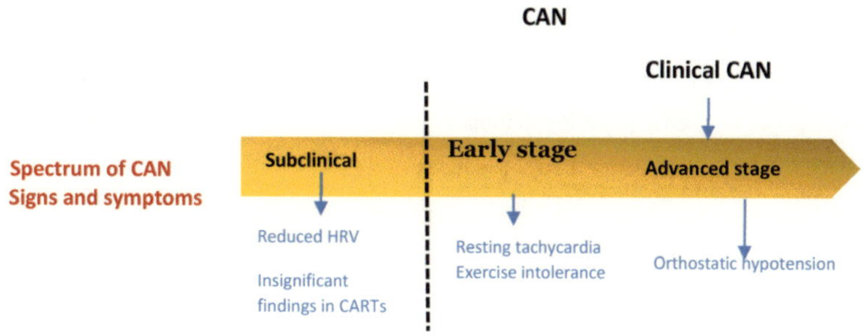


**Figure 2.**
*Progression of CAN with signs and symptoms [9, 22].*

into clinical CAN, sympathetic tone augments during early stage and followed by sympathetic denervation in later stage (**Figure 2**). This denervation begins at the apex of the heart and advances towards the base of the heart. This disproportionate sympathetic denervation of ventricles predisposes to the development of cardiac arrhythmias. CAN is also associated with silent myocardial infarction (MI) and sudden death. CAN is highly associated with cardiovascular morbidity and mortality and thus, it is crucial to be diagnosed at its early stage to prevent these complications [25].

Clinical CAN is usually diagnosed and its severity is assessed by autonomic score obtained through five standard cardiovascular autonomic reflex tests (CARTs): (1) the HR response to deep breathing (2) the HR response to standing (3) the Valsalva maneuver (4) the blood pressure response to standing and (5) the blood pressure response to sustained handgrip [26]. Whereas, subclinical CAN is diagnosed based on changes in HRV, baroreflex sensitivity, and cardiac imaging showing increased torsion of the left ventricle [26]. Sensitivity of standards CARTs to detect subclinical CAN is very limited as no significant changes are seen on standard CARTs [26]. Detecting CAN at subclinical stage is of paramount importance to provide early intervention on modifiable risk factors of CAN to prevent progression CAN to its severe or advanced form [24, 26].

## 4. Heart rate variability

Heart rate is controlled by changes in sympathetic and parasympathetic influences, neurohumoral factors (epinephrine and thyroid hormones), ionic concentrations (calcium and potassium) and local temperature of SA node [27]. But, the HRV measured over short period of time (5 minutes) at rest is largely determined by changes of autonomic nervous system control (predominantly by the vagal tone) and the stretch of SA node [22]. On the contrary, long-term measurement of HRV obtained through 24-hour Holter ECG can be influenced by concomitant illness, use of medications, and lifestyle factors (exercise, stress, smoking, etc.) in addition to afore mentioned factors [22]. HRV is also varies due to other physiological factors (**Table 1**). Short-term HRV (5 minutes) measurement is a reliable technique to detect autonomic dysfunction [9]. HRV describes the variations of both instantaneous heart rate and RR intervals which in turn reflect the cardiac autonomic nervous control (**Figure 3**) [13]. HRV measurement obtained from 5 min-ECG recording represents marker for the measurement of resting autonomic tonic activity; the balance between sympathetic & parasympathetic nervous activity at any instant. Thus, alteration of HRV can detect the impairment of resting sympathetic and parasympathetic activity individually and shift of the normal sympathovagal

| Physiological factors influencing on HRV | | |
|---|---|---|
| • Age | • Circadian rhythm | • Body position |
| • Gender | • Respiration | • Physical fitness |
| • Food ingestion | • Body mass index | |

**Table 1.**
*Physiological factors to be considered while measuring HRV.*

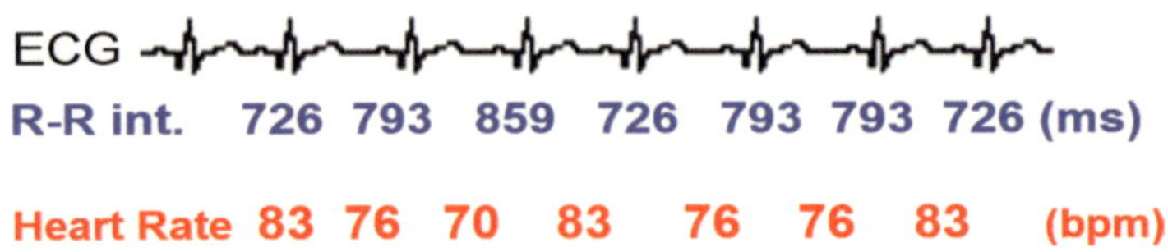


**Figure 3.**
*Heart rate variability (HRV). Ms: Milliseconds, bpm: Beats per minute, R-R int.: R-R interval.*

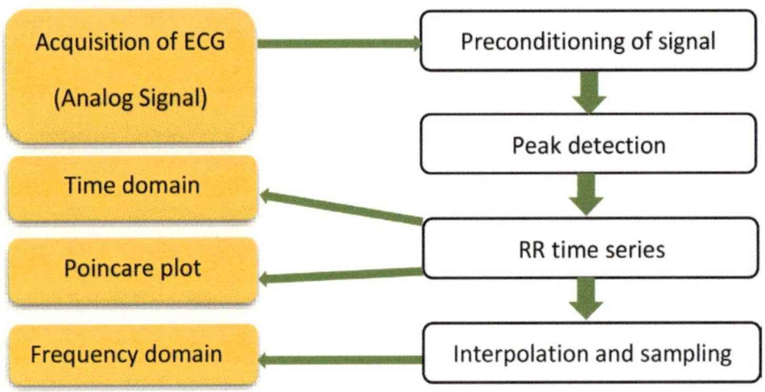


**Figure 4.**
*Quantification of HRV into time domain and frequency parameters along with Poincare plot.*

balance. HRV is quantified or measured by three methods; time domain, frequency domain and nonlinear analysis of short-term (5 mins) and long-term ECG (24 hrs.) recording (**Figure 4**). HRV test is an accurate quantitative and reproducible measurement of autonomic nerve function [13].

### 4.1 Time and frequency domain, and non-linear analysis of HRV

The time domain method measures the heart rate at any point either in time or in the intervals between successive QRS complex of a continuous ECG record. The interval between adjacent QRS complexes is known as normal-to normal (NN) interval. HRV time-domain indices quantify the amount of HRV observed during monitoring periods that may range from <1 min to >24 h. Time domain variables include the SDNN, SDANN, SDNNI, RMSSD, NN50, pNN50, HR Max – HR Min (**Table 2**) [28] (**Figure 5**).

Frequency domains variables (**Table 3**) are derived through many methods. Fast Fourier Transformation (FFT) is one the commonest methods to derive frequency components of HRV. Power spectrum derived through FFT is subsequently categorized into different bands of frequencies: VLF- (0.0033 to 0.04) Hz, LF- (0.04 to 0.15) Hz and HF- (0.15 to 0.4) Hz. Power spectral densities (PSD) are then plotted

| Variable | Unit | Description | Physiological correlates |
|---|---|---|---|
| SDNN* | Ms | Standard deviation of NN intervals | Reflects PNS function |
| SDANN | ms | Standard deviation of the average NN intervals for each 5 min segment of a 24 h HRV recording | " |
| SDNN index | Ms | Mean of the standard deviations of all the NN intervals for each 5 min segment of a 24 h HRV recording | " |
| NN50 | Ms | Number of R-R interval differences ≥50 ms | " |
| pNN50 | % | Percentage of successive RR intervals that differ by more than 50 ms | " |
| RMSSD | Ms | The Root square of the mean of the sum of the squares of differences between adjacent RR intervals. | " |
| Max HR-Min HR | Bpm | The average difference between the highest and lowest HRs during each respiratory cycle | Mediated by RSA |

**It is more accurate when measured from 24 h-ECG recording than that measured from shorter period.*
*"Reflects PNS function. RSA: respiratory sinus arrhythmia. Bpm: beats per minute. PNS: parasympathetic nervous system.*

**Table 2.**
*Time domain variables of HRV with physiological significance.*

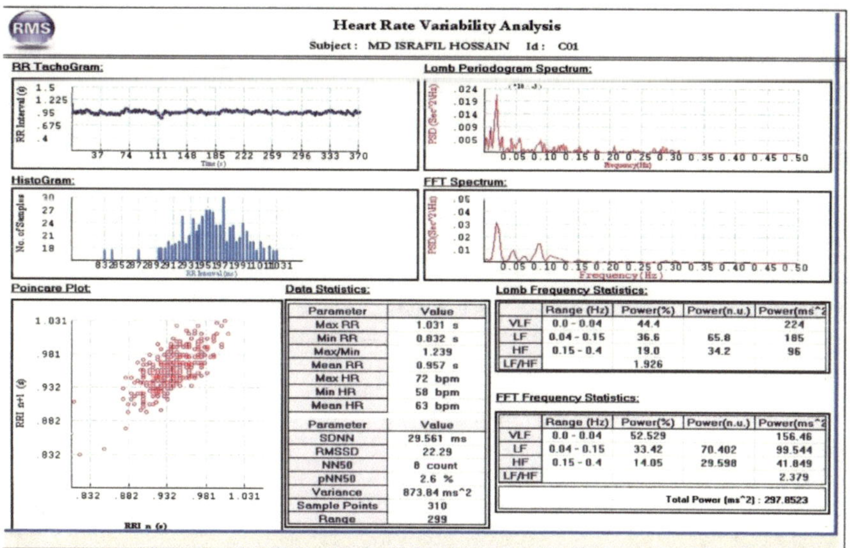


**Figure 5.**
*Time domain, frequency domain measurements and Poincare plot of HRV obtained through RMS Polyrite.*

in $ms^2$/Hz against preset frequencies. Power of the spectral bands are calculated in $ms^2$ (absolute power) and in normalized units (n.u). For example, normalize unit of LF is calculated by the formula: [LF/total power-VLF] × 100. Power of LF and HF are established in short term analysis of HRV. Nonlinear method of HRV analysis (**Table 4**) through Poincare plot is done by plotting every RR interval against the prior interval consequently forming a scatter plot.

| Variable | Unit | Description | Physiological correlates |
|---|---|---|---|
| *VLF power | $ms^2$ | Absolute power of the very-low-frequency band (0.0033–0.04 Hz) | Mediated renin-angiotensin system |
| LF peak | Hz | Peak frequency of the low-frequency band (0.04–0.15 Hz) | PNS and SNS influences |
| LF power | $ms^2$ | Absolute power of the low-frequency band (0.04–0.15 Hz) | " |
| LF power | Nu | Relative power of the low-frequency band (0.04–0.15 Hz) in normal units | " |
| HF peak | Hz | Peak frequency of the high-frequency band (0.15–0.4 Hz) | PNS influences |
| HF power | $ms^2$ | Absolute power of the high-frequency band (0.15–0.4 Hz) | # |
| HF power | Nu | Relative power of the high-frequency band (0.15–0.4 Hz) in normal units | # |
| LF/HF | % | Ratio of LF to HF power | Sympatho-vagal balance |

**It is not well defined in short-term recording.*
*"PNS AND SNS influences.*
*#PNS influences.*

**Table 3.**
*Frequency domain variables of HRV with physiological significance.*

| Variable | Unit | Description | Physiological correlates |
|---|---|---|---|
| SD1 | Ms | Poincaré plot standard deviation perpendicular the line of identity | PNS influences |
| SD2 | Ms | Poincaré plot standard deviation along the line of identity | SNS influences |
| SD1/SD2 | % | Ratio of SD1- to – SD2 power | Sympatho-vagal balance |

**Table 4.**
*Non-linear variables of HRV and physiological significance.*

## 4.2 HRV in type 2 diabetes mellitus

Reduced HRV is the earliest of sign CAN, reflecting impaired sympathetic and parasympathetic activity without apparent clinical signs and symptoms of CAN [29]. T2DM causes decrease in almost all HRV variables. In a systematic review and meta-analysis performed on 25 studies analyzing HRV in T2DM showed overall decrease in the HRV in patients with T2DM owing to reduction both sympathetic and parasympathetic nerve function [30]. In another systematic review done on eight studies showed SD1/SD2, SDANN, and HF to have more sensitivity and specificity to detect autonomic dysfunction in diabetic patients indicating their potentials to be better diagnostic markers [31].

Abnormal nonlinear HRV variables are associated with diabetes or with the risk of development of T2DM [32]. Likewise, a review study revealed reduction in HRV variables, obtained through short-term and 24-hour ECG recording, in metabolic syndrome and T2DM [29].

There are no standard reference values for HRV variables to diagnose CAN [22]. However, Breder and Sposito proposes the diagnosis of CAN could be made on obtaining abnormal result in at least two of the following six parameters:

SDNN <50 ms, RMSSD <15 ms, PNN50 < 0.75%, LF < 300 $ms^2$, HF < 300 $ms^2$ derived from 24-hour Holter ECG recording [33].

## 5. Conclusion

HRV displays beat-to-beat variations caused predominantly by the interplay of PNS and SNS control on SA node. Decline in HRV is seen even before manifesting signs and symptoms of diabetic CAN. Reduced HRV is the earliest sign of CAN. CAN is one of the under diagnosed microvascular complications of T2DM caused by hyperglycemia induced neuronal damage. Almost all HRV variables are decreased in T2DM.

## Conflict of interest

The authors declare no conflict of interest.

## Author details

Sultana Ferdousi[1]* and Phurpa Gyeltshen[2]

1 Department of Physiology, Bangbandhu Sheikh Mujib Medical University, Shahbag, Dhaka, Bangladesh

2 Khesar Gyalpo University of Medical Sciences of Bhutan, Thimphu, Bhutan

*Address all correspondence to: sferdousiratna@bsmmu.edu.bd

## References

[1] Mellitus D. Diagnosis and classification of diabetes mellitus. Diabetes care. 2005 Jan 1;28(S37):S5-10.

[2] World Health Organization, 2016. Global report on diabetes.

[3] Kaiser AB, Zhang N, Van Der Pluijm W. Global prevalence of type 2 diabetes over the next ten years (2018-2028).

[4] World Health Organization, 2019. Classification of diabetes mellitus.

[5] Pinhas-Hamiel O, Zeitler P. Acute and chronic complications of type 2 diabetes mellitus in children and adolescents. The Lancet. 2007 May 26;369(9575):1823-31.

[6] Chawla A, Chawla R, Jaggi S. Microvasular and macrovascular complications in diabetes mellitus: distinct or continuum?. Indian journal of endocrinology and metabolism. 2016 Jul;20(4):546.

[7] Vinik AI, Maser RE, Mitchell BD, Freeman R. Diabetic autonomic neuropathy. Diabetes care. 2003 May 1;26(5):1553-79.

[8] Vinik AI, Ziegler D. Diabetic cardiovascular autonomic neuropathy. Circulation. 2007 Jan 23;115(3):387-97.

[9] Dimitropoulos G, Tahrani AA, Stevens MJ. Cardiac autonomic neuropathy in patients with diabetes mellitus. World journal of diabetes. 2014 Feb 15;5(1):17.

[10] Clemente de Souza Pereira Rolim L, de Sá JR, Chacra AR, Dib SA. Diabetic cardiovascular autonomic neuropathy: Risk factors, clinical impact and early diagnosis. Arq Bras Cardiol 2008;90(4): 23-31.

[11] Trivedi GY, Saboo B, Singh RB, Maheshwari A, Sharma K, Verma N. Can decreased heart rate variability be a marker of autonomic dysfunction, metabolic syndrome and diabetes?. Journal of Diabetology. 2019 May 1;10(2):48.

[12] Buccelletti E, Gilardi EM, Scaini E, Galiuto LE, Persiani RO, Biondi AL, Basile FL, Silveri NG. Heart rate variability and myocardial infarction: systematic literature review and metanalysis. Eur Rev Med Pharmacol Sci. 2009 Jul 1;13(4):299-307.

[13] Malik M. Heart rate variability: Standards of measurement, physiological interpretation, and clinical use: Task force of the European Society of Cardiology and the North American Society for Pacing and Electrophysiology. Annals of Noninvasive Electrocardiology. 1996 Apr;1(2):151-81.

[14] Cha SA, Park YM, Yun JS, Lee SH, Ahn YB, Kim SR, Ko SH. Time-and frequency-domain measures of heart rate variability predict cardiovascular outcome in patients with type 2 diabetes. Diabetes research and clinical practice. 2018 Sep 1;143:159-69.

[15] Olshansky B, Sabbah HN, Hauptman PJ, Colucci WS. Parasympathetic nervous system and heart failure: pathophysiology and potential implications for therapy. Circulation. 2008 Aug 19;118(8):863-71.

[16] Giacco F, Brownlee M. Oxidative stress and diabetic complications. Circulation research. 2010 Oct 29;107(9):1058-70.

[17] Fisher VL, Tahrani AA. Cardiac autonomic neuropathy in patients with diabetes mellitus: current perspectives. Diabetes, metabolic syndrome

and obesity: targets and therapy. 2017;10:419.

[18] Chaudhuri A, Umpierrez GE. Oxidative stress and inflammation in hyperglycemic crises and resolution with insulin: implications for the acute and chronic complications of hyperglycemia. Journal of Diabetes and its Complications. 2012 Jul;26(4):257.

[19] Oguntibeju OO. Type 2 diabetes mellitus, oxidative stress and inflammation: examining the links. International journal of physiology, pathophysiology and pharmacology. 2019;11(3):45.

[20] Vinik AI, Erbas T, Casellini CM. Diabetic cardiac autonomic neuropathy, inflammation and cardiovascular disease. Journal of diabetes investigation. 2013 Jan;4(1):4-18.

[21] Bandeira DM, Da Fonseca LJ, Guedes DS, Rabelo LA, Goulart MO, Vasconcelos SM. Oxidative stress as an underlying contributor in the development of chronic complications in diabetes mellitus. International journal of molecular sciences. 2013 Feb;14(2):3265-84.

[22] Serhiyenko VA, Serhiyenko AA. Cardiac autonomic neuropathy: risk factors, diagnosis and treatment. World journal of diabetes. 2018 Jan 15;9(1):1.

[23] Spallone V, Ziegler D, Freeman R, Bernardi L, Frontoni S, Pop-Busui R, Stevens M, Kempler P, Hilsted J, Tesfaye S, Low P. Cardiovascular autonomic neuropathy in diabetes: clinical impact, assessment, diagnosis, and management. Diabetes/ metabolism research and reviews. 2011 Oct;27(7):639-53.

[24] Spallone V. Update on the impact, diagnosis and management of cardiovascular autonomic neuropathy in diabetes: what is defined, what is new, and what is unmet. Diabetes & metabolism journal. 2019 Feb 1;43(1):3-0.

[25] Williams SM, Eleftheriadou A, Alam U, Cuthbertson DJ, Wilding JP. Cardiacautonomicneuropathyinobesity, the metabolic syndrome and prediabetes: a narrative review. Diabetes Therapy. 2019 Dec 1:1-27.

[26] Agashe S, Petak S. Cardiac autonomic neuropathy in diabetes mellitus. Methodist DeBakey cardiovascular journal. 2018 Oct;14(4):251.

[27] Guyton A, Hall J. Textbook of Medical Physiology. 13th ed.New Delhi: ELSEVIER;2011.p.121

[28] Shaffer F, Ginsberg JP. An overview of heart rate variability metrics and norms. Frontiers in public health. 2017 Sep 28;5:258.

[29] Trivedi GY, Saboo B, Singh RB, Maheshwari A, Sharma K, Verma N. Can decreased heart rate variability be a marker of autonomic dysfunction, metabolic syndrome and diabetes?. Journal of Diabetology. 2019 May 1;10(2):48.

[30] Benichou T, Pereira B, Mermillod M, Tauveron I, Pfabigan D, Maqdasy S, Dutheil F. Heart rate variability in type 2 diabetes mellitus: A systematic review and meta–analysis. PloS one. 2018 Apr 2;13(4):e0195166.

[31] Franca da Silva AK, Penachini da Costa de Rezende Barbosa M, Marques Vanderlei F, DestroChristofaro DG, Marques Vanderlei LC. Application of heart rate variability in diagnosis and prognosis of individuals with diabetes mellitus: systematic review. Annals of Noninvasive Electrocardiology. 2016 May;21(3):223-35.

[32] Vinik AI, Casellini C, Parson HK, Colberg SR, Nevoret ML. Cardiac autonomic neuropathy in diabetes:

a predictor of cardiometabolic events. Frontiers in neuroscience. 2018 Aug 27;12:591.

[33] Breder IS, Sposito AC. Cardiovascular autonomic neuropathy in type 2 diabetic patients. Revista da AssociaçãoMédicaBrasileira. 2019 Jan;65(1):56-60.

Section 4

# Lifestyle and Diabetes - Nutritional Intervention

Chapter 13

# The Role of Lifestyle Medicine in the Management of Diabetes Mellitus

*Dabota Yvonne Buowari*


## Abstract

Lifestyle medicine is a medical specialty that involves the use of lifestyle in the prevention and management of non-communicable diseases like diabetes mellitus and cardiovascular diseases. Recent studies have shown that diabetes mellitus can be prevented following lifestyle modifications. Lifestyle medicine is a branch of medicine that promotes lifestyle modifications as a way of life. This includes promoting healthy eating which includes a whole plant-based diet, low fat, low sugar and low salt. It also includes exercises, sleeping healthy and reducing stress. This is involved in the management of diabetes mellitus. Diabetic management is expensive especially in low and middle-income countries where health insurance is not available for the entire populace and diabetics have to pay out of pocket for their medications.


**Keywords:** lifestyle medicine, diabetes mellitus, exercise, physical activity, whole plant based diet

## 1. Introduction

Globally, there is an increase in the prevalence of non-communicable diseases such as Type 2 Diabetes Mellitus, cancer, hypertension, other cardiovascular diseases and stroke. Most of these illnesses are related to a modification in the lifestyle worldwide costs of healthcare leading to morbidity and mortality are diseases linked to environmental factors and lifestyle modification [1]. There has been a steady increase worldwide in the prevalence of non-communicable diseases to an alarming rate including diabetes mellitus which is becoming an epidemic [2–4] as this increase has been on for the past 20 years [5–7]. According to the International Diabetes Federation (IDF), it is estimated that 387 million adults are diabetic with either type 1 or type 2 diabetes mellitus [3] and this number is predicted to rise to 392 million by 2035 [3, 8]. This predicted increase is due to globalization and urbanization [2]. Urbanization is affected by modifications in lifestyle with physical inactivity and sedentary lifestyle from various epidemiological and interventional studies have revealed that the majority of chronic illnesses such as diseases that affect the cardiovascular system such as hypertension, cancer and Type 2 Diabetes Mellitus result due to lifestyle behavior and habits that are caused by improper eating habits, eating unhealthy foods, and lack of physical activity [9–11]. In primary and specialist health facilities, the majority of the consultations are related to highly preventable lifestyle.



IntechOpen

Lifestyle modification is the first line of treatment in the management of non-communicable diseases [12, 13]. The commonest form of diabetes mellitus affecting 90% of diabetics is Type 2 Diabetes Mellitus. Diabetes mellitus is an economic and health burden to the sufferer and health systems as it also affects the quality of life especially when complications occur [2, 4, 8, 9, 14].

Diabetes mellitus is a risk factor for cardiovascular disease, a common cause of blindness due to diabetic retinopathy, amputation of the lower limb following diabetic neuropathy and diabetic foot ulcer and other life-threatening complications such as end-stage kidney disease (ESKD) [9, 15, 16]. Globally, diabetes mellitus is the second leading cause of blindness and renal disease [17]. Therefore it is important to prevent diabetes mellitus as it causes loss of working hours due to the impact they have on the economy and the individual. This is worst in the low and middle-income countries with the poor healthcare system and lack of health insurance for the entire populace where people have to pay out of pocket when seeking healthcare.

Diabetes mellitus is a chronic non-communicable metabolic disease in which the plasma glucose is elevated [12], characterized by insulin resistance and deficiency in insulin secretion and it may be acquired or hereditary [17, 18]. Obesity and overweight are risk factors for diabetes mellitus [17]. This is because insulin resistance and metabolic syndrome are promoted by obesity and overweight [8, 17]. For the primary prevention of diabetes mellitus, a 5-10 kg weight loss is recommended [6, 8].

Sensitivity to insulin and glycaemic control is improved by engaging in moderate weight loss and increased physical activity [6]. Obesity is a risk factor for diabetes mellitus [6]. Ignoring lifestyle medicine leads to an increased workload on the healthcare system. Globalization and adaptation of the Western lifestyle are some of the reasons for the increasing numbers of chronic diseases including Type 2 Diabetes Mellitus. Making good choices in lifestyle can significantly help in lowering the risk of these chronic diseases as most of the risk factors for these diseases are related to lifestyle behavior [2].

The history of lifestyle is very important in history taking [7]. The component of lifestyle medicine which promotes weight loss and prevents obesity is essential in the management and prevention of diabetes mellitus [8, 19, 20]. Therefore diabetes mellitus can be prevented by maintaining an ideal weight, therefore, modification in lifestyle does not only prevent diabetes mellitus but also prevents other non-communicable diseases [3, 8, 21].

## 2. Research methodology

This is review article on the role of lifestyle medicine in the management of Type 2 Diabetes Mellitus. A search was done using Google scholar, and PubMed using the key words lifestyle medicine and diabetes, the role of the pillars of lifestyle and management of Type 2 Diabetes Mellitus. Articles that highlighted the management of Type 2 Diabetes Mellitus using hypoglycaemic agents were excluded in this study.

## 3. What is lifestyle medicine

Lifestyle medicine is a relatively new medical specialty yet to be established in most countries. Lifestyle medicine has been defined by various scholars. Lifestyle medicine is the use of interventions and integration of lifestyle practices within conventional medicine to lower the risk of disease. It serves as an adjunct to the management of illnesses [22, 23]. The practice of lifestyle medicine is evidence-based in scientific research and it addresses the root and underlying causes of diseases by empowering individuals with life skills and knowledge through a behavioral change in making healthy choices [24]. In this new medical discipline, it uses daily habits and practice impacts on both the prevention and treatment of diseases to improve the overall health of the individual in conjunction with both pharmaceutical and surgical therapy [3, 25]. All pharmaceutical agents have side effects as most drugs are metabolized in the liver and excreted by the kidneys. Hence it is very important to prevent them like diabetes mellitus. The Canadian Academy of Lifestyle Medicine defines lifestyle medicine as an evidence-based branch of medicine in which there is a comprehensive change in lifestyle including nutrition, physical activity, stress management, social connectedness and exposure to harmful environmental factors [26]. Lifestyle medicine is used to prevent and treat lifestyle-related diseases but it does not tell patients to abandon and stop their medications.

Lifestyle-related diseases (LRD) are illnesses in which lifestyle factors significantly influence the pathophysiology of the disease as there can be a significant improvement in the prevention and treatment of the disease following a change in the aetiological factors. Travel medicine and sports medicine, lifestyle medicine is a novel branch in the clinical practice of medicine [8] but it is gaining grounds due to its benefits. The prevention and reversal of chronic diseases linked to lifestyle can be done using evidence-based lifestyle therapeutic approaches. Lifestyle interventions affect physical and mental health positively, including a better quality of life [13]. The focus of lifestyle medicine programmes in the management of diabetes mellitus is to change the eating habits and physical activity behavior, especially in obese patients with type 2 diabetes mellitus is very important to control symptoms and it reduces the risk of cardiovascular-related morbidity and diabetic complications [27].

## 4. The pillars of lifestyle medicine

The components of lifestyle medicine are interventions that when they are practised lead to improvement in health and overall wellbeing. The modalities of lifestyle medicine are (**Figure 1**) [3, 13, 28]:

1. Increased physical activity and exercise.

2. Stress management.

3. Healthy eating by promoting consumption of whole plant-based diet.

4. Adequate sleep and good sleep hygiene.

5. Avoid consumption of tobacco and alcohol.

6. Increased mental and emotional wellbeing by having good social connectedness.

## 5. The role of lifestyle medicine in the management of diabetes mellitus

All the components of lifestyle medicine are important and play necessary roles in the prevention of Type 2 Diabetes Mellitus and management of Type 1 & 2 Diabetes Mellitus. This is because Type 1 Diabetes Mellitus has a strong

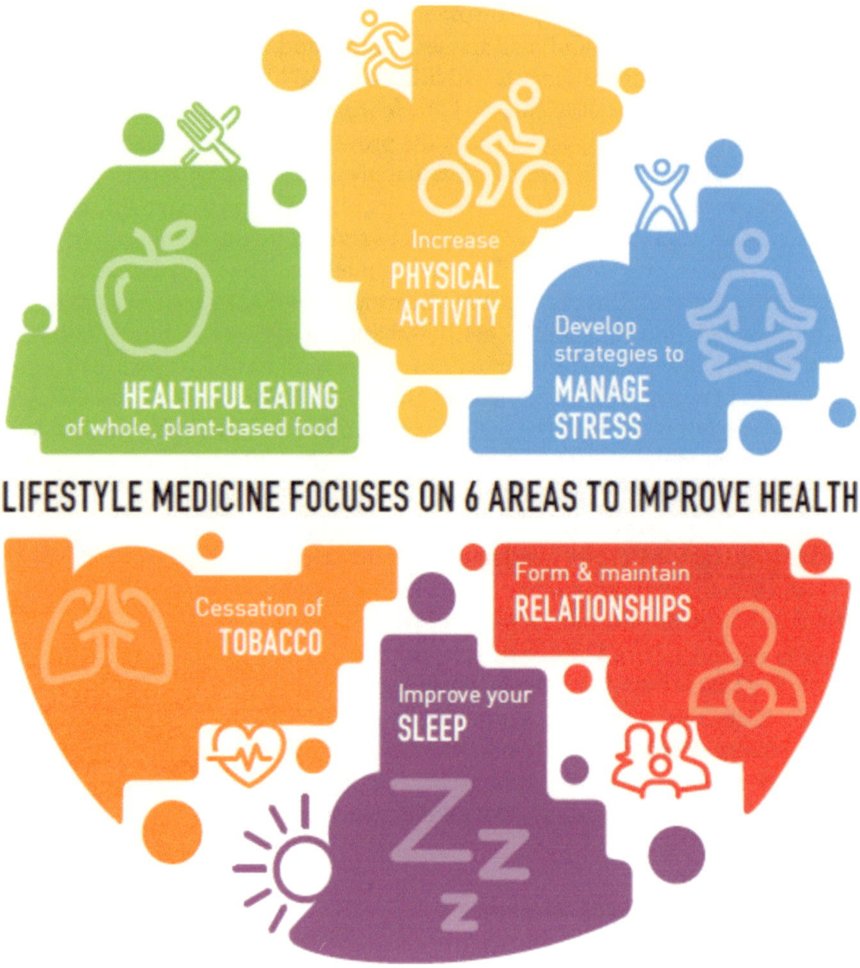
Increase
PHYSICAL
ACTIVITY
HEALTHFUL EATING
of whole, plant-based food
Develop
strategies to
MANAGE
STRESS
LIFESTYLE MEDICINE FOCUSES ON 6 AREAS TO IMPROVE HEALTH
Cessation of
TOBACCO
Form & maintain
RELATIONSHIPS
Improve your
SLEEP

**Figure 1.**
*Courtesy American College of Lifestyle Medicine.*

relationship with genetics but lifestyle modification guides its management in the long-term to prevent diabetic complications such as diabetic neuropathy, retinopathy including diabetic foot ulcer. This is very important as it affects the overall wellbeing of the individual especially in developing countries where amputees are shamed and have general poor wellbeing and economic power. Type 2 Diabetes Mellitus can be prevented through modification in lifestyle by healthy living on a whole plant-based diet, prevention of obesity by weight control, having good sleep hygiene and avoiding unnecessary stress as much as possible [8, 12, 19]. This is because the risk factors of diabetes mellitus are related to modifiable lifestyle such as obesity [14]. The practice of lifestyle medicine is cost-effective in the management and prevention of diabetes mellitus because no special equipment is really necessary as what is involved is to be disciplined which has to be enforced by individuals on themselves [14]. Good healthy eating of a whole plant-based diet and increased physical activity is aimed at increasing energy uptake, reducing energy intake in food thereby preventing overweight and obesity which is a key risk factor for Type 2 Diabetes Mellitus and gestational diabetes mellitus [6]. Evidence from research has shown that remission of Type 2 Diabetes Mellitus with bariatric surgery can occur following intensive interventions in lifestyle but with few untoward adverse effects [11].

According to the American College of Lifestyle Medicine [11]:

1. Significant clinical improvement in patients with type 2 diabetes mellitus can occur following adequate intensive interventions in modifications of lifestyle.

2. Consumption of a whole plant-based diet in addition to participating in moderate exercise can lead to remission of diabetes mellitus and should be added to the optimal treatment of diabetes mellitus.

Lifestyle modification is also important in the prevention of pre-diabetes Mellitus before it progresses to diabetes mellitus [3]. In the Heart of New Ulm (HONU) Project, the heart screening programme showed that a decline in lifestyle modification especially increased body weight (overweight and obesity) and consumption of alcohol as well as a reduction in the consumption of fruits and vegetables over two years is associated with a higher incidence of metabolic syndrome including diabetes mellitus [11].

The result of this project showed a strong association between body mass index and metabolic syndrome [11]. In another study conducted in Nepal, there was a statistical relationship between type 2 diabetes mellitus and hypertension, dyslipidaemia, alcohol and tobacco use [14]. All these are diseases related to harmful healthy habits which can be prevented by modification in lifestyle. Evidence from other research has shown that remission of type 2 diabetes mellitus is possible with non-pharmacological interventions which include lifestyle modification that translates to the practice of lifestyle medicine [8, 11], increasing physical activity in the form of exercise and engaging in healthy dietary habits and reduction in weight is the primary goal of prevention of Type 2 Diabetes Mellitus [11].

Modification in lifestyle is the first line of management of diabetes mellitus. Weight loss is necessary for Type 2 Diabetes Mellitus and hypertension related to obesity. Exercise and healthy eating are necessary to lose weight and there are some of the pillars lifestyle medicine [29]. The reduction in weight is important as a preventive measure of cardiovascular disease and non-communicable disease as obesity serves as a risk factor for these diseases. The modification in lifestyle required for the management of diabetes mellitus are Medical Nutrition Therapy (MNT), Diabetes Self-Management Education and Support (DSMES), physical activity, cessation of the use of tobacco and counseling [30]. The results of the study conducted by Johansen et al. [31] in which 98 participants were randomized. There was a change in the level of glycosylated hemoglobin ($HbA_{1c}$) from 6.65 to 6.34% in the group where there was an intervention in the modification of their lifestyle, there was a reduction in the dose of oral hypoglycaemic agents in 73.5% of the study participants [31].

## 6. The role of the pillars of lifestyle medicine in the management of diabetes mellitus

### 6.1 The role of stress management in the management of diabetes mellitus

Stress management is one of the pillars of lifestyle medicine. Stress can be defined as the response the body makes to any demand that is made on it. Being a diabetic is stressful already and diabetes mellitus is also stressful to the body; the worst is when there are diabetic complications. During stress, several hormones are released such as cortisol and other hormones that mobilized energy [32]. These hormones lead to hyperglycaemia as stress affects the endocrine system leading to changes in the mechanism of metabolism of glucose. Chronic exposure to stress has several deleterious effects on the body [33]. The rise in the blood glucose following stress is not associated with physical stress alone but with any form of stress including emotional and psychosocial stress [34], which may be experienced daily.

There is an undiagnosed and underestimated incidence of depression, anxiety, the stress in diabetics [32], and there is a correlation between these mental problems with non-communicable diseases including diabetes mellitus. Some diabetics have co-morbid mental health disorders that are not recognized by the physician hence they are not diagnosed [32]. In a case–control study conducted by Krishna [34] among Type 2 diabetics on depression, anxiety and stress, there was a lower level of depression, anxiety and stress in the healthy controls compared to those diagnosed with diabetes mellitus as the diabetics had a higher incidence of depression, anxiety and stress. Hence, stress management is key in diabetes mellitus management.

Emotional problems are common in diabetics and diabetics are at risk of various emotional and psychological problems such as depression, anxiety and diabetes-specific distress [35]. One of the sources of distress in diabetes is the lifelong treatment which is required [36]. Faridah et al. [36] in their study on the relationship between emotional distress and quality of life of patients with Type 2 Diabetes Mellitus used the diabetes distress scale for their study. In this study, a significant relationship was observed using linear regression between emotional distress characteristics p-value >0.05 [36]. There was a positive relationship between glycaemic control and emotional distress in another study conducted by Strandberg et al. (2019) [37] where 319 adults with Type 1 diabetes mellitus were studied. This study proposed that during every clinical consultation with a diabetic, depression and diabetes specific emotional distress should be watched out for [37].

In a South African cohort study conducted to investigate distress related to diabetes mellitus in patients with Type 2 Diabetes Mellitus, diabetes distress scale was used for this study. Distress was seen in 44% of the study participants [38]. This study recommends that attention should be paid to the psychological requirements of the patients as it has a great impact on the outcome of the disease [38]. In a randomized trial of Type 2 Diabetes Mellitus by Survit et al. [39], a significant reduction in $HbA_{1c}$ occurred following education on stress management (0.5%). There was a lower level of the HbA1c after one year in subjects who were educated on stress management [39].

### 6.2 The role of adequate sleep and good sleep hygiene in the management of diabetes mellitus

Sleep is important for good health and adequate sleep is important for the management of sleep. Sleep may be defined as a state of unconsciousness in which the body rejuvenates itself and the soul is also nourished [15]. During sleep there is a healing of the physical body leading to the enhancement of health. The prescribed amount of sleep required daily is eight hours within 24 hours and at least 30 minutes of nap in the afternoon [15]. When sleeping, stress reduces including regaining energy and strength after tiredness as there is a reduction in the levels of hormones released during stress such as cortisol. Poor sleep or insufficient sleep can cause deleterious effects on the body, especially mental and physical health. Sleep is necessary for the regulation of several physiologic functions and processes. Some of these processes are related to the regulation of metabolism including the metabolism of glucose in the body [40]. The human mind and body need sleep to function healthily [41]. Several factors affect sleep including stress. In the management of diabetes mellitus, adequate sleep is important [42] as it is required for the effective maintenance of good glycaemic control [33]. In Type 2 diabetes mellitus, there is a correlation between glycaemic control and disturbances. In sleep, as evidenced by epidemiologic studies, although the extent remains unclear [42]. Results of some studies have shown that loss of sleep causes an increase in calorie intake within 24 hours [40]. Although there is a novel discovery that insufficient sleep has been associated as an important risk factor for the development of diabetes mellitus, these studies are not yet conclusive [40].

Some other studies have investigated the association between diabetes mellitus and sleep apnoea, have revealed that autonomic neuropathy may be the reason for a dysfunction in the central respiration control of the diaphragm and also a decrease in the upper airway [16]. Also sleep apnoea in diabetes mellitus may also be related to obesity, as obesity is a risk factor for diabetes mellitus and sleep apnoea in a study by Bing-Qian et al. [33] on the impact of the quality of sleep on glycaemic control on patients with Type 2 Diabetes Mellitus, there was no significant relationship seen between the sleep efficiency and glycaemic control [1] although the researchers acknowledged that good sleep is necessary for improving the quality of life of diabetics. In a systematic review and meta-analysis on the impact of the amount of sleep and quality of sleep on glycaemic control in Type 2 Diabetes Mellitus, there was not enough evidence to conclude to relate the quality of sleep and the level of glycosylated hemoglobin although it was found that higher levels of glycosylated hemoglobin were seen in diabetics with sleep disturbances the glycosylated hemoglobin was not affected by disturbed sleep [42]. However glycaemic control in patients with Type 2 Diabetes Mellitus is disrupted with too much or too little sleep.

According to Surani et al. [41], there is a disruption in the glycaemic control following impaired quality of sleep which may have some deleterious effects on the body and the quality of life [42] as poor sleep leads to impaired decision making, loss of concentration. This will affect taking decisions on healthy food choices hence patients will choose unhealthy habits that will worsen the glycaemic control and overall management of the patients. In diabetics, there is speculation that reduced quality and duration of sleep can affect glucose control negatively [41, 43]. Also poor sleep in diabetics may be due to poor glycaemic control leading to poor quality of sleep which is required for the general wellbeing of every human being [43]. Hence for good glycaemic control, good sleep hygiene is necessary [15]. As sometimes disturbance of sleep may be an unrecognized health issue in diabetics.

### 6.3 The role of increased physical activity and exercise in the management of diabetes mellitus

Physical inactivity and sedentary lifestyle are one of the risk factors for noncommunicable diseases and obesity and obesity is a risk factor for diabetes mellitus. There are short and long term advantages of physical activity including exercise and this cause a reduction of illnesses with obesity and physical inactivity as its predisposing factors including diabetes mellitus [24]. According to the results of several meta-analytical epidemiological studies on physical exercise including the Diabetes Prevention Programme (DPP) in the United States, diet and exercise and other components of lifestyle medicine causes a reduction in the progression of impaired glucose tolerance (IGT) in Type 2 Diabetes Mellitus [44].

During physical activity and exercise, it acts as physical stress on the body thereby leading to changes in the transportation of glucose thereby satisfying the increased energy demand that occurs during exercise [8]. Hence among the core components of lifestyle medicine in the management of diabetes mellitus [12]. Results of some observational studies have revealed that one of the non-invasive therapies for the prevention and management of diabetes mellitus is exercise; this extends to pregnant women, hence exercise also serves as a preventive measure and for management of gestational diabetes mellitus [45] low impact exercises can be done by pregnant women.

In diabetes mellitus, there is an inadequate amount of insulin and hyperglycaemia also results from increased insulin resistance [19]. Insulin resistance is promoted by obesity and physical inactivity. In the muscles that are not exercised, deposition of visceral fat and also deposition of fat in the liver and muscle occurs by the sequestration of glucose transporter 4 (GLUT-4) [8]. This deposition of fat increases obesity and also worsens insulin resistance. Exercise burns off deposited fat which will definitely in turn positively affect insulin resistance. Improvement of the tolerance of glucose, reduction of insulin resistance and improvement in the lipid profile occurs during exercise thereby increasing and improving cardiovascular and cardiopulmonary function [10]. This improves the sensitivity of insulin and also helps in weight loss, which in turn improves the overall wellbeing of the diabetic and also serves as a preventive measure of other non-communicable diseases [5, 10, 45]. It also stimulates the uptake of glucose. In a study conducted by Miyauch et al. [46], the levels of glycosylated hemoglobin were decreased was seen in patients who engage in an exercise regimen [46]. The aims of exercise in both the prevention and management of Type 2 Diabetes Mellitus are to achieve good metabolic control of diabetes mellitus, weight reduction, increased physical activity, improvement of the cardiovascular function, improvement in dyslipidaemia by reduction of the blood lipids and the general sense of wellbeing and quality of life [10]. Exercise is also necessary for the management of Type 1 Diabetes Mellitus.

Mechanism of improvement of blood glucose through exercise therapy [18]:

- Increased intake of glucose
- Increased utilization of glucose
- Improved insulin sensitivity
- Protection of the function of beta cells of the pancreas

The recommended international guidelines for exercise for adults 18 years and above is to engage in an exercise of moderate intensity for 150 minutes or aerobic exercise and physical activity of vigorous activity for 15 minutes weekly. This can be done as episodes of ten minutes including exercises that strengthen the body involving the major groups of muscles performed on two or more days per week [8]. An exercise regimen begins with a warm-up exercise to stimulate the muscles followed by the conditioning phase and ending with the cooling-down phase. All the phases of exercise are important to prevent injury and muscle soreness. Exercise can act as medicine to the body but diabetics should still be counseled on taking their medications and not to avoid regular check-ups. Diabetics should avoid high impact and vigorous exercises except under the guidance of a physician. Diabetics who should not participate in exercises:

1. Diabetics with retinopathy
2. Diabetics with neuropathy
3. Recurrent hypoglycaemia
4. Recurrent hyperglycaemia

Exercise is very important in the prevention of Type 2 Diabetes Mellitus, it is also important in the management of Type 1, 2 and gestational diabetes mellitus [10, 18, 38].

### 6.4 The role of eating whole plant-based diet in the prevention and management of diabetes mellitus

Eating a whole plant-based diet involves eating meals composed of plants and removing processed meals, animal and animal products, high salt, sugar and fat. This is because they are all risk factors for non-communicable diseases and diabetes mellitus. These meals are referred to as unhealthy foods because of the negative effects. Consumption of a whole plant-based diet involves eating food rich in fruits, vegetables, and legumes. Fruits, vegetables and legumes are available globally and should be encouraged. Good nutrition is very important in any lifestyle intervention [24]. In whole food plant-based diet, consumption of fruits, legumes, whole grains, including nuts and seeds are emphasized. Also, the consumption of animal products and unhealthy foods such as red and white meat, poultry, fish, eggs, dairy products, refined and processed meal, added sugars and oils are minimized and if possible eliminated from the diet [11]. It has been shown that vegetarians who do not eat any animal product have a low prevalence of diabetes mellitus 2.9% with omnivores having a prevalence of 7.6%. Various data have shown between the consumption of processed meat such as bacon, sausage, and hot dog including consumption of eggs and diabetes mellitus [9]. Counseling patients on nutrition is very important in the management of diabetes mellitus. Every diabetic should always have a counseling session during their follow-up visit which should include diet from food available in the locality. The etiology of a wide range of diseases is linked to diet. One of the fundamental determinants of human health is the amount and type of food consumed [5].

It is very important to balance calorie intake and physical activity as a strategy to maintain an ideal weight and preventing overweight obesity and chronic diseases [3]. To fill up the satiety while consuming low calories, complex carbohydrates with a low glycaemic index should be consumed. Other dietary restrictions such as fasting improve the blood glucose but it should be done under the supervision of a physician preferably an endocrinologist and a diabetologist if available to avoid rebound hyperglycaemia which can lead to non-diabetic ketoacidosis and hyperglycemic hyperosmolar state. Intermittent fasting can be practised by diabetics as it is effective but not strict fasting [11].

Decreased consumption of fruits and vegetables is associated with metabolic syndrome [11]. Nutrition is very important in the practice of lifestyle medicine, various guidelines on nutrition for diabetes mellitus have recommended diets lows in red and processed meat, refined grains, added sugar, food sweetened with sugar and salts and saturated and trans-fat [3].

Lifestyle medicine promotes the eating of whole plant based diet which is one of the pillars of lifestyle medicine. There are various other diets plans that has been found to be beneficial in the management of diabetes mellitus such as the low glycaemic diet, dietary approaches to stop hypertension diet (DASH) and the Mediterranean diet.

In a study conducted by Paula et al. [47], they found out when the DASH diet was combined with walking, the result is a reduction in the ambulatory blood pressure monitoring in hypertensive patients with diabetes mellitus [47].

## 7. Conclusion

Diabetes mellitus is a non-communicable disease that can be prevented and managed using lifestyle modification which involves eating a diet that is rich in complex carbohydrates and roughage. People with a family history of diabetes mellitus can prevent it from manifesting in them by modifying it. Good glycaemic control in diabetics can be achieved through good dietary control. This is because of financial commitment to diabetic management in patients without access to health insurance. It also helps to eliminate the psychosocial aspect diabetics go through having to take drugs throughout their lifetime.

## Author details

Dabota Yvonne Buowari
Department of Accident and Emergency, University of Port Harcourt Teaching Hospital, Port Harcourt, Rivers State, Nigeria

*Address all correspondence to: dabotabuowari@yahoo.com

## References

[1] Sagner Mikatz D, Egger G, Liannow I, Schulz KLT, Braman M, et al. Lifestyle medicine potential for reversing a world of chronic disease epidemics: from cell to community. The International Journal of Clinical Practice. 2014, 68, 11, 1289-1292. Doi.10.1111/ijcp.12509

[2] Bodai BI, Nlakata TE, Wong WT, Clark DP, Lawenda S, Tson C, et al. Lifestyle medicine: a brief review of its dramatic impact on health and survival. Perm J. 2018, 22; 17-25. Doi. 10.7818/TPP/17-25

[3] Rippe JM. Lifestyle medicine: the health-promoting power of daily habits and practices. American Journal of Lifestyle Medicine. 2018, 12, 12(6), 499-512 doi.10.1177/15598276185554

[4] Nwatu CB, Onyekonwu CI, Unaogu NN, Ijeoma UN, Onyeka TC, et al. Health-related quality of life in Nigerians with complicated diabetes mellitus. A study from Enugu, South-East Nigeria. Nigerian Journal of Medicine. 2019, 28(2) 138-147

[5] Asif M. The prevention and control of type 2 diabetes by changing lifestyle and dietary pattern. J Educ Health Promot. 2014, 3:1, doi.10.41031/2277-9531.127541

[6] Yin-Ming L, Chin-Hsiae T. Lifestyle modification to manage type 2 diabetes. Tznchi Medical Journal. 2013, 25, 254-255

[7] Houlden RL, Yen HH, Mirranlinu A. The lifestyle history: a neglected but essential component of the medical history. American Journal of Lifestyle Medicine. 2018, 12(5), 404-415

[8] Galariz KI, Narayan V, Lobelo F, Weber WB. Lifestyle and the prevention of type 2 diabetes: a static report. American Journal of Lifestyle Medicine. 2018, 12(1), 4-20

[9] Bodai BI, Nlakata TE, Wong WT, Clark DP, Lawenda S, Tson C, et al. Lifestyle medicine: a brief review of its dramatic impact on health and survival. Perm J. 2018, 22; 17-25. Doi. 10.7818/TPP/17-25

[10] Khan S. Exercise for the management of diabetes mellitus: a review of the evidence. Journal of xxx Medical College. 2013, 3(2), 99-108

[11] Kelly J, Karlson M, Steinke G. Type 2 diabetes remission and lifestyle medicine: a position statement from the American College of Lifestyle Medicine. American Journal of Lifestyle Medicine. 2020.DOI;10.10.1177/1559827620930962

[12] Mekonnem OK, Abate HK, Fegeane ET. Modification among diabetes mellitus patients attending the University of Gondar. Comprehensive Specialized Metabolic Syndrome and Obesity Targets and Therapy. 2020, 13, 1969-1977

[13] Ripal RM. Lifestyle medicine: the importance of considering all the causes of disease. Revista de Psiquiatria Salud Menta. 2012, 5(1), 48-52

[14] Shrestha B, Nepal B, Shakya YL, Reyni B. Lifestyle factors associated with the risk of type 2 diabetes mellitus. Grande Medical Journal. 2019, (2), 77-83

[15] Dricy A, Baba V, Durai S, Asha HS, Belavendra A. A relationship between sleep quality and glycaemic control among subjects with type 2 diabetes mellitus. Indian Journal of Continuing Nursing Education. 2017m 18(2), 39-49

[16] Bopparu S, Surani S. Sleep and diabetes. International Journal of Endocrinology. 2010 doi.10.1155/2010/759505

[17] Riaz S. Diabetes Mellitus. Scientific Research and Essay. 2009, 4(5), 367-373

[18] Yang D, Yang Y, Li Y, Han R. Physical exercise as therapy for type 2 diabetes mellitus: from mechanism to orientation. Annals of Nutrition and Metabolism. 2015, 74, 313-321 doi.10.1159/000500110

[19] Olokoba AB, Obaterus OA, Olokoba CB. Type 2 diabetes mellitus: a review of current trends. Oman Medical Journal. 2012, 27(4), 269-273

[20] Mimich DM, Bland JS. Personalised lifestyle medicine: relevance for nutrition and lifestyle recommendations. The Scientific World Journal. 2013. Doi. http://dx.doi.org/10.1155/2013/129841

[21] Pok GK, Battjes-Fries MCE, Patjo ON, Vanderzji N, Piji H, Voshol P. Lifestyle medicine for type 2 diabetes: practice-based evidence for long-term efficacy of a multi-component lifestyle intervention (Reverse diabetes 2 Now). BMJ. Doi: 10.1136/bmjnph-2020-00081

[22] American College of Preventive Medicine, 2009, Lifestyle Medicine Evidence Review

[23] Yeh B, Kong D. The advent of lifestyle medicine. J Lifestyle Medicine. 2013, 13(1), 1-8

[24] Rooke J (Ed). Gobble J, Ballard T, Oglesby W, Guttrie G, Howard C, Newsam RJ. Lifestyle medicine standards task force. Lifestyle medicine standards. American College of Lifestyle Medicine. www.lifestylemedicine.org. ACCM-Standard

[25] Egger G. Defining a structure and methodology for the practice of lifestyle medicine. American Journal of Lifestyle Medicine. 2016, DOI, 10,1177/155982 7616669327, XX(X), 1-8

[26] Canadian academy of lifestyle medicine. www.canadalifesty lemedicine.ca

[27] Forey JP, Posha WSC. The challenge of diet, exercise and lifestyle modification in the management of the obese diabetic patient. International Journal of Obesity. 1999, 23 Suppl 7,S5-S12

[28] Lindetrom J, Laicheranti TA, Mameli M, et al. Finnish diabetes prevention study group. The Finnish Diabetes Prevention Study Group (DPS): lifestyle intervention and 3-year results on diet and physical activity. Diabetes Care. 2003, 26, 3230-3236

[29] Masuo K. Lifestyle modification is the first line treatment for Type 2 Diabetes. www.intechopen.com 2003. http://dx.doi.org/10.5772/56377

[30] American Diabetes Association. Lifestyle management standards of medical care in diabetes. Diabetes Care. 2018, 14(1), s38-s50.

[31] Johansen MY, MacDonald CS, Hansen KB, Karstoft K, Christensen R, Peterson M et al. Effect of an intensive lifestyle intervention on glycaemic control in patients with Type 2 Diabetes, a randomized clinical trial. JAMA. 2017, 318(77), 637-646.

[32] Kaur H, Kocher R. Stress and diabetes mellitus. International Journal of Health Sciences and Research. www.ijhsr.org. 2017, 7(7), 265-272

[33] Bing – Qian Z, Xiao – Mei L, Dan W, Xing – Feng Y. Sleep quality and its impact on glycaemic control in patients with type 2 diabetes mellitus. International Journal of Nursing Science. 2014(1), 260-265

[34] Krishna P. Depression, anxiety and stress levels in patients with type 2 diabetes mellitus. National Journal of

Physiology, Pharmacy and Pharmacology. 2018,8(1),1570-1571

[35] Pouver F. Should we screen for emotional distress in Type 2 Diabetes Mellitus? Nat Rev Endocrinol. 2009, 5, 665-671.

[36] Faridah IN, Perwitasari DA, Pusfita M, Jasman H. Relationship between emotional distress and quality of life on Type 2 Diabetes Mellitus patients in Merati Island, Regency Hospital. IOP Conference Series Materials: Science and Engineering. 259,2017.0.2002. doi: 10.1088/1757-899x/259/1/012002

[37] Strandberg RM, Graue M, Wentzel-Carson T, Peyrot M, Rokne B. relationships of diabetes-specific emotional distress, depression, anxiety and overall well-being with $HbA_{1c}$ in adult persons with Type 1 Diabetes. Journal of Psychosomatic Research. 2014, 77(3), 174-179

[38] Ramkisson S, Pillary BJ, Sartorius B. Diabetes distress and related factors in South African adults with Type 2 Diabetes. Journal of Endocrinology, Metabolic and Diabetes of South Africa. 2016, 21(2), 35-39.

[39] Survit RS, Triburg MAL, Zucker N, McCaskill MC, Parekh P, Feinglos MN et al. Stress management improves long-term glycaemic control in Type 2 Diabetes. Diabetes

[40] Grandner MA, Seixas A, Shetty S, Shenoy S. Sleep duration and diabetes risk: population trends and potential mechanisms. Current Diabetic Reports. 2016, 16(11), 106. Doi.10.1007/S/1892-016-0805-8

[41] Surani S, Biito V, Surani A, Ghamande S. Effect of diabetes mellitus on sleep quality. World Journal of Diabetes. 2015, 6(6), 865-874

[42] Lee SWH, Ng. KY, Chin WK. The impact of sleep amount and sleep quality on glycaemic control in type 2 diabetes: a systematic review and meta-analysis. Sleep Medicine Reviews. 2017, 31, 91-101

[43] Knutson KL, Ryden AM, Mander BA, Cauter EV. Role of sleep duration and quality in the risk and severity of type 2 diabetes mellitus. Arch Intern Med. 2006,166: 1768-1774

[44] Sati T. Physical exercise for diabetes mellitus: the effective programmes for treatment. JMAS: 2003, 46(7), 314-320

[45] Wang C, Gyelfi KJ, Hiu-Xia Y. Exercise and its role in gestational diabetes mellitus. Chronic Diseases and Translational Medicine. 2016, 2, 208-214

[46] Miyauchi M, Toyoda M, Kaneyema N, Miyatake H, Tanaka E, Kimura M, Umezono T, et al. Exercise therapy for the management of type 2 diabetes mellitus: superior efficacy of activity monitors over pedometers. Journal of Diabetes Research. 2016. http://dx.doi-org/10.1155/2016/5043964

[47] Paula TP, Viana LV, Neto ATZ, Leitao C, Gross JL, Azevedo MJ. Effects of DASH diet and walking on blood pressure in patients with Type 2 Diabetes and uncontrolled hypertension: a randomized trial. The Journal of Clinical Hypertension. 2015, 17(1), 895-901

Chapter 14

# Nutritional Interventions: Diet Modifications, Nutritional Supplements, Complementary and Alternative Medicine

*Jameela Banu*


## Abstract

Type 2 diabetes (T2DM) is characterized by increased circulating blood glucose levels. Several therapies are available to control glucose levels. However, nutritional choices play a major role in managing diabetes. Nutritional supplements can help in reducing the side effects of medicines on the individual so, this chapter will not only discuss several nutritional choices but also available nutritional supplements to control T2DM. Keeping in mind the traditional belief that food is medicine and as therapies are often associated with deleterious side effects, this chapter will discuss alternative and herbal medicines. In addition, life style alterations with proper nutritional choices is also important and will be touched upon in this chapter.


**Keywords:** diet modifications, nutritional supplements, complementary and alternative medicine

## 1. Introduction

Diabetes Mellitus (DM) is a chronic metabolic medical condition that is diagnosed in 422 million people globally and every year 1.6 million deaths are attributed to this condition [1]. It is a disease that can lead to many other severe medical problems and affects almost all the different systems in the body. Diabetes as a result of autoimmune condition, where the pancreatic β-cells are destroyed compromising insulin production, is referred to as Type 1 Diabetes Mellitus (T1DM), while diabetes caused by several other factors including increasing insulin resistance is referred to as Type 2 Diabetes Mellitus (T2DM). As the classic symptom of diabetes is increase in circulating blood glucose, one of the important treatment criteria is focused on food consumption and the type of nutrients consumed. Several diets have been advocated to patients, in addition to life style changes such as increased physical activity and an organized exercise regimen. As carbohydrates are the main source of glucose, diets closely look at reducing carbohydrate intake followed by fat consumption. A major risk factor for developing diabetes is being obese. So many diet plans for diabetic patients focus on weight loss. We will discuss the different diets, nutritional supplements and any alternative and complementary medical choices the patients can opt for.



IntechOpen

## 2. Diets

Several diets have been available for patients with diabetes. Some of them are tested in randomized clinical trials while others have been put forth by nutritionists or other professionals. The main focus of these diets is weight loss as obesity is also a growing global pandemic and is a major risk factor for several severe medical conditions including T2DM. Large randomized controlled studies such as Look Action for Health in Diabetes (Look AHEAD) study, Finnish Diabetes Prevention study and Diabetes Prevention Program Research group had focused on reducing body weight and incidence of diabetes.

### 2.1 Look AHEAD study

This study included 5145 patients and continued for eleven years (2001–2012) in the US [2]. The major goals for this study were to reduce body weight by 7% and increasing physical activity to ≥175 mins/week. Participants of this study were ethnically diverse (African Americans, Hispanic and Native American/Alaskan native) and were diabetic. Co morbidities included hypertension and cardiovascular disease (CVD) [2]. There were three phases of the study with nutritional interventions, lifestyle and behavioral modifications. The nutritional interventions were as follows: Phase I (1–12 months) patients were encouraged to replace two of their meals with shakes, one snack with a bar and consume low energy dense foods. The energy goals were dependent on the body weight of the individuals: <250 lbs. were limited to 1200-1500Kcal and those ≥250 lbs. were limited to 1500-1800 kcal/day [2]. Medications were given to patients who failed to show weight reduction in the first 6 months. Physical activity goals were set at moderately intense activity for 175 minutes/week. Either self monitoring or in person monitoring was conducted at regular intervals. Weight regain was addressed by further counseling and replanning the diet. In Phase 2 (2 years –4 years) and Phase 3 (5 years and above) patients were monitored and were expected to maintain the goal of 10% body weight loss following the diet and activity [2]. Patients successfully lost weight and were physically fit with this diet lifestyle change, however, they could not maintain the weight loss [3]. Patients also improved some of the conditions for diabetic patients [3].

### 2.2 Finnish diabetes prevention study

This study was started in 1998 to determine if an intensive exercise-diet program can prevent or delay the onset of T2DM [4]. A total of 522 patients were in the study and divided into the control and intervention groups. The diet modification included reduction of total fat consumption to <30% with less than 10% saturated fats and high fiber intake [4]. The physical activity goal was 4 hours/week of walking, bicycling or other exercise [5]. The focus of this study was to follow patients to see if there was decrease in the development of diabetes and reported that there was 43% decrease in the risk of development of diabetes. After thirteen years, this study reported that the recommended interventions successfully prevented the progression of T2DM on a long term basis [6].

### 2.3 Diabetic prevention program research group

This study was conducted across 27 clinics in the US. There were 1079 ethnically diverse patients [7]. The goal was to reduce body weight by 7% in the first 6 months by increasing physical activity and consuming a diet with less fats and saturated fats. They reported a 58% reduction in the incidence rate of diabetes [7].

Other long term randomized clinical trials like Da Qing IGT and Diabetes Study have also shown that diet and exercise interventions are very efficient in reducing the risk of developing diabetes [8].

### 2.4 Low carbohydrate diet

The recommended intake of carbohydrate is 45% - 65% per day. Choices with decreased refined carbohydrates, no added sugar, increased intake of grains, legumes, vegetables and fruits were recommended along with limiting high fructose syrup and sucrose. The sources of carbohydrates are not a major factor in the glycemic response as randomized trials showed no difference in glycemic response when sources of carbohydrates was substituted [9]. However, it is important to note that complex sources of carbohydrates are beneficial in determining the circulating glucose levels after meals. Post prandial glucose levels are reflective of the amount of sugar not the type of sugar [10, 11]. Fructose is metabolized in the liver and can affect lipid metabolism so limiting fructose consumption is recommended. Low carbohydrate diet is very effective in decreasing body weight [12, 13]. Patients on this diet not only lost body weight but also decreased HbA1C, however, they were prone to gain weight very quickly. Low carbohydrate diet maybe a short term solution to manage T2DM and can comprise of fiber, vitamins and minerals. Patients on such diet have to be checked for their lipid profile, renal function and protein intake regularly [14].

### 2.5 Low glycemic index diet

Glycemic Index (GI) rises with increase in glucose levels [10]. Factors affecting GI are rate of digestion, cooking method, type of carbohydrate, fat content, protein content and acidity of the food. High starchy foods digest faster so there is high and quick release of glucose. Lower GI foods does not rise the blood glucose levels as quickly. Insulin response and glucagon inhibitors are also affected. High fiber delays the digestion process, increases CCK, incretins and satiety. Lower glycemic diet does not reduce body weight but reduces HbA1c and improves insulin sensitivity [15, 16]. This diet can only have moderate effects in controlling postprandial hyperglycemia. It did not have any effect on the body weight but decreased HbA1C by 0.5% [10].

### 2.6 Low fat diet

Fat consumption is targeted by this diet as diets high in fats can reduce insulin sensitivity and increase endogenous production of glucose by the liver and production of proinflammatory cytokines [10, 17]. This diet focuses more on consumption of ≤30% calories from fat which would be around 50 g of fat for 1500Kcal/day diet. The type of fat consumed determines the damage caused more than the quantity of fat especially with respect to glycemic control [18]. It induced weight loss and had very little effect on glycemic control [10]. However, the long term effects of weight loss may reduce or delay the onset of T2DM.

### 2.7 Very low calorie diet

Decreasing calories is another method to reduce body weight, thereby, decreasing the risk of developing T2DM. The recommendation for those seeking this diet option consumed 400 to 800 calories/d of high quality protein and carbohydrates fortified with vitamins, minerals and trace elements. Decreased body weight and HbA1C were reported with high rate of body weight regain [10].

### 2.8 Mediterranean diet

This diet is more popular and 30–40% of the diet consists of monounsaturated fats. Legumes, fruits, vegetables, nuts, whole grain, fish and moderate ingestion of wine. Has a positive effect on glycemic control and reduces the incidence of diabetes by 52% (**Figure 1**). The body weight regain with this diet was low. The major problem is that adherence rate was low [10].

### 2.9 Protein sparing modified diet

Combination of low carbohydrate ketogenic diet and very low calorie diet. Patients prescribed this diet are started off on a very low calorie diet (800 calories/day) for the first six months and then the calories are increased gradually. At the beginning carbohydrate intake is limited to 20-50 g/day with 1.2–1.5 g/Kg of proteins [19]. Successful in weight loss and lowering HbA1C and fasting glucose. However, there is a low adherence rate among patients and they may increase weight regain quickly [10].

### 2.10 Vegetarian and vegan diet

Both vegetarian and vegan diets are centered around cereal, fruits, vegetables, legume and nuts. However, vegetarian diets may include dairy products and/or

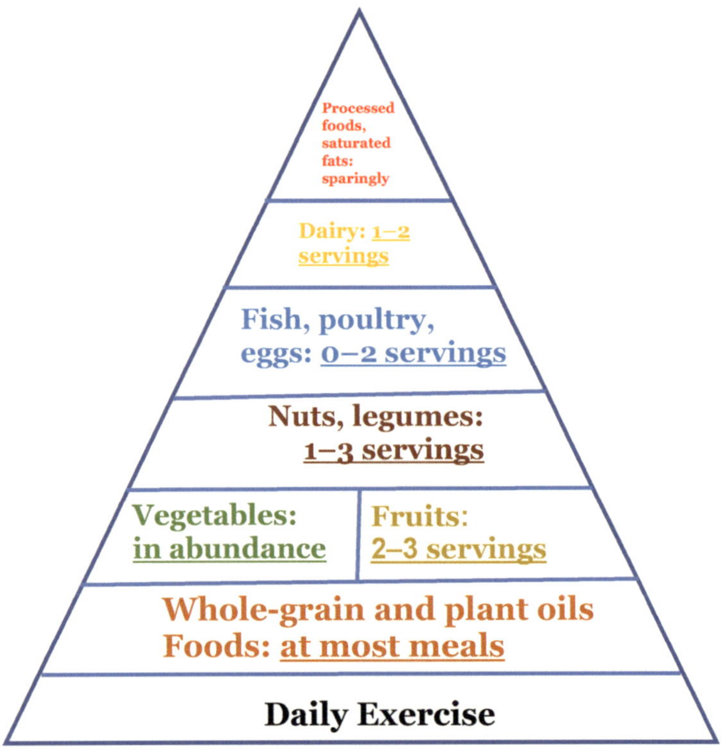


**Figure 1.**
*Mediterranean diet: Recommends consumption of mainly whole grains, vegetables, fruits, nuts and legumes. Limiting animal protein to 0–2 servings and one serving of dairy (as a source of calcium). Consumption of red meat, saturated fats and processed foods is not encouraged and recommended to consume only sparingly. Moderate consumption of wine is now recognized as part of this diet.*

eggs. It reduced body weight, but reduction of HbA1C was not significant. There is very little research on the long term effects of these diets. And it is known that patients on these diets may lack in essential nutrients [10].

### 2.11 High protein diet

A major portion of the calories in this diet is protein with 30% of energy from proteins. Weight loss occurred with females losing total fat and abdominal fat mass. But total lean mass also decreased. Although it improved glucose control and decreased HbA1C (0.28%) [20]. Low fat cottage cheese, cheese tofu, red meat, chicken, peanut butter, fish and lentils were some of the constituents of this diet. Diet should be individualized and patients must account for cardiometabolic risk and renal profile, long term effects are not known [10].

### 2.12 Other diets

Based on the knowledge about the effects of different macronutrients on circulating glucose levels many other popular diets have been introduced. These diets have not been studied using controlled trials so the outcomes are not authenticated. These diets include the Paleo diet, Atkins diet/keto diet, Nutrisystems etc. They are all focused on weight loss. It is important to account for the different macro and micronutrients on maintaining normal metabolism in the body. Therefore, a carbohydrate free or a fat free diet or vegan diet can be very deleterious to health, unless there is a balance in the nutrient intake.

#### *2.12.1 Paleo diet*

Paleo diet also referred to as the Hunter-Gatherer diet or Stone Age diet became popular as the evolution of human diets was recognized from simple diets to complex highly processed diets in the modern world. The Paleo diet simulates diet eaten by the Stone Age humans who were hunters and collected food that was readily available in nature like meat (mainly lean), organ meats, fish, vegetables, fruits, nuts and seeds [21]. This diet is reported to improve insulin resistance and showed significant decrease in HbA1C, body weight and BMI is a small clinical trial [22, 23]. The main issues with this diet is that patients have low vitamin D and calcium [24].

#### *2.12.2 Atkins/keto diet*

The Atkins diet was promoted by Dr. Robert C Atkins, a cardiologist and recommended a low carbohydrate with high protein and fat diet. There are several modifications now available and are referred to as Keto diet. This diet shifts the energy needs of the body from carbohydrate to fats, therefore, The diet includes sources of high fat content like butter, nuts and cream [25]. The low carbohydrate diet recommends the use of 100 g/d of carbohydrates with 50–60% fat and 20–30% protein and the very low carbohydrate diet recommends <50 g/d of carbohydrates. Weight loss, low insulin levels, deceased hunger are some of the benefits reported [26, 27]. In T1DM patients the carbohydrate levels have to be adjusted to the insulin levels to maintain post prandial glucose levels and reduce hypoglycemia [28]. The preferred source of energy in the body is glucose, restricting this macronutrient forces the body to use fats for energy production. Unfortunately, when this happens many ketone bodies are produced and this is deleterious to the metabolism especially in the long run.

#### *2.12.3 Nutrisystems*

A meal plan for losing weight was proposed by Nutrisystems. This diet is customized to individuals for three meals and snacks per day. These diets are balanced and claims to be easy to prepare. The foods used are low glycemic carbohydrates, high fiber and lean proteins with no artificial sweeteners or flavors. Customers are expected to pick from basic, vegetarian, uniquely your, uniquely your ultimate, basic diabetss, diabetes-uniquely yours, ultimate diabetes as well as diet for men. Customers are given the option of picking their own meals or from customized meals. A couple of small (10 and 69 participants) short term (three months) studies used a portion controlled Nutrisystem diabetic diet to determine the effects on weight loss and diabetes. They reported that obese T2DM patients may show significant improvements in weight and glycemic control [29, 30]. A slightly larger study (100 participants) conducted for six months using Nutrisystem diabetes diet reported significantly increased weight loss with statistically insignificant reduction of HbA1C [31]. As this diet is more flexible than the other diets, it may be beneficial to individuals who carefully adhere to the diet and instructions.

Many other modified diets such as South Beach Diet, Zone diet, Macrobiotics, Blood group diet, Ayurvedic diets, Raw food diets, Cleansing diet, Crash diets, Calorie restricted diet are also available. These diets focus on reducing body weight and the major recommendations include decreased or no processed foods, more fiber, vegetables and fruits and decreased total fat intake [32, 33]. Care has to be taken to avoid any vitamins and mineral deficiencies.

## 3. Nutritional supplements

The use of natural products as therapy was in practice for many centuries in different parts of the world. This practice relates very well with the idea that food is medicine. Some of these practices are classified as traditional medicine. Around the world there is an increase interest in using these medicines which are categorized under complementary and alternative medicines. In developing countries, 90% of the population seek plant products as alternative treatment options [34]. The most important benefit could be that there are less or even no side effects and is cost effective. However, the main constraint for these products not being popularly recommended, is the limited scientific evidence about the efficacy, mechanism and side effects. But this is slowly changing as in the past few decades, scientific literature with information on the efficacy, side effects and mechanism of action of several natural products and their compounds has increased. Some of these different natural products that are not only implicated in controlling diabetes but also decrease other medical complications that arise due to diabetes [35].

Plant products are unique in that they have several ingredients and the active ingredient(s)/compound(s) are attributed to having the main effect. This has led the pharmaceutical industry to use some of these active ingredients in currently available allopathic drugs [36]. It is important to identify these active ingredients and study their effects to understand their mechanisms of action. However, it has been observed that when these compounds are isolated, they are sometimes not as efficient when compared to the whole extracts and this maybe because the other ingredients, although in small quantities, may influence the activity of the main compound.

High blood glucose can be due to several different factors apart from consumption of high levels of carbohydrates and inactivity. When the patient is diagnosed with hyperglycemia, they are advised about food intake and increasing physical activity by entering an exercise program. There are drugs and nutritional supplements that will reduce the absorption of glucose in the intestines by inhibiting enzymes such as α amylase and α glucosidase, thereby, lowering postprandial glucose [37]. However, it has been recognized that there are many other factors such as pancreatic dysfunction, insulin resistance, imbalanced rate of glycogenolysis and gluconeogenesis and increased glucagon production result in increased production of endogenous glucose [38]. In addition, these patients may also have less insulin production with progressive β-cell dysfunction [39]. Therefore, diabetic patients may benefit more with plant products as these have multiple compounds that may affect multiple targets [40–43].

Traditional medicines have been popular in different parts of the world and some of them have been traced back to thousands of years - Chinese traditional medicine and Ayurveda. Many cultures around the world such as the American Indians, Mexican, Chinese, Indian subcontinent, various parts of Europe, Africans, Australians have incorporated locally available plants to treat diabetes [36]. Chinese traditional medicine describes bitter flavor and plants that release heat as the most important factors for treating T2DM [44]. Bitter flavor can consolidate the body, remove dampness and purge heat while cold property removes heat syndrome which is seen in T2DM patients during the initial and middle stages of the condition [44]. Ayurvedic treatment uses different approaches including plant medicines incorporated in the diet, exercise, medications, massage, sunlight, controlled breathing and detoxification [45].

There are hundreds of plants that are used in different traditional medicines to treat diabetes. We have listed a few of the most promising common plants that have anti-diabetic activity in animal models and human studies with minimum side effects in **Table 1**. A commonly used vegetable in Asia and Africa is bitter melon (*Momordica charantia*) (**Figure 2A**). This has multiple anti diabetic properties when consumed as fresh juice or eaten regularly. Side effects reported so far is diarrhea [44, 46–51]. Spices used in a wide variety of cuisines around the world like cinnamon (*Cinnamomum*) and some used in the Indian subcontinent such as fenugreek (*Trigonella foenum*) are also implicated in controlling hyperglycemia (**Figure 2B** and **C**). They are widely used in North Africa, Asia and South Europe to treat diabetes. Prolonged use of cinnamon may cause gastrointestinal problems, allergic reactions and liver disease in sensitive people due to the presence of coumarin. Little is known about the side-effects of fenugreek and is safe in amounts that are used for cooking, however, large doses may cause diarrhea, nausea and gastrointestinal issues [46, 52–64]. Green tea (*Camellia sinensis*) is now a common beverage around the world, although it has been used in East Asia for centuries. It has some benefits to diabetic patients and the side effects include insomnia, nausea and heartburn [65, 66] (**Figure 2D**). Basil (*Oscimum basilicum*) and gurmar (*Gymnema sylvestre*) are used in Ayurvedic medicine. Gurmar has many anti-diabetic properties compared to basil. Consumption of high levels of basil may cause liver damage, while Gurmar may cause hypoglycemia headache and nausea [46, 67–72]. Prickly pear (*Opuntia ficus-indica, Opuntia matudae*) is used widely in Central and South America as a vegetable. The health benefits of this fruit include anti-diabetic properties. Mild diarrhea with nausea when consumed in large quantities are the reported side-effects [73–76]. Chinese rhubarb (*Rheum palmatum*) has been studied for its anti-diabetic properties and has been in use in Chinese traditional medicine for a long time. Side effects reported are constipation, diarrhea, stomach pain and inflammation of the pancreas. [44, 77]. Overall, these plants have been part of cuisines for centuries. More long term randomized trials in different ethnic populations will be more informative. The side-effects should be considered, as understanding and keeping track of the side-effects will help in dose determination and sensitivity among patients. Another important factor to consider is the ethnic

| Plant | Common name | Part of the plant used | Anti-diabetic properties | Area traditionally used as medicine | References |
|---|---|---|---|---|---|
| *Momordica charantia* | Bitter melon | Fruit | • ↓Glucose, HbA1C, fasting and PP glucose, PEPCK.<br>• ↑Glucose uptake in cells, insulin signaling, GLUT4, PI3K, PPAR.<br>• Antioxidative and anti inflammatory | Africa, China, India, | [26, 28–33] |
| *Cinnamomum* sp. | Cinnamon | Bark | • ↓Fasting glucose, HbA1C, PEPCK.<br>• Mimics insulin in rodents, anti inflammatory, improves insulin sensitivity | China, India, Persia | [36–40, 42, 46] |
| *Trigonella fienum-graecum* | Fenugreek | Seeds, Leaves | • ↓Glucose, HbA1C, PP glucose.<br>• ↑Insulin secretion<br>• Renew pancreatic b cells | India, South Europe, Mediterranean | [34, 35, 41, 43–45] |
| *Camellia sinensis* | Tea- green | Leaves | • ↓HbA1C<br>• Improves insulin sensitivity, glucose tolerance | Global | [47–48] |
| *Gymnea sylvestre* | Gurmar | Leaves | • ↓Glucose levels<br>• ↑Insulin secretion, promotes islet cell regeneration, delays glucose absorption<br>• binds to the receptors for sweet in the taste buds and inhibit sugar from binding | India | [28, 52–54] |
| *Opuntia ficus-indica, O. matudkae* | Nopal | Fruit | • ↓Intestinal absorption of glucose, PP glucose<br>• Improves insulin sensitivity, anti-oxidative | Central and South America | [55–58] |
| *Oscimum basilicum* | Basil, Tulsi | Leaves | • ↓A glucosidase, a amylase, hyperglycemia<br>• ↑Insulin stimulated glucose metabolism, GLUT4 translocation, liver glycogen content | South East Asia | [49–51] |
| *Rheum palmatum* | Chinese Rhubarb | Root | • ↓HbA1C, glucose, insulin resistance | Chinese | [26, 59] |

*PP = post prandial, HbA1C = Hemoglobin A1C, GLUT4 = Glucose transporter 4, PEPCK = Phosphoenol pyruvate carboxy kinase, PI3K = Phosphoinositide 3-kinase, PPAR = Peroxisome proliferator-activated receptor. ↓ = decrease, ↑ = increase.*

**Table 1.**
*List of some plants beneficial to diabetic patients.*

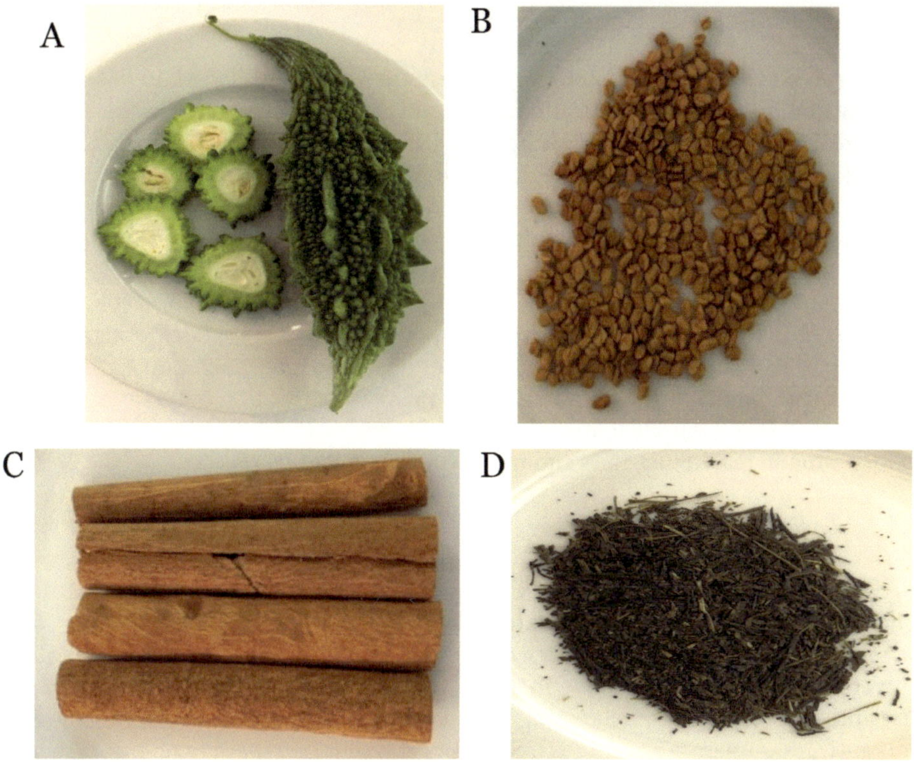


**Figure 2.**
*Some herbal products beneficial to diabetic patients. (A) Bitter melon, (B) Fenogreekseeds and leaves, (C) cinnamon sticks, (D) driedgreentea.*

background of the patient and their family history. This is very critical, as the response of patients to any therapy is dependent on these factors. This also calls for any medicine or diet prescription/counseling to be more individual specific.

Different parts of the plants are used – roots, stem, flowers, fruits and seeds. Each part of the plant may have different concentrations of phytochemicals which are the main players in the health benefits they show. Different compounds have been isolated from the potential medicinal plants and studied for their effects on the different pathways that are involved in the medical condition of interest.

### 3.1 Active ingredients/compounds

Some of the active ingredients have been characterized in either *in vitro* or *in vivo* studies including randomized control trials (RCT) for their anti-diabetic properties. Some of the common compounds studied are saponins, flavones, and polyphenols.

#### *3.1.1 Saponins*

Saponins increase liver glycogen synthesis, inhibit glycogen breakdown and promote insulin sensitivity in the peripheral tissues by increasing Glut 4 expression [78, 79]. Saponins also decrease body weight and inhibit enzymes that breakdown glucose [79, 80]. Found in legumes such as broad beans and lentils, bitter melon, asparagus, spinach and tea.

#### *3.1.2 Flavonoids*

Flavonoids are a group of compounds that are widely found in plant products and are implicated in several health benefits including T2DM. They inhibit enzymes that breakdown glucose and protect pancreatic β-cell damage, stimulate insulin secretion, promote glucose uptake in peripheral tissues, inhibit α amylase and α glucosidase and stimulate glycogenesis [43, 46, 80, 81]. Kaempferol inhibits hepatic inflammation, protects β cells by inhibiting apoptosis, lowers fasting glucose and improves insulin sensitivity [82–84]. They exhibit anti oxidative and anti-inflammatory properties as well [85]. Present in *Gingko biloba*, grapefruit broccoli, kale and tea. Anthocyanin also improves insulin sensitivity, decrease fasting sugar, in addition, it increases adiponectin and regulates glucose internalization via PPARγ, upregulates Glut4 and translocates Glut4 to membrane [86, 87]. It also increases AMPK in liver and muscle to increase glucose uptake and inhibit gluconeogenesis [88]. Found in tea, honey, nuts and many vegetables and fruits.

#### *3.1.3 Polyphenols*

Polyphenols are another group of compounds which include resveratrol, quercetin, epigallocathechin-3 gallate and triterpenoids have multiple targets in reducing hyperglycemia. Resveratrol reduces blood glucose, increases insulin secretion and modulates the enzymes of carbohydrate metabolism [89–91]. It also has anti-oxidative and by decreasing the production of proinflammatory cytokines it is anti-inflammatory as well [82]. Resveratrol is found in the skin of grapes, peanuts, coca, and berries like blueberries, bilberries and cranberries. Quercetin lowers body weight and decreases proinflammatory cytokines [92–94]. Onion has high quantities of quercetin but is also found in a variety of other vegetables and fruits including green leafy vegetable, apples, raspberries, red grapes and cherries. Epigallocathechin 3 gallate alters insulin secretion by increasing it and lowers glucose levels and body weight [95]. High levels are found in tea especially green tea. Triterpenoids can modulate insulin resistance [46, 49]. Found in bitter melon, olives, grapes, mango, apples, tomatoes and many other vegetables.

Alkaloids and polysaccharides present in plants may also control hyperglycemia [96].

## 4. Micronutrients

### 4.1 Minerals

Minerals like chromium magnesium and vanadium can influence hyperglycemia and are used in medications to treat T2DM. Chromium is poorly absorbed with age and T2DM patients have decreased levels of chromium [97]. Studies have shown that chromium deficiency causes reversible insulin resistance and when supplemented improves glycemic control [57]. Another mineral that most T2DM patients show low levels is magnesium [36]. Magnesium is a cofactor for many enzymes in glucose oxidation and it modulates glucose across cell membranes. Mg deficiency causes insulin resistance. It may increase insulin secretion and increase uptake of glucose in peripheral tissues [36]. Vanadium was used in certain insulin preparations and in animal models has shown increased uptake of glucose and its metabolism. It is also reported to increase insulin sensitivity. It may modulate glucose oxidation, glycogen synthesis and hepatic glucose output modulation [98].

### 4.2 Vitamins

Vitamins like vitamin C and E may also help T2DM patients. Vitamin C can improve glycemic control [99] while vitamin E, as an anti-oxidant, may influence protein glycation, insulin sensitivity and secretion [36].

## 5. Conclusions

Several diets have been studied to reduce the risk of developing diabetes and to control hyperglycemia. Almost all of them focus on decreasing body weight so they reduce body fat content as well. Many of the diets are beneficial in delaying the onset of diabetes and to diabetic patients. However, some of the diets require for the patients to be monitored constantly. Many plant products used in traditional medicine around the world have been scientifically studied to determine the efficacy, mechanism and side effects with focus of their effects on hyperglycemia. Diabetes being a complicated disease, T2DM patients may benefit more if multi targeted therapy is given. In addition to diet, another important factor that will help T2DM is the level of physical activity and exercise. Any diet with exercise is more beneficial than either one alone.

Mayo clinic recommends diet rich in fiber, vegetables, fruits and whole grain with low fat dairy products [100]. The American Diabetic Association and The American Heart Association recommend a balanced plate similar to that of USDA (**Figures 3** and **4**) with half plate of vegetables, a quarter plate of healthy carbohydrates such as brown rice, whole wheat couscous, whole grain pasta or plain sweet potato and some less than a quarter plate of protein [101, 102]. Fats are essential to the body as they are integral part of the cell membrane and hormones. They are required to digest any fat that is consumed. However, there has been a debate whether saturated fats are required for the body or not. The importance of having less than 10% saturated fat in the diet is now recognized although instead of saturated fatty acids, mono and poly unsaturated fatty acids are recommended. With respect to nutritional supplements there is no recommendation from American Diabetes Association. However, there is an increase in the number of patients seeking complementary and alternative medicine due to lower side effects and cost effectiveness. With a steady increase in scientific authentication of plant products for preventing and treating medical conditions nutritional supplements may become more popular. Interestingly, many of the plant products are consumed almost everyday in many cultures and these population also report diabetes. One reason maybe because they do not eat it everyday at the required dosage in addition to major change in lifestyle from an active on to a more sedentary one, as seen in any developed societies.

With many options for diets to choose from for patients, it is important to remember that as individuals differ among themselves, a individualized diet is important and equally important is adhering to the diet [103]. For diabetic patients to help control the progression of the disease, it is important to consider bio individual needs of each patients. Whether it is the choice of drugs, nutrition therapy or life style changes, it is important to have individually tailored treatment regimens for diabetic patients based on several factors including the ethnicity, life style, choice of foods etc. Other important factors to consider, in T2DM patients, are how much endogenous insulin is produced, and the level of insulin resistance to recommend diets that can target β-cell function and tissue-specific insulin sensitivity [104]. In T1DM patients it is critical to monitor the insulin that is administered and adjust

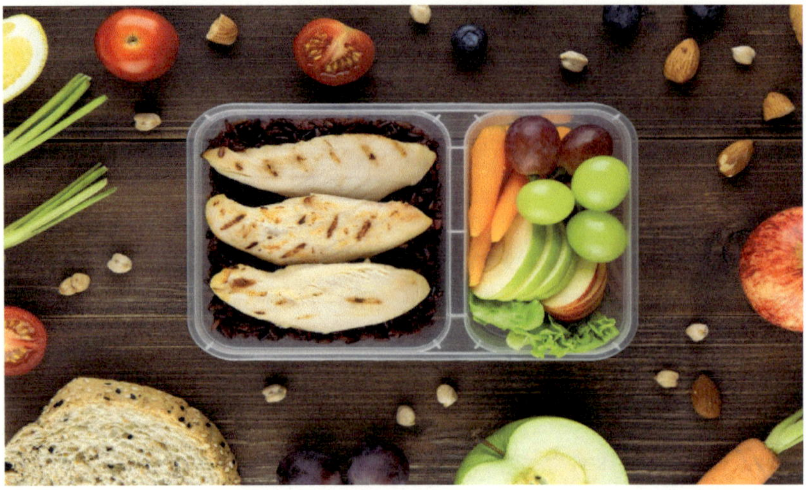

**Figure 3.**
*USDA recommended 'my plate' showing recommended portions of each macronutrients: Carbohydrates (40–60%); proteins (10–35% for males; 13–15% for females), fats (20–35%). (fiber 25 g) https://www.fns.usda.gov/cnpp.*

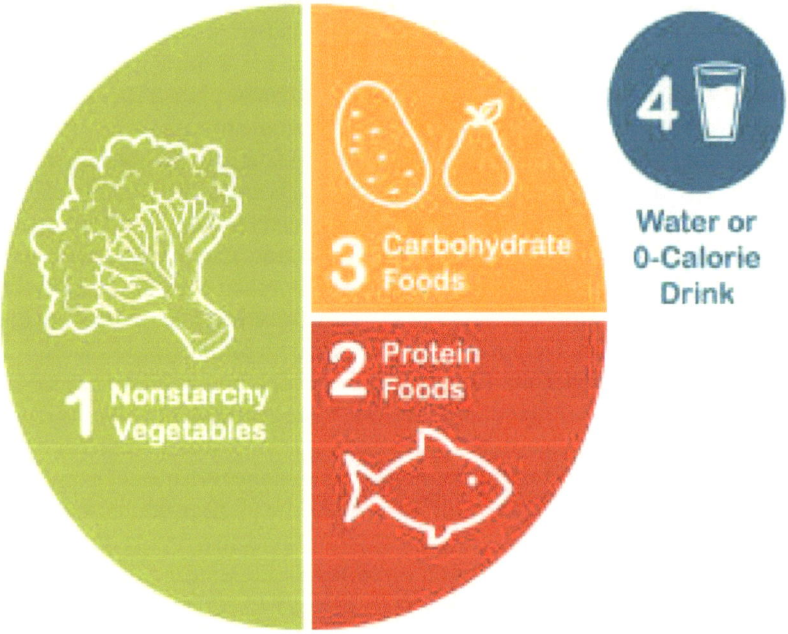


**Figure 4.**
*ADA recommended plate model for balanced food intake. %0% vegetables, 25% protein and 25% carbohydrate is recommended with a glass of water or no calories drink. https://diabetes.org/nutrition.*

the macronutrients to avoid hypoglycemic condition. Most of the time carbohydrate counting in the diet is recommended for T1DM patients.

## Conflict of interest

The author declares no conflict of interest.

## Author details

Jameela Banu
Department of Health and Biomedical Sciences and Department of Biology, University of Texas Rio Grande Valley, Edinburg, Texas, USA

*Address all correspondence to: jameela.banu@utrgv.edu

## References

[1] WHO. *Diabetes Overview*. 08/20/2020]; Available from : https://www.who.int/health-topics/diabetes/diabetes#tab=tab_1.

[2] Look, A.R.G., et al., *The Look AHEAD study: a description of the lifestyle intervention and the evidence supporting it.* Obesity (Silver Spring), 2006. **14**(5): p. 737-52.

[3] Steinberg, H., C. Jacovino, and A.E. Kitabchi, *Look inside Look AHEAD: why the glass is more than half-full.* Curr Diab Rep, 2014. **14**(7): p. 500.

[4] Uusitupa, M., et al., *The Finnish Diabetes Prevention Study.* Br J Nutr, 2000. **83 Suppl 1**: p. S137-42.

[5] Lindstrom, J., et al., *Sustained reduction in the incidence of type 2 diabetes by lifestyle intervention: follow-up of the Finnish Diabetes Prevention Study.* Lancet, 2006. **368**(9548): p. 1673-9.

[6] Lindstrom, J., et al., *Improved lifestyle and decreased diabetes risk over 13 years: long-term follow-up of the randomised Finnish Diabetes Prevention Study (DPS).* Diabetologia, 2013. **56**(2): p. 284-93.

[7] Diabetes Prevention Program Research, G., *The Diabetes Prevention Program (DPP): description of lifestyle intervention.* Diabetes Care, 2002. **25**(12): p. 2165-71.

[8] Pan, X.R., et al., *Effects of diet and exercise in preventing NIDDM in people with impaired glucose tolerance. The Da Qing IGT and Diabetes Study.* Diabetes Care, 1997. **20**(4): p. 537-44.

[9] Bantle, J.P., et al., *Metabolic effects of dietary sucrose in type II diabetic subjects.* Diabetes Care, 1993. **16**(9): p. 1301-5.

[10] Sandouk, Z. and M.C. Lansang, *Diabetes with obesity--Is there an ideal diet?* Cleve Clin J Med, 2017. **84**(7 Suppl 1): p. S4-S14.

[11] Malik, V.S., et al., *Sugar-sweetened beverages and risk of metabolic syndrome and type 2 diabetes: a meta-analysis.* Diabetes Care, 2010. **33**(11): p. 2477-83.

[12] Samaha, F.F., et al., *A low-carbohydrate as compared with a low-fat diet in severe obesity.* N Engl J Med, 2003. **348**(21): p. 2074-81.

[13] Vetter, M.L., et al., *Long-term effects of low-carbohydrate versus low-fat diets in obese persons.* Ann Intern Med, 2010. **152**(5): p. 334-5.

[14] Association, A.D., *Introduction.* Diabetes Care, 2017. **40**(Suppl 1): p. S1-S2.

[15] Thomas, D., Elliott, E.J., *Low glycemic index or low glycemic load, diets for diabetes mellitus.* Cocharane Database Syst Rev, 2009. **1:CD006296**: p. 29.

[16] Braunstein, C.R., Meija, S.B., Stoiko, E., Noronha J.C., Choo, V., Ha, V., Augustin, L., Jenkins, D.J.A., Kendall, C.W.C., Sievenpiper, J.L. *Effect of low-glycemic index/load diets on body weight: A systemic Review and Meta-Analysis*. in *Experimental Biology*. 2016. San Diego: The FASEB Journal.

[17] Savage, D.B., K.F. Petersen, and G.I. Shulman, *Disordered lipid metabolism and the pathogenesis of insulin resistance.* Physiol Rev, 2007. **87**(2): p. 507-20.

[18] Evert, A.B., et al., *Nutrition therapy recommendations for the management of adults with diabetes.* Diabetes Care, 2014. **37 Suppl 1**: p. S120-43.

[19] Chang, J. and S.R. Kashyap, *The protein-sparing modified fast for obese patients with type 2 diabetes: what to expect.* Cleve Clin J Med, 2014. **81**(9): p. 557-65.

[20] Ajala, O., P. English, and J. Pinkney, *Systematic review and meta-analysis*

*of different dietary approaches to the management of type 2 diabetes.* Am J Clin Nutr, 2013. **97**(3): p. 505-16.

[21] Staff, M.C. *Paleo diet: What is it and why is it so popular?* 10/08/2020]; Available from: https://www.mayoclinic.org/healthy-lifestyle/nutrition-and-healthy-eating/in-depth/paleo-diet/art-20111182.

[22] Tarantino, G., V. Citro, and C. Finelli, *Hype or Reality: Should Patients with Metabolic Syndrome-related NAFLD be on the Hunter-Gatherer (Paleo) Diet to Decrease Morbidity?* J Gastrointestin Liver Dis, 2015. **24**(3): p. 359-68.

[23] Jonsson, T., et al., *Beneficial effects of a Paleolithic diet on cardiovascular risk factors in type 2 diabetes: a randomized cross-over pilot study.* Cardiovasc Diabetol, 2009. **8**: p. 35.

[24] Jew, S., S.S. AbuMweis, and P.J. Jones, *Evolution of the human diet: linking our ancestral diet to modern functional foods as a means of chronic disease prevention.* J Med Food, 2009. **12**(5): p. 925-34.

[25] Freeman, J.M., E.H. Kossoff, and A.L. Hartman, *The ketogenic diet: one decade later.* Pediatrics, 2007. **119**(3): p. 535-43.

[26] Hamdy, O., et al., *Fat Versus Carbohydrate-Based Energy-Restricted Diets for Weight Loss in Patients With Type 2 Diabetes.* Curr Diab Rep, 2018. **18**(12): p. 128.

[27] Bolla, A.M., et al., *Low-Carb and Ketogenic Diets in Type 1 and Type 2 Diabetes.* Nutrients, 2019. **11**(5).

[28] Nielsen, J.V., et al., *Low carbohydrate diet in type 1 diabetes, long-term improvement and adherence: A clinical audit.* Diabetol Metab Syndr, 2012. **4**(1): p. 23.

[29] Fabricatore, A.N., Herron, L.A., Wadden, T.A., *Reduction in glycemic variability and hyperglycemia with a low-glycemic index portion controlled diet in persons with type 2 diabetes.*, in *American Diabetes Association*. 2012: Philadelphia.

[30] Foster, G.D., et al., *The effects of a commercially available weight loss program among obese patients with type 2 diabetes: a randomized study.* Postgrad Med, 2009. **121**(5): p. 113-8.

[31] Foster, G.D., Wadden, T.A., LaGrotte, C.A., Hesson, L.A., Komaroff, E., VanderVeur, S.S., Homko, C.J., Maschak-Carry, B.J., Reyner, N., Diewald, L.K., Kiotz, A.L., Wojtanowski, A., Herring, S., Tioxon, D.A., Vetter, M., Sanders, T., *The effects of a portion controlled meal plan versus a diabetes self-management program on weight and glycemic control among obese patients with type 2 diabates.*, in *American Scientific Meeting of the Obesity Society*. 2011: Orlando, FL.

[32] Rosenthal, J., *Integrative Nutrition*. 2014, New York: Institute for Integrative Nutrition.

[33] Marian M.J. & Mullin, G.E., *Integrative Nutrition Therapy*. 2016, Boca Raton, FL: CRC Press.

[34] Organization, W.H., *Traditional medicine - growing needs and potential, WHO policy persespective on medicine.* 2002. **2**: p. 1-6.

[35] Rizvi, S.I. and N. Mishra, *Traditional Indian medicines used for the management of diabetes mellitus.* J Diabetes Res, 2013. **2013**: p. 712092.

[36] Yeh, G.Y., et al., *Systematic review of herbs and dietary supplements for glycemic control in diabetes.* Diabetes Care, 2003. **26**(4): p. 1277-94.

[37] Senthil, S.L., Raghu, C., Arjun, H., Anantharaman, P., *In vitro and in silico inhibition properties of fucoidan against α-amylase and α-D-glucosidase*

*with relevance to type 2 diabetes mellitus.* Carbohydrate Polymers, 2019. **209**: p. 350-355.

[38] Van Poelje, P.D., Dang, Q., Erion, M.D., *Fructose-1, 6 bisphosphatase as a therapeutic target for type 2 diabetes.* Drug Discovery Today Therapeutic Strategies, 2007. **4**: p. 103-109.

[39] Fryirs, M., P.J. Barter, and K.A. Rye, *Cholesterol metabolism and pancreatic beta-cell function.* Curr Opin Lipidol, 2009. **20**(3): p. 159-64.

[40] Csermely, P., V. Agoston, and S. Pongor, *The efficiency of multi-target drugs: the network approach might help drug design.* Trends Pharmacol Sci, 2005. **26**(4): p. 178-82.

[41] Peters, J.U., *Polypharmacology - foe or friend?* J Med Chem, 2013. **56**(22): p. 8955-71.

[42] Reddy, A.S. and S. Zhang, *Polypharmacology: drug discovery for the future.* Expert Rev Clin Pharmacol, 2013. **6**(1): p. 41-7.

[43] Pereira, A.S.P., et al., *Evaluation of the Anti-Diabetic Activity of Some Common Herbs and Spices: Providing New Insights with Inverse Virtual Screening.* Molecules, 2019. **24**(22).

[44] Chen, H., et al., *Application of Herbal Medicines with Bitter Flavor and Cold Property on Treating Diabetes Mellitus.* Evid Based Complement Alternat Med, 2015. **2015**: p. 529491.

[45] Shekelle, P.G., Hardy, M., Morton, S.C., Coulter, I., Venuturnpalli, S., Favreau, J., Hilton, L.K. , *Are Ayurvedic herbs for diabetes effective?* The Journal of Family Practice, 2005. **54**: p. 876-886.

[46] Ota, A., Ulrih, N.P., *An overview of herbal products and secondary metabolites used for managemnent of type two diabete.* Frontiers in Pharmacology, 2017. **8**: p. 1-14.

[47] Sun, F.Q., Zhang, G., Huang, B., Bai, J., Yu, X. , *Clinical observation of using bitter melon to treat DM.* Lisoning J of PRactical Diabetaology, 2000. **8**: p. 34-35.

[48] Kumar, R., et al., *Fruit extracts of Momordica charantia potentiate glucose uptake and up-regulate Glut-4, PPAR gamma and PI3K.* J Ethnopharmacol, 2009. **126**(3): p. 533-7.

[49] Giovannini, P., M.J. Howes, and S.E. Edwards, *Medicinal plants used in the traditional management of diabetes and its sequelae in Central America: A review.* J Ethnopharmacol, 2016. **184**: p. 58-71.

[50] Leatherdale, B.A., et al., *Improvement in glucose tolerance due to Momordica charantia (karela).* Br Med J (Clin Res Ed), 1981. **282**(6279): p. 1823-4.

[51] Omokhua-Uyi, A.G. and J. Van Staden, *Phytomedicinal relevance of South African Cucurbitaceae species and their safety assessment: A review.* J Ethnopharmacol, 2020. **259**: p. 112967.

[52] Al-Habori, M., Al-Aghbari, AM. Al-Mamary, E., *Antidiabetic and hypocholestrolaemic effects of fenugreek.* Phytother Res, 1998. **12**: p. 233-242.

[53] Valette, G., et al., *Hypocholesterolaemic effect of fenugreek seeds in dogs.* Atherosclerosis, 1984. **50**(1): p. 105-11.

[54] Sheng, X., et al., *Improved Insulin Resistance and Lipid Metabolism by Cinnamon Extract through Activation of Peroxisome Proliferator-Activated Receptors.* PPAR Res, 2008. **2008**: p. 581348.

[55] Khan, A., et al., *Cinnamon improves glucose and lipids of people with type 2 diabetes.* Diabetes Care, 2003. **26**(12): p. 3215-8.

[56] Crawford, P., *Effectiveness of cinnamon for lowering hemoglobin A1C in patients with type 2 diabetes: a randomized, controlled trial.* J Am Board Fam Med, 2009. **22**(5): p. 507-12.

[57] Nahas, R. and M. Moher, *Complementary and alternative medicine for the treatment of type 2 diabetes.* Can Fam Physician, 2009. **55**(6): p. 591-6.

[58] Mang, B., et al., *Effects of a cinnamon extract on plasma glucose, HbA, and serum lipids in diabetes mellitus type 2.* Eur J Clin Invest, 2006. **36**(5): p. 340-4.

[59] Madar, Z., et al., *Glucose-lowering effect of fenugreek in non-insulin dependent diabetics.* Eur J Clin Nutr, 1988. **42**(1): p. 51-4.

[60] Akilen, R., et al., *Glycated haemoglobin and blood pressure-lowering effect of cinnamon in multi-ethnic Type 2 diabetic patients in the UK: a randomized, placebo-controlled, double-blind clinical trial.* Diabet Med, 2010. **27**(10): p. 1159-67.

[61] Gupta, A., R. Gupta, and B. Lal, *Effect of Trigonella foenum-graecum (fenugreek) seeds on glycaemic control and insulin resistance in type 2 diabetes mellitus: a double blind placebo controlled study.* J Assoc Physicians India, 2001. **49**: p. 1057-61.

[62] Kochhar, A. and M. Nagi, *Effect of supplementation of traditional medicinal plants on blood glucose in non-insulin-dependent diabetics: a pilot study.* J Med Food, 2005. **8**(4): p. 545-9.

[63] NCCIH. *Fenugreek*. 08/22/2020]; Available from: https://www.nccih.nih.gov/health/fenugreek.

[64] NCCIH. *Cinnamon*. 08/22/2020]; Available from: https://www.nccih.nih.gov/health/cinnamon.

[65] Fukino, Y., et al., *Randomized controlled trial for an effect of green tea-extract powder supplementation on glucose abnormalities.* Eur J Clin Nutr, 2008. **62**(8): p. 953-60.

[66] Venables, M.C., et al., *Green tea extract ingestion, fat oxidation, and glucose tolerance in healthy humans.* Am J Clin Nutr, 2008. **87**(3): p. 778-84.

[67] Broadhurst, C.L., M.M. Polansky, and R.A. Anderson, *Insulin-like biological activity of culinary and medicinal plant aqueous extracts in vitro.* J Agric Food Chem, 2000. **48**(3): p. 849-52.

[68] El-Beshbishy, H., Bahashwan, S., *Hypoglycemic effect of basil (Ocimum basilicum) aqueous extract ismediated through inhibition of α-glucosidase and a-amylase activities: An invitro study.* Toxicol Ind Health, 2012. **28**: p. 42-50.

[69] Ezeani, C., et al., *Ocimum basilicum extract exhibits antidiabetic effects via inhibition of hepatic glucose mobilization and carbohydrate metabolizing enzymes.* J Intercult Ethnopharmacol, 2017. **6**(1): p. 22-28.

[70] Baskaran, K., et al., *Antidiabetic effect of a leaf extract from Gymnema sylvestre in non-insulin-dependent diabetes mellitus patients.* J Ethnopharmacol, 1990. **30**(3): p. 295-300.

[71] Li, Y., et al., *Effect of-Gymnema Sylvestre, Citrullus colocynthis and Artemisia absinthium on Blood Glucose and Lipid Profile in Diabetic Human.* Acta Pol Pharm, 2015. **72**(5): p. 981-5.

[72] Kamble, B., et al., *Effects of Gymnema sylvestre extract on the pharmacokinetics and pharmacodynamics of glimepiride in streptozotocin induced diabetic rats.* Chem Biol Interact, 2016. **245**: p. 30-8.

[73] McKennon, S.A., *Non-Pharmaceutical Intervention Options For Type 2 Diabetes: Diets And Dietary*

*Supplements (Botanicals, Antioxidants, and Minerals)*, in *Endotext*, K.R. Feingold, et al., Editors. 2000: South Dartmouth (MA).

[74] Frati, A.C., et al., *Acute hypoglycemic effect of Opuntia streptacantha Lemaire in NIDDM.* Diabetes Care, 1990. **13**(4): p. 455-6.

[75] Lopez-Romero, P., et al., *The effect of nopal (Opuntia ficus indica) on postprandial blood glucose, incretins, and antioxidant activity in Mexican patients with type 2 diabetes after consumption of two different composition breakfasts.* J Acad Nutr Diet, 2014. **114**(11): p. 1811-8.

[76] Zhao, L.Y., et al., *Antidiabetic effect of a newly identified component of Opuntia dillenii polysaccharides.* Phytomedicine, 2011. **18**(8-9): p. 661-8.

[77] Wang, S.F., *The experimental study of the effect of alcohol extract from Rhenum palmatum L on diabetes type 2 rats with insulin resistance.* Modern J of Integrated Traditional Med and Western Med, 2007. **16**: p. 1606-1719.

[78] Ma, C.-Y., Yu, H.-Y., Wang, H.-J, Geng, L.-J., Guan, H.-Y, *Hypoglycemic mechanism of total saponins of Momordica charantia in typer 2 diabetes mellitus rats.* Tianjin Medical J, 2014. **42**: p. 321-324.

[79] Ma, C.Y., Yu, H.Y., Wang, H.J., Guan, H.Q., *Effects of total saponins of Momordica charantia on plasma lipids and adipocyte factors in type 2 diabetes rats.* Pharmacology and Clinics of Chinese Materia Medica, 2013. **29**: p. 56-59.

[80] Chen, L.H., Pan, Z.H., Cao, Y.L. Ma, Q.Y. , *A screen of α-glucosidase inhibitors from rhizoma anemarrhenae.* Food & Machinery, 2013. **29**: p. 147.

[81] Chen, J., et al., *Natural flavonoids as potential herbal medication for the treatment of diabetes mellitus and its complications.* Nat Prod Commun, 2015. **10**(1): p. 187-200.

[82] Luo, C., et al., *Kaempferol alleviates insulin resistance via hepatic IKK/NF-kappaB signal in type 2 diabetic rats.* Int Immunopharmacol, 2015. **28**(1): p. 744-50.

[83] Zhang, Y. and D. Liu, *Flavonol kaempferol improves chronic hyperglycemia-impaired pancreatic beta-cell viability and insulin secretory function.* Eur J Pharmacol, 2011. **670**(1): p. 325-32.

[84] Vinayagam, R. and B. Xu, *Antidiabetic properties of dietary flavonoids: a cellular mechanism review.* Nutr Metab (Lond), 2015. **12**: p. 60.

[85] Calderon-Montano, J.M., et al., *A review on the dietary flavonoid kaempferol.* Mini Rev Med Chem, 2011. **11**(4): p. 298-344.

[86] Stull, A.J., et al., *Bioactives in blueberries improve insulin sensitivity in obese, insulin-resistant men and women.* J Nutr, 2010. **140**(10): p. 1764-8.

[87] Scazzocchio, B., et al., *Cyanidin-3-O-beta-glucoside and protocatechuic acid exert insulin-like effects by upregulating PPARgamma activity in human omental adipocytes.* Diabetes, 2011. **60**(9): p. 2234-44.

[88] Kurimoto, Y., et al., *Black soybean seed coat extract ameliorates hyperglycemia and insulin sensitivity via the activation of AMP-activated protein kinase in diabetic mice.* J Agric Food Chem, 2013. **61**(23): p. 5558-64.

[89] Palsamy, P. and S. Subramanian, *Resveratrol, a natural phytoalexin, normalizes hyperglycemia in streptozotocin-nicotinamide induced experimental diabetic rats.* Biomed Pharmacother, 2008. **62**(9): p. 598-605.

[90] Palsamy, P. and S. Subramanian, *Ameliorative potential of resveratrol on proinflammatory cytokines, hyperglycemia mediated oxidative stress, and pancreatic beta-cell dysfunction in streptozotocin-nicotinamide-induced diabetic rats.* J Cell Physiol, 2010. **224**(2): p. 423-32.

[91] Palsamy, P., S. Sivakumar, and S. Subramanian, *Resveratrol attenuates hyperglycemia-mediated oxidative stress, proinflammatory cytokines and protects hepatocytes ultrastructure in streptozotocin-nicotinamide-induced experimental diabetic rats.* Chem Biol Interact, 2010. **186**(2): p. 200-10.

[92] Cherniack, E.P., *Polyphenols: planting the seeds of treatment for the metabolic syndrome.* Nutrition, 2011. **27**(6): p. 617-23.

[93] Rivera, L., et al., *Quercetin ameliorates metabolic syndrome and improves the inflammatory status in obese Zucker rats.* Obesity (Silver Spring), 2008. **16**(9): p. 2081-7.

[94] Yin, J., H. Zhang, and J. Ye, *Traditional chinese medicine in treatment of metabolic syndrome.* Endocr Metab Immune Disord Drug Targets, 2008. **8**(2): p. 99-111.

[95] Li, C., et al., *Green tea polyphenols modulate insulin secretion by inhibiting glutamate dehydrogenase.* J Biol Chem, 2006. **281**(15): p. 10214-21.

[96] Chen, Z.H., *Advances on hypoglycemic functions of bitter gourd components.* J Food Industry, 2014. **35**: p. 250-252.

[97] *A scientific review: the role of chromium in insulin resistance.* Diabetes Educ, 2004. **Suppl**: p. 2-14.

[98] O'Connell, B., *Select vitamins and minerals in the management of diabetes.* Diabetes Spectrum, 2001. **14**: p. 133-148.

[99] Eriksson, J. and A. Kohvakka, *Magnesium and ascorbic acid supplementation in diabetes mellitus.* Ann Nutr Metab, 1995. **39**(4): p. 217-23.

[100] Staff, M.C. *Diaetes diet: Create your healthy-eating plan*. [cited 2020 08/30/2020]; Available from: https://www.mayoclinic.org/diseases-conditions/diabetes/in-depth/diabetes-diet/art-20044295.

[101] Association, A.H. *The Diabetic Diet*. [cited 2020 9/27/2020]; Available from: https://www.heart.org/en/health-topics/diabtes/prevention-treatment-of-diabtes/the diabetic diet.

[102] Association, A.D. *Nutrition Eating does not have to be boring*. 8/30/2020]; Available from: https://diabetes.org/nutrition.

[103] Khazrai, Y.M., G. Defeudis, and P. Pozzilli, *Effect of diet on type 2 diabetes mellitus: a review.* Diabetes Metab Res Rev, 2014. **30 Suppl 1**: p. 24-33.

[104] Guess, N.D., *Dietary Interventions for the Prevention of Type 2 Diabetes in High-Risk Groups: Current State of Evidence and Future Research Needs.* Nutrients, 2018. **10**(9).

Chapter 15

# Role of Nutrient and Energy Sensors in the Development of Type 2 Diabetes

*Verónica Hurtado-Carneiro, Ana Pérez-García, Elvira Álvarez and Carmen Sanz*


## Abstract

Cell survival depends on the constant challenge to match energy demands with nutrient availability. This process is mediated through a highly conserved network of metabolic fuel sensors that orchestrate both a cellular and whole-body energy balance. A mismatch between cellular energy demand and nutrient availability is a key factor in the development of type 2 diabetes, obesity, metabolic syndrome, and other associated pathologies; thus, understanding the fundamental mechanisms by which cells detect nutrient availability and energy demand may lead to the development of new treatments. This chapter reviews the role of the sensor PASK (protein kinase with PAS domain), analyzing its role in the mechanisms of adaptation to nutrient availability and the metabolic response in different organs (liver, hypothalamus) actively cooperating to control food intake, maintain glycaemia homeostasis, and prevent insulin resistance and weight gain.


**Keywords:** PASK, mTOR, AMPK, obesity, food intake, fasting/feeding, GLP-1

## 1. Introduction

Nutrients such as carbohydrates, amino acids, fats, vitamins, minerals, etc. are supplied at regular intervals by food intake and are necessary for the normal functioning of cells and a healthy physiology [1]. They act as metabolic substrates for energy production and as building blocks for the synthesis of macromolecules and cellular components. Accordingly, organisms have developed mechanisms to detect levels of specific nutrients in the extra- and intracellular compartments to ensure rates of growth, proliferation, and function coordinate properly and adjust to nutrient availability.

## 2. Nutrients and energy sensors: importance in glucose and energy homeostasis

Nutrient-sensing mechanisms are found in all organisms, from yeast through to mammals. Importantly, some of these mechanisms in multicellular organisms have also evolved for regulation by the endocrine system, allowing the coordination of nutrient-sensing activity among different cells/tissues in the body [2].



IntechOpen

Nutrient sensors are proteins that detect fluctuations in nutrient levels or products of their metabolism within the physiological range, and induce a cellular response, leading to changes in the nutrient distribution or in feeding behavior [1]. These sensors respond to alterations in nutrient levels through diverse mechanisms, including the activation of phosphorylation cascades, changes in gene transcription, and enzymatic activities, among others [2].

The sensing of a nutrient may involve the direct binding of its molecule to the sensor or an indirect mechanism relying on the detection of a surrogate molecule that reflects nutrient abundance. There are homeostatic responses in multicellular eukaryotes to maintain nutrient levels circulating within a narrow range, such as hormone release, which act as signals to facilitate the coordination of consistent responses in the whole organism [3].

An effective and adequate response to changes in nutrient availability is vital in the human body, and its alteration triggers pathologies such as obesity, metabolic syndrome, and aging-related diseases (e.g. cancer and neurodegeneration).

Some situations in which nutrient sensors are chronically affected by excessive amounts of certain nutrients (e.g. carbohydrates and some fats) lead to the development of common characteristics of obesity and type 2 diabetes mellitus (T2D), such as insulin resistance, oxidative stress, and the dysfunction of organelles including the endoplasmic reticulum and mitochondria [4].

The increasing number of overweight and obese people, and associated diseases such as T2D, is driving research to explore the basic mechanisms that maintain nutrient homeostasis in a healthy state and the molecular mechanisms disrupted in T2D and obesity, as well as the neural and molecular underpinnings of feeding behavior. A central role in these disease-related mechanisms corresponds to nutrient sensing and the regulation of feeding behavior [1].

Glucose is a critical nutrient in mammals, with extracellular and intracellular mechanisms to maintain its levels within a narrow physiological band.

Glucose is an energy substrate, but it is also a key molecule in the control of glucose-dependent insulin secretion by the pancreas. The increase in insulin in the blood as glycaemia facilitates the uptake of glucose by the liver and skeletal muscle, highlighting the cooperation and retro-regulation between glucose and insulin signaling. In short, circulating and intracellular glucose, acting as a signaling molecule, is detected by different glucose sensors that modulate eating behavior and the release of counter-regulatory hormones in response to hypoglycemic states. The answer is therefore to maintain glucose and energy homeostasis [5], avoiding the development of T2D and other diseases. Some of the main nutrient sensors described are the following:

- **Glucokinase (GCK)**: It is an enzyme that catalyzes the phosphorylation of glucose to glucose-6-phosphate. GCK is expressed in hepatocytes, pancreatic α and β cells, entero-endocrine cells, and specialized brain cells in humans and most other vertebrates. It is considered a true glucose sensor due to its kinetic properties that ensure that the rate of glucose phosphorylation is proportional to blood glucose levels. For example, pancreatic GCK connects glucose sensing to insulin secretion by the pancreatic β-cell, and so regulates blood glucose homeostasis.
  GCK in the liver is also a glucose sensor (**Figure 1**). Its activity regulates the rate of glycogen accumulation and hepatic glucose production [6].
  Mutations in the GCK gene that increase enzyme activity lead to hypoglycemia due to hyperinsulinism, while mutations that decrease enzyme activity lead to hyperglycemia or diabetes. Due to its importance in glucose homeostasis, this enzyme is one of the main study targets for the development of a new antidiabetic therapy strategy [7].

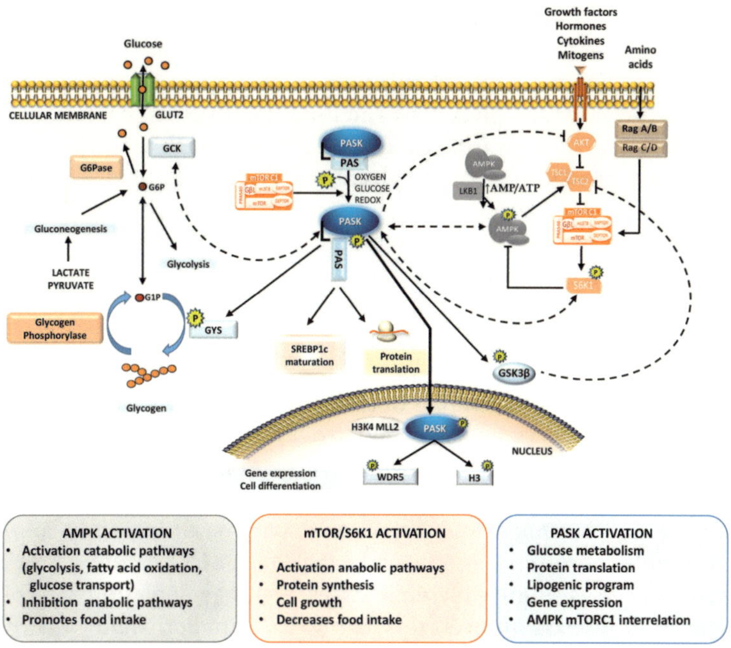


**Figure 1.**
*PASK signaling interaction with other nutrient sensors. PAS domains detect environmental parameters (light, oxygen and redox state). A metabolite or protein binds to the PAS domain after transient activation auto- or transphosphorylation stabilizes and activates PASK. Physiological effects of PASK in other nutrient sensors (glucose transporter (GLUT2), glucokinase (GCK), AMP-activated kinase (AMPK) and mammalian target of rapamycin (mTOR))/S6K pathway due to activation or inhibition (direct: solid lines; indirect: dashed lines)*

Additionally, GCK is a key component in glucose-sensing neurons located in the hypothalamus [8–10].

- **Glucose transporter GLUT-2**: It is a glucose transporter that acts as a sensor of changes in extracellular glucose levels. This is due to a high Km (more than other glucose transporters of the same family) and thus a very low affinity for glucose, allowing a rapid equilibrium between the glucose concentration on both sides of the membrane, independently of the action of insulin [11]. GLUT2 is expressed mainly in hepatic cells, pancreatic β cells, basolateral membranes of intestinal, renal epithelial cells, and in specific brain nuclei. In hepatic cells, GLUT2 involves an efficient transport of glucose across the plasmatic membrane only when intra- or extra-cellular glucose is high, being a key controller of glucose homeostasis (**Figure 1**). β-pancreatic cells take up glucose through the GLUT-2 transporter and carry out insulin synthesis and secretion. Glucose transport by GLUT-2 and then GCK facilitates oxidation by increasing intracellular ATP, which leads to signaling via ATP-dependent $K^+$ channels [1]. Decreased GLUT2 levels in pancreatic β cells have been detected in cases of diabetes in both animals and human patients.
GLUT2 is also found in neurons located in certain glucose-sensing brain regions involved in controlling feeding behavior [9, 12, 13].

- **AMP activated protein kinase (AMPK):** It is a heterotrimeric complex with a serine/threonine kinase domain [14, 15]. AMPK perceives cellular energy availability by detecting the AMP/ATP ratio (**Figure 1**). This kinase is activated in states of low energy availability or metabolic stress that reduces

ATP production (e.g. heat shock, hypoxia, ischemia and fasting conditions) or accelerates its consumption (muscle contraction). Once active, AMPK acts by inhibiting the anabolic pathways responsible for the synthesis of macromolecules (proteins and glycogen) and lipids (fatty acids, triglycerides and cholesterol), and by activating catabolic pathways, such as the β-oxidation of fatty acids, glucose uptake and glycolysis. The net result of AMPK activity is the restoration of the energy balance, as the main energy sensor [16]. The AMPK pathway at central level integrates peripheral information through nutrients and hormones. Hypothalamic AMPK is involved in feeding behavior, the thermogenesis of brown adipose tissue (BAT) and browning of white adipose tissue (WAT) [17, 18].

- **Mammalian Target of Rapamycin (mTOR)**: The mTORC1 complex is a serine/threonine kinase which forms part of the mTOR/S6K pathway integrating nutrients, hormones, growth factors and cellular energy levels to control protein transcription and synthesis and cell size, growth, metabolism, autophagy and thermogenesis [19]. Growth factors, amino acids, mitogens, and favorable energy states activate the mTORC1/S6K1 pathway, promoting anabolic processes (**Figure 1**), while states of energy depletion and cellular stress such as hypoxia suppress this pathway. The hypothalamic mTORC1 complex is an energy sensor involved in food intake and body weight control [20, 21]. AMPK and mTORC1 act together in food intake regulation, as low nutrient levels during fasting activate AMPK, although the mTORC1 complex remains inactive, while the activity of these sensors is reversed after food ingestion, indicating that AMPK and mTORC1 could have opposite functions in the control of feeding behavior [22].

- **PAS kinase (PASK):** It is also called PASKIN, and is defined as the protein kinase that contains an N-terminal Per-Arnt-Sim (PAS) domain and a C-terminal serine/threonine kinase catalytic domain [23]. Like AMPK and mTORC1, it is a nutrient-responsive protein that regulates glucose metabolism and cellular energy, and is also responsive to a variety of intracellular cues, including light, oxygen, and redox state, among many others [24]. In mammals, PASK may be activated by small metabolites, and could regulate glycogen synthesis and protein translation (**Figure 1**), in addition to being involved in the regulation of glucose homeostasis and energy metabolism [25–27], and epigenetics and differentiation [28].

This chapter will focus on the study of this last sensor, and like AMPK and mTORC1, it can be considered a pharmacological target for diseases, such as obesity and diabetes.

### 2.1 Neuronal and peripheral regulation of homeostasis by nutrient sensing

The key to maintaining homeostatic and energy control is a balanced food intake and energy expenditure, whereas altered regulation leads to obesity and T2D. The regulation of the energy balance is controlled by the hypothalamus, as the central organ that integrates nutrient levels and hormonal changes. The hypothalamic response to regulate glucose and whole-body energy homeostasis is to control food intake and several physiological functions in peripheral organs, such as lipid metabolism and thermogenesis [29, 30]. The brain receives inputs from nutrients, adiposity signals, and hormonal neural and metabolic signaling from the gastrointestinal tract. The gut-brain and gut-brain-liver axes act to regulate energy and glucose homeostasis, respectively [31–33]. The brain likewise controls energy-consuming processes such as skeletal muscle fatty acid oxidation, thermogenesis, and locomotor activity [34]. Deficient intercommunications between the brain and peripheral organs may contribute to the appearance of obesity and T2D [30, 33].

The hypothalamus is a key brain area for maintaining an energy balance and homeostasis. Hypothalamic areas thereby play a key role in the control of food intake and energy homeostasis. The mid-20th century recorded the first indications that the electrical stimulation of the ventromedial hypothalamus (VMH) suppresses food intake, and that bilateral lesions of these areas induce hyperphagia and obesity. The VMH has therefore been called the satiety center. By contrast, alterations in the lateral hypothalamic area (LH) induce the opposite set of responses, and the LH is hence called the hunger center. Changes in blood glucose levels can be monitored by neuronal cells located in the hypothalamus or the brain stem [35]. They can therefore act as a true glucose sensor in the control of food intake and energy homeostasis. In fact, the first brain glucose sensors were discovered in the VMH and LH nucleus, where circulating glucose concentrations drive changes in neuronal electrical activity [36, 37]. This means glucose would act mainly as an excitatory molecule in certain VMH neurons, and as an inhibitory molecule in those of LH and the nucleus of the tractus solitarius (NTS) [38]. This is due to at least two kinds of glucose sensor neurons: glucose-excited neurons (GE) are located mainly in the VMH (as well as the arcuate nucleus, ARC, and the paraventricular nucleus PVN), and are excited by increased glucose levels in the extracellular space, while glucose-inhibited neurons (GI) are present mainly in the LH, median ARC, and PVN, and are excited by decreases in glucose concentrations [10, 37, 39]. It has been suggested that the activation of the firing rate of GE neurons depends on the closure of the ATP-sensitive $K^{+}_{ATP}$ channels by increases in extracellular glucose (similar electrophysiological pattern to β-pancreatic cells), whereas GI neurons may increase their firing rate in response to hypoglycemia following the inactivation of the $Na^{+}$/$K^{+}$-ATPase pump (similar electrophysiological pattern to α-pancreatic cells) [40].

Some of the component molecules responsible for the hypothalamic glucose sensing systems are as follows: GCK, GLUT-2, and the GLP-1 receptor, which are co-expressed in areas involved in energy homeostasis regulation, food intake, and glucose metabolism [9, 12, 41, 42]. The most glucose-sensitive regulator seems to be the GCK, which is present in both GE and GI neurons (albeit to a lesser extent) [43]. However, glucose transporters such as GLUT-2, GLUT-3, the insulin-dependent transporter (GLUT-4), and the sodium-glucose transporter (SGLT) do not seem to have a predominant role in the response by GE and GI neurons to alterations in glucose levels [10]. GE neurons are known to use GLUT-2 for glucose uptake, then GCK mediates the phosphorylation, and the glucose oxidation increases ATP/ADP, leading to the closure of ATP-sensitive $K^{+}_{ATP}$ channels and depolarization, promoting $Ca^{2+}$ influx and neurotransmitter release [33, 44, 45].

Hypothalamic sensing neurons also use fatty acids (FA) as signaling molecules [46]. Some of these sensing neurons respond to both FA and glucose, whereby these neurons distinguish between fasting and feeding states. When the effect of glucose is excitatory, FA tend to inhibit those neurons [46]. A deficiency of fatty acid translocator/receptor CD36 in VMH neurons stimulates food intake, enhances insulin resistance, and increases body weight and fat mass in lean and obese rats [47]. FA sensing therefore plays a key role in integrating signals for regulating glucose and energy homeostasis and fat deposition.

It has also been reported that FA are oxidized by astrocytes in VMH under a low-fat diet, while under a high-fat diet (HFD) astrocytes in this area generate ketone bodies that can be exported to neurons and signal a decrease in short-term food intake and protect against obesity. However, this effect is lost when besides

HFD there is a resistance to leptin. Animals in these cases remain hyperphagic and exposed to obesity [48].

Additionally, with changes in nutrient concentrations some neurons located in hypothalamic nuclei secrete and respond to the hormones and neuropeptides involved in the control of food intake and energy homeostasis.

For example, the ARC secretes hormones and detects inputs from the peripheral signals involved in the control of feeding behavior. There are two important subpopulations of secretory neurons in ARC: one synthetizes the α-melanocyte-stimulating hormone (α-MSH) derived from pro-opiomelanocortin (POMC), as well as the cocaine- and amphetamine-regulated transcript (CART); both of which are anorexigenic peptides. The second subpopulation of neurons secretes the agouti-related protein (AgRP) and neuropeptide Y (NPY) orexigenic peptides [49]. These peptides are directed by nerve fibers to other important hypothalamic regions, and their synthesis and release coordinate with metabolic sensors to accurately control eating behavior and energy metabolism. Additionally, these two populations and other neurons located in different hypothalamic nuclei have receptors for hormones secreted peripherally, such as leptin, insulin, ghrelin, and other gastrointestinal peptides, such as glucagon like peptide (GLP-1), which in turn are being secreted under the control of changes in nutrient availability.

AMPK is another hypothalamic molecule responsible for energy sensing. It has been reported to act as an "energy integrator", and not only perceives the cellular energy state, but also has a role in the regulatory mechanisms of body energy homeostasis [50, 51]. It has a mainly neuronal distribution [52], highly expressed in ARC, PVN, VMH and LH, with AMPKα2 being the most predominant isoform [53].

Fasting increases and feeding decreases AMPK activity in various hypothalamic nuclei [18, 53]. Several studies have shown that hypothalamic AMPK is regulated by blood glucose levels. Peripheral or central hyperglycemia inhibits AMPK in several hypothalamic nuclei. Furthermore, the anorexigenic neuronal signaling (NPY/AgRP) is AMPK-dependent in the hypothalamus. Thus, AMPK mutants have suppressed the NPY/AgRP response, and therefore food intake, reducing body weight. However, elevated AMPK increases NPY/AgRP expression, food intake and body weight [53, 54].

Fasting and feeding are accompanied by hormonal and nutrient changes both in peripheral tissues and in the CNS, which can lead to variations in AMPK activity. Accordingly, AMPK integrates nutritional information and hormonal signals. Several studies have shown that fasting and orexigenic signals (e.g. ghrelin, adiponectin, cannabinoids and glucocorticoids) increase hypothalamic AMPK activity, contributing to an increase in food intake; by contrast, food and anorectic signals such as leptin, insulin, resistin, GLP-1 and α-MSH decrease this kinase's activity, helping to generate a state of satiety. AMPK activation therefore promotes food intake, while the decrease in its enzymatic activity is associated with hypophagia. This effect is due, at least in part, to an increase in the expression of NPY and AgRP in the arcuate nucleus, and of MCH in the lateral hypothalamus [17, 18, 54].

AMPK activity can induce appetite via the inhibition of malonyl-CoA and the activation of carnitine palmitoyltransferase-1 (CPT-1). The inhibition of malonyl-CoA leads to decreased fatty acid synthesis and increased $\beta$-oxidation. Furthermore, increased $\beta$-oxidation could induce orexigenic gene expression. In addition, AMPK activation through the sympathetic nerve can reduce thermogenesis and energy expenditure. Additionally, activated hypothalamic AMPK may prompt enhanced glucose production [55].

Besides AMPK, mTORC1 is another hypothalamic metabolic sensor regulator of feeding behavior and body weight [20]. mTORC1 and the downstream target S6K1 are widely distributed in the brain, mainly in the PVN and ARC. Their signaling responds to nutrient availability and is colocalized with NPY/AgRP and POMC/CART neurons in the ARC [20]. mTORC1 activation decreases food intake and body weight [56]. mTORC1 integrates signals from nutrients, adiposity signals, and gut hormones [21]. Hypothalamic AMPK and mTORC1 respond to nutrient levels in opposite ways [57, 58]. Additionally, mTORC1 is inhibited by AMPK activation via the tuberous sclerosis complex 2 (TSC2) [59, 60]. Moreover, AMPK is also a substrate for the mTOR-S6K1 pathway (**Figure 1**) [22].

In short, the interplay between both hypothalamic pathways plays an important role in regulating food intake and body weight.

Several peripheral signals are involved in controlling food intake and energy homeostasis. Moreover, changes in nutrient levels involving glucose [61] and FA [62, 63] or ketone bodies [48], adiposity signals (leptin, insulin) [64], and gastrointestinal (ghrelin [65], GLP-1 [57, 58, 66]) signals, alter the activity of sensing neurons located in the VMH and other brain areas.

Two peripheral hormones, leptin and insulin, provide the brain with information about the energy stored as adipose tissue [64]. Leptin and insulin levels in plasma correlate with adipose mass and body weight. Insulin levels correlate better with visceral adiposity [67]. Its plasma levels also reflect changes, decreasing during fasting and increasing during feeding; glucose-induced insulin secretion is also dependent on body fat (review by Benoit et al.) [64]. Obesity is frequently related to insulin resistance as higher insulin levels are required to maintain suitable levels of blood glucose. The administration of insulin to the brain reduces food intake and increases energy expenditure [68]. Impaired insulin signaling due to neuronal deletion of the insulin receptor and insulin receptor substrate 2 (IRS2) increases food intake [69]. Leptin is secreted by adipose tissue, and blood levels correlate directly with adiposity [70]. Leptin receptor deficiency has been related to hyperphagia and obesity [71]. However, leptin supplied to the ARC reduces food intake and body weight, and promotes locomotor activity [72].

Hormones secreted in the gut after feeding as cholecystokinin and GLP-1 promote satiety when administered centrally and peripherally [66]. By contrast, ghrelin released under fasting conditions by the stomach acts as an orexigenic signal inducing food intake [31].

The liver plays a vital role in regulating whole-body glucose and lipid homeostasis. It is the main site for the synthesis, metabolism, storage and redistribution of carbohydrates, proteins and lipids, especially during the adjustment periods in fasting and feeding. In postprandial states, the liver is exposed to more ingested nutrients and to higher levels than other tissues. The liver is especially responsible for much of glucose uptake when hyperinsulinemia and hyperglycemia coincide, storing it as a glycogen and associated to a reduction in muscle glucose uptake [73]. The efficiency of hepatic glucose uptake is coordinated neurally, depending also on diet components and high-fat and high-fructose decreases in glycogen storage. Glucose transport is facilitated by GLUT2, with the intrahepatic glucose concentration being similar to that of blood glucose. Its metabolism therefore depends on GCK activity, which in part determines glycogen synthesis [74]. By contrast, when blood glucose drops, and other organs require energy, the liver produces glucose by glycogenolysis and/or gluconeogenesis. Gluconeogenesis is responsible for half of the total glucose produced by the liver during an overnight fast, so this contribution is essential for glucose homeostasis [75]. Therefore, hepatic metabolism is critical for proper glucose homeostasis in response to insulin and for preventing diabetes [73, 75]. Insulin in the hypothalamic nuclei regulates hepatic glucose production [76, 77]. Insulin acts on the brain (hypothalamus and brain stem), also modulating pancreatic insulin and glucagon secretion [78]. The close coordination between the brain and peripheral organs helps to maintain whole-body glucose and energy homeostasis.

In turn, there is a close relationship between the appearance of insulin resistance in the liver and the development of T2D [79, 80]. Decreased hepatic insulin sensitivity contributes to postprandial hyperglycemia and enhances hepatic glucose production, leading to exacerbated hyperglycemia and chronic hyperinsulinemia in diabetics [81]. There is evidence to suggest that impairing insulin hypothalamic signaling [82] or an HFD [83] contributes to the appearance of diabetes.

## 3. PASK: a new nutrient sensor

PASK is an evolutionarily conserved nutrient-responsive protein kinase that regulates glucose homeostasis, senses a cell's energy or nutrient status, and suitably regulates cellular metabolism. PASK responds to glucose availability and regulates glucose homeostasis in yeast, rodents and mammals. Despite this pivotal role, the molecular mechanisms of PASK regulation and function are largely unknown [84].

PAS domains (see Section 2) are versatile sensors designed to detect environmental parameters, such as light, oxygen and redox state [24]. These domains are often regulated by the binding of a diverse group of small ligands, including ATP, heme or flavins, within the hydrophobic pocket at the core of the domain (review by Henry et al.) [85]. As with other PAS domains, the PASK adopts this characteristic fold and binds small organic molecules within its hydrophobic core [86]. Unlike other PAS domains, however, the physiological ligand(s) for PASK remain unknown. *In vitro* experiments performed indicate that this domain should inhibit kinase activity [84].

In a hypothetical activation model, a metabolite or protein activates PASK by binding to the PAS domain and relieving PAS domain inhibition. This transient activation may subsequently be stabilized through auto- or transphosphorylation (**Figure 1**). PASK can then phosphorylate several substrates (**Figure 2**) [23, 27, 86, 87].

PASK is known to be a physiological regulator of glucose metabolism, functioning in pancreatic islet cells regulating glucagon and insulin secretion [88, 89]; several translation factors and glycogen synthase are PASK substrates [90, 91], suggesting its implication in the control of protein synthesis and glycogen metabolism.

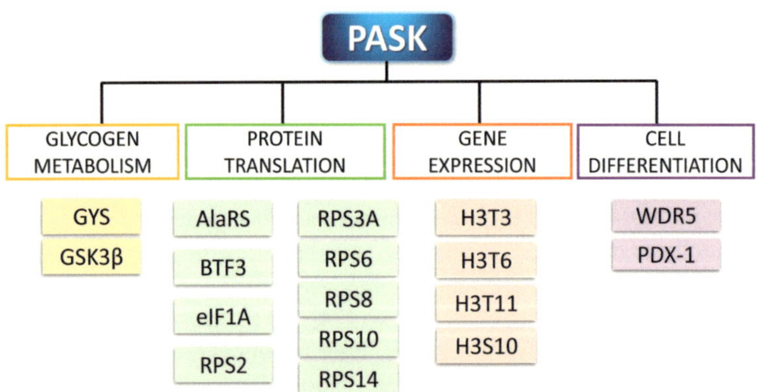


**Figure 2.**
*PAS Kinase substrates in mammals. Cellular process regulated by PAS kinase and* in vitro *or* in vivo *substrates identified in mammals. Glycogen metabolism: Glycogen synthase (GYS), Glycogen synthase kinase 3 beta (GSK3β). Protein translation: Alanine-tRNA ligase (AlaRS); Basic transcription factor 3 (BTF3); Eukaryotic translation elongation factor (eIF1A); Ribosomal proteins S2, S3A, S6, S8, S10 and S14 (RPS2), (RPS3A), (RPS6), (RPS8), (RPS10) and (RPS14). Gene expression: Histone H3 tails residues threonine 3, 6, 11 and serine 10 (H3T3), (H3T6), (H3T11) and (H3S10); Cell differentiation: WD repeat-containing protein 5 (WDR5) and Pancreatic Duodenal Homeobox 1 (PDX1).*

Katschinski et al. [92] have been the first to inactivate mouse gene coding to PASK. These PASK-deficient mice (PASK$^{-/-}$) recorded normal development, growth and reproduction. It was subsequently found that PASK$^{-/-}$ male mice are resistant to weight gain, hepatic triglyceride accumulation, and insulin resistance when placed on an HFD [93]. Without a change in food intake or exercise, these PASK$^{-/-}$ male mice also record a hypermetabolic phenotype, giving off more $CO_2$ and taking in more $O_2$. PASK is involved in the proteolytic maturation of the sterol regulatory binding protein (SREBP1c), the main lipogenic transcription factor [94, 95]. SREBP1c activity and target genes decreased in PASK$^{-/-}$ mice, with an associated decrease in hepatic lipid deposits [96].

Lipids are important substances that store energy for oxidation and metabolism. As the main cause of imbalanced lipid metabolism, excessive lipid accumulation in the liver has been involved in the development of metabolic syndromes, such as T2D, obesity, hepatic adipose infiltration and unpredicted morbidity. It is therefore extremely important to maintain a balance between lipid synthesis and catabolism. PASK has been reported to regulate many of the phenotypes.

PASK deficiency decreases insulin production, insulin resistance, body weight and hepatic triglyceride accumulation, while leading to increased glycogen storage, as well as metabolic rate [97]. Some of the effects observed in PASK$^{-/-}$ have also been confirmed using PASK pharmacologic inhibitors [98].

Our studies have been based on this mouse model. PASK$^{-/-}$ mice have been described by Hao et al. [93], and generously donated to us by Dr. Roland H. Wegner (Veterinary Department of the canton of Zurich).

New PASK functions have recently been described, including the unexpected role it has in promoting the differentiation of myogenic progenitor cells, embryonic stem cells, and adipogenic progenitor cells. This PASK function is dependent upon its ability to phosphorylate WD repeat-containing protein 5 (WDR5), which is a member of several protein complexes, including those that catalyze histone H3 Lysine 4 trimethylation (H3K4me3) during transcriptional activation. Thus, as an upstream kinase of WDR5, PASK integrates signaling cues with the transcriptional network to regulate the differentiation of progenitor cells [99]. In addition, the phosphorylation of PASK by mTORC1 is required for the activation of myogenin transcription, exiting from self-renewal, and the induction of the myogenesis program. mTORC1-PASK signaling is required for increasing myogenin-positive committed myoblasts (early stage of myogenesis) [100].

Moreover, it has been confirmed that the metabolic sensor PASK could affect both the phosphorylation and the methylation of histone H3 tails. It contributes to the methylation of H3 lysine 4 (H3K4) di- and tri-methylation through its association with the H3K4 MLL2 methyltransferase complex and to the phosphorylation of several threonine residues (T3, T6 and T11) and serine (S10) on H3 as a histone kinase [101]. The methylation of histone H3 lysine 4 H3K4 has been linked to transcriptional activation.

## 4. PASK hypothalamic function in food intake and energy homeostasis

The hypothalamus is the key to controlling food intake. The identification of hypothalamic glucose sensing systems and neuronal populations expressing and responding to orexigenic and anorexigenic peptides (see Section 2.1) has focused the studies on the hypothalamic nuclei. They have been specifically directed toward identifying the mechanisms involved in controlling nutrient sensing, feeding behavior and its relationship with insulin actions in the central nervous system in order to regulate energy and glucose homeostasis. Hypothalamic metabolic sensors respond in opposite ways to changes in nutrients and orexigenic or anorexigenic peptides, and their activation/inhibition regulates food intake. For example, the hypothalamic AMPK is activated by fasting and inhibited by refeeding [53, 57, 102], and the mTORC1/S6K pathway is activated by glucose and amino acids, inhibiting food intake [20, 57, 103]. Both pathways are involved in controlling feeding and regulating the energy balance.

In 2013, PASK was identified in the hypothalamic areas involved in feeding behavior, and its expression was regulated under fasting/refeeding conditions [104, 105]. It was proposed as a hypothalamic and liver nutrient sensor and a general regulator of glucose metabolism and cellular energy. Moreover, $PASK^{-/-}$ mice resist diet-induced obesity [93]; it might therefore be understood that PASK could control the hypothalamic function related to intake control. For example, elevated glucose levels decrease mRNA coding to PASK in VMH and LH areas in hypothalamic organotypic cultures and in neuroblastoma N2A cells [104]. The PASK expression is also regulated *in vivo* in response to fasting/refeeding conditions. This effect is clearer in LH: mRNA coding to PASK is lower under fasting conditions and increases in response to refeeding conditions [105]. The effect observed after refeeding *in vivo* is the opposite to the glucose effect found in VMH and LH in hypothalamic organotypic cultures and neuroblastoma N2A cells. However, the effect is similar to those produced in the presence of both glucose and the anorexigenic peptide GLP-1 (an incretin release from intestinal L-cells in response to feeding) [106, 107]. The role of PASK in the hypothalamus would be similar to other well-known metabolic sensors, such as AMPK and mTORC1. The activation of AMPK and mTORC1 is coordinated and antagonistic. While AMPK is activated by a fall in energy, mTORC1 is activated by its increase. Hypothalamic metabolic sensors, such as AMPK and mTORC1, therefore play an important role in feeding behavior, body weight homeostasis, and energy balance (see Section 2.1). These sensors respond to changes in nutrient levels in the VMH and LH (hypothalamic areas involved in feeding behavior) and in neuroblastoma N2A cells, and those effects are modulated by the GLP-1 in lean and obese rats [57].

Studies in $PASK^{-/-}$ mice have indicated that PASK-deficiency involves a downregulation of mRNA levels coding to AMPKα2 in VMH, and slightly so in LH [105], while impairing the coordination of the AMPK and mTORC1/S6K1 pathways. Thus, both the AMPK and mTORC1/S6K1 pathways are surprisingly activated at the same time under fasting and feeding conditions in $PASK^{-/-}$ mice [105]. This finding could mean that the inhibition of mTORC1/S6K through AMPK activation requires the coordinated phosphorylation of TSC2 by Glycogen synthase kinase 3β (GSK3β) [59], which is a PASK substrate *in vitro,* and PASK deficiency could therefore alter hypothalamic GSK3β activity [108]. Additionally, this study has found that the exendin-4 regulatory effect on metabolic sensor activity is lost in $PASK^{-/-}$ mice, and the anorexigenic properties of exendin-4 significantly reduced, suggesting that PASK could be a mediator in the brain GLP-1 signaling pathway. Some of the antidiabetogenic effects of exendin-4 might be modulated through these processes. This means that hypothalamic PASK, interacting with AMPK and mTORC1 pathways, and in coordination with anorexigenic/orexigenic peptides, could be a key enzyme in food intake control, and in peripheral tissue functions, such as brown adipose tissue thermogenesis, pancreatic insulin secretion, etc. However, more studies are needed to clarify this hypothesis and the putative molecular mechanism of PASK actions in whole-body physiology.

The downregulation of mRNA coding to AMPKα2 and the modulation of the GLP-1 effects in hypothalamus in $PASK^{-/-}$ mice suggest that both effects may also be regulating thermogenesis in BAT and the browning of white fat, as both processes are mediated by the inhibition of hypothalamic AMPK [109, 110].

As well as acting in hypothalamic functions, PASK also has key functions in the peripheral tissues. For example, diabetes and PASK have been linked, as a human mutation of the *PASK* gene has been correlated with maturity-onset diabetes of the young (MODY). This mutation increases kinase activity and decreases glucose-stimulated insulin secretion by the pancreas [111]. In addition, decreased PASK expression in pancreatic islets has been reported in human T2D [88]. The PASK function in peripheral tissues could be crucial for maintaining metabolic and energy homeostasis.

## 5. PASK contribution to hepatic adaptation to fasting/feeding

The liver maintains metabolic homeostasis, and it is especially essential in the proper control of glucose during fasting and feeding periods. In particular, the liver is one of the main insulin-responsive organs, so it records a greater glucose uptake when glycaemia rises, storing it as glycogen (see Section 2.1). By contrast, when blood glucose falls, and other organs require energy, the liver produces glucose by glycogenolysis and gluconeogenesis. Therefore, the correct hepatic response to insulin and hepatic metabolism are critical for maintaining glycaemia within physiological ranges, and therefore for the proper control of diabetes.

Studies with PASK$^{-/-}$ mice have reported the critical role PASK plays in hepatic adaptation to fasting/feeding periods, especially under an HFD [93, 112]. It is interesting that PASK expression is regulated in the liver by fasting/feeding, with fasting downregulating it [112]. Moreover, Perez-Garcia et al. [113] have found that PASK deficiency alters the complex hepatic response to fasting/feeding. The expression of the transcription factors and key enzymes that regulate gluconeogenesis and mitochondrial fatty acid transport under fasting conditions is altered in PASK$^{-/-}$ mice, with lower forkhead box protein O1 (*Foxo 1*) and carnitine palmitoyltransferase 1A (*Cpt1a*) and higher peroxisome proliferator-activated receptor alpha (*Ppara*). Similarly, PASK deficiency modifies the activity of the protein kinase B (AKT) overactivated under fasting and the stability of phosphoenolpyruvate carboxykinase (PEPCK) [113], while no detectable changes have been observed in the maintenance of blood glucose homeostasis during prolonged fasting periods [105].

A good example of PASK deficiency effects under feeding involves the changes recorded in GCK, which is a critical enzyme in the hepatic function. GCK is an enzyme involved in hepatic glucose sensing (see Section 2). This enzyme is activated by the increase in blood glucose which occurs in feeding periods. It therefore adjusts hepatic glucose phosphorylation to blood glucose levels, acting as a glucose sensor. The importance of GCK in maintaining glucose homeostasis is evidenced by the severe impacts caused by mutations in the GCK gene. The loss of GCK function in the human body causes maturity-onset diabetes of the young type 2 (MODY2) [114]. By contrast, activating mutations generate persistent hyperinsulinemia [115]. Many liver functions are controlled by GCK, which acts together with insulin in the maintenance of blood glucose homeostasis [116], and the activation of glycolytic and lipogenic gene expression. GCK is also involved in glycogen synthesis and storage in the liver [117]. The enzymatic activity of GCK is controlled by transcriptional and posttranscriptional mechanisms. While the transcriptional regulation of the GCK gene is basically insulin-dependent [118], the posttranscriptional mechanisms of regulation involve interaction with other proteins, highlighting the glucokinase regulatory protein (GCKR). GCKR modulates GCK activity when glucose levels decline by binding and sequestering it in the nucleus, and thus avoiding its function in the cytoplasm [116, 119].

Studies relating the role of PASK to the GCK function [113] have revealed that GCK activity is reduced in PASK$^{-/-}$ mice for two reasons: on the one hand, the lower protein expression, and on the other, its mainly nuclear location. It cannot be ruled out that the decrease in GCK may be partly due to the blocking of lipogenesis that characterizes PASK$^{-/-}$ mice. In addition, the conversion of excess carbohydrates into lipids might also be limited by the low levels of acetyl CoA carboxylase (ACC) and fatty acid synthase (FAS), although the gene coding to ACC and liver pyruvate kinase (LPK) is overexpressed under non-fasted conditions in PASK$^{-/-}$ mice. Additionally, glycogen metabolism could also be modified because glycogen synthase is a PASK substrate [90].

The hepatic PASK role in the control of hepatic adaptation to fasting/feeding becomes more important under an HFD because it dysregulates hepatic metabolic responses to fasting and feeding, leading to a non-alcoholic fatty liver, obesity, insulin resistance, diabetes, and associated cardiovascular problems. Some studies have evidenced that PASK$^{-/-}$ mice fed with a HFD resist the development of obesity and hepatic steatosis, with improved insulin sensitivity [93, 96, 112]. A consequence of an HFD for the liver is that it alters the downregulation of the *Pask* expression produced by fasting, as normally happens in a standard-fat diet [112]. Interestingly, PASK$^{-/-}$ mice with an HFD record improved parameters for the following: body weight, glucose tolerance, insulin resistance (see Section 6.1.), and serum lipid parameters [112]. Some of the PASK effects are due to changes in the proteolytic maturation of SREBP1c, others by regulating transcription factors and enzymes that play a key role in the hepatic response to fasting/feeding. Thus, PASK deficiency compensates for gene expression altered by an HFD. For example, it decreases the expression of genes overexpressed in HFD-fed mice (transcription factors involved in the regulation of gluconeogenic enzymes, the transport of fatty acid into mitochondria, β-oxidation, and *de novo* lipogenesis). PASK also modifies the expression of the short noncoding RNAs involved in lipid metabolism and glucose homeostasis. Such is the case of miR-33a and miR-143, whose expression in HFD-fed mice is controlled by PASK. Thus, PASK deficiency improves the hepatic adaptation to feeding/fasting, especially under pathogenic situations such as an HFD, through a highly regulated molecular mechanism that controls the expression and function of the transcription factors, enzymes and miRNAs involved in glucose and insulin signaling.

PASK deficiency also improves oxidative metabolism and mitochondrial biogenesis [120], increasing the ROS-detoxifying enzymes and the expression of *FoxO3a* and PTEN-induced kinase 1 (PINK1) involved in cell survival and mitophagy, respectively. All of these are interesting effects of PASK deficiency for states that increase oxidative stress, such as aging, diabetes, and obesity.

In sum, there are several results that highlight PASK's role in the control of the key genes and proteins that lead to hepatic metabolic adaptation to fasting or feeding situations.

Accordingly, PASK has been proposed as one of the possible targets for the treatment of the metabolic syndrome.

## 6. PASK and insulin resistance

The growing interest in the PASK function began with the finding that its deficiency prevents many of the deleterious effects of HFDs [93, 112], with a highlight being the insulin resistance that accompanies these diets, and which has been widely associated with the development of T2D [121, 122].

The same level of PASK is expressed in pancreatic α and β cells, and it is involved in insulin and glucagon secretion [88]. PASK promotes insulin expression [108], while PASK deficiency decreases the expression of preproinsulin at high glucose concentrations [123]. As for glucagon, PASK regulates its secretion by glucose [88].

PASK is also important in the development of pancreatic α and β cells, reflecting its key role in diabetes [89]. Thus, even though PASK deletion does not affect glucose-stimulated insulin secretion or insulin levels in response to fasting and feedback, it does decrease pancreatic β-cell mass in specific KO animals. By contrast, the deletion of PASK in pancreatic α cells improves glucagon secretion both *in vivo* and *in vitro*. PASK therefore plays a clear role in glucagon secretion and in the development of β-cell precursors.

There are two determining factors that promote the onset of T2D, dysfunctions in insulin secretion and peripheral resistance to the action of insulin. We cannot speak of a single class of T2D because there is considerable heterogeneity. In general, obesity prompts the metabolic syndrome [124], which in addition to obesity includes other pathologies such as hypertension, hypertriglyceridemia, elevated fasting glucose levels, and dyslipidemia. T2D is associated with insulin resistance (**Figure 3**), and over long periods it can lead to hyperinsulinemia. Finally, the pancreas fails and hypoinsulinemia sets in.

Insulin signaling activates the PI3K/AKT pathway that controls most metabolic effects (**Figure 3**) [125]. Insulin stimulates glucose uptake in muscle and adipose tissue, promoting glucose transporter type 4 (GLUT4) expression and translocation to the cell membrane [126, 127]. In turn, insulin decreases lipolysis in adipose tissue,

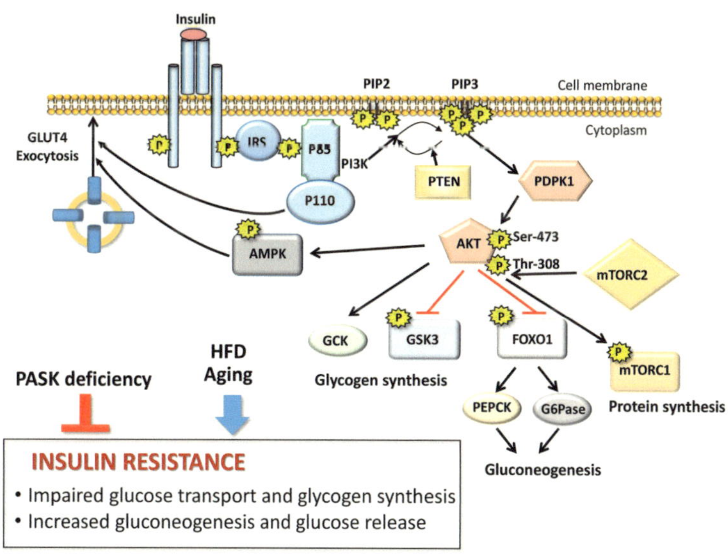


**Figure 3.**
*Insulin signaling and insulin resistance. Insulin signaling recruit insulin receptor substrates (IRS) activates the phosphoinositide 3-kinase (PI3K)/AKT pathway that controls most metabolic effects. In muscle and adipose tissue this pathway activates AMP-activated protein kinase (AMPK) promoting glucose transporter type 4 (GLUT4) expression and translocation to the cell membrane. In the liver this pathway activates glucokinase (GCK) and glycogen synthase kinase (GSK) inducing glycogen synthesis and suppresses gluconeogenesis inhibiting the expression of phosphoenolpyruvate carboxykinase (PEPCK) and glucose-6-phosphatase (G6Pase). Arrow stimulates, T bar red inhibits. Insulin resistance impairs the activation of PI3K/Akt pathway. In the skeletal muscle and adipose tissue impairs glucose uptake decreasing GLUT4 expression and translocation. In the liver insulin resistance suppresses glycogen synthesis and promotes gluconeogenesis through the expression of PEPCK and G6P genes.*

reducing the level of circulating free FA [128]. Insulin in the liver induces glycogen synthesis and suppresses gluconeogenesis [75].

The loss of sensitivity to insulin, generally called insulin resistance, affects this hormone's main peripheral target organs [125]. Insulin resistance could increase the concentration of free FA in the blood [129], decrease glucose uptake in skeletal muscle, and stimulate gluconeogenesis, increasing glucose release in the liver, thereby contributing to the metabolic syndrome [130, 131]. Abdominal obesity releases an excess of free FA, and the associated inflammation may interfere with insulin signaling [132].

### 6.1 Obesity, insulin resistance and PASK

Obesity in humans is defined as a body mass index (BMI = weight/height$^2$) of more than 30 kg/m$^2$. There are numerous studies linking fat intake and the onset of T2D, but it has not been possible to establish a consensus on the relationship between fat intake and obesity. A positive correlation has nonetheless been established between fat consumption and the BMI by Nagao et al. [121]. Moreover, the effect of consuming animal fats that contain high amounts of saturated fatty acids (SFAs) has also been compared with the consumption of fat with monounsaturated (MUFA) or polyunsaturated fatty acids (PUFA). PUFA intake is reported to reduce the risk of T2D. The variability detected also depends on the genetic factors that contribute 40% to the development of T2D [121].

Genetic variability is also considered in studies on the effect of an HFD in mice [121, 133]. In sum, a diet containing high amounts of animal or vegetable fat rich in saturated or unsaturated FA ω6/ω9 increases body weight and resistance to insulin appears, and to compensate there is an increase in insulin levels. These effects are not observed when using oils rich in unsaturated FA ω3 [134].

The liver's key function of maintaining metabolic homeostasis in both fasting and a postprandial state makes it one of the main organs affected by an HFD. It has been posited that a long-term HFD induces lipid (triglycerides) accumulation in hepatocytes as a result of insulin resistance. Nonalcoholic fatty liver disease (NAFLD) is the first step toward the onset of a chronic condition. This first step is followed by oxidative stress and impairment of the mitochondrial function, which triggers associated inflammation, hepatic damage and fibrosis [135, 136].

PASK$^{-/-}$ mice are protected against hepatic steatosis and the insulin resistance induced by an HFD [93]. We have reported that a long-term HFD severely alters the liver response needed to maintain metabolic homeostasis during fasting and feeding periods [112]. Firstly, the hepatic *Pask* expression is stimulated by feeding [96]. By contrast, HFD-fed mice have similar levels of hepatic *Pask* gene expression under fasting and feeding conditions [112]. Our results suggest that this effect might be responsible for some of the metabolic changes associated with this diet.

An HFD has a drastic effect on the expression of transcription factors that regulate the adaptation to fasting/feeding conditions. For instance, the transcription factors (FOXO1, peroxisome proliferator-activated receptor γ coactivator 1α (PGC1α) and PPARα) stimulated under fasting to promote the expression of the gluconeogenic enzymes (PEPCK and glucose 6-phosphatase (G6Pase)) and the genes that support fatty acid transport into mitochondria and β-oxidation are significantly overstimulated in HFD-fed mice. However, PASK deficiency blocks or diminishes the expression of all these genes under an HFD.

Similarly, the adaptation to a postprandial state is regulated by glucose and insulin through the expression of transcriptional factors (carbohydrate-responsive element-binding protein (CHREBP), liver X receptor alpha (LXRα) and *SREBP1*) [137, 138]. They promote the expression of lipogenic genes (*Acc1*, *Fas* and stearoyl-CoA desaturase-1 (*Scd1*)), stimulating the conversion of excess carbohydrates into FA and triglycerides. An HFD also overexpresses both *Lxrα* and peroxisome proliferator-activated receptor gamma (*Pparγ*) but this effect is diminished in PASK$^{-/-}$ mice [112]. The overexpression of *Lxrα* [139] and *Pparγ* [140, 141] has previously been associated with liver steatosis in human and mouse models of obesity and diabetes.

The effects of an HFD cause multiple changes in transcription factors and the key enzymes of the main hepatic metabolic pathways that allow metabolic adaptation. Genes promoting de novo lipogenesis that are expressed only under feeding conditions with a standard diet can also be overexpressed under fasting conditions with an HFD, which induces the overexpression of transcription factors and metabolic enzyme genes controlling de novo lipogenesis (*Chrebp*, *Lxrα*, *Srebp1c*, *Acc1* and *Scd1*) under a fasted state [112].

PASK deficiency eliminates many harmful effects that HFDs cause in the liver (**Figure 3**), also decreasing the lipid depots that over time can develop hepatic steatosis. Thus PASK$^{-/-}$ mice under an HFD have lower blood glucose levels, improve their sensitivity to the action of insulin, preventing the appearance of insulin resistance, which in turn is correlated with smaller increases in body weight and improved lipid profile [112]. PASK pharmacologic inhibition likewise confirms its key role for restoring insulin sensitivity, and for reducing hepatic fat content and the fibrosis caused by an HFD [98].

### 6.2 Aging, insulin resistance and PASK

The risk of T2D increases in aging due to the many imbalances that characterize this stage of life, which are often associated with overweight, impaired glucose metabolism, hypertension and dyslipidemia [142].

The aging process is characterized metabolically by the following: the development of insulin resistance (**Figure 3**), changes in body composition and mitochondrial dysfunction. In addition, hyperinsulinemia and glucose intolerance develop during aging [143, 144]. There are numerous metabolic changes in peripheral tissues that affect the uncontrolled gluconeogenesis of the liver, accompanied by an increase in lipogenesis in adipose tissue, and by defects in glycogen synthesis and glucose uptake in skeletal muscle [144]. Glucose metabolic dysfunction is closely correlated with oxidative stress, as occurs in diabetic or obese patients [145, 146].

Aging is normally accompanied by an increase in visceral fat, which is one of the main contributors to insulin resistance and the development of T2D. Likewise, it leads to an increase in proinflammatory cytokines, which interfere with insulin activity [144].

Another consequence of aging is the progressive loss of mitochondrial function in various tissues such as the liver or skeletal muscle. Thus, certain studies affirm that there is an association in aging between insulin resistance and glucose intolerance, together with a reduction in oxidative activity and mitochondrial ATP synthesis [144]. With aging, the liver undergoes molecular changes such as an increased inflammatory response, dysregulation of the genetic expression of antioxidant enzymes, and mitochondrial dysfunction, significantly altering redox homeostasis. It is also accompanied by the liver's reduced capacity for regeneration, which greatly affects liver function [147].

The nutrient sensing mechanisms needed to detect and respond to variations in their levels are dysregulated by aging [148]. So both nutrient sensor pathways, AMPK and mTORC1, are involved in a lifespan [149]. PASK senses intracellular oxygen, redox state and various metabolites [100]. Additionally, PASK regulates both AMPK and mTORC1 pathways [104, 105]. The aging process at cellular level is regulated by insulin/IGF signaling and both AMPK and mTORC1 pathways, which are in turn regulated by nutrient levels, whose signals converge on several targets: FOXO, nuclear factor: erythroid-derived 2-like 2 (NRF2), tumor protein p53, and sirtuins (SIRT) in order to control metabolic homeostasis, oxidative stress, and quality cellular housekeeping [150].

PASK$^{-/-}$ mice may avoid several of the deleterious defects induced by the aging process [151]. Aged PASK$^{-/-}$ mice maintain both low blood glucose values and insulin concentrations similar to young WT mice. They do not develop glucose intolerance or insulin resistance, as confirmed by a normal HOMA-IR index. These effects correlate with a high expression of the longevity gene *FoxO3a* and the transcription factor NRF2, as the main regulator of the redox balance [151]. Signaling through the system NRF2/KEAP1: kelch-like ECH-associated protein 1 regulates the transcription of enzymes that protect cells against oxidative stress [152]. An elevated expression of glutamate-cysteine ligase modifier subunit (GCLm) and heme oxygenase-1 (HO1) have been found in aged PASK$^{-/-}$ mice under fasted conditions. The efficiency of this redox system decreases in step with aging in WT mice, significantly diminishing the antioxidant response [153]. Likewise, PASK deficiency prevents the drastically age-related decrease in the expression of several antioxidant enzymes under basal conditions, such as catalase (CAT) and glutathione peroxidase (GPx) [151].

In relation to the maintenance of the mitochondrial function and energy homeostasis, we have confirmed that the expression of the several transcription factors and nuclear receptors needed to maintain mitochondrial biogenesis (*Ppargc1a, Sirt1* and *Nrf2)* are affected in fasted aged WT mice [151] in accordance with the previous literature that relates aging to a decrease in cellular energy input [154], an increase in oxidative stress [155], and the mitochondrial dysfunction of cellular redox homeostasis [156, 157]. However, the expression of *Nrf2, Ppargc1a, Ppar*$\gamma$ and *Sirt1* increases under fasting in aged PASK$^{-/-}$ mice. This means they maintain lower levels of ROS/RNS, while aged WT mice record a lower expression of antioxidant enzymes and increased levels of ROS/RNS [151].

We might therefore contend that some of the dysfunctions produced during aging in PASK$^{-/-}$ mice could be related to hormetic responses. Slight toxic effects can generate beneficial actions that compensate for the initial damage and even improve cellular health [158]. Aging decreases *Pask* expression in the liver of WT mice perhaps as a compensatory mechanism. PASK$^{-/-}$ mice maintain the same blood glucose values as young WT mice, and do not develop insulin resistance.

## 7. Conclusions

PASK function could be critical for preserving the nutrient effect on hypothalamic AMPK and mTORC1/S6K1 pathways and maintain the regulatory role of GLP1/exendin-4 in food intake.

PASK regulates the hepatic glucose sensor GCK and AKT, an insulin signaling intermediators, and glucose and lipidic metabolism through the regulation of the key genes and proteins required during hepatic fasting/feeding adaptation. Moreover, PASK deficiency improves mitochondrial biogenesis and antioxidant mechanisms.

HFDs alter the adaptive response of *Pask* gene expression to fasting/feeding. PASK deficiency eliminates many of the harmful effects HFDs have on the liver, thereby decreasing the lipid depots. PASK deficiency decreases the expression of several transcription factors stimulated under fasted conditions to promote the expression of the gluconeogenic enzymes and those promoting the expression of lipogenic genes after feeding that are significantly overstimulated in wild type HFD-fed mice.

PASK deficiency avoids insulin resistance and glucose intolerance during aging, preventing an age-related decrease in the expression of several antioxidant enzymes and improving mitochondrial function.

All these actions make PASK a significant pharmacological target for diseases, such as obesity and diabetes, and for preventing some of the more harmful effects of aging.

## Acknowledgements

This work was supported by grants from the Complutense University-Banco Santander Funding Programme for the Creation and Consolidation of Research Teams.

We thank Pilar Dongil for their contribution to this work.

## Conflict of interest

The authors declare no conflict of interest.

## Author details

Verónica Hurtado-Carneiro[1,3]*, Ana Pérez-García[1], Elvira Álvarez[1] and Carmen Sanz[1,2]

1 Department of Biochemistry and Molecular Biology, Faculty of Medicine, University Complutense of Madrid, Madrid, Spain

2 Department of Cellular Biology, Faculty of Medicine, University Complutense of Madrid, Madrid, Spain

3 Department of Physiology, Faculty of Medicine, University Complutense of Madrid, Madrid, Spain

*Address all correspondence to: verohur@ucm.es

## References

[1] Miyamoto T, Wright G, Amrein H. Nutrient sensors. Curr Biol. 2013;23(9):R369-73.

[2] Chantranupong L, Wolfson RL, Sabatini DM. Nutrient-sensing mechanisms across evolution. Cell. 2015;161(1):67-83.

[3] Efeyan A, Comb WC, Sabatini DM. Nutrient-sensing mechanisms and pathways. Nature. 2015;517(7534):302-10.

[4] Yamashita AS, Belchior T, Lira FS, Bishop NC, Wessner B, Rosa JC, et al. Regulation of Metabolic Disease-Associated Inflammation by Nutrient Sensors. Mediators Inflamm. 2018;2018:8261432.

[5] Ruud J, Steculorum SM, Bruning JC. Neuronal control of peripheral insulin sensitivity and glucose metabolism. Nat Commun. 2017;8:15259.

[6] Matschinsky FM, Magnuson MA, Zelent D, Jetton TL, Doliba N, Han Y, et al. The network of glucokinase-expressing cells in glucose homeostasis and the potential of glucokinase activators for diabetes therapy. Diabetes. 2006;55(1):1-12.

[7] Osbak KK, Colclough K, Saint-Martin C, Beer NL, Bellanne-Chantelot C, Ellard S, et al. Update on mutations in glucokinase (GCK), which cause maturity-onset diabetes of the young, permanent neonatal diabetes, and hyperinsulinemic hypoglycemia. Hum Mutat. 2009;30(11):1512-26.

[8] Roncero I, Alvarez E, Vazquez P, Blazquez E. Functional glucokinase isoforms are expressed in rat brain. J Neurochem. 2000;74(5):1848-57.

[9] Alvarez E, Martinez MD, Roncero I, Chowen JA, Garcia-Cuartero B, Gispert JD, et al. The expression of GLP-1 receptor mRNA and protein allows the effect of GLP-1 on glucose metabolism in the human hypothalamus and brainstem. J Neurochem. 2005;92(4):798-806.

[10] Levin BE, Routh VH, Kang L, Sanders NM, Dunn-Meynell AA. Neuronal glucosensing: what do we know after 50 years? Diabetes. 2004;53(10):2521-8.

[11] Williams TF, Exton JH, Park CR, Regen DM. Stereospecific transport of glucose in the perfused rat liver. Am J Physiol. 1968;215(5):1200-9.

[12] Roncero I, Alvarez E, Chowen JA, Sanz C, Rabano A, Vazquez P, et al. Expression of glucose transporter isoform GLUT-2 and glucokinase genes in human brain. J Neurochem. 2004;88(5):1203-10.

[13] Jurcovicova J. Glucose transport in brain - effect of inflammation. Endocr Regul. 2014;48(1):35-48.

[14] Hardie DG, Ross FA, Hawley SA. AMPK: a nutrient and energy sensor that maintains energy homeostasis. Nat Rev Mol Cell Biol. 2012;13(4):251-62.

[15] Garcia D, Shaw RJ. AMPK: Mechanisms of Cellular Energy Sensing and Restoration of Metabolic Balance. Mol Cell. 2017;66(6):789-800.

[16] Hardie DG. AMP-activated protein kinase: maintaining energy homeostasis at the cellular and whole-body levels. Annu Rev Nutr. 2014;34:31-55.

[17] Lopez M. Hypothalamic AMPK and energy balance. Eur J Clin Invest. 2018;48(9):e12996.

[18] Andersson U, Filipsson K, Abbott CR, Woods A, Smith K, Bloom SR, et al. AMP-activated protein kinase plays a role in the control

of food intake. J Biol Chem. 2004;279(13):12005-8.

[19] Saxton RA, Sabatini DM. mTOR Signaling in Growth, Metabolism, and Disease. Cell. 2017;168(6):960-76.

[20] Cota D, Proulx K, Smith KA, Kozma SC, Thomas G, Woods SC, et al. Hypothalamic mTOR signaling regulates food intake. Science. 2006;312(5775):927-30.

[21] Hu F, Xu Y, Liu F. Hypothalamic roles of mTOR complex I: integration of nutrient and hormone signals to regulate energy homeostasis. Am J Physiol Endocrinol Metab. 2016;310(11):E994-E1002.

[22] Dagon Y, Hur E, Zheng B, Wellenstein K, Cantley LC, Kahn BB. p70S6 Kinase Phosphorylates AMPK on Serine 491 to Mediate Leptin's Effect on Food Intake. Cell Metab. 2012;16(1):104-12.

[23] Kikani CK, Antonysamy SA, Bonanno JB, Romero R, Zhang FF, Russell M, et al. Structural bases of PAS domain-regulated kinase (PASK) activation in the absence of activation loop phosphorylation. J Biol Chem. 2010;285(52):41034-43.

[24] Moglich A, Ayers RA, Moffat K. Structure and signaling mechanism of Per-ARNT-Sim domains. Structure. 2009;17(10):1282-94.

[25] DeMille D, Grose JH. PAS kinase: a nutrient sensing regulator of glucose homeostasis. IUBMB Life. 2013;65(11):921-9.

[26] Zhang DD, Zhang JG, Wang YZ, Liu Y, Liu GL, Li XY. Per-Arnt-Sim Kinase (PASK): An Emerging Regulator of Mammalian Glucose and Lipid Metabolism. Nutrients. 2015;7(9):7437-50.

[27] Grose JH, Rutter J. The role of PAS kinase in PASsing the glucose signal. Sensors (Basel). 2010;10(6):5668-82.

[28] Hurtado-Carneiro V, Perez-Garcia A, Alvarez E, Sanz, C. PAS kinase: A nutrient and energy sensor "master key" in the response to fasting/feeding conditions. Front Endocrinol. 2020; 11(999).

[29] Morton GJ, Cummings DE, Baskin DG, Barsh GS, Schwartz MW. Central nervous system control of food intake and body weight. Nature. 2006;443(7109):289-95.

[30] Lam TK. Neuronal regulation of homeostasis by nutrient sensing. Nat Med. 2010;16(4):392-5.

[31] Cummings DE, Overduin J. Gastrointestinal regulation of food intake. J Clin Invest. 2007;117(1):13-23.

[32] Pena-Leon V, Perez-Lois R, Seoane LM. mTOR Pathway is Involved in Energy Homeostasis Regulation as a Part of the Gut-Brain Axis. Int J Mol Sci. 2020;21(16).

[33] Roh E, Song DK, Kim MS. Emerging role of the brain in the homeostatic regulation of energy and glucose metabolism. Exp Mol Med. 2016;48:e216.

[34] Spiegelman BM, Flier JS. Obesity and the regulation of energy balance. Cell. 2001;104(4):531-43.

[35] Anand BK, Chhina GS, Sharma KN, Dua S, Singh B. Activity of Single Neurons in the Hypothalamic Feeding Centers: Effect of Glucose. Am J Physiol. 1964;207:1146-54.

[36] Ashford ML, Boden PR, Treherne JM. Glucose-induced excitation of hypothalamic neurones is mediated by ATP-sensitive K+ channels. Pflugers Arch. 1990;415(4):479-83.

[37] Song Z, Levin BE, McArdle JJ, Bakhos N, Routh VH. Convergence of pre- and postsynaptic influences

on glucosensing neurons in the ventromedial hypothalamic nucleus. Diabetes. 2001;50(12):2673-81.

[38] Mizuno Y, Oomura Y. Glucose responding neurons in the nucleus tractus solitarius of the rat: in vitro study. Brain Res. 1984;307(1-2):109-16.

[39] Oomura Y, Yoshimatsu H. Neural network of glucose monitoring system. J Auton Nerv Syst. 1984;10(3-4):359-72.

[40] Silver IA, Erecinska M. Glucose-induced intracellular ion changes in sugar-sensitive hypothalamic neurons. J Neurophysiol. 1998;79(4):1733-45.

[41] Alvarez E, Roncero I, Chowen JA, Thorens B, Blazquez E. Expression of the glucagon-like peptide-1 receptor gene in rat brain. J Neurochem. 1996;66(3):920-7.

[42] Navarro M, Rodriquez de Fonseca F, Alvarez E, Chowen JA, Zueco JA, Gomez R, et al. Colocalization of glucagon-like peptide-1 (GLP-1) receptors, glucose transporter GLUT-2, and glucokinase mRNAs in rat hypothalamic cells: evidence for a role of GLP-1 receptor agonists as an inhibitory signal for food and water intake. J Neurochem. 1996;67(5):1982-91.

[43] Dunn-Meynell AA, Rawson NE, Levin BE. Distribution and phenotype of neurons containing the ATP-sensitive K+ channel in rat brain. Brain Res. 1998;814(1-2):41-54.

[44] Schuit FC, Huypens P, Heimberg H, Pipeleers DG. Glucose sensing in pancreatic beta-cells: a model for the study of other glucose-regulated cells in gut, pancreas, and hypothalamus. Diabetes. 2001;50(1):1-11.

[45] Marty N, Dallaporta M, Thorens B. Brain Glucose Sensing, Counterregulation, and Energy Homeostasis. Physiology. 2007;22(4):241-51.

[46] Le Foll C, Irani BG, Magnan C, Dunn-Meynell AA, Levin BE. Characteristics and mechanisms of hypothalamic neuronal fatty acid sensing. Am J Physiol Regul Integr Comp Physiol. 2009;297(3):R655-64.

[47] Le Foll C, Dunn-Meynell AA, Levin BE. Role of FAT/CD36 in fatty acid sensing, energy, and glucose homeostasis regulation in DIO and DR rats. Am J Physiol Regul Integr Comp Physiol. 2015;308(3):R188-98.

[48] Le Foll C, Levin BE. Fatty acid-induced astrocyte ketone production and the control of food intake. Am J Physiol Regul Integr Comp Physiol. 2016;310(11):R1186-92.

[49] Cone RD, Cowley MA, Butler AA, Fan W, Marks DL, Low MJ. The arcuate nucleus as a conduit for diverse signals relevant to energy homeostasis. Int J Obes Relat Metab Disord. 2001;25 Suppl 5:S63-7.

[50] Blanco Martinez de Morentin P, Gonzalez CR, Saha AK, Martins L, Dieguez C, Vidal-Puig A, et al. Hypothalamic AMP-activated protein kinase as a mediator of whole body energy balance. Rev Endocr Metab Disord. 2011;12(3):127-40.

[51] Ramamurthy S, Ronnett G. AMP-Activated Protein Kinase (AMPK) and Energy-Sensing in the Brain. Exp Neurobiol. 2012;21(2):52-60.

[52] Turnley AM, Stapleton D, Mann RJ, Witters LA, Kemp BE, Bartlett PF. Cellular distribution and developmental expression of AMP-activated protein kinase isoforms in mouse central nervous system. J Neurochem. 1999;72(4):1707-16.

[53] Minokoshi Y, Alquier T, Furukawa N, Kim YB, Lee A, Xue B, et al. AMP-kinase regulates food intake by responding to hormonal and nutrient

signals in the hypothalamus. Nature. 2004;428(6982):569-74.

[54] Claret M, Smith MA, Batterham RL, Selman C, Choudhury AI, Fryer LG, et al. AMPK is essential for energy homeostasis regulation and glucose sensing by POMC and AgRP neurons. J Clin Invest. 2007;117(8):2325-36.

[55] Huynh MK, Kinyua AW, Yang DJ, Kim KW. Hypothalamic AMPK as a Regulator of Energy Homeostasis. Neural Plast. 2016;2016:2754078.

[56] Blouet C, Ono H, Schwartz GJ. Mediobasal hypothalamic p70 S6 kinase 1 modulates the control of energy homeostasis. Cell Metab. 2008;8(6):459-67.

[57] Hurtado-Carneiro V, Sanz C, Roncero I, Vazquez P, Blazquez E, Alvarez E. Glucagon-like peptide 1 (GLP-1) can reverse AMP-activated protein kinase (AMPK) and S6 kinase (P70S6K) activities induced by fluctuations in glucose levels in hypothalamic areas involved in feeding behaviour. Mol Neurobiol. 2012;45(2):348-61.

[58] Hurtado-Carneiro V, Roncero, I., Blazquez, E., Alvarez, E., Sanz, C. Glucagon-like peptide-1 and its implications in obesity. HOT TOPICS IN ENDOCRINE AND ENDOCRINE-RELATED DISEASES. 2013(Chap 7):165-95.

[59] Inoki K, Zhu T, Guan KL. TSC2 mediates cellular energy response to control cell growth and survival. Cell. 2003;115(5):577-90.

[60] Byfield MP, Murray JT, Backer JM. hVps34 is a nutrient-regulated lipid kinase required for activation of p70 S6 kinase. J Biol Chem. 2005;280(38):33076-82.

[61] Blouet C, Schwartz GJ. Hypothalamic nutrient sensing in the control of energy homeostasis. Behav Brain Res. 2010;209(1):1-12.

[62] Le Foll C, Dunn-Meynell AA, Miziorko HM, Levin BE. Regulation of hypothalamic neuronal sensing and food intake by ketone bodies and fatty acids. Diabetes. 2014;63(4):1259-69.

[63] Migrenne S, Magnan C, Cruciani-Guglielmacci C. Fatty acid sensing and nervous control of energy homeostasis. Diabetes Metab. 2007;33(3):177-82.

[64] Benoit SC, Clegg DJ, Seeley RJ, Woods SC. Insulin and leptin as adiposity signals. Recent Prog Horm Res. 2004;59:267-85.

[65] Chen X, Ge YL, Jiang ZY, Liu CQ, Depoortere I, Peeters TL. Effects of ghrelin on hypothalamic glucose responding neurons in rats. Brain Res. 2005;1055(1-2):131-6.

[66] Rodriquez de Fonseca F, Navarro M, Alvarez E, Roncero I, Chowen JA, Maestre O, et al. Peripheral versus central effects of glucagon-like peptide-1 receptor agonists on satiety and body weight loss in Zucker obese rats. Metabolism. 2000;49(6):709-17.

[67] Woods SC, Seeley RJ, Porte D, Jr., Schwartz MW. Signals that regulate food intake and energy homeostasis. Science. 1998;280(5368):1378-83.

[68] Air EL, Benoit SC, Blake Smith KA, Clegg DJ, Woods SC. Acute third ventricular administration of insulin decreases food intake in two paradigms. Pharmacol Biochem Behav. 2002;72(1-2):423-9.

[69] Bruning JC, Gautam D, Burks DJ, Gillette J, Schubert M, Orban PC, et al. Role of brain insulin receptor in control of body weight and reproduction. Science. 2000;289(5487):2122-5.

[70] Considine RV, Sinha MK, Heiman ML, Kriauciunas A,

Stephens TW, Nyce MR, et al. Serum immunoreactive-leptin concentrations in normal-weight and obese humans. N Engl J Med. 1996;334(5):292-5.

[71] Coppari R, Ichinose M, Lee CE, Pullen AE, Kenny CD, McGovern RA, et al. The hypothalamic arcuate nucleus: a key site for mediating leptin's effects on glucose homeostasis and locomotor activity. Cell Metab. 2005;1(1):63-72.

[72] Oswal A, Yeo G. Leptin and the control of body weight: a review of its diverse central targets, signaling mechanisms, and role in the pathogenesis of obesity. Obesity (Silver Spring). 2010;18(2):221-9.

[73] Moore MC, Coate KC, Winnick JJ, An Z, Cherrington AD. Regulation of hepatic glucose uptake and storage in vivo. Adv Nutr. 2012;3(3):286-94.

[74] Gomis RR, Ferrer JC, Guinovart JJ. Shared control of hepatic glycogen synthesis by glycogen synthase and glucokinase. Biochem J. 2000;351 Pt 3:811-6.

[75] Petersen MC, Vatner DF, Shulman GI. Regulation of hepatic glucose metabolism in health and disease. Nat Rev Endocrinol. 2017;13(10):572-87.

[76] Schwartz MW, Seeley RJ, Tschop MH, Woods SC, Morton GJ, Myers MG, et al. Cooperation between brain and islet in glucose homeostasis and diabetes. Nature. 2013;503(7474):59-66.

[77] Obici S, Zhang BB, Karkanias G, Rossetti L. Hypothalamic insulin signaling is required for inhibition of glucose production. Nat Med. 2002;8(12):1376-82.

[78] Thorens B. Brain glucose sensing and neural regulation of insulin and glucagon secretion. Diabetes Obes Metab. 2011;13 Suppl 1:82-8.

[79] Fisher SJ, Kahn CR. Insulin signaling is required for insulin's direct and indirect action on hepatic glucose production. J Clin Invest. 2003;111(4):463-8.

[80] Tripathy D, Eriksson KF, Orho-Melander M, Fredriksson J, Ahlqvist G, Groop L. Parallel manifestation of insulin resistance and beta cell decompensation is compatible with a common defect in Type 2 diabetes. Diabetologia. 2004;47(5):782-93.

[81] Michael MD, Kulkarni RN, Postic C, Previs SF, Shulman GI, Magnuson MA, et al. Loss of insulin signaling in hepatocytes leads to severe insulin resistance and progressive hepatic dysfunction. Mol Cell. 2000;6(1):87-97.

[82] Gelling RW, Morton GJ, Morrison CD, Niswender KD, Myers MG, Jr., Rhodes CJ, et al. Insulin action in the brain contributes to glucose lowering during insulin treatment of diabetes. Cell Metab. 2006;3(1):67-73.

[83] Ono H, Pocai A, Wang Y, Sakoda H, Asano T, Backer JM, et al. Activation of hypothalamic S6 kinase mediates diet-induced hepatic insulin resistance in rats. J Clin Invest. 2008;118(8):2959-68.

[84] Rutter J, Michnoff CH, Harper SM, Gardner KH, McKnight SL. PAS kinase: an evolutionarily conserved PAS domain-regulated serine/threonine kinase. Proc Natl Acad Sci U S A. 2001;98(16):8991-6.

[85] Henry JT, Crosson S. Ligand-binding PAS domains in a genomic, cellular, and structural context. Annu Rev Microbiol. 2011;65:261-86.

[86] Amezcua CA, Harper SM, Rutter J, Gardner KH. Structure and interactions of PAS kinase N-terminal PAS domain: model for intramolecular kinase regulation. Structure. 2002;10(10):1349-61.

[87] Schlafli P, Troger J, Eckhardt K, Borter E, Spielmann P, Wenger RH. Substrate preference and phosphatidylinositol monophosphate inhibition of the catalytic domain of the Per-Arnt-Sim domain kinase PASKIN. FEBS J. 2011;278(10):1757-68.

[88] da Silva Xavier G, Farhan H, Kim H, Caxaria S, Johnson P, Hughes S, et al. Per-arnt-sim (PAS) domain-containing protein kinase is downregulated in human islets in type 2 diabetes and regulates glucagon secretion. Diabetologia. 2011;54(4):819-27.

[89] Semplici F, Mondragon A, Macintyre B, Madeyski-Bengston K, Persson-Kry A, Barr S, et al. Cell type-specific deletion in mice reveals roles for PAS kinase in insulin and glucagon production. Diabetologia. 2016;59(9):1938-47.

[90] Wilson WA, Skurat AV, Probst B, de Paoli-Roach A, Roach PJ, Rutter J. Control of mammalian glycogen synthase by PAS kinase. Proc Natl Acad Sci U S A. 2005;102(46):16596-601.

[91] Rutter J, Probst BL, McKnight SL. Coordinate regulation of sugar flux and translation by PAS kinase. Cell. 2002;111(1):17-28.

[92] Katschinski DM, Marti HH, Wagner KF, Shibata J, Eckhardt K, Martin F, et al. Targeted disruption of the mouse PAS domain serine/threonine kinase PASKIN. Mol Cell Biol. 2003;23(19):6780-9.

[93] Hao HX, Cardon CM, Swiatek W, Cooksey RC, Smith TL, Wilde J, et al. PAS kinase is required for normal cellular energy balance. Proc Natl Acad Sci U S A. 2007;104(39):15466-71.

[94] Rosen ED, Walkey CJ, Puigserver P, Spiegelman BM. Transcriptional regulation of adipogenesis. Genes Dev. 2000;14(11):1293-307.

[95] Horton JD, Goldstein JL, Brown MS. SREBPs: activators of the complete program of cholesterol and fatty acid synthesis in the liver. J Clin Invest. 2002;109(9):1125-31.

[96] Wu X, Romero D, Swiatek WI, Dorweiler I, Kikani CK, Sabic H, et al. PAS kinase drives lipogenesis through SREBP-1 maturation. Cell Rep. 2014;8(1):242-55.

[97] Pape JA, Newey CR, Burrell HR, Workman A, Perry K, Bikman BT, et al. Per-Arnt-Sim Kinase (PASK) Deficiency Increases Cellular Respiration on a Standard Diet and Decreases Liver Triglyceride Accumulation on a Western High-Fat High-Sugar Diet. Nutrients. 2018;10(12).

[98] Swiatek W, Parnell KM, Nickols GA, Scharschmidt BF, Rutter J. Validation of PAS Kinase, a Regulator of Hepatic Fatty Acid and Triglyceride Synthesis, as a Therapeutic Target for Nonalcoholic Steatohepatitis. Hepatol Commun. 2020;4(5):696-707.

[99] Kikani CK, Wu X, Paul L, Sabic H, Shen Z, Shakya A, et al. Pask integrates hormonal signaling with histone modification via Wdr5 phosphorylation to drive myogenesis. Elife. 2016;5.

[100] Kikani CK, Wu X, Fogarty S, Kang SAW, Dephoure N, Gygi SP, et al. Activation of PASK by mTORC1 is required for the onset of the terminal differentiation program. Proc Natl Acad Sci U S A. 2019;116(21):10382-91.

[101] Karakkat JV, Kaimala S, Sreedharan SP, Jayaprakash P, Adeghate EA, Ansari SA, et al. The metabolic sensor PASK is a histone 3 kinase that also regulates H3K4 methylation by associating with H3K4 MLL2 methyltransferase complex. Nucleic Acids Res. 2019;47(19):10086-103.

[102] Lee K, Li B, Xi X, Suh Y, Martin RJ. Role of neuronal energy status in the regulation of adenosine 5'-monophosphate-activated protein kinase, orexigenic neuropeptides expression, and feeding behavior. Endocrinology. 2005;146(1):3-10.

[103] Cota D, Matter EK, Woods SC, Seeley RJ. The role of hypothalamic mammalian target of rapamycin complex 1 signaling in diet-induced obesity. J Neurosci. 2008;28(28):7202-8.

[104] Hurtado-Carneiro V, Roncero I, Blazquez E, Alvarez E, Sanz C. PAS kinase as a nutrient sensor in neuroblastoma and hypothalamic cells required for the normal expression and activity of other cellular nutrient and energy sensors. Mol Neurobiol. 2013;48(3):904-20.

[105] Hurtado-Carneiro V, Roncero I, Egger SS, Wenger RH, Blazquez E, Sanz C, et al. PAS kinase is a nutrient and energy sensor in hypothalamic areas required for the normal function of AMPK and mTOR/S6K1. Mol Neurobiol. 2014;50(2):314-26.

[106] Drucker DJ, Nauck MA. The incretin system: glucagon-like peptide-1 receptor agonists and dipeptidyl peptidase-4 inhibitors in type 2 diabetes. Lancet. 2006;368(9548):1696-705.

[107] Malik J, Roohi N. GLP-1, a powerful physiological incretin: an update. J Biol Regul Homeost Agents. 2018;32(5):1171-6.

[108] Semache M, Zarrouki B, Fontes G, Fogarty S, Kikani C, Chawki MB, et al. Per-Arnt-Sim kinase regulates pancreatic duodenal homeobox-1 protein stability via phosphorylation of glycogen synthase kinase 3beta in pancreatic beta-cells. J Biol Chem. 2013;288(34):24825-33.

[109] Beiroa D, Imbernon M, Gallego R, Senra A, Herranz D, Villarroya F, et al. GLP-1 agonism stimulates brown adipose tissue thermogenesis and browning through hypothalamic AMPK. Diabetes. 2014;63(10):3346-58.

[110] Lopez M, Dieguez C, Nogueiras R. Hypothalamic GLP-1: the control of BAT thermogenesis and browning of white fat. Adipocyte. 2015;4(2):141-5.

[111] Semplici F, Vaxillaire M, Fogarty S, Semache M, Bonnefond A, Fontes G, et al. Human mutation within Per-Arnt-Sim (PAS) domain-containing protein kinase (PASK) causes basal insulin hypersecretion. J Biol Chem. 2011;286(51):44005-14.

[112] Perez-Garcia A, Dongil P, Hurtado-Carneiro V, Blazquez E, Sanz C, Alvarez E. High-fat diet alters PAS kinase regulation by fasting and feeding in liver. J Nutr Biochem. 2018;57:14-25.

[113] Perez-Garcia A, Dongil P, Hurtado-Carneiro V, Blazquez E, Sanz C, Alvarez E. PAS Kinase deficiency alters the glucokinase function and hepatic metabolism. Sci Rep. 2018;8(1):11091.

[114] Vionnet N, Stoffel M, Takeda J, Yasuda K, Bell GI, Zouali H, et al. Nonsense mutation in the glucokinase gene causes early-onset non-insulin-dependent diabetes mellitus. Nature. 1992;356(6371):721-2.

[115] Christesen HB, Jacobsen BB, Odili S, Buettger C, Cuesta-Munoz A, Hansen T, et al. The second activating glucokinase mutation (A456V): implications for glucose homeostasis and diabetes therapy. Diabetes. 2002;51(4):1240-6.

[116] Iynedjian PB. Molecular physiology of mammalian glucokinase. Cell Mol Life Sci. 2009;66(1):27-42.

[117] Dentin R, Pegorier JP, Benhamed F, Foufelle F, Ferre P, Fauveau V, et al. Hepatic glucokinase is required for the synergistic action of ChREBP and SREBP-1c on glycolytic and lipogenic gene expression. J Biol Chem. 2004;279(19):20314-26.

[118] Magnuson MA, Andreone TL, Printz RL, Koch S, Granner DK. Rat glucokinase gene: structure and regulation by insulin. Proc Natl Acad Sci U S A. 1989;86(13):4838-42.

[119] Agius L. Glucokinase and molecular aspects of liver glycogen metabolism. Biochem J. 2008;414(1):1-18.

[120] Dongil P, Perez-Garcia A, Hurtado-Carneiro V, Herrero-de-Dios C, Blazquez E, Alvarez E, et al. Pas Kinase Deficiency Triggers Antioxidant Mechanisms in the Liver. Sci Rep. 2018;8(1):13810.

[121] Nagao M, Asai A, Sugihara H, Oikawa S. Fat intake and the development of type 2 diabetes. Endocr J. 2015;62(7):561-72.

[122] Thanopoulou AC, Karamanos BG, Angelico FV, Assaad-Khalil SH, Barbato AF, Del Ben MP, et al. Dietary fat intake as risk factor for the development of diabetes: multinational, multicenter study of the Mediterranean Group for the Study of Diabetes (MGSD). Diabetes care. 2003;26(2):302-7.

[123] da Silva Xavier G, Rutter J, Rutter GA. Involvement of Per-Arnt-Sim (PAS) kinase in the stimulation of preproinsulin and pancreatic duodenum homeobox 1 gene expression by glucose. Proc Natl Acad Sci U S A. 2004;101(22):8319-24.

[124] Reaven GM. The insulin resistance syndrome: definition and dietary approaches to treatment. Annu Rev Nutr. 2005;25:391-406.

[125] Boucher J, Kleinridders A, Kahn CR. Insulin receptor signaling in normal and insulin-resistant states. Cold Spring Harb Perspect Biol. 2014;6(1).

[126] Bogan JS. Regulation of glucose transporter translocation in health and diabetes. Annu Rev Biochem. 2012;81:507-32.

[127] Leto D, Saltiel AR. Regulation of glucose transport by insulin: traffic control of GLUT4. Nat Rev Mol Cell Biol. 2012;13(6):383-96.

[128] Haemmerle G, Zimmermann R, Strauss JG, Kratky D, Riederer M, Knipping G, et al. Hormone-sensitive lipase deficiency in mice changes the plasma lipid profile by affecting the tissue-specific expression pattern of lipoprotein lipase in adipose tissue and muscle. J Biol Chem. 2002;277(15):12946-52.

[129] Bederman IR, Previs SF. Hormonal regulation of intracellular lipolysis in C57BL/6J mice: effect of diet-induced adiposity and data normalization. Metabolism. 2008;57(10):1405-13.

[130] Alberti KG, Zimmet P, Shaw J, Group IDFETFC. The metabolic syndrome--a new worldwide definition. Lancet. 2005;366(9491):1059-62.

[131] Eckel RH, Grundy SM, Zimmet PZ. The metabolic syndrome. Lancet. 2005;365(9468):1415-28.

[132] Xu H, Barnes GT, Yang Q, Tan G, Yang D, Chou CJ, et al. Chronic inflammation in fat plays a crucial role in the development of obesity-related insulin resistance. J Clin Invest. 2003;112(12):1821-30.

[133] Burcelin R, Crivelli V, Dacosta A, Roy-Tirelli A, Thorens B. Heterogeneous

metabolic adaptation of C57BL/6J mice to high-fat diet. Am J Physiol Endocrinol Metab. 2002;282(4):E834-42.

[134] Buettner R, Scholmerich J, Bollheimer LC. High-fat diets: modeling the metabolic disorders of human obesity in rodents. Obesity (Silver Spring). 2007;15(4):798-808.

[135] Tilg H, Moschen AR. Evolution of inflammation in nonalcoholic fatty liver disease: the multiple parallel hits hypothesis. Hepatology. 2010;52(5):1836-46.

[136] Yilmaz Y. Review article: is non-alcoholic fatty liver disease a spectrum, or are steatosis and non-alcoholic steatohepatitis distinct conditions? Aliment Pharmacol Ther. 2012;36(9):815-23.

[137] Hegarty BD, Bobard A, Hainault I, Ferre P, Bossard P, Foufelle F. Distinct roles of insulin and liver X receptor in the induction and cleavage of sterol regulatory element-binding protein-1c. Proc Natl Acad Sci U S A. 2005;102(3):791-6.

[138] Ono H, Shimano H, Katagiri H, Yahagi N, Sakoda H, Onishi Y, et al. Hepatic Akt activation induces marked hypoglycemia, hepatomegaly, and hypertriglyceridemia with sterol regulatory element binding protein involvement. Diabetes. 2003;52(12):2905-13.

[139] Lima-Cabello E, Garcia-Mediavilla MV, Miquilena-Colina ME, Vargas-Castrillon J, Lozano-Rodriguez T, Fernandez-Bermejo M, et al. Enhanced expression of pro-inflammatory mediators and liver X-receptor-regulated lipogenic genes in non-alcoholic fatty liver disease and hepatitis C. Clin Sci (Lond). 2011;120(6):239-50.

[140] Rahimian R, Masih-Khan E, Lo M, van Breemen C, McManus BM, Dube GP. Hepatic over-expression of peroxisome proliferator activated receptor gamma2 in the ob/ob mouse model of non-insulin dependent diabetes mellitus. Mol Cell Biochem. 2001;224(1-2):29-37.

[141] Bedoucha M, Atzpodien E, Boelsterli UA. Diabetic KKAy mice exhibit increased hepatic PPARgamma1 gene expression and develop hepatic steatosis upon chronic treatment with antidiabetic thiazolidinediones. J Hepatol. 2001;35(1):17-23.

[142] Lechleitner M. Obesity and the metabolic syndrome in the elderly--a mini-review. Gerontology. 2008;54(5):253-9.

[143] Catalano KJ, Bergman RN, Ader M. Increased susceptibility to insulin resistance associated with abdominal obesity in aging rats. Obes Res. 2005;13(1):11-20.

[144] Barzilai N, Huffman DM, Muzumdar RH, Bartke A. The critical role of metabolic pathways in aging. Diabetes. 2012;61(6):1315-22.

[145] Dandona P, Thusu K, Cook S, Snyder B, Makowski J, Armstrong D, et al. Oxidative damage to DNA in diabetes mellitus. Lancet. 1996;347(8999):444-5.

[146] Goodarzi MT, Navidi AA, Rezaei M, Babahmadi-Rezaei H. Oxidative damage to DNA and lipids: correlation with protein glycation in patients with type 1 diabetes. J Clin Lab Anal. 2010;24(2):72-6.

[147] Kim IH, Kisseleva T, Brenner DA. Aging and liver disease. Curr Opin Gastroenterol. 2015;31(3):184-91.

[148] Kenyon C. The plasticity of aging: insights from long-lived mutants. Cell. 2005;120(4):449-60.

[149] Solon-Biet SM, Mitchell SJ, de Cabo R, Raubenheimer D, Le Couteur DG, Simpson SJ. Macronutrients and caloric intake in health and longevity. J Endocrinol. 2015;226(1):R17-28.

[150] Salminen A, Kaarniranta K. AMP-activated protein kinase (AMPK) controls the aging process via an integrated signaling network. Ageing Res Rev. 2012;11(2):230-41.

[151] Dongil P, Perez-Garcia A, Hurtado-Carneiro V, Herrero-de-Dios C, Alvarez E, Sanz C. PAS kinase deficiency reduces aging effects in mice. Aging (Albany NY). 2020;12.

[152] Taguchi K, Motohashi H, Yamamoto M. Molecular mechanisms of the Keap1-Nrf2 pathway in stress response and cancer evolution. Genes Cells. 2011;16(2):123-40.

[153] Zhang H, Davies KJA, Forman HJ. Oxidative stress response and Nrf2 signaling in aging. Free Radic Biol Med. 2015;88(Pt B):314-36.

[154] Ziegler DV, Wiley CD, Velarde MC. Mitochondrial effectors of cellular senescence: beyond the free radical theory of aging. Aging Cell. 2015;14(1):1-7.

[155] Cui H, Kong Y, Zhang H. Oxidative stress, mitochondrial dysfunction, and aging. J Signal Transduct. 2012;2012:646354.

[156] Colantoni A, Idilman R, de Maria N, Duffner LA, Van Thiel DH, Witte PL, et al. Evidence of oxidative injury during aging of the liver in a mouse model. J Am Aging Assoc. 2001;24(2):51-7.

[157] Castro Mdel R, Suarez E, Kraiselburd E, Isidro A, Paz J, Ferder L, et al. Aging increases mitochondrial DNA damage and oxidative stress in liver of rhesus monkeys. Exp Gerontol. 2012;47(1):29-37.

[158] Calabrese EJ, Dhawan G, Kapoor R, Iavicoli I, Calabrese V. What is hormesis and its relevance to healthy aging and longevity? Biogerontology. 2015;16(6):693-707.

Chapter 16

# Therapeutic Effect of Folate and Cobalamin in Diabetics

*Farah Qudsia and Samreen Riaz*


## Abstract

Diabetes Mellitus type 2 is a metabolic ailment. It is a condition when insulin is produced by our body but, it is not used properly by us. The number of diabetic patients is increasing in the whole world. The problem of obesity is also very closely related to it, which itself is expanding. The individuals diagnosed with type 2 Diabetes Mellitus have high chance of microvascular problems (like nephropathy, retinopathy and neuropathy). They are also at the verge of facing macrovascular ailments (like cardiovascular comorbidities). This indicates that many antidiabetic agents should be administered in combination, to maintain normal sugar level in blood. The management for the patients suffering from diabetes should be effective and harmless for them. It should also improve the general well-being of the patients. So many remedies have been developed for the management of diabetes. Several of them are being developed. We should enhance insulin sensitivity to let our body use insulin effectively. We also must stop the increasing pancreatic β-cell failure which is a specific characteristic of Diabetes Mellitus type 2. The microvascular complications must also be avoided or revoked. Our direst need is to develop agents which may help us in achieving goals mentioned earlier. Many micronutrients are involved in combating the Diabetes Mellitus and complication associated to the malady. These micronutrients are vitamins. Our main focus in this chapter are Vitamins B9 (Folate) and B12 (Cobalamin). Many researches have shown that the said parameters were decreased in patients suffering from Diabetes Mellitus. The level of these two vitamins should be maintained to the normal level and not toward the border line. The maintained level of these vitamins will help in controlling the main problems in patients suffering from Diabetes Mellitus like neuropathy, anemia and many others. By taking these vitamins along with other preventive measures, Diabetes Mellitus can be controlled and can be less dangerous.


**Keywords:** diabetes mellitus, cobalamin, folic acid, microvascular complications, micronutrients

## 1. Introduction

The permanent harm, dysfunction, and failure of multiple human body parts, like eyes, kidneys, heart, nerves and blood vessels could be caused by persistent hyperglycemia [1].

### 1.1 Preventing the development of diabetes mellitus

The risk of the diabetes raises seven times in older age (55+) than it is in younger age (20 to 34 years old). So, it is really important to gear up to control diabetes in midlife. Specially minimizing the spread of type 2 Diabetes Mellitus is crucial for individuals and even the societies. The importance of eradication of *type 2 Diabetes Mellitus* is even because of its harmful side effects.

Healthy lifestyle and body-weight control in midlife plays a crucial role in avoiding or postponing manifestation of type 2 Diabetes Mellitus since lifestyle interventions seem more durable concerning their protective potential in this part of life. The different pharmaceutical approaches to eradicate type 2 Diabetes Mellitus are not effective after they root out the disease for the first time. Also, such approaches have so many side effects on the patients going through such techniques. Therefore, for the time being, no drug is licensed for diabetes prevention.

Nonetheless, novel medicaments' attempts for diabetes prevention and supporting healthy aging are under scientific investigation. The diabetes can result in severe hypoglycemia, premature cardiovascular complications, other severe problems and even death. So, every possible step should be taken in order to eradicate this. The lifestyle of the patient should be changed to fight diabetes. All possible pharmaceutical techniques should also be applied to control the ailment. Diabetes prevention has a vital influence in the making of health policy [2].

### 1.2 Pathophysiology of diabetes

Numerous pathogenic processes are responsible of the growth of diabetes. These range from autoimmune demolition of the pancreatic β-cells with subsequent insulin shortage to anomalies that result in confrontation to insulin action. Lacking insulin action results from insufficient insulin emission and/or reduced tissue responses to insulin at one or more points in the complex paths of hormone action. The basis of the abnormalities in carbohydrate, fat, and protein metabolism in diabetes is deficient action of insulin on target tissues. Weakening of insulin secretion and defects in insulin action frequently coexist in the same patient, and it is mostly uncertain which anomaly, if either alone, is the main reason of the glucose excess in blood [1].

When we take the meal, the glucose levels in blood rise that activates insulin secretion. This results in a rise in biotransformation, transport and storage of insulin in fat tissues and muscles. During fasting, liver provides the glucose in blood that is used by the brain, without any dependence on insulin. Besides storing glucose, insulin also hinders the secretion of glucagon and drops the quantity of serum fatty acids resulting in a downfall in production of glucose in liver [3]. Inadequate insulin or confrontation to insulin in the body results in lessened uptake of glucose by tissues that has intracellular hypoglycemia and extracellular hyperglycemia as its outcome. The glucogenesis is caused by intracellular hypoglycemia and gluconeogenesis that results in breakdown of fats (resulting in diabetic ketoacidosis) and reduces synthesis of gamma globulins and protein (resulting in polyphagia, cachexia and reduced wound healing), while osmotic dieresis and hyperglycemic coma are caused by the extracellular hyperglycemia [4].

### 1.3 Pathogenesis about type 1 diabetes mellitus

A deficiency of insulin secretion occurs in Insulin dependent Diabetes Mellitus (IDDM). It is because of the autoimmune demolition of pancreatic beta cells that results in metabolic disorders associated with Insulin Dependent Diabetes Mellitus [4]. The last stage of β-cell demolition shows the beginning of clinical ailment resulting in type 1 diabetes mellitus. There the infiltrating lymphocytes, monocytes and a blend of pseudo atrophic islets form along with a few cells emitting glycogen, somatostatin and polypeptide from pancreas. This results in an immunogenic process whose outcome is the ailment [5–7]. Genetic makeup, autoimmunity and environmental factors are accountable for islets cell demolition [8].

### 1.4 Pathogenesis about type 2 diabetes mellitus

Many healthy operations are impaired in Non-Insulin dependent diabetes mellitus (NIDDM). This lessens the adjustment of tissue acceptance to insulin which results in reduced insulin influence via insulin confrontation and reduced insulin emission by the beta cells of pancreas [9].

Several genetic imperfections, and some environmental factors like overweightness are important in this type of diabetes. They are accountable for peripheral tissue insulin reluctance and beta cell problems [8].

## 2. Therapy of diabetes mellitus

As indicated by ongoing appraisals, the human populace overall seems, by all accounts, to be amidst a pestilence of diabetes. Notwithstanding the incredible steps that have been made in the comprehension and the executives of diabetes, the infection and sickness related difficulties are expanding continuously. Along with this, ongoing improvements in comprehension of the pathophysiology of the ailment procedure has unlocked a few new roads to distinguish and create novel treatments to battle the epidemic of diabetes [10]. The cure of diabetes with artificial medications is expensive and odds of reactions are so many. Phytomedicine has been utilized since old occasions in different regions around the globe where access to up-to-date drugs is restricted. Therapeutic plants and phytochemicals assume a significant job in the administration of diabetes mellitus particularly in underdeveloped nations where assets are small. Utmost pervasive amongst phytochemical bunches are the glycosides, alkaloids, polysaccharides and phenolics, for example, terpenoids, steroids and flavonoid. Regardless of impressive advancement in the improvement of artificial medications, the disclosure of phytomedicine as an elective treatment is increasing [11]. Simultaneously, phytochemicals recognized from customary medical plants are exhibiting an energizing open door for the improvement of new kinds of therapeutics. This has quickened the worldwide exertion to saddle and gather those restorative plants that bear significant number of potential phytochemicals appearing advantageous impacts in battling diabetes and diabetes-related entanglements. In this manner, as the malady is advancing continuously, there is a critical need of recognizing native resources occurring in nature so as to get them, and concentrate in detail, their potential on various recently distinguished focuses so as to create them as new treatments [10]. The improvement of type 2 diabetes might be decreased by the admission of cancer prevention agents in the eating routine [12].

### 2.1 Vitamins and diabetes mellitus type 2

Nutrients are the natural mixes needed by our body which are termed as mandatory ingredients required in definite quantities. They cannot be made in adequate quantity by the human body, and thus, should be gotten from the eating routine. Thirteen distinct kinds of vitamins are found that are ordered by their organic and substance action; every one of them keeps a particular job in human body [13].

Vitamins are termed as either fat-dissolvable or water-solvent. There are thirteen vitamins found in nature. Nine of them could dissolve in water (8 B Vitamins and Vitamin C) whereas, four of them could dissolve in fat (A, D, E, and K). The water-solvent Vitamins effectively make solution in water and are discharged from the body quickly since they could not be kept for quite a while, aside from nutrient B12 [14]. Whereas, fat-solvent Vitamins are caught up in the digestive system within the existence of lipid and they are bound to be kept in the body. As they are kept for quite a while, they can prompt hypervitaminosis more than the water-dissolvable vitamins; a few nutrients are necessary for the body cell development and improvement (for instance folate and vitamin B12).

**Vitamin B6 also play a crucial role in diabetics as it is a cofactor for approximately 150 reactions that regulate the metabolism of glucose, lipids, amino acids, DNA, and neurotransmitters. In addition, it plays the role of antioxidant by counteracting the formation of reactive oxygen species (ROS) and advanced glycation end-products (AGEs). Epidemiological and experimental studies indicated an evident inverse association between vitamin B6 levels and diabetes, as well as a clear protective effect of vitamin B6 on diabetic complications. Interestingly, by exploring the mechanisms that govern the relationship between this vitamin and diabetes, vitamin B6 can be considered both a cause and effect of diabetes** [15]**.**

Folate is known as vitamin B9 which has significant functionality in human body. We need folate for the repair, creation and methylation of DNA [16]. In a study in America, it was seen that the **intake of folate in young adulthood was inversely associated with diabetes incidence in midlife amongst Americans. The observed association may be partially explained by mechanisms related to homocysteine level, insulin sensitivity, and systemic inflammation** [17]**.**

Besides, it goes about as a helper in numerous fundamental natural responses. Folic Acid has a significant job in cell division and it is particularly required amid early stages and pregnancy. Our body needs folic acid so as to avoid iron deficiency and create sound RBCs (Red Blood Cells), while Vitamin B12 assumes a significant job in providing basic methyl bunches for protein and DNA amalgamation. Vitamin B12 is bound to the protein in our meal and hydrochloric acid in the stomach discharges B12 from it amid ingestion. Once discharged, vitamin B12 consolidates with an ingredient known as intrinsic factor [18].

The type 2 Diabetes Mellitus is a heterogenous malady which is usually connected to vital chemical reactions, especially starch and fat administration in the living being. Be that as it may, most micronutrients are likewise associated with some route either as a component of the reason or impact of this perpetual pathology. The outcomes and problems of diabetes are the aftereffect of a disparity between free radical development and their control by common cancer prevention agents [19]. Thus, those micronutrients that have an antioxidant function are very important in the development of the disease and its complications, while other non-antioxidant vitamins have also shown a relationship.

Vitamins A, C and E, which have antioxidant properties are discovered diminished in diabetic patients, may be because of an expanded need to limit the extraordinary oxidative pressure created by irregularities in glucose digestion. Then again, retinol binding protein applies a tweaking impact, as it has adipokine capacities. As for the B complex Vitamins, pyridoxine, thiamin and biotin have been discovered diminished though the systems are not obvious, whereas using its supplements has demonstrated some betterment of the metabolic control in individuals suffering from diabetes. The assimilation of folate and Vitamin B12 is critically diminished by the prolonged utilization of metformin, which is the most used medicine in simple diabetes, subsequently these two supplements have been discovered insufficient in the ailment and most presumably should be administered consistently. Whereas, Vitamin D is viewed as a hazard for the improvement of diabetes just as its difficulties, especially those related to heart and blood vessels. Though a few examinations have discovered a relationship of Vitamin K admission with sugar digestion which require more research. Research on the utilization of multivitamin supplements have indicated uncertain outcomes. The individuals utilizing metformin amid delayed periods may require folate and Vitamin B12 [20].

### 2.2 Cobalamin or B12 vitamin

Vitamin B12 is a non-protein ingredient in the single-carbon metabolic pathways, engaged with the making of methionine, pyrimidine and purine bases. Its deficiency due to DNA damage or faulty repair is involved in cancer, vascular diseases and some birth defects, while a consequent hyperhomocysteinemia, also related to folic acid deficiency; it has been recognized as a risk for hypertension and atherosclerosis [21].

The water-soluble vitamin is *Vitamin B12*. It is found within many foodstuffs as well as exists in nutritional medicines. It is present with many types as well as has mineral cobalt [22–25], thus compounds having vitamin B12 features may together know as "Cobalamins".

#### *2.2.1 Forms of vitamin B12*

These compounds are listed as [26].

- Hydroxocobalamin
- Methyl cobalamin
- 5-deoxyadenosylcobalamin and Adenosyl cobalamin
- Cyanocobalamin

#### *2.2.2 Functions of vitamin B12*

- It is essential of the suitable RBCs development, neurological role, and DNA synthesis. Vitamin B12 acts as a cofactor for methionine synthase and L-methyl malonyl-CoA mutase. Methionine synthase activates the alteration of homocysteine to methionine [26, 27]. Methionine is vital for the development of S-adenosylmethionine which is a general methyl donor for roughly 100 different substrates, including RNA, DNA, hormones, lipids and proteins. L-methyl malonyl-CoA mutase transforms L-methyl malonyl-CoA to succinyl-CoA during destruction of propionate [22, 26, 27], which is an important biochemical reaction in metabolism of protein and fat. Succinyl-CoA is also necessary for the making of hemoglobin.

- It is present within the protein of food and may be free through action of gastric protease and HCl during digestion. When artificial vitamin B12 is mixed in prepared meals and nutritional supplements, it is now in free form and, therefore, does not involve this detachment process. Free vitamin B12 joins with intrinsic factor which is a glycoprotein released by the gastric tube's parietal cells. The complex formed as a consequence experiences ingestion inside the distal ileum by the help of receptor-mediated endocytosis [26, 28].

- It can be in particular main component to keep strong nerve cells as well as this assists for making of RNA and DNA hereditary matter of body [28].

- Its mechanism is directly with vitamin B9 as well-known as folic acid or folate, to aid build RBCs and hence keep anemic conditions from building up in the body. Folic acid and Vitamin B12 play role jointly for making S-adenosylmethionine (SAMe), a chemical compound concerned in immunity related functions and person's mood changes.

- Vitamins B12, Vitamin B6 as well as B9 act mutually for the management of status of the homocysteine amino acid. Elevated status for homocysteine is linked by heart disease. Though, scientists do not have confidence that homocysteine can be reason for heart disease otherwise only an indicator which shows the risk of heart attack.

- Vitamin B12 has a key role in the production of energy in the body. It keeps the cells fit. Without it, cells become weak.

- The heart as well as whole cardiovascular system requires B12. It has functions of eliminate hazardous protein known as homocysteine. When homocysteine becomes tolerable so that it stays throughout blood, this devastates arteries results in swelling as well as heart disease.

- Research works explain people having osteoporosis can contain elevated status for homocysteine as well as decreased status for B12 as compared to persons having strong and fit bones [29].

- Nerves contain defensive cover for their protection from pollutants as well as free radicals within blood. Devoid of casing, known as myelin sheaths, bare nerves are injured as well as might expire. Such deceased nerves disturb signals toward and away from brain as well as might take part in function in nerve associated circumstances. Vitamin B12 assists approach by which the body replenishes this defending casing [30].

#### *2.2.3 Sources of vitamin B12*

The Vitamin B12 is found within organic foodstuffs, as well as in meat, fish, eggs, poultry, milk products and milk itself. It does not find within plants and its products only in very small quantity, but prepared breakfast cereals may be easily accessible resource for vitamin B12 having elevated availability for vegetarians [26]. Some dietary yeast foodstuffs also have vitamin B12.

Prepared foodstuffs have different formulation and this may be essential understand tags of manufactured goods find out the nutritional ingredients. Various food origins of vitamin B12 are enlisted in the **Table 1** [31].

#### *2.2.4 Metabolism of vitamin B12*

The Vitamin B12 is utilized by us in two ways, as methyl cobalamin or 5-deoxyadenosyl cobalamin. Methionine synthase is an enzyme which needs methyl cobalamin as a cofactor. It is usually responsible of the transformation of the amino acid homocysteine to methionine, whereas methionine, is needed for the methylation of DNA. 5-Deoxyadenosyl cobalamin is a helper enzyme needed by those enzymes which transform l-methyl malonyl CoA into succinyl CoA. This transformation is a primary point in the taking out of energy from fats and proteins. Additionally, succinyl CoA is needed for the making of hemoglobin which is the compound that is a carrier of oxygen molecules in red blood cells [32].

| Food | Micrograms (mcg) per serving | Percent DV* |
|---|---|---|
| Beef | 70.7 | 1,178 |
| Breakfast cereals, fortified with 100% of the DV for vitamin B12, 1 serving | 6.0 | 100 |
| Trout | 5.4 | 90 |
| Salmon | 4.8 | 80 |
| Tuna fish | 2.5 | 42 |
| Cheeseburger, twofold pastry as well as bread roll, 1 sandwich | 2.1 | 35 |
| Milk | 1.2 | 18 |
| Yogurt, fruit | 1.1 | 18 |
| Cheese, Swiss | 0.9 | 15 |
| Egg | 0.6 | 10 |
| Chicken | 0.3 | 5 |

** Percent Daily Value. A guide to the nutrients in one serving of food*

**Table 1.**
*Different sources of vitamin B12 [31].*

## 3. Vitamin B12 and diabetes

The connection between diabetes and vitamin B12 can be explained as:

### 3.1 Vitamin B12 deficiency and type 1 diabetes mellitus

Diabetes Type 1 is an automatic immune state which is the outcome from auto immune devastation for insulin releasing from beta cells of pancreas. This can be consistently related to new organ as well as non-organ particular auto immune plus endocrine situations results in growth of autoimmune polyglandular disorders [33].

Pernicious anemia due to chronic autoimmune gastritis can be very much widespread amongst people having type 1 diabetes. Pernicious anemia and Chronic autoimmune gastritis are present within almost 2% as well as up to 1% common people correspondingly. Amongst people having type 1 diabetes, incidence raises 3 to 5 times [34]. vitamin B12 shortage because of pernicious anemia present repeatedly amongst individuals having type 1 diabetes.

Individuals suffering from type 1 diabetes show parietal cell antibodies (PCA) plus auto antibodies to intrinsic factor (AIF) type 1 as well as 2 (De Block *et al.*, 1999) in particular people having antibodies of glutamate decarboxylase-65 (GAD-65) as well as HLA-DQA1*0501-B1*0301 haplotype [35]. The PCA hampers release for intrinsic factor leading to pernicious anemia, state that can be 10 times further prevailing amongst people having type 1 DM as well as people do not have DM. Type 1 AIF lead to vitamin B12 deficit inhibiting attachment of vitamin B12 to IF. This inhibits transport toward assimilation spot, terminal ileum. Such auto antibodies can be present within 70% people suffering from pernicious anemia.

Main autoimmune hypothyroidism as well as celiac ailment is common comorbidities between people having type 1 diabetes [36] and directly influence vitamin B12 metabolism. Vitamin B12 shortage between people having autoimmune hypothyroidism is described as existence of gastric parietal cell antibodies as well as intrinsic factor, decreased ingestion by mouth because of thyroid hormone insufficiency as well as flawed assimilation because of bowel wall edema, decreased bowel motility and increased growth of bacteria [37]. Celiac disease can be greatly widespread autoimmune mediated gastrointestinal state happen within 1–16% people having type 1 diabetes in contrast to 0.3–1% of common people. Intake for wheat gluten as well as further associated proteins is recognized as activator for situation within genetically liable persons. Because of linked enteropathy, people frequently stop to thrive, anemia and chronic diarrhea owing to micronutrient (mainly folate, vitamin B12) malabsorption [38].

### 3.2 Metformin stimulated vitamin B12 deficiency amongst patients with T2DM

Due to lack for contradictions such as renal as well as hepatic dysfunction, current guiding principles support utilization of metformin like primary line glucose reducing mediator parallel to changes in way of life [39]. Regardless of better glycemic reducing influence, metformin is revealed for reduction of vitamin B12 status. The possibility for having metformin coupled vitamin B12 deficit can be deeply affected of growing age, metformin dosage as well as period of use. The given methods for clarification of metformin induced vitamin B12 shortage amongst people having type 2 diabetes comprise: variations of small bowel motility that induces increased growth of bacteria as well as resulting vitamin B12 deficit, viable reduction and vitamin B12 malabsorption, changes within intrinsic factor status as well as contact to tubulin endocytic receptor. Metformin hamper calcium bound assimilation for complex of vitamin B12-IF at the terminal ileum. Such inhibition consequence could be inverted using calcium medication [40].

## 4. Folate, folic acid or B9

The term folate includes 150 components of the family of pteroilglutamate, which participate in cell replication by enzymatic activity in purine base synthesis for DNA and are a primary co-factor for transamination in the transformation of amino acids, particularly homocysteine into methionine. Folates are present in animal tissue, leafy vegetables, legumes and nuts and their deficiency has been associated to megaloblastic anemia, neural tube defects, cardiovascular disease, cancer and senile dementia [41].

Implication of folate in pathogenesis of type 2 DM is linked with vitamin B12 shortage and its consequent hyperhomocysteinemia, and although its deficiency is not widespread, supplementation trials have been carried out in diabetic patients [42].

Folates are made up of 4[(2-amino-4-oxo-1,4-dihydropteridin-6-yl) methylamino] benzoic acid, pteroic acid which is bonded with multiple or single monomers of L-glutamate. They lie in the family of heterocyclic organic compounds group [43].

There are eight different types of B vitamins. They are collectively called as B complex vitamins. Folate i.e., Vitamin B9 is also one of them. The naturally present folate forms are also based on vitamin B9. Many of the foods contain B vitamins. Many of folates are also taken from foods. They are generally made up of a mix of reduced folates. Reduced folates are any type of pteroyl mono glutamates, or an amalgam of pteroyl glutamates. They have a peculiar degree of pteridine ring reduction. Also, they have a different number of glutamates remains and one-carbon replacements [44]. The seven of total eight B vitamins can dissolve in water and hence cannot be kept by our body. We must constantly get their supply in our daily diet. Folates (vitamin B9) have that property. We can get them from foods like beans (and other legumes), salmon, citrus fruits, whole grains, leafy vegetables, meat and dairy etc. If we fail to fulfill our need of folate form our daily diet then we can take supplements which contain artificially synthesized folate to fulfill our needs. Folate fortification is also done to increase the folic acid intake by people. A number of commercially sold synthetic forms of folates are even better as compared to the natural ones [45]. They could be easily broken down chemically, especially reduced type of unsubstituted tetra and di-hydro forms are chemically stable. Tetrahydrofolates are usually found as the unsubstituted poly glutamates and tetrahydrofolates, that is, 5-methyl, 5,10-methylene, and 10-formyl etc. [46]. Reduced substituted forms of vitamins are prone to the chemical changes. Oxidative reactions occur in them which results in the activeness loss of vitamins. There are no acknowledged undesired effects of folates. An excess intake of them is not dangerous for human beings. The maximum usage limit of synthetic folates is capped to 1 mg daily. It is advised because excessive administration of folates may cover up the vitamin B12 deficiency [47].

### 4.1 Roles

Folic acid is considered to be an essential nutrient for our body. Folic Acid derivatives are necessary components for the DNA production. They are also needed for the erythrocyte synthesis. The biosynthesis of some amino acids needs tetrahydrofolates as a crucial ingredient. They are needed in the biosynthesis of precursors of DNA also [48]. Folic acid is necessary for the production of deoxyribose nucleic acid (DNA). They even aid maintenance of the process of methylation [49]. They also participate as helper molecules in some biological reactions. The cell division in our body essentially needs folate. We need it even more during pregnancy and infancy. It is needed in multiple crucial processes like quick cell growth and proliferation. The production of RBCs also needs folate. This acts to keep from anemia [50]. Nucleotide synthesis is the most important function of folate. It is required for the production and repair of DNA. Folates are also responsible of the production of methionine by alteration of Homocysteine in the procedure of re-methylation. Methionine is a useful amino acid which is in turn used to produce other necessary proteins. It may get converted to an important methyl donor i.e., S-adenosylmethionine [51].

### 4.2 Inadequacy

The deficiency of folate is not common in developed countries. But it is reported in many of the third-world countries. Folate deficiency could be due to multiple reasons. The poor diet and erroneous metabolism of vitamins could be responsible for it [52]. The US government along with that of many other countries has made fortification of food with folate to be mandatory for their nationals. This helps in eradication of NTDs worldwide. Mostly they use floor for the fortification because it is widely used by the public. The routine ingestion of folate is examined by taking the blood samples and measuring the folate levels in them. If the level of folate is low in blood samples then it means the folate is not taken up to required level [51].

We can fulfill our folate requirement by taking folate fortified diet. Artificial folate supplements are also available in the market which can serve the purpose. But the availability of any of the options of folate intake vary in different regions of world. The folate absorption also differs for every supplement used. Dietary Folate Equivalent (DFE) is the amount of folate our body can absorb out of the supplement taken per serving. Every DFE unit is considered to be one micro gram of folates or 0.6 micro grams of artificially made folate [50].

Loss of appetite along with decrease in body weight may occur due to deficiency in folate. The deficiency might be faced when one's need of folate increases or diet is reduced from a certain level. It is reported as a key health issue in some countries. Though it is rare in developed countries which enforce folate fortification of foods. Folate and vitamin B12 deficiency impacts all public of all ages. It is related to many diseases like neural tube defects in infants, diarrhea, anemia and other birth defects etc. [52].

The loss of methyl groups from DNA is termed as DNA hypomethylation. This could be affected by the deficiency of folate. The folate ingestion can fix such problems [53]. The overall methylation and DNA synthesis processes could also be negatively affected by the deficiency of folate in human body. Thymidyl acid, dTMP (Deoxythymidine monophosphate), is used as a monomer in DNA. Its supply in body becomes limited due to increased rate of removal of dUMP (Deoxy uridine Monophosphate) from the molecule of DNA. This is increased due to defective methylation cycle as a result of folate deficiency. DNA repair reactions start due to these problems which in turn declines the required cell division [45].

### 4.3 Metabolism of folate (vitamin B9)

Folic acid is inactive biochemically, it is transformed by dihydrofolate reductase into methyl tetrahydrofolate and tetrahydro folic acid. These folate congeners are carried by receptor-mediated endocytosis through body cells. There they are required to generate and use format, and synthesize thymidylate nucleic acids and purine, methylate tRNA, keep general erythropoiesis, interconvert amino acids. Utilizing vitamin B12 as a helper enzyme, folate can standardize high homocysteine quantities by re-methylation of homocysteine to methionine via methionine synthetase [16].

## Author details

Farah Qudsia* and Samreen Riaz
Department of Microbiology and Molecular Genetics, University of the Punjab, Quaid-e-Azam Campus, Lahore, Pakistan

*Address all correspondence to: farah.qudsiaa@gmail.com

## References

[1] American Diabetes Association. (2018). 2. Classification and diagnosis of diabetes: standards of medical care in diabetes—2018. *Diabetes care*, *41*(Supplement 1), S13-S27.

[2] Fasching, P. (2019). The New Ways of Preventing and Treating Diabetes Mellitus. In *Prevention of Chronic Diseases and Age-Related Disability* (pp. 71-81). Springer, Cham.

[3] Kangralkar, V. A., Patil, S. D., & Bandivadekar, R. M. (2010). Oxidative stress and diabetes: a review. *International Journal of Pharmaceutical Applications*, *1*(1), 38-45.

[4] Ozougwu, J. C., Obimba, K. C., Belonwu, C. D., & Unakalamba, C. B. (2013). The pathogenesis and pathophysiology of type 1 and type 2 diabetes mellitus. *Journal of Physiology and Pathophysiology*, *4*(4), 46-57.

[5] Al Homsi, M. F., & Lukic, M. L. (1992). An Update on the pathogenesis of Diabetes Mellitus. *Department of Pathology and medical microbiology (Immunology Unit) faculty of medicine and health sciences, UAE University, Al Ain, United Arab Emirates*.

[6] Gill, R. G., & Haskins, K. (1993). Molecular mechanisms underlying diabetes and other autoimmune diseases. *Immunology today*, *14*(2), 49-51.

[7] Yagi, H., Matsumoto, M., Kunimoto, K., Kawaguchi, J., Makino, S., & Harada, M. (1992). Analysis of the roles of CD4+ and CD8+ T cells in autoimmune diabetes of NOD mice using transfer to NOD athymic nude mice. *European journal of immunology*, *22*(9), 2387-2393.

[8] Van der Gaag, N. A., Rauws, E. A., van Eijck, C. H., Bruno, M. J., van der Harst, E., Kubben, F. J., ... & Klinkenbijl, J. H. (2010). Preoperative biliary drainage for cancer of the head of the pancreas. *New England Journal of Medicine*, *362*(2), 129-137.

[9] DeFronzo, R. A., Ferrannini, E., Zimmet, P., & Alberti, G. (Eds.). (2015). *International Textbook of Diabetes Mellitus, 2 Volume Set* (Vol. 1). John Wiley & Sons.

[10] Tiwari, A. K., & Madhusudanarao, J. (2002). Diabetes mellitus and multiple therapeutic approaches of phytochemicals: Present status and future prospects.

[11] B Gaikwad, S., Krishna Mohan, G., & Sandhya Rani, M. (2014). Phytochemicals for diabetes management. *Pharmaceutical Crops*, *5*(1).

[12] Montonen, J., Knekt, P., Järvinen, R., & Reunanen, A. (2004). Dietary antioxidant intake and risk of type 2 diabetes. *Diabetes Care*, *27*(2), 362-366.

[13] Combs Jr, G. F., & McClung, J. P. (2016). *The vitamins: fundamental aspects in nutrition and health*. Academic press.

[14] Chatterjea, M. N., & Shinde, R. (2011). *Textbook of medical biochemistry*. Wife Goes On.

[15] Mascolo E, Vernì F. Vitamin B6 and Diabetes: Relationship and Molecular Mechanisms. International journal of molecular sciences. 2020 Jan;21(10):3669.

[16] Krebs, M. O., Bellon, A., Mainguy, G., Jay, T. M., & Frieling, H. (2009). One-carbon metabolism and schizophrenia: current challenges and future directions. *Trends in molecular medicine*, *15*(12), 562-570.

[17] Zhu J, Chen C, Lu L, Yang K, Reis J, He K. Intakes of Folate, Vitamin

B6, and Vitamin B12 in Relation to Diabetes Incidence Among American Young Adults: A 30-Year Follow-up Study. Diabetes Care. 2020 Oct 1;43(10):2426-34.

[18] Aghajanian, G. K., & Marek, G. J. (2000). Serotonin model of schizophrenia: emerging role of glutamate mechanisms. *Brain Research Reviews*, *31*(2-3), 302-312.

[19] Zatalia, S.R. and Sanusi, H. (2013) The role of antioxidants in the pathophysiology, complications and management of diabetes mellitus. Acta. Med. Indones., 45(2), 141-147.

[20] Valdés-Ramos, R., Ana Laura, G. L., Beatriz Elina, M. C., & Alejandra Donaji, B. A. (2015). Vitamins and type 2 diabetes mellitus. *Endocrine, Metabolic & Immune Disorders-Drug Targets (Formerly Current Drug Targets-Immune, Endocrine & Metabolic Disorders)*, *15*(1), 54-63.

[21] O'Leary, F. and Samman, S. (2010) Vitamin B12 in Health and Disease. Nutrients, 2, 299-316.

[22] Combs, G. (1992). Vitamin B12 in The Vitamins New York. Academic Press, Inc.

[23] Herbert, V. and Das, K. (1994). Vitamin B12 in Modern Nutrition in health and disease. Baltimore, MD: Williams & Wilkins.

[24] Herbert, V. (1996). Vitamin B12 in Present Knowledge in Nutrition 17th ed Washington. DC: International Life Sciences Institute Press.

[25] Zittoun, J. and Zittoun, R. (1999). Modern clinical testing strategies in cobalamin and folate deficiency. *Seminars in hematology.* pp. 35-46.

[26] Intakes, I. o. M. S. C. o. t. S. E. o. D. R. (1998). *Dietary reference intakes for thiamin, riboflavin, niacin, vitamin B6, folate, vitamin B12, pantothenic acid, biotin, and choline.* National Academies Press (US).

[27] Clarke, R. (2008). B-vitamins and prevention of dementia. *Proceedings of the Nutrition Society*, **67**:75-81.

[28] Biemans, E., Hart, H. E., Rutten, G. E., Renteria, V. G. C., Kooijman-Buiting, A. M. and Beulens, J. W. (2015). Cobalamin status and its relation with depression, cognition and neuropathy in patients with type 2 diabetes mellitus using metformin. *Acta diabetologica*, **52**:383-393.

[29] Ebesunun, M., Umahoin, K., Alonge, T. and Adebusoye, L. (2014). Plasma homocysteine, B vitamins and bone mineral density in osteoporosis: a possible risk for bone fracture. *African journal of medicine and medical sciences*, **43**:41-47.

[30] Osimani, A., Berger, A., Friedman, J., Porat-Katz, B.-S. and Abarbanel, J. M. (2005). Neuropsychology of Vitamin $B_{12}$ Deficiency in Elderly Dementia Patients and Control Subjects. *Journal of geriatric psychiatry and neurology*, **18**:33-38.

[31] File, C. N. (2015). Nutrient Profile: Beets, raw.

[32] He, M., & Dowd, P. (1998). Mechanism of action of vitamin b12. Ultrafast radical clocks provide no evidence for radical intermediates in cyclopropane models for the methylmalonyl-coa to succinyl-coa carbon skeleton rearrangement. *Journal of the American Chemical Society*, *120*(6), 1133-1137.

[33] Van den Driessche, A., Eenkhoorn, V., Van Gaal, L. and De Block, C. (2009). Type 1 diabetes and autoimmune polyglandular syndrome: a clinical review. *Neth J Med*, **67**:376-387.

[34] De Block, C. E., De Leeuw, I. H. and Van Gaal, L. F. (2008). Autoimmune

gastritis in type 1 diabetes: a clinically oriented review. *The Journal of Clinical Endocrinology & Metabolism*, **93**:363-371.

[35] De Block, C. E., De Leeuw, I. H. and Van Gaal, L. F. (1999). High Prevalence of Manifestations of Gastric Autoimmunity in Parietal Cell Antibody-Positive Type 1 (Insulin-Dependent) Diabetic Patients 1. *The Journal of Clinical Endocrinology & Metabolism*, **84**:4062-4067.

[36] Joffe, B., Distiller, L., Landau, S., Blacking, L. and Klisiewicz, A. (2010). Spectrum of Autoimmune Disorders in Type 1 Diabetes–A Cross-Sectional Clinical Audit. *Journal of Diabetes & Metabolism*, **1**:1-2.

[37] Fein, H. G. and Rivlin, R. S. (1975). Anemia in thyroid diseases. *Medical Clinics of North America*, **59**:1133-1145.

[38] Selimoglu, M. A. and Karabiber, H. (2010). Celiac disease: prevention and treatment. *Journal of clinical gastroenterology*, **44**:4-8.

[39] Day, C. (2012). ADA-EASD diabetes guidance: individualised treatment of hyperglycaemia. *The British Journal of Diabetes & Vascular Disease*, **12**:146-151.

[40] Bauman, W. A., Shaw, S., Jayatilleke, E., Spungen, A. M. and Herbert, V. (2000). Increased intake of calcium reverses vitamin B12 malabsorption induced by metformin. *Diabetes care*, **23**:1227-1231.

[41] Crider, K.S.; Yang, T.P.; Berry, R.J. and Bailey, L.B. (2012) Folate and DNA Methylation: A Review of Molecular Mechanisms and the Evidence for Folate's Role. Adv. Nutr., 3, 21-38.

[42] Sasaki, Y.; Sone, H.; Kamiyama, S.; Shimizu, M.; Shirakawa, H.; Kagawa, Y.; Komai, M. and Furukawa, Y. (2012) Administration of biotin prevents the development of insulin resistance in the skeletal muscles of Otsuka Long-Evans Tokushima Fatty rats. Food Funct., 3(4), 414-419.

[43] Rittner, Don, & Bailey, Ronald Albert. (2005). Encyclopedia of Chemistry (Science Encyclopedia).

[44] Cheung, Evelyn Ning Man. (2010). *Synthesis and Application of Polymer Stabilized Lanthanide Fluoride Nanoparticles.* University of Toronto.

[45] Laanpere, Margit, Altmäe, Signe, Stavreus-Evers, Anneli, Nilsson, Torbjörn K, Yngve, Agneta, & Salumets, Andres. (2010). Folate-Mediated One-Carbon Metabolism and Its Effect on Female Fertility and Pregnancy Viability. *Nutrition Reviews, 68*(2), 99-113.

[46] Joint, FAO, & Organization, World Health. (2005). Vitamin and Mineral Requirements in Human Nutrition.

[47] Beaudin, Anna E., & Stover, Patrick J. (2007). Folate-Mediated One-Carbon Metabolism and Neural Tube Defects: Balancing Genome Synthesis and Gene Expression. *Birth Defects Research Part C: Embryo Today: Reviews, 81*(3), 183-203. doi: 10.1002/bdrc.20100.

[48] Rittner, Don, & Bailey, Ronald Albert. (2005). Encyclopedia of Chemistry (Science Encyclopedia).

[49] Nazki, F. H., Sameer, A. S., & Ganaie, B. A. (2014). Folate: Metabolism, Genes, Polymorphisms and the Associated Diseases. *Gene, 533*(1), 11-20. doi: 10.1016/j.gene.2013.09.063.

[50] Riaz, Samreen. (2014). Evaluation and Analysis of Human Folate Levels in Pakistani Diabetic Population. *International Journal of S cientific & Engineering Research, 5*(12), 1572.

[51] Chan, Y. M., Bailey, R., & O'Connor, D. L. (2013). Folate. *Adv Nutr, 4*(1), 123-125. doi: 10.3945/an.112.003392

[52] Barnabé, Aline, Aléssio, Ana Cláudia Morandi, Bittar, Luis Fernando, de Moraes Mazetto, Bruna, Bicudo, Angélica M, de Paula, Erich V, Höehr, Nelci Fenalti, & Annichino-Bizzacchi, Joyce M. (2015). Folate, Vitamin B12 and Homocysteine Status in the Post-Folic Acid Fortification Era in Different Subgroups of the Brazilian Population Attended to at a Public Health Care Center. *Nutrition journal, 14*(1), 1.

[53] Zheng, Miaoyan, Zhang, Meilin, Yang, Juhong, Zhao, Shijing, Qin, Shanchun, Chen, Hui, Gao, Yuxia, & Huang, Guowei. (2014). Relationship between Blood Levels of Methyl Donor and Folate and Mild Cognitive Impairment in Chinese Patients with Type 2 Diabetes: A Case-Control Study. *Journal of clinical biochemistry and nutrition, 54*(2), 122-128.

Section 5

# Machine Learning and Cyber Systems for Diabetes

Chapter 17

# Selecting Intermittent Fasting Type to Improve Health in Type 2 Diabetes: A Machine Learning Approach

*Shula Shazman*


## Abstract

Intermittent fasting (IF) is the cycling between periods of eating and fasting. The two most popular forms of IER are: the 5: 2 diet characterized by two consecutive or non-consecutive "fast" days and the alternate-day energy restriction, commonly called alternate-day fasting (ADF). The second form is time-restricted feeding (TRF), eating within specific time frames such as the most prevalent 16: 8 diet, with 16 hours of fasting and 8 hours for eating. It is already known that IF can bring about changes in metabolic parameters related with type 2 diabetes (T2D). Furthermore, IF can be effective in improving health by reducing metabolic disorders and age-related diseases. However, it is not clear yet whether the age at which fasting begins, gender and severity of T2D influence on the effectiveness of the different types of IF in reducing metabolic disorders. In this chapter I will present the risk factors of T2D, the different types of IF interventions and the research-based knowledge regarding the effect of IF on T2D. Furthermore, I will describe several machine learning approaches to provide a recommendation system which reveals a set of rules that can assist selecting a successful IF intervention for a personal case. Finally, I will discuss the question: Can we predict the optimal IF intervention for a prediabetes patient?


**Keywords:** machine learning, decision tree, type 2 diabetes, insulin resistance, precision medicine, intermittent fasting

## 1. Introduction

Obesity is an epidemic in developed countries. The obesity epidemic is increasing its magnitude and its public health impact. In 2017–2018, 67% of the population in Australia were overweight or obese [1]. In the United States, only minority of the individuals have a healthy weight (body mass index (BMI) of 18.5–25 kg/m$^2$, [2]. Furthermore, according to the World Health Organization (WHO), nearly 2 billion adults are overweight and more than 600 million patients are obese [3]. Type 2 Diabetes (T2D) is one of the chronical diseases associated with Obesity. T2D is usually characterized by insulin resistance (IR) [4]. Insulin resistance (IR) happens when the body does not fully respond to insulin. IR level can be used as a filtering index for primary T2D prevention.



IntechOpen

IR can be measured by using the homeostatic model assessment of insulin resistance (HOMA-IR) equation. HOMA-IR can be evaluated by fasting glucose and insulin levels. People with T2D commonly have High HOMA-IR score, which indicates significant insulin resistance [5–7].

As little as 3% weight reduction produces clinically significant effects to reduce HOMA-IR [8, 9]. The most widely prescribed strategy to induce weight loss is to reduce the daily calory intake [10]. Current guidelines recommended continuous energy restriction (CER) along with comprehensive lifestyle intervention, as the cornerstone of obesity treatment [11]. For some individuals CER are effective for weight loss. However, many people realize that this type of diet is difficult to follow, as it requires robust calorie counting, and frustration is caused be owing to the feeling of never being able to eat freely.

There has been increased interest in identifying alternative dietary weight loss strategies, because of the relative ineffectiveness of traditional CER approaches for achieving and sustaining weight loss. One such approach is intermittent fasting (IF) also called intermittent energy restriction (IER) which encompasses various diets that cycle between periods of fasting and no fasting, these diets do not necessarily specify what to eat. The regimens of IER may be easier to follow and maintain over time than CER. Furthermore, people do not fully compensate during fed periods for the lack of energy created during prolonged periods of fasting. Therefore, IER may lead to metabolic adjustments that prefer greater fat mass loss, better maintaining of lean mass, and weight loss [12–13].

The IER regimens range from fasting the whole days at a time to fasting for several hours during the day. IER paradigms involve recurring periods with little or no energy intake with intervening periods of ad libitum food intake. The two most popular forms of IER are: the 5: 2 diet characterized by two consecutive or non-consecutive "fast" days and the alternate-day energy restriction, commonly called alternate-day fasting (ADF). The second form is time-restricted feeding (TRF), eating within specific time frames such as the most prevalent 16: 8 diet, with 16 hours of fasting and 8 hours for eating.

Previous studies and systematic reviews provide an overview of IER regimes [14–34]. Those studies report the health benefits leading by IER regimes and discuss the physiological mechanisms by which health outcomes might be improved [35]. However, the question of whether IER is always able to reduce HOMA-IR is not answered by the latter studies; In other words, what are the conditions (age, gender, basal fasting glucose level, etc.) needed to make the IER effective for reducing HOMA-IR have not yet been deciphered. Moreover, results of previous studies are reported on a group level only rather than report per individual.

In today's era of precision medicine, we can be motivated to answer the question Can we predict who will be Successful on an IMF or TRF Diet or CER? For example, a patient with prediabetes or diabetes comes to see his physician to ask for advice. Could such patient benefit from a specific IF intervention? Benefit in terms of reducing HOMA-IR or even eliminating the T2D altogether. A recommendation system which suggest effective IF intervention for a certain patient is found in a new study [36]. The recommendation system is based on individual data from human fasting intervention studies. The system presented in the study, predicts which type of IF treatment can improve an individual's health and preventing or curing T2D. A machine learning approach is used to develop the recommendation system while a set of rules which can assist individual patients and their physicians in selecting the best IF intervention is provided by the results of the study.

A further question will be discussed in this chapter: Can we predict the optimal intervention IMF or TRF Diet or CER or other for a prediabetes patient? and what is the accuracy of such prediction?

## 2. Type 2 diabetes (T2D)

Diabetes is a chronic, metabolic disease characterized by elevated levels of blood glucose (or blood sugar). Our metabolism converts food into energy for our bodies to use. One of the things needed for this process is insulin. The pancreas makes a hormone called insulin. The insulin helps the cells turn glucose from the food we eat into energy. After we eat, the sugar levels in our blood rise and insulin is released into the bloodstream. The insulin then makes the cells absorb sugar from the blood. If this process does not work properly, the blood sugar levels rise. The medical term for blood sugar levels that are too high is hyperglycemia.

According to the International Diabetes Federation in 2017 there were 425 million people in the world with diabetes. That is close to 1 in 11 people [37].

### 2.1 Main types of diabetes

There are two main types of diabetes: type 1 and type 2. Glucose gives the body cells energy, but to enter the cells it needs insulin. People with type 1 diabetes do not produce insulin; while people with T2D do not respond to insulin as well as they should. Both types of diabetes can lead to chronically high blood sugar levels. Type 1 diabetes usually develops in childhood or teenage years. This disease is a result of damage to the pancreas that leaves it producing either very little insulin or none. Type 1 diabetes is caused by an autoimmune reaction where the body's defense system attacks the cells that produce insulin. Things are different in T2D, where insulin is made by the pancreas, but the body's cells lose the ability to absorb and use the insulin. In people who have T2D, the pancreas produces enough insulin, but it no longer influences the body's cells. The medical term for this is "insulin resistance" (IR). The pancreas can compensate for this for a while by producing more insulin. But at some point, it can no longer keep up, and then blood sugar levels start to rise. T2D is characterized by (IR), where the body does not fully respond to insulin. In the past, T2D was often referred to as "adult-onset" diabetes because it is commonly diagnosed later in life. T2D is much more common than type 1 diabetes. Among all the people living with diabetes, 90–95% percent have T2D. This chapter focuses on T2D.

### 2.2 Causes and risk factors

Usually, a combination of things causes T2D. There are several gene mutations linked to diabetes. Not everyone who carries a mutation will get diabetes. However, many people with diabetes do have one or more of these mutations. Being overweight or obese can cause IR. People with insulin resistance often have a group of conditions commonly called "Metabolic syndrome", including high blood sugar, extra fat around the waist, high blood pressure, high cholesterol and high triglycerides. Another cause can be bad communication between cells. Sometimes, cells send the wrong signals or do not pick up messages correctly. When these problems affect how cells make and use insulin or glucose, a chain reaction can lead to diabetes. Finally, broken beta cells can cause diabetes since if the cells that make insulin send out the wrong amount of insulin at the wrong time, blood sugar is not controlled properly.

Various factors can increase the likelihood of developing T2D. They can be described using 3 categories. The category of risk factors is who you are: age of 45 or older, a family relative with diabetes or ethnicity. The second category is health and medical history: being prediabetes can increase the risk for diabetes, heart and blood vessel disease, high blood pressure, low HDL ("good") cholesterol, high triglycerides, being overweight or obese, Gestational diabetes while you were pregnant and finally depression. The last category of risk factors is the daily habits and lifestyle. Among this category we can find factors such as getting little or no exercise, smoking, stress or sleeping too little or too much.

### 2.3 Symptoms and complications

T2D can evolve moderately during several years. Blood sugar levels stay high all the time when T2D is untreated. High blood sugar levels may cause the following symptoms: thirstiness, frequent urination, tiredness and apathy, fulsomeness and dizziness or even lose consciousness. In addition to T2D symptoms there are complications of T2D containing, five times more likely to get heart disease or have a stroke, dialysis, or kidney replacement in case the kidneys are damaged. Furthermore, high blood sugar can damage the small blood vessels in the backs of the eyes and in cases of neglect, it can cause blindness. Digestive disorders, not feeling of the feet and sexual response are considered as T2D complications as well. Lesions cure slower and can become infected when blood does not circulate well. Miscarriage are more likely in women with diabetes. A condition in which breathing stops and starts while you sleep might developed. It is more likely to have hearing problems. Finally, high blood sugar can damage your brain and might put you at higher risk of Alzheimer's disease.

### 2.4 How does T2D diagnosed?

Hemoglobin is a protein that transports oxygen to the body cells. It can be found inside red blood cells. In cases of high glucose level in the blood glucose can attach the hemoglobin. Hemoglobin that is attached to glucose is called glycated hemoglobin. T2D diabetes is usually diagnosed using the A1C test. A1C test measures the amount of hemoglobin in the blood that has glucose attached to it.

Red blood cells are constantly dying and regenerating. Their lifespan is approximately three months. Glucose attaches (glycates) to hemoglobin inside the red blood cells, so the record of how much glucose is attached to the hemoglobin also lasts for about three months. Normally, about 6 percent of hemoglobin has glucose attached. If there is too much glucose attached to the hemoglobin cells, the test results will be high A1C. If the amount of Glycated hemoglobin amount is normal, the A1C results will be normal. An A1C level of 6.5 percent or higher on two separate tests means you have diabetes.

The symbol A1C represents a specific type of hemoglobin. The "A" in Hemoglobin A (HgbA) stands for "adult." HgbA can be found in two types HgbA1 and HgbA2. In individuals from six months old about 98% of HgbA is type 1 (HgbA1). Type A1 has subtypes A1A, A1B, A1C, and others. Two-thirds of hemoglobin with glucose attached is type A1C [38]. Therefore, HgbA1C is a good marker for glucose control. Larger amount of hemoglobin will be glycated when more glucose is circulating in the blood.

However, the A1C test results are not always meaningful. For example, when we want to measure A1C difference before and after an intervention that is shorter than three months. The difference of A1C before and after the intervention will not tell us the accurate result because it is an average calculation. In such case we need another test to diagnose the glucose level in blood. Fasting blood glucose test is a blood sample which is taken after an overnight fast. A normal level of fasting glucose is a reading of less than 100 mg/dL (5.6 mmol/L). If the fasting blood glucose is 126 mg/dL (7 mmol/L) or higher, it considered diabetes. Values between 100 to 125 considered prediabetes. T2D is generally characterized by insulin resistance, where the body does not fully respond to insulin.

HOMA-IR stands for Homeostatic Model Assessment of Insulin Resistance. Using HOMA-IR equation insulin resistance can be estimated from fasting glucose and insulin levels. High score of HOMA-IR indicates a significant Insulin resistance which usually found in people with Diabetes Type 2. An updated HOMA model (HOMA2) was published by Jonathan Levy in 1998. HOMA2 model took account of variations in hepatic and peripheral glucose resistance, increases in the insulin secretion curve for plasma glucose concentrations above 10 mmol/L (180 mg/dL) and the contribution of circulating proinsulin [39]. In 2004, the HOMA2 Calculator [40] was released by Oxford university UK. This provides quick and easy access to the HOMA2 model for researchers who wish to use model-derived estimates of Insulin resistance, rather than linear approximations as provided by HOMA-IR model. There are additional tests to diagnose Diabetes type 2,beside those mentioned here, however those methods will not be discussed further in this chapter.

### 2.5 How is T2D treated?

There are two approaches to treat T2D. The first is lifestyle changes and the second is medications. Adopting a healthy lifestyle can help lower the risk of diabetes. Healthy life style contains: lose weight, get active, eat right, avoid highly processed carbs, sugary drinks, and trans and saturated fats, limit red and processed meats, quit smoking and finally work to keep from gaining weight after you quit smoking, so you do not create one problem by solving another. It is possible to reach your target blood sugar levels with diet and exercise alone. However, if changing lifestyle is not enough several medicines exist to treat diabetes. Among the medicine functions are: Lowering the amount of glucose your liver makes and helps your body responding better to the insulin. Helping your body make more insulin, making you more sensitive to insulin. Causing slow digestion and lowering blood sugar levels and finally help your kidneys filter out more glucose.

## 3. Intermittent fasting

In historical periods in the past when food was not always available fasting was sure to happen. Many religious philosophies have practiced fasting for centuries; however, cyclically restricting or reducing calories has recently taken off as a way to lose weight and improve health outcomes. Intermittent fasting (IF) is proposed as an alternative dieting strategy. IF includes cycles of fasting and unrestricted eating periods, which may allow more flexibility and thereby enhance devoutness [41]. Intermittent fasting is generally grouped into two main categories: whole-day fasting and time-restricted feeding. Both categories range in flexibility of time spent fasting. The details of intermittent fasting interventions which participate in the research described in this chapter are found in the following subsections.

### 3.1 Continuous energy restriction (CER)

In a paper from 2011 [42] Michelle Harvie describes a randomized controlled trial to compare the feasibility and effectiveness of intermittent continuous energy (IER) with continuous energy restriction (CER) for weight loss, insulin sensitivity and other metabolic disease risk markers. The CER involved a 25% energy restriction from estimated baseline energy requirements using reported metabolic energy turnovers estimated basal metabolic rate [43] for 7 days per week. The CER group was prescribed a daily 25% restriction based on a Mediterranean-type diet (30% fat, 15% monounsaturated, 7.5% saturated fat, 7.5% polyunsaturated fatty acids, 45% low glycemic load carbohydrate and 25% protein) [44].

### 3.2 Intermittent energy restriction (IER)

The IER group from the randomized controlled trial in Harvie's paper [42] took a very low-calorie diet (VLCD) (75% restriction) on two consecutive days and for the remaining 5 days consume food for weight maintenance. The VLCD provided 2700 kJ of energy and 50 g protein per day, four portions of vegetables (~80 g per portion), one portion of fruit, a salty low-calorie drink and a multivitamin and mineral supplement. The duration of the intervention was six months.

### 3.3 Daily morning fasting (DMF)

Daily morning fasting is based on the Bath Breakfast Project (BBP) [45]. BBP is a randomized controlled trial comparing the effects of daily breakfast consumption relative to extended fasting on energy balance and human health. In a randomized cross-over design, obese men and women extended their overnight fast by omitting breakfast consumption or ingesting a typical carbohydrate-rich breakfast of (521 ± 94 kcal), before an ad libitum pasta lunch 3 h later. The duration of intervention was 4 weeks.

### 3.4 Fasting every second day (FESD)

Fasting every second day (FESD) was experienced in a paper of Nils Halberg [46]. The duration of the intervention was 14 days of fasting every second day for 20 h, giving seven fasting periods. Each fasting period started at 22:00 and ended at 18:00 the following day. During the fasting periods, the subjects could drink water and were instructed to maintain habitual activities.

### 3.5 Intermittent energy and carbohydrate restriction (IECR)

Another IER approach is tested in the paper of Michelle Harvie from 2013 [47]. The test in latter paper included two intermittent energy and carbohydrate restriction (IECR) regimens, including one which allowed ad libitum protein and fat (IECR PF). Overweight 115 women were randomized to an overall 25% energy restriction, either as an IECR (2500–2717 kJ/d,40 g carbohydrate/d for 2 d/week) or a 25% daily energy restriction (DER – which is type of CER - approximately 6000 kJ/d for 7 d/week) or an IECR PF for a 3-month weight-loss period and 1 month of weight maintenance (IECR or IECR PF for 1 d/week).

## 4. The steps in machine learning

This study described in this chapter aims to predict whether a specific IF intervention would reduce the insulin resistance of an individual with prediabetes. The approach to answer this question is machine learning. The process of machine learning is composed of 5 major steps: The first is identifying the required data and gathering data from various sources. The next step is preparing and Pre-processing the data to have homogeneity. Then the model must be built by selecting the right Machine Learning classifier. The fourth step is to train and test the data and gain insights from the model results. Finally, we might want to improve results by feature selection for example.

## 4.1 Identifying required data

In order to answer the question of this study, authors of 25 published papers that performed randomized clinical trials investigating the IF effects on T2D parameters were asked for the individual data. I received the individual data from 5 out 25 papers [42, 45–48]. The other authors replied that they could not submit the data due to the confidentiality of the participants.

## 4.2 Processing the data

### *4.2.1 Choosing people*

The selection criteria for this research were: basal fasting glucose above 5 mmol/L (90 mg/dL) or BMI (Body Mass Index) above or equal to 25. Those criteria were established since they indicate possible prediabetes [49]. The IDF's 2019 cutoff for fasting glucose indicating prediabetes is 100 mg/dL; we set the cutoff at 90 mg/dL. Finally, 254 individuals who answered the criteria were selected. **Table 1** contains the average values of the numerical attributes of the data. The average values show decrease in weight, BMI, fasting glucose and fasting insulin however we should remember that those are averages therefore we cannot conclude that all the interventions work all the time for all the people. This would be the query that the machine learning approach will investigate.

### *4.2.2 HOMA-IR equation*

The Homeostatic Model Assessment of Insulin Resistance (HOMA-IR) has been proven to be a very sensitive test for indicating prediabetes [8]. Insulin resistance can be estimated from fasting glucose and insulin levels. This is shown in the HOMA-IR equation presented as follows:

$$\mathrm{HOMA} - IR - \mathrm{Fasting\ Glucose} * \mathrm{Fasting\ Insulin} \tag{1}$$

Prediabetes people or people with T2D usually have a significant insulin resistance. A high score of HOMA-IR indicates a significant insulin resistance. To learn the difference of HOMA-IR before and after the intervention the HOMA-IR using (Eq. (1)) was calculated twice for each of the 254 individuals. Once HOMA-IR was calculated for the basal values of fasting glucose and insulin and once for the values after the intervention. The difference between them represents the insulin resistance reduction.

### *4.2.3 Types of intermittent fasting interventions*

This study contains 9 different types of interventions, starting from continuous energy restriction – through intermittent energy restriction for two days a week, or

| Age | Weight | | BMI | | Fasting glucose (mmol/liter) | | Fasting insulin (pmol/liter) | |
|---|---|---|---|---|---|---|---|---|
| | Basal | After | Basal | After | Basal | After | Basal | After |
| 44.3 | 87.5 | 81.1 | 32.1 | 31 | 4.99 | 4.93 | 61.1 | 53.6 |

**Table 1.**
*Average values of attribute in selected data.*

daily morning fasting or fasting every second day. Part of the interventions contained specific diets. The names of the different types of the interventions and their description are found in **Table 2** below.

**Table 2** summarizes the different IF regimens included in this study. The reference to each regimen is also shown in **Table 2** for further details.

#### *4.2.4 Individual's features*

The data collected for each individual in this study contained details regarding the age, gender, weight, ethnicity, basal BMI, basal fasting glucose, fasting glucose after intervention, basal fasting insulin and fasting insulin after intervention. Details of the intervention such as intervention's name and duration were also included for each individual. For being able to train and learn from the data the features 'fasting glucose after intervention' and 'fasting insulin after intervention' must be excluded. A calculated feature named 'HOMA-IR difference' was added to the training vector. This feature was calculated as follows: if the intervention is successful we expect a reduction in HOMA-IR; thus, if the HOMA-IR difference is greater than zero the assignment in the 'HOMA-IR difference' column is set to TRUE otherwise it is FALSE. The final training vector included the ten following features: age, gender, weight, ethnicity, basal BMI, basal fasting glucose, basal fasting insulin, intervention's name, intervention's and HOMA-IR difference.

### 4.3 Building a model from the data

The problem of the study describe here is a classification question. Can we predict whether an intermittent fasting intervention will be useful to improve T2D risk parameters for a certain individual? Classification is a data mining technique which solve problems by analyzing large volumes of data. Furthermore, classification is the process of finding a model that describes and differentiates data classes, where the ultimate goal is being able to use the model to predict the class of an instance whose label is unknown. Decision trees are kind of algorithm that can be used for classification, while additional algorithms which can be used for this purpose are

| Intervention name | Details | CER\ IER | Duration | Reference |
|---|---|---|---|---|
| CER | Continuous energy restriction - 7 days a week trail | CER | 24 weeks | [42] |
| IER | Intermittent energy restriction - 2 days a week trail | IER | 24 weeks | [42] |
| DMF | Daily Morning Fasting | IER | 4 weeks | [45] |
| FESD | Fasting Every Second | IER | 2 weeks | [46] |
| IECR | Intermittent Energy and Carbohydrate Restriction | IER | 24 weeks | [47] |
| IECR+PF | Intermittent Energy and Carbohydrate Restriction + free protein and fat | IER | 24 weeks | [47] |
| DER | Daily Energy Restriction | CER | 24 weeks | [47] |
| High Carb | High Carbohydrate weight loss diet | CER | 12 weeks | [48] |
| High Mono | High Monounsaturated weight loss diet | CER | 12 weeks | [48] |

**Table 2.**
*IF regimens.*

neural networks, naïve bayes, logistic regression and others. However, the decision tree classification with the Waikato Environment for Knowledge Analysis (Weka) is the simplest way to mine information from a database. Furthermore, decision trees can deal with a large variety of feature types like binary, nominal, ordinal, categorial and numeric like those found in our mixed dataset [50]. Finally, decision trees are an intuitive way of representing a sequence of rules that lead to a class or value. The decision tree output is a flowchart-like tree structure. The decision tree algorithms J48, LMT (Logistic Model Tree), Random Forest and Random Tree as well as the Logistic Regression and Naïve Bayes classifiers were tested on the data in this study.

### 4.4 Training and testing

The next step was training the dataset (254 individuals) and building models using six different classifiers: J48 decision tree, Logistic Model Tree, Random forest, Random tree, Logistic and Naïve Bayes. The optimal number of features as a function of sample size is proportional to $\sqrt{n}$ (n is the sample size) for highly correlated features [51]. The features in the study shown here are highly correlated and $\sqrt{254} = 15.9$ while the number of features is 9 (i.e. 9 attributes for 254 individuals is reliable). Following the training comes the testing. Two test approaches were selected to validate the model – the leave-one-out and the 10-fold cross validations. In the leave-one-out approach you test every individual by excluding it from the training set, train the 253 left individuals and then test the excluded one. This happens 254 times, namely for every individual in the dataset. The 10-fold cross validation test approach divide the dataset into 10 groups equal in size. Then for ten times train and build the model with nine of the groups together and test the individual found in the 10th excluded group.

## 5. Decision rules for health benefit due to intermittent fasting

### 5.1 Prediction whether HOMA-IR decreases

When measuring performance of machine learning classifiers, accuracy is not enough. For comparing results from different classifiers, we need an additional measure. The additional measure is based on the definition of four groups resulted when solving a classification. For example, in our case when the case is that there is a reduction in HOMA-IR then the TRUE-POSITIVE (TP) group is when the prediction is correct, while the FALSE-POSITIVE (FP) group is when the prediction is not correct. The two additional groups found when the case is that there is no HOMA-IR reduction then TRUE-NEGATIVE (TN) will be when the prediction is false in other words the prediction is correct; however, when the prediction is not correct we say it is the FALSE-NEGATIVE (FN). The additional measure to compare between different classifiers is Area Under Curve (AUC) measure. AUC presents the relation between the TP rate and the FP rate and it is a very useful in the comparison between classifiers. The value of AUC ranges between 0 to 1. AUC equals 1 means a perfect classifier TP = 1 and FP = 0, while random classifier is when AUC is equal approximately to 0.5.

The AUC of the six different classifiers – J48, LMT, Random Forest, Random Tree, Logistic Regression and Naïve Bayes using the two test methods mentioned in the previous paragraph – are shown in **Table 3**. The AUC of the 10-Fold test is shown in the first row of **Table 3** while the Leave-One-Out test is found in the second row. For both tests the AUC differences between the classifiers are very small (0.67 to 0.75 in the 10-fold and 0.65–0.8 in the leave-one-out); we therefore conclude that all six classifiers perform similarly. The advantage of Random Forest is to prevent overfitting by creating random subsets of the features and building smaller trees and then combining the subtrees, however J48 is shown to yield the most accurate prediction within the decision tree algorithms [50]. In addition, J48 explains itself and easy to follow. In the J48 decision tree, the internal nodes are the different features (age, gender, weight, etc.), the branches between the nodes represent the possible values that these features may have (age: lower than 18 or equal higher than 18, gender: male/female, etc.). The terminal nodes tell us the final value of the prediction(TRUE or FALSE assigned for HOMA-IR difference). As shown in **Table 3** using J48 classifier and the 10-fold cross validation test the model AUC is 0.7. Furthermore, the Leave-One-Out test achieves AUC of 0.8. Therefore, the J48 model successfully predicts whether an intervention would help an individual improve his T2D risk parameters by reducing HOMA-IR.

The visualization of the J48 decision tree is found in **Figures 1–4**. Interestingly the attribute gender is the first node in the tree, as shown in **Figures 1** and **2**. Having the gender as the first splitting attribute indicates that this attribute is the most informative one for the decision. Moreover, for males the duration of the intervention is the most important attribute to decide the effectiveness of the intervention (**Figure 1**); while for females the basal fasting insulin level is reported as the most important feature (**Figure 2**). Green in **Figures 1–4** represents TRUE which indicates success in reducing HOMA-IR while red represents FALSE which indicates no reduction.

Analyzing the sub-decision tree of the males' side shown **Figure 1**, brings to the conclusion that men are indifferent to the type of the intervention rather they affected by the duration of the intervention. Success of intervention defined by reducing HOMA-IR, can be achieved by short duration of fasting (less or equal to 2.5 weeks) and lower BMI (less or equal to 25.8) or long duration of intervention and age 41 years and younger. Reasonably, attributes like lower BMI and younger age make it easier to reduce HOMA-IR.

| | J48 | LMT | Random Forest | Random Tree | Logistic | Naive Bayes |
|---|---|---|---|---|---|---|
| 10-Fold | 0.7 | 0.75 | 0.75 | 0.67 | 0.79 | 0.73 |
| Leave-One- Out | 0.8 | 0.74 | 0.74 | 0.66 | 0.79 | 0.72 |

**Table 3.**
*AUC for different classifiers.*

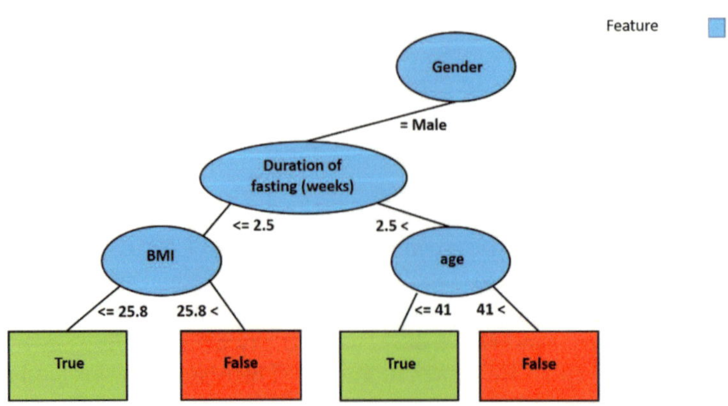


**Figure 1.**
*Sub-decision tree – Male side.*

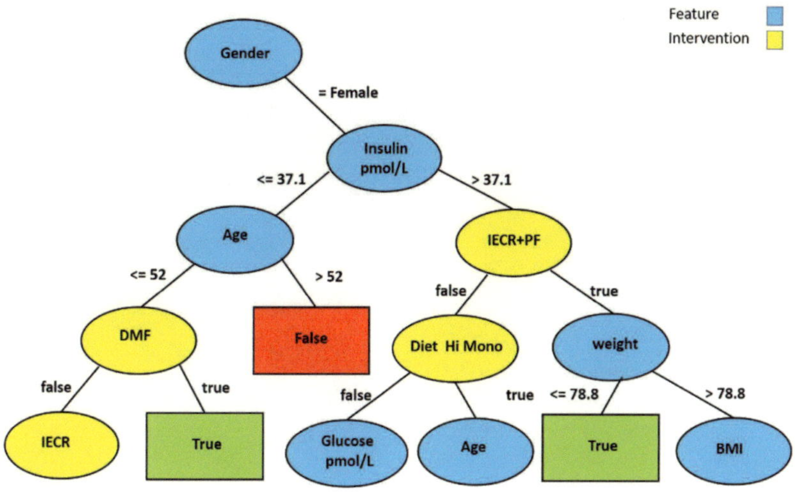


**Figure 2.**
*Sub-decision tree – Female side.*

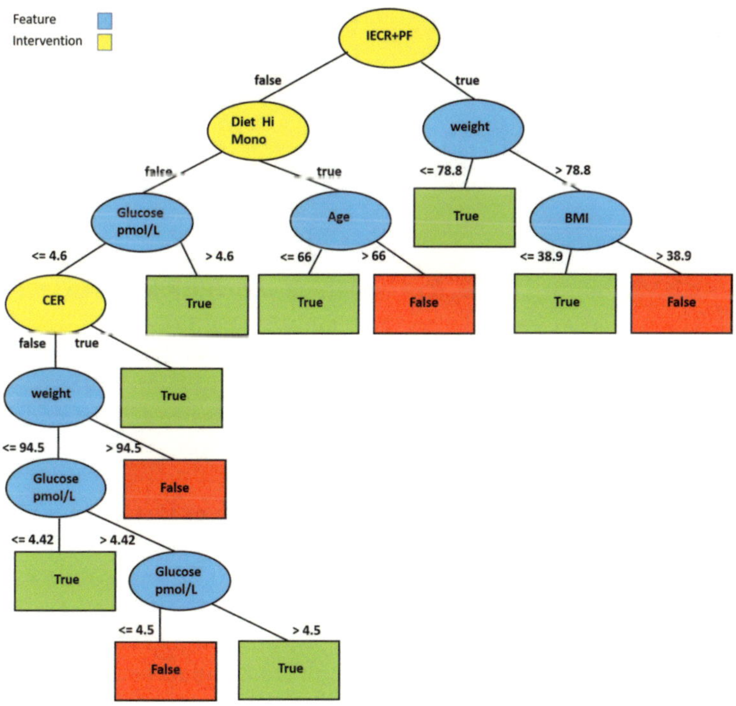


**Figure 3.**
*Sub-decision tree – Female left side.*

Unlike the male side of the decision tree, in the female side the type of intervention is part of the tree and is represented by the nodes of the tree. As shown in **Figure 2** the intervention are nodes of the tree which are colored yellow while the nodes that represent attributes are colored blue. Moreover, the view of the tree on the female side consist of many different and connected parts compared with the male side of the tree. The fact that there are more women in the dataset than men can be the reason for this complexity view. The different interventions are part of the decision nodes as shown in **Figure 2**. The different interventions are arranged hierarchically

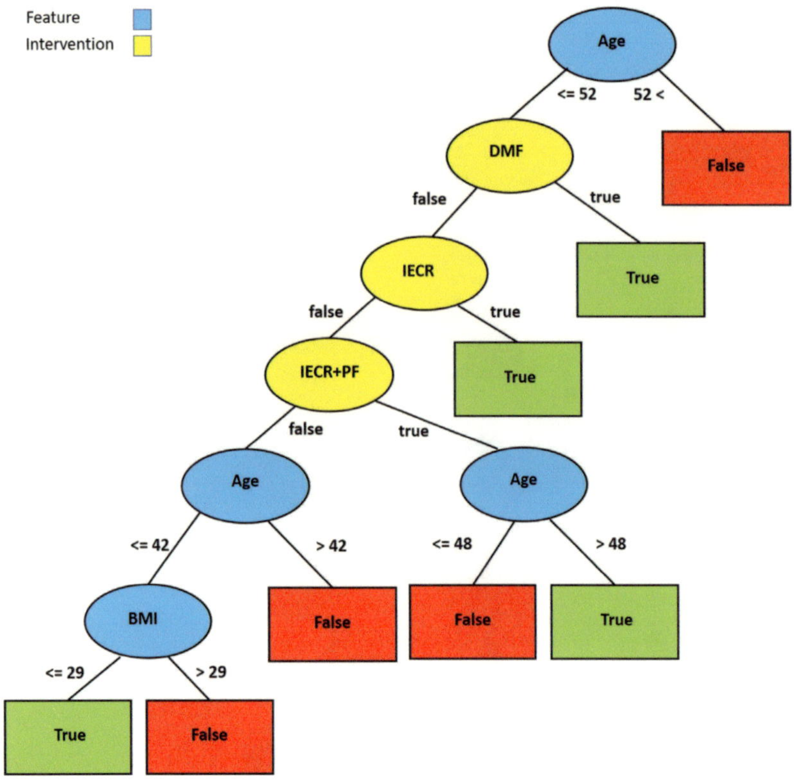


**Figure 4.**
*Sub-decision tree – Female right side.*

starting with DMF followed by IECR or beginning with IECR followed by the Hi Mono diet. The success of the different interventions in improving HOMA-IR is shown in **Figure 3**. The hierarchical structure of the interventions is organized by their success, beginning with DMF, IECR and then IECR+PF. An interesting evidence which should be further investigated is found in **Figure 4**. That evidence is the node where lower BMI leads to an unsuccessful intervention.

### 5.2 Testing separately the reduction of fasting glucose or fasting insulin

To find out whether only fasting glucose reduction or fasting insulin reduction taken separately instead of HOMA-IR can be used to predict the usefulness of an intervention two additional train and test process were done. **Table 4** summarizes the results of the predictions based once only on fasting glucose reduction and once only on fasting insulin reduction.

As shown in **Table 4** the prediction of improvement in T2D based on HOMA-IR is more effective than the prediction based on fasting glucose or the fasting insulin separately. As shown in Eq. 1, the HOMA-IR calculation is based on both fasting glucose and fasting insulin.

### 5.3 Comparing results with random classification

An interesting question would be would these results based on HOMA-IR obtain on random? To answer this question, I reordered the values in the HOMA-IR column in an arbitrary way. The ratio between the TRUE values and the FALSE values was identical to the original column. The AUC results of training and testing

| | HOMA-IR reduction | FASTING Glucose reduction | FASTING Insulin reduction |
|---|---|---|---|
| 10-Fold Cross Validation test | 0.7 | 0.6 | 0.55 |
| Leave- One-Out test | 0.8 | 0.6 | 0.6 |

**Table 4.**
*Summary of AUC results for improving T2D risk parameters.*

| Excluded Feature | 10-Fold Cross Validation test | Leave-One-Out test |
|---|---|---|
| None | 0.7 | 0.8 |
| Age | 0.68 | 0.7 |
| Gender | 0.68 | 0.62 |
| Weight | 0.64 | 0.73 |
| Ethnic | 0.68 | 0.74 |
| Basal BMI | 0.69 | 0.77 |
| Fasting Glucose – basal | 0.65 | 0.73 |
| Fasting Insulin – basal | 0.62 | 0.6 |

**Table 5.**
*Features selection – AUC results of J48 Decision tree.*

with random data were much lower compared with the original data. The 10-Fold cross validation test yields 0.56 AUC compared with 0.7 in the original data. The Leave-One-Out test difference in AUC between the random and the original data was even more significant – 0.61 AUC in the random data compared with 0.8 in the original data. Those results answer the question asked above and suggest that the model predictions cannot be obtain in random.

### 5.4 Testing features redundancy

Another interesting question is whether all the features mentioned in 4.2.4 are needed for the prediction. To test this a feature selection test was performed on the data. In each test a different feature was excluded. The AUC results are shown in **Table 5**.

The feature in every row of **Table 5** except of the first row, is excluded and AUC is calculated without this feature. None of the features is redundant since as shown in **Table 5** the highest AUC is shown when all features are trained.

## 6. Conclusions

To achieve steady-state fasting levels for many metabolic substrates which are found in blood draws taken from patients, the patients are required to fast 8–12 hours. This evidence can show us that even a single fasting interval in humans (e.g., overnight) can reduce basal concentrations of metabolic biomarkers related with T2D, such as insulin and glucose. Intermittent fasting regimens may be a promising approach to losing weight and improving metabolic health. Moreover, these eating regimens may offer promising nonpharmacological approaches to improving health in general and specifically improve T2D condition.

The question in this study is not how to lose weight but to answer the question of which of the people suffering from T2D can benefit through an intermittent fasting approach and what is the best type of intermittent fasting for a particular person. This it offers a recommendation system based on data from several clinical trials for answering those questions. The recommendation system selects the optimal intervention to improve the health of prediabetes individuals or people with T2D. The improvement in health reflected in reducing their glucose and insulin levels which are considered T2D risk parameters and composed the HOMA-IR equation. The procedure in this study is built using a machine learning approach and is the results are presented by a decision tree. The conclusions from the decision rules derived from the tree are that males and females have a different set of rules because the node gender comes first in the tree. The success of intervention in males depends on the duration of the IF. Therefore, males are indifferent to the type of intervention. Moreover, males with a smaller BMI will be more likely to have a successful intervention in case the duration of intervention is equal or less than 2.5 weeks. On the other hand, if the duration of the intervention is more than 2.5 weeks for males than age will be important to its success. Reasonably, younger age will serve as a benefit. The level of basal fasting insulin is the most important attribute for a successful intervention in female. There are some cases where no intervention within the dataset of this study can assist in improving HOMA-IR for example if a female with a basal fasting insulin equal or less than 37.1 pmol/L (for moderate insulin resistance the fasting insulin should be in the range of 18–48 pmol/L) and age exceeding 52.

To apply for a wider population additional clinical trail's data should be used. Moreover, a larger dataset will make it possible, to build a software which would assist physicians in advising an optimal intervention to their patients and by that providing a better personalized medical service to their patients.

## Acknowledgments

I wish to thank Michelle Harvie, Nils Halberg, Flemming Dela, Peter M. Clifton, Eric Ravussin, Leonie Kaye Heilbronn and Enhad Chowdhury for their assistance in this study by sending the individual data from their published clinical trial papers.

## Author details

Shula Shazman
The Open University, Raanana, Israel

*Address all correspondence to: shulash@openu.ac.il

## References

[1] Australian Bureau of Statistics. National Health Survey: First Results, 2017-2018 [Internet]. Canberra (ACT): Commonwealth of Australia; 2018 [cited 2019 Oct 25]. ABS cat. no. 4364.0.55.001. Available from: https://www.abs.gov.au/ausstats/

[2] Ogden, C.L., Carroll, M.D., Kit, B.K., Flegal, K.M. Prevalence of childhood and adult obesity in the United States 2011-2012. JAMA. 2014; 311, 806-814. DOI: 10.1001/jama.2014.732

[3] WHO. 2017. 10 facts on obesity, Accessed September 17, 2019. Available from: https://www.who.int/features/factfiles/obesity/en/

[4] Roy Taylor. Insulin Resistance and Type 2 Diabetes. Diabetes 2012 Apr; 61(4):778-779. https://doi.org/10.2337/db12-0073

[5] Tang, Q., Li, X., Song, P. and Xu. L. Optimal cut-off values for the homeostasis model assessment of insulin resistance (HOMA-IR) and pre-diabetes screening: Developments in research and prospects for the future. Drug Discoveries & Therapeutics. 2015; *9(6):380-385.* DOI: 10.5582/ddt.2015.01207

[6] Sharma, S. and Fleming, E. Use of HbA1C testing to diagnose pre-diabetes in high risk African American children: A comparison with fasting glucose and HOMA-IR. Diabetes & Metabolic Syndrome: Clinical Research & Reviews 6 (2012): 157-162. DOI: 10.1016/j.dsx.2012.09.004

[7] Dagmar Horáková, Ladislav Štěpánek, Vladimír Janout, Jana Janoutová, Dalibor Pastucha, Helena Kollárová, Alena Petráková, Lubomír Štěpánek, Roman Husár and Karel Martiník. Optimal Homeostasis Model Assessment of Insulin Resistance (HOMA-IR) Cut-Offs: A Cross-Sectional Study in the Czech Population. Medicina (Kaunas). 2019 May; 55(5): 158. DOI: 10.3390/medicina55050158

[8] National Institute for Health and Care Excellence. Weight management: lifestyle services for overweight or obese adults [Internet]. [London]: NICE; 2014 [updated May 2017; cited 2020 Jan 16]. [Public health guideline [PH53]). Available from:https://www.nice.org.uk/guidance/ph53/chapter/1-Recommendations.

[9] M.D. Jensen, D.H. Ryan, C.M. Apovian, J.D. Ard, A.G. Comuzzie, K.A. Donato, et al.,2013 AHA/ACC/TOS guideline for the management of overweight and obesity in adults: a report of the american college of cardiology/american heart association task force on practice guidelines and the obesity society, J Am Coll Cardiol. 63 (25, Part B) (2014) 2985-3023.

[10] Julia C., Peneau S., Andreeva V.A., Mejean C.; Fezeu L., Galan P., Hercberg S. Weight-loss strategies used by the general population: How are they perceived? PLoS ONE **2014**, 9, e97834. DOI: 10.1371/journal.pone.0097834

[11] Jensen M.D., Ryan D.H., Apovian C.M., Ard J.D., Comuzzie A.G., Donato K.A., Hu F.B., Hubbard V.S., Jakicic J.M., Kushner R.F., et al. 2013 AHA/ACC/TOS guideline for the management of overweight and obesity in adults: A report of the American College of Cardiology/American Heart Association Task Force on Practice Guidelines and The Obesity Society. Circulation 2014, 129, S102–S138. DOI: 10.1161/01.cir.0000437739.71477.ee

[12] Mattson M.P., Longo V.D., Harvie M. Impact of intermittent fasting on health and disease processes. Ageing Res. Rev. 2017, 39, 46-58. DOI: 10.1016/j.arr.2016.10.005

[13] Ana Luísa and Kremer Faller. Impact of intermittent fasting on the body weight of overweight and obese individuals. http://dx.doi.org/10.1590/1806-9282.66.2.237

[14] Lukas Schwingshackl, Jasmin Zähringer, Kai Nitschke, Gabriel Torbahn, Szimonetta Lohner, Tilman Kühn, Luigi Fontana, Nicola Veronese, Christine Schmucker and Joerg J Meerpohl. Impact of intermittent energy restriction on anthropometric outcomes and intermediate disease markers in patients with overweight and obesity: systematic review and meta analyses. Critical Reviews in Food Science and Nutrition. 2020. DOI: 10.1080/10408398.2020.1757616

[15] Kai Liu, Bo Liu, Leonie K. Heilbronn. Intermittent fasting: What questions should we be asking? Physiology & Behavior 218. 2020. DOI: 10.1016/j.physbeh.2020.112827

[16] Stephen D. Anton, Stephanie A. Lee, William T. Donahoo, Christian McLaren, Todd Manini, Christiaan Leeuwenburgh and Marco Pahor. The Effects of Time Restricted Feeding on Overweight, Older Adults: A Pilot Study. Nutrients 2019, 11, 1500; DOI:10.3390/nu11071500

[17] Surabhi Bhutani, Monica C. Klempel, Cynthia M. Kroeger, John F. Trepanowski and Krista A. Varady. Alternate Day Fasting and Endurance Exercise Combine to Reduce Body Weight and Favorably Alter Plasma Lipids in Obese Humans. Obesity, 2013, 21, 1370-1379. DOI:10.1002/oby.20353

[18] Jane Bowen , Emily Brindal, Genevieve James-Martin and Manny Noakes. Randomized Trial of a High Protein, Partial Meal Replacement Program with or without Alternate Day Fasting: Similar Effects on Weight Loss, Retention Status, Nutritional, Metabolic, and Behavioral Outcomes. Nutrients 2018, 10, 1145; DOI:10.3390/nu10091145 www.mdpi

[19] S. Carter, P.M. Clifton, J.B. Keogh. The effects of intermittent compared to continuous energy restriction on glycaemic control in type 2 diabetes; a pragmatic pilot trial. Diabetes research and clinical practice 122 ( 2016 ) 106-112. http://dx.doi.org/10.1016/j.diabres.2016.10.010

[20] Sharayah Carter, Peter *M. Clifton*, Jennifer B. Keogh. Effect of Intermittent Compared With Continuous Energy Restricted Diet on Glycemic Control in Patients With Type 2 Diabetes A Randomized Noninferiority Trial. JAMA Network Open. 2018;1(3):e180756. DOI:10.1001/jamanetworkopen.2018.0756

[21] Rachel Leah Taft. Intermittent Fasting for Weight Loss: Pros and Cons for People with Diabetes. AADE in Practice. 2019. Volume: 7 issue: 4, page(s): 42-46.

[22] Corey A. Rynders, Elizabeth A. Thomas, Adnin Zaman, Zhaoxing Pan, Victoria A. Catenacci and Edward L. Melanson. Effectiveness of Intermittent Fasting and Time-Restricted Feeding Compared to Continuous Energy Restriction for Weight Loss. Nutrients. 2019. 14;11(10):2442. DOI: 10.3390/nu11102442

[23] Victoria A. Catenacci, Zhaoxing Pan, Danielle Ostendorf, Sarah Brannon, Wendolyn S. Gozansky, Mark P. Mattson, Bronwen Martin, Paul S. MacLean, Edward L. Melanson, and William Troy Donahoo. A Randomized Pilot Study Comparing Zero-Calorie Alternate-Day Fasting to Daily Caloric Restriction in Adults with Obesity. Obesity (2016) 24, 1874-1883. DOI:10.1002/oby.21581

[24] Samira Eshghinia, Michael Gadgevich Gapparov. Effect of Short-Term Modified Alternate-Day Fasting

on the Lipid Metabolism in Obese Women. IRANIAN JOURNAL OF DIABETES AND OBESITY, VOLUME 3, NUMBER 1, SPRING 2011.

[25] Michelle Louise Headland, Peter Marshall Clifton, Jennifer Beatrice Keogh. Effect of intermittent compared to continuous energy restriction on weight loss and weight maintenance after 12 months in healthy overweight or obese adults. International Journal of Obesity (2019) 43:2028-2036. https://doi.org/10.1038/s41366-018-0247-2

[26] Amy T. Hutchison, Bo Liu, Rachel E. Wood, Andrew D. Vincent, Campbell H. Thompson, Nathan J. O'Callaghan, Gary A. Wittert, and Leonie K. Heilbronn. Effects of Intermittent Versus Continuous Energy Intakes on Insulin Sensitivity and Metabolic Risk in Women with Overweight. Obesity (2019) 27, 50-58. DOI:10.1002/oby.22345.

[27] Hana Kahleova, Lenka Belinova, Hana Malinska, Olena Oliyarnyk, Jaroslava Trnovska, Vojtech Skop, Ludmila Kazdova, Monika Dezortova, Milan Hajek, Andrea Tura, Martin Hill and Terezie Pelikanova. Eating two larger meals a day (breakfast and lunch) is more effective than six smaller meals in a reduced-energy regimen for patients with type 2 diabetes: a randomised crossover study. Diabetologia (2014) 57:1552-1560. DOI 10.1007/s00125-014-3253-5

[28] Cynthia M Kroeger, John F Trepanowski, Monica C Klempel, Adrienne Barnosky, Surabhi Bhutani, Kelsey Gabel, Krista A Varady. Eating behavior traits of successful weight losers during 12 months of alternate-day fasting: An exploratory analysis of a randomized controlled trial. Nutr Health. 2018 March ; 24(1): 5-10. DOI:10.1177/0260106017753487

[29] Iolanda Cioffi, Andrea Evangelista, Valentina Ponzo, Giovannino Ciccone, Laura Soldati, Lidia Santarpia, Franco Contaldo, Fabrizio Pasanisi, Ezio Ghigo and Simona Bo. Intermittent versus continuous energy restriction on weight loss and cardiometabolic outcomes: a systematic review and meta-analysis of randomized controlled trials. J Transl Med. 2018 Dec 24;16(1):371. DOI: 10.1186/s12967-018-1748-4

[30] Stephanie Welton, Robert Minty, Teresa O'Driscoll, Hannah Willms Denise Poirier, Sharen Madden and Len Kelly. Intermittent fasting and weight loss. Canadian Family Physician Vol 66. 2020.

[31] Patterson and Sears. Metabolic Effects of Intermittent Fasting. Annu Rev Nutr. 2017 Aug 21;37:371-393. DOI: 10.1146/annurev-nutr-071816-064634

[32] Bartosz Malinowski, Klaudia Zalewska, Anna Węsierska, Maya M. Sokołowska, Maciej Socha, Grzegorz Liczner, Katarzyna Pawlak-Osińska and Michał Wiciński. Intermittent Fasting in Cardiovascular Disorders-An Overview. Nutrients. 2019 Mar 20;11(3):673. DOI: 10.3390/nu11030673

[33] Kavitha Ganesan, Yacob Habboush and Senan Sultan. Intermittent Fasting: The Choice for a Healthier Lifestyle. Cureus. 2018 Jul 9;10(7):e2947. DOI: 10.7759/cureus.2947

[34] Adrienne R Barnosky, Kristin K Hoddy, Terry G Unterman and Krista A Varady. Intermittent fasting vs daily calorie restriction for type 2 diabetes prevention: a review of human findings. Transl Res. 2014 Oct;164(4):302-11. DOI: 10.1016/j.trsl.2014.05.013

[35] Stephen D. Anton, Keelin Moehl, William T. Donahoo, Krisztina Marosi, Stephanie A. Lee, Arch G. Mainous, Christiaan Leeuwenburgh, and Mark P. Mattson. Flipping the Metabolic Switch: Understanding and Applying the Health Benefits of Fasting. Obesity. 2017. DOI:10.1002/oby.22065

[36] Shula Shazman. A Machine Learning Approach to Select the Type of Intermittent Fasting in Order to Improve Health by Effects on Type 2 Diabetes. Conference: 11th International Conference on Bioinformatics Models, Methods and Algorithms. Bioinformatics 2020. DOI: 10.5220/0008950201310137

[37] International Diabetes Federation 2017. Diabetes Atlas 8th edition.

[38] McCulloch DK, Nathan DM, Wolfsdorf JI, Mulder JE, eds. Estimation of blood glucose control in diabetes mellitus. Wolters Kluwer Health. Accessed at: www.uptodate.com. 2013. -- 2. A1C test and diabetes. National Diabetes Information Clearinghouse (NDIC). Available at: http://diabetes.niddk.nih.gov/dm/pubs/A1CTest/A1C_Test_DM_508.pdf. Accessed 011414. -- 3. American Diabetes Association. Standards of Medical Care in Diabetes—2014. Diabetes Care 2014;37:S14-S80.

[39] Levy J. C, Matthews D. R, Hermans M.P. Correct homeostasis model assessment (HOMA) evaluation uses the computer program. Diabetes Care 1998; 21: 2191-92. DOI: 10.2337/diacare.21.12.2191

[40] HOMA2 Calculator. Oxford University. Available at: https://www.dtu.ox.ac.uk/homacalculator/download.php

[41] Heilbronn L.K, Smith S.R, Martin C.K, Anton S.D. and Ravussin E. Alternate-day fasting in nonobese subjects: effects on body weight, body composition, and energy metabolism. Am. J. Clin. Nutr. 81 (1) (2005) 69-73. DOI: 10.1093/ajcn/81.1.69

[42] Harvie M.N, Pegington M, Mattson M.P, Frystyk J, Dillon B, Evans G, Cuzick J, Jebb S.A, Martin B, Cutler R.G, Son T.G, Maudsley S, Carlson O.D, Egan J.M, Flyvbjerg A. and Howell A. The effects of intermittent or continuous energy restriction on weight loss and metabolic disease risk markers: a randomized trial in young overweight women. International Journal of Obesity (2011) 35, 714-727. DOI: 10.1038/ijo.2010.171

[43] Schofield W.N. Predicting basal metabolic rate, new standards and review of previous work. Hum Nutr Clin Nutr 1985; 39 (Suppl 1): 5-41.

[44] Shai I, Schwarzfuchs D, Henkin Y, Shahar DR, Witkow S, Greenberg I et al. Weight loss with a low-carbohydrate, Mediterranean, or low-fat diet. N Engl J Med 2008; 359: 229-241. DOI: 10.1056/NEJMoa0708681

[45] Chowdhury E.A, Richardson J.D, Holman G.D, Tsintzas K, Thompson D. and Betts J.A. The causal role of breakfast in energy balance and health: a randomized controlled trial in obese adults. Am J Clin Nutr. 2016 Mar;103(3):747-56. DOI: 10.3945/ajcn.115.122044

[46] Halberg N, Morten H, Nathalie S, Bente S, Thorkil P, Peter S and Flemming D. Effect of intermittent fasting and refeeding on insulin action in healthy men. J Appl Physiol 99: 2128-2136, 2005. DOI:10.1152/japplphysiol.00683

[47] Harvie M, Wright C, Pegington M, McMullan D, Mitchell E, Martin B, Cutler R.G, Evans G, Whiteside S, Maudsley S, Camandola S, Wang R, Carlson O.D, Egan J.M, Mattson M.P. and Howell A. The effect of intermittent energy and carbohydrate restriction v. daily energy restriction on weight loss and metabolic disease risk markers in overweight women. British Journal of Nutrition (2013), 110, 1534-1547. DOI:10.1017/S0007114513000792

[48] Clifton P. M., Noakes M. and Keogh J. B. 2004. Very Low-Fat (12%) and High Monounsaturated Fat (35%)

Diets Do Not Differentially Affect Abdominal Fat Loss in Overweight, Nondiabetic Women. Very Low-Fat (12%) and High Monounsaturated Fat (35%) Diets Do Not Differentially Affect Abdominal Fat Loss in Overweight, Nondiabetic Women. J Nutr. 2004 Jul;134(7):1741-5. DOI: 10.1093/jn/134.7.1741

[49] IDF Diabetes Care. Volume 42, Supplement 1, January 2019.

[50] Sewaiwar P. and Verma K.K. Comparative Study of Various Decision Tree Classification Algorithm Using WEKA. International Journal of Emerging Research in Management &Technology 2015. ISSN: 2278-9359 (Volume- 4, Issue-10) .

[51] Hua J., Xiong Z., Lowey J., Suh E. and Dougherty E. R. Optimal number of features as a function of sample size for various classification rules. Bioinformatics. 2004. 21(8):1509-15. DOI: 10.1093/bioinformatics/bti171

Chapter 18

# Integrated Cyber-Physical System to Support Early Diagnosis and Prevention of Prediabetes and Complications of Type 2 Diabetes

*Zsolt P. Ori*

## Abstract

Dietary and exercise interventions are the mainstay of prevention, and they constitute important part in the treatment of type 2 diabetes (DM2) and its complications. Automated, continuous, individualized non-invasive measurement of pathological processes leading to DM2 and complications are needed in terms of self-explaining metrics for improved individualized lifestyle management. Our company, the Ori Diagnostic Instruments, LLC is using tools of Medical Cybernetics (MC) to monitor non-invasive indicators of insulin resistance, exercise capacity, and autonomic dysfunction. The MC approach utilizes mathematical process and measurement models which are connected to a wearable sensor system. This chapter has the purpose to show how already widely available information technologies like smart phones, cloud computing, and sensor devices of the fitness industry could be put together into an integrated cyber-physical system (ICPS) to support fitness goals like fighting cardiometabolic conditions including high insulin resistance and low level of cardiorespiratory fitness and help building resilience with improved physiological reserve capacity. We want to demonstrate also how ICPS can be not only used for fitness self-management but can be extended to become a platform of noninvasive monitoring devices and become a medical software to support person-centered, outcome driven treatments for DM2 and complications in primary care.

**Keywords:** medical cybernetics, non-invasive monitoring, insulin resistance, exercise capacity, cardiorespiratory fitness, cardio-vegetative stress, metabolic syndrome, atherosclerotic disease, autonomic dysfunction, anemia, heart failure

## 1. Introduction

This chapter envisions the possibility of continuous risk assessment with non-invasive monitoring using tools of Medical Cybernetics (MC) facilitating early diagnosis and prevention of type 2 diabetes (DM2) and its complications including cardiovascular disease (CVD), chronic kidney disease (CKD) and heart failure (HF). MC offers a suitable conceptual framework to make the pathological processes of DM2, CVD, CKD, and HF observable and controllable through appropriate interventions facilitated by mathematical modeling. Utilizing principles of MC has the potential to enable primary care to help more beyond current standard of care and to make Digital Health more accessible to our patients. Moving away from traditional reductionism and embracing holistic approaches will certainly help fulfill the promise of Medical Cybernetics (MC) and help find workable solutions to tackle the ever growing health related challenges of humanity and introduce new approaches to manage and self-manage chronic non-communicative conditions or diseases in the 21st century. Already available information technologies like smart phones, cloud computing and the widely available sensor devices of the fitness industry could be put together into a cyber-physical system (CPS) to gain needed data and tools and to provide a holistic approach. The principle idea behind using MC [1–9] and developing a CPS [5, 6] is to gain deep insight and make so far unmeasurable phenomena indirectly calculable in the users' natural environment and put these unknown phenomena in the appropriate context for improved control. The plethora of new data gained with such CPS will lead to the creation of needed metrics and open opportunities for optimized self-control and dynamic behavior interventions based on the targeted metrics, leading to self-healing and cyber-therapy supervised by health care providers.

Ori Diagnostic Instruments, LLC (ODI) has been conducting R&D [1–11] and recently we introduced a CPS [5, 6]. CPS is a mobile technology integrating sensory data from various mobile devices into individualized dynamic mathematical models of physiological processes allowing for analysis and prediction using the models and allowing for quasi-real time feedback to the user (and optionally the primary provider). We have developed several technical and medical innovations allowing for creation of a CPS: 1. Self-adaptive models of the human energy metabolism (SAM-HEM) [1–11]; 2. Self-improving measurement models to amend validity, reliability, consistency, and accuracy of bioelectrical measurements [7–9]; 3. Using the minimum variance Kalman filter along with state space modeling technique [1–11] where process models of state variables work in unison with measurement models, mutually updating each other's *a priori* and *a posteriori* model calculations with the help of the minimum variance Kalman filter; 4. Utilizing principles of "least action/stationary action" to obtain essential practically unmeasurable parameters of the human energy metabolism [5–6]; 5. Applying principles of "maximum information entropy" to evaluate stochastic processes and perform parameter estimations with constraints or subsidiary conditions [7–10]; 6. Feasibility demonstration of our process modeling technologies in simulation studies using published trial data [1–6, 11]; 7. Innovations using a CPS to reenergize primary care and facilitate goals of Global Health [4, 10, 11].

Some important advantages of ODI's innovations to combat noncommunicable cardiometabolic diseases are the following. 1. An important aspect of ODI's innovations is the integration of self-adapting models into a cloud based cyber-physical system [5, 6] that provides user feedback and allows for truly individualized patient-oriented approaches. 2. Further it is anticipated that ODI's holistic and data driven individualized diagnostic approach will allow not just to help prevention and improve management and self-management of chronic conditions related to DM2 but also to lend help during emerging medical emergencies [7, 10]. 3. It is envisioned here that as more and more wearable physiological sensors become available, the sensors can be integrated with our cyber-physical system platform and their respective self-adaptive pathophysiological process models and self-learning measurement models [10, 11]. 4. A user's individual dynamic mathematical models provide feedback and prediction to assist behavior modification by supporting and maximizing control [10, 11]. 5. A CPS can realize not just a complex adaptive system at the individual level, but also through interconnections a network of individualized cyber-physical systems can be realized, allowing for network analysis and machine learning/artificial intelligence. Global Health goals [10, 11] could be approached at a community or even societal level.

This chapter consists of two parts. In part I, we will show how already widely available information technologies like smart phones, cloud computing, and sensor devices of the fitness industry could be put together into an integrated cyber-physical system (ICPS) to support fitness goals like fighting increased insulin resistance and low level of cardiorespiratory fitness and help in building resilience with improved physiological reserve capacity. This form of ICPS supports fitness goals without the wider scope of a "medical software "i.e. without the intention of medical treatment. This non-medical software ICPS focuses on three interlinked physiological/pathophysiological processes: 1. Cardiometabolic Functioning and Disease (CMD), 2. Cardiovascular Functioning and Disease (CVD), and 3. Cardio-vegetative Functioning and Stress (CVS). We will show how representative metrics reflecting health in these areas of physiological functioning and early disease can be created using MC modeling using data from a wearable sensor system (SS). Regarding CMD, the reader will be informed about how the non-invasive measurement of insulin resistance is possible with the R- or Rw-ratio which follows changes of the invasively measured HOMA-IR. R- or Rw-ratio related estimates are derived from serially measured weight, fat weight by bioimpedance measurement, and energy balance related data [3–6]. The CVD health status is assessed by indirectly estimating maximal oxygen uptake (VO2max) from daily physical activity and heart rate related data [5]. Indices of CVS health are obtained from time and frequency domain analysis of heart rate variability (HRV) [12, 13].

In part II an upgraded version of ICPS to medical software will be outlined which still has to be developed and clinically tried and properly examined and verified according to applicable rules and regulations by FDA. The major reason for distinction between non-medical software and FDA approved medical software is that the former primarily serves the purpose of prevention of prediabetes, DM2 and complications as opposed to the latter where medical diagnosis is made requiring active therapeutic interventions by health professionals. The part II subchapter is inspired also by the most recent summary recommendation for person-centered, outcomes-driven treatments of DM2 in primary care by leading academic authors [14]. One of the key points of this article is to call for "a patient-centered approach that addresses patients' multimorbidities, needs, preferences, and barriers and includes diabetes education and lifestyle interventions as well as pharmacologic treatment...". The medical software version of ICPS could be complementary to key points in [14]. We introduce here to the reader how the following comorbid conditions could be observed non-invasively and how metrics can be created to see outcomes objectively. We will discuss here the following pathological processes as targets of monitoring, tracking and metric creation for outcome measures: 1. CMD and Metabolic Syndrome (MS), 2. Atherosclerotic Cardiovascular Disease (ASCD), 3. Autonomic Dysfunction (AD), 4. Chronic Anemia due to CKD, and 5. Heart failure (HF). Here we want to point out that [14] puts great emphasis on ASCD, CKD and HF as a targeted outcome measure for interventions. It is envisioned here that self-explaining metrics regarding disease processes 1–5 can be displayed quasi real time on the patient's smart phone app giving tremendous opportunity for patients to educate themselves and learn more about their diseases and ask appropriate questions. The feedback of information may help improve self-management in a non-judgmental manner. The self-explaining nature of metrics may also point out individual responsibilities to fight modifiable risk factors. Having quantifiable metrics allows for dynamic lifestyle interventions which could be managed, self-managed or helped with automated feedback of information. Further, the response to pharmacological interventions could be gauged, helping to track results of treatment and recognize inadvertent side effects.

To our knowledge there is no noninvasive tool or monitoring device available to measure increased oxidative stress, inflammation, or insulin resistance in the user's natural environment. However, these pathological processes are strongly interlinked, leading to among others DM2, CMD, MS, CVD, ASCD, AD, Chronic Anemia of CKD, and HF. Importantly, ICPS is built on the holistic modeling approach of considering the entire human energy metabolism and insulin resistance. The latter can be viewed also as a surrogate marker for whole body oxidative stress and inflammation [15]. The bio-physical principle behind the proposed conceptual framework of ICPS and for process models is the recognition that the changes of the body composition (lean mass and fat mass) and the energy flow in and out of the body are governed by the fat vs. carbohydrate burning ratio and are strongly linked to insulin resistance [16, 17]. The significance of this is that an impaired mitochondrial lipid oxidation is a major anomaly in the chain of metabolic events leading to obesity and increase of insulin resistance [18]. High insulin resistance is associated with high respiratory quotient (RQ) reflecting lower fat burning than normal [19]. We have no non-invasive measuring technique for Oxidative Stress. However, there is a strong connection between Oxidative Stress and Insulin Resistance [20]. Similarly, there are strong connections between inflammation and insulin resistance [21] but there is no non-invasive tool available currently to monitor whole body inflammation. Therefore, we intend to use the R- and Rw ratio to give at least a qualitative signal tool if the trends of changes in the metabolism are in the right or wrong direction in terms oxidative stress and inflammation. *Our central hypothesis is that by improving insulin resistance with the use of ICPS, we can ameliorate the condition of oxidative stress, overall inflammation, fat vs. carbohydrate oxidation, and cardiovascular disease progression*.

To our knowledge ODI is the first in using the principle of "least action/stationary action" as a principle for finding key physiological parameters of the energy metabolism [5, 6]. This is instrumental to estimate noninvasively the HOMA- IR linked marker of insulin resistance R- or Rw-ratio which are defined as $R = \Delta L/\Delta F$ and $Rw = \Delta W/\Delta F$ where $\Delta L$, $\Delta W$ and $\Delta F$ are lean mass, weight and fat mass change over 24 hrs. For monitoring of insulin resistance, we were able to prove the feasibility of this concept [5–6]. Further, we have shown that our Weight, Fat weight, Energy Balance (WFE) model can estimate changes of Rw without mandatory calorie counting by serially measuring weight, fat weight, and energy balance [6]. Our extended model of WFE calculation is called WFE-DNL-AT [6] and allows also for estimating for the first time noninvasively in the user's natural environment the otherwise difficult or impossible to measure changes of state variables (SV's) of the metabolism such as 24 h nonprotein respiratory quotient (24hRQ), utilized macronutrient energy intake, fat vs. carbohydrate oxidation rate (Fox/Cox), de novo lipogenesis (DNL), and adaptive thermogenesis (AT). However, WFE-DNL-AT calculations require knowledge of the daily macronutrient calorie intake.

For measuring daily changes of fat mass F, lean body mass L, the measurement of intracellular water mass (ICW) as well as extracellular water mass (ECW) are also needed. Unfortunately, bioimpedance measurement technologies are not suitable for clinical use in current form due to significant interindividual variations mainly due to lack of reliable bio-electrical modeling of electrical properties of a body segment. On the other hand, bioimpedance measurements are quite well suited for individualized measurements or serial measurement as the intraindividual variation is small. The electrical modeling issue can be improved with using the principle of "maximum information entropy" [9, 10]. Therefore, ODI developed a Body Composition and Hydration Status Analyzer stand up scale (BC-HS-A) [7–10]. We use here several innovations for creating individualized bioimpedance measurement models [7–10].

A general principle of the development of ICPS as medical software is that we want to connect the calculated SV's to morbidity and mortality risks. An example is given in [22] where cumulative incidence of various CVD events is compared in people with and without diabetes. The hazard ratio for CVD in view of HOMA-IR is published in [23]. CVD mortality and all-cause mortality is investigated with low cardiorespiratory fitness according to weight categories in [24]. Waist circumference is connected to mortality in [25]. Mortality is evaluated according to weight status with incidence of diabetes in [26]. CVD and mortality as a function of BMI is published in [27]. Heart Rate Variability and Risk of All-Cause Death and Cardiovascular Events are investigated in [28]. All these published morbidity/mortality studies allow us to assess the time trajectory of likelihood of morbidity and mortality as a function of the individually calculated SV's.

ICPS generates SV's and metrics in each domain of use (1–5) and displays the results quasi real time on the screen of a mobile app, the Metabolic Health Monitoring (MHM) Mobile app or on the Metabolic Manager Software Tool (MST) Web app. MHM is designed for displaying the SV's quasi real time and for entering input data and providing feedback that is either machine generated or from MST by personal trainer or primary provider. MST is a web app designed for use by personal trainer/primary provider (s) or the user himself/herself for analysis and prediction of the calculated SV's and metrics. MST enables also planning for lifestyle change and evaluating progress and outcome.

## 2. ICPS non-medical software (ORI FIT-MET™)

### 2.1 Description of the process models

Here we introduce ICPS ORI FIT-MET™ for the purpose to achieve fitness and prevent prediabetes, DM2 and complications such as CVD and AD. Uniquely, ICPS can construct trajectories of SV's (metrics) quasi real time in three domains of health: 1. Cardiometabolic Functioning and Disease (CMD), 2. Cardiovascular Functioning and Disease (CVD), and 3. Cardio-vegetative Functioning and Stress (CVS) with major implications to morbidity/mortality risks. Each of these domains have their mathematical process models to estimate the SV's (metrics). ICPS uses the predictive Kalman filter to predict future changes based on serially measured input data and using the respective predictive model calculation.

Ad 1. For CMD we use our Cardiometabolic Function Model (CMFM) which utilizes our Self-Adaptive Model of the Human Energy Metabolism (SAM-HEM) [1–4]; the Weight, Fat weight, Energy Balance model calculation (WFE); and the de novo lipogenesis, adaptive thermogenesis, and 24 hr. respiratory quotient model calculation WFE-DNL-AT [6]. The metric for insulin resistance in terms of R- or Rw-ratio carries the power of allowing to estimate the fat vs. carbohydrate burning and it is reflective of overall oxidative stress and inflammation. The CMFM modeling can calculate and predict the following physiological SV's: weight, fat mass, lean mass, ECW, ICW, R-ratio, Rw-ratio, Fat vs. Carbohydrate Oxidation, and 24 h non-protein respiratory quotient. With precise calorie counting the estimations of utilized macronutrient energy intake, de novo lipogenesis DNL and adaptive thermogenesis AT is possible.

Ad 2. For CVD process modeling ODI uses a cardiovascular fitness model (CVFM) in which the maximum oxygen uptake capacity ($VO_2max$) is estimated from heart rate and measuring maximal activity energy expenditure (aEEmax) during graded exercise. The $VO_2max$ calculation model uses multiple linear regression with data on age, sex, height, percent body fat, aEEmax, and the slope between HR and physical activity as in [29]. CVFM is self-adapting (self-learning) from the daily incoming data and assesses changes of $VO_2max$, exercise capacity, and heart rate reserve. We adopted the Critical Power model from [30] which is defined as the maximal sustainable aerobic power not causing "fatigue" to measure exercise capacity.

Ad 3. For CVS modeling ODI uses its Cardio-vegetative Stress Model (CVSM) which calculates the state variables (SV's) measuring functioning of the autonomous nervous system and estimating imbalance between sympathetic vs. parasympathetic activity. The time domain measure is the standard deviation of R-R intervals (SDNN) and the frequency domain power spectrum indicators are the low frequency spectral power of HRV (LFr), the high frequency spectral power of HRV (HFr), and their ratio LFr/HFr [12–13, 28].

## 2.2 Data flow

The usage of ICPS ORI FIT-MET™ is centered around data flowing in and out of the system. ICPS works with a wearable Sensor System (SS) to provide input data for the process models to arrive at metrics regarding CMD, CVD, CVS. The heart rate and physical activity energy expenditure related input data come from a wearable wristwatch-type fitness tracker like Garmin's smart watch. The body composition and hydration status related input data come from Garmin's Index scale. Alternatively, ODI developed its own fitness tracker, the sensor belt (SB) [7], and the BC-HS-A stand up scale [8, 9]. During regular use, ICPS updates every day the SV's and creates metrics allowing for trend prediction. The input and result data can be displayed on MHM or MST.

## 2.3 Analysis and interpretation

ODI's proposition is that MC modeling can provide special insight into physiological/ pathophysiological processes. MC modeling gives the expected direction of change of a variable in the future i.e. by connecting the data points and drawing a trajectory of the predicted changes. The benefit is that instead of comparing the user's data against a group average, the individualized modeling and data trajectory creation allows for self-comparison to historical data, capturing individual characteristics and facilitating individualized interventions. The MC models are generating metrics and trajectories allowing for tracking progress and facilitating dynamic behavioral changes. The undeniable advantage of modern portable electronics is that they can provide the resources and powerful data for self-healing in a non-judgmental way. The self-explaining context of SV's have the potential to raise self-awareness and draw attention to risk reduction and individual responsibility in the fight against modifiable noncommunicative disease processes. The derived metrics provided by ICPS have the potential to give the opportunity for education and learning about risks for health, development of new skills to fight risks, building motivation, as well as measuring self-efficacy in the fight against modifiable risks. The same ICPS metrics can be used by a personal trainer/primary provider for teaching and guiding needed changes of lifestyle or behavior. Importantly, it must be emphasized that the most important tool in our armamentarium to enhance insulin sensitivity and along with-it fat burning is endurance training [31] and it works even if no weight loss is achieved.

## 3. ICPS medical software

### 3.1 Description of the process models

Inspired by the call for person-centered, outcome-driven treatment as a new paradigm for treatment of type 2 diabetes in primary care [14] we present here our vision of how MC type approaches could significantly help goals set forth by the academic authors in [14]. Target points for outcome in [14] are ASCD, CKD, and HF. For a practicing primary physician, it is desirable to offer non-invasive monitoring for patients in their natural environment not just for early detection of deterioration but also to improve patients' handling of rising issues with appropriate behaviors.

Here we offer a preview about ICPS as a Medical Software and show how we can construct trajectories of SV's quasi real time in five domains of disease processes: 1. CMD and Metabolic Syndrome (MS), 2. Atherosclerotic Cardiovascular Disease (ASCD), 3. CVS and Autonomic Dysfunction (AD), 4. Chronic Anemia due to CKD, and 5. Heart failure (HF). It appears natural to extend the use of ICPS non-Medical Software with the areas of Chronic Anemia due to CKD and Heart failure. The respective process models are the following:

Ad1. The MC model for CMD and MS remains the same Cardiometabolic Function Model (CMFM) as in ICPS ORI FIT-MET™. Response to the therapies of metabolic syndrome could be tracked and compared with baseline for de novo lipogenesis DNL, Fat vs. Carbohydrate Oxidation, and 24 h non-protein respiratory quotient. These metrics can supply valuable feedback in terms of ongoing diet and exercise habits with implications to spur needed change.

Ad 2. For ASCD we want to extend CVFM. In the modeling of the maximum oxygen uptake capacity ($VO_2max$) we also want to consider modeling oxygen delivery which depends on hemoglobin concentration (Hb), total hemoglobin mass due to chronic anemia of CKD and cardiac output. For modeling of oxygen delivery and oxygen consumption we use the model equations in [32]. For process modeling of hemoglobin concentration, total hemoglobin mass, and cardiac output see also Ad 4. and 5.

Ad 3. For CVS modeling ODI uses CVSM. For quantifying AD, the rationale is that there are strong associations between central adiposity (which is a marker of insulin resistance) and autonomic dysfunction [33] and there is an increased sympathetic system activity in metabolic syndrome [34]. We plan on using promising markers beyond SDNN, LFr, and HFr to recognize AD such as heart rate recovery time [33]. For the prediction of sudden cardiac death, we want to also use the correlation dimension of R-R intervals D2 [35].

Ad 4. We want to build a modeling platform for Chronic Anemia due to CKD. The main rationale is that anemia is a recognized risk factor for cardiovascular disease [36]. This is potentially important because iron deficiency anemia, if corrected, may in fact improve endothelial function and potentially improve morbidity and mortality [36]. Not surprisingly, anemia and insulin resistance and type 2 diabetes are interlinked [37] through various inflammatory processes which play crucial roles in the development of insulin resistance. There is also an inverse correlation between iron levels and HbA1c [38]. The reasons for this include kidney complications, neuropathy, and malabsorption occurring in the setting of advanced DM2. The elevated blood sugar will, over time, damage small blood vessels in the kidneys leading also to CKD. The erythropoietin production by the kidney goes down and along with it the production of red blood cells by bone marrow. Several studies show that diabetics with reduced renal function are more likely to end up with iron deficiency anemia than those without reduced renal function [38]. The significance of monitoring hemoglobin concentration and mass is that it determines exercise performance, surgical outcome [39], and impacts heart failure [40].

The self-adapting process model of anemia of CKD (SAM-AC) will predict future hemoglobin concentration and total hemoglobin mass based on non-invasively measured hemoglobin concentration (Hb), extracellular water (ECW), and intracellular water (ICW). The ECW and ICW comes from ICPS ORI FIT-MET™. For capturing and predicting dynamics of changes of hemoglobin concentration ( $Hb_k$ ) and hemoglobin mass ( $tHbmass_k$) for day $k$ we use the following process models (Eqs. (1–3 and 5)) and measurement model (Eq. (4)). Hb concentration measurement comes from a non-invasive hemoglobin concentration measuring device like in [41, 42]. Data of daily *a posteriori* estimates of $ECW_k^{(+)}$ and $ICW_k^{(+)}$ will come from ODI's ICPS ORI FIT-MET™. We assume that 7.4% of the total body water constitutes the plasma volume (PV). Further we assume that the plasma albumin concentration is semi-constant, and it is not changing as rapidly as ECW and ICW, then the following formula could be used for plasma volume as in Eq. (1):

$$PV_k^{(+)} = \left(ECW_k^{(+)} + ICW_k^{(+)}\right).0.074; \tag{1}$$

The initial hemoglobin mass is calculated as $tHbmass_0 = Hb_0 .PV_0$ . The process equation for *a priori* (denoted as ( − )) hemoglobin mass on day $k$ is in Eq. (2):

$$tHbmass_k^{(-)} = Hb_{k-1}^{(+)} . PV_k^{(+)} + u_k; \tag{2}$$

The process equation for *a priori* (denoted as ( − )) hemoglobin concentration prediction is in Eq. (3):

$$Hb_k^{(-)} = \frac{tHbmass_k^{(-)}}{PV_k^{(+)}} + w_k; \tag{3}$$

The measurement model with the measured hemoglobin concentration $Hb_k$ on day $k$ is in Eq. (4):

$$Hb_k = Hb_k^{(-)} + v_k; \tag{4}$$

The process equation for *a posteriori* (denoted as ( + )) hemoglobin concentration is in Eq. (3):

$$Hb_k^{(+)} = Hb_k^{(-)} + K_k.\left(Hb_k - Hb_k^{(-)}\right); \tag{5}$$

Here $K_k$ symbolizes the Kalman gain provided by the Kalman filter. The random terms $u_k$ , $w_k$ , and $v_k$ represent errors and are assumed to be normally distributed with expectancy value and initial value of zero and estimated variance values with assumed non-zero initial value which is updated throughout the time of observation by the Kalman filter algorithm. Applying the Kalman filter guarantees minimum variance for errors. We use the maximum information entropy principle with

Lagrange multipliers and the Kalman filter with constraint as in (1) for minimizing error in Eqs. (4) in the estimation/ prediction process. The modeling calculation allows recognition of the significant deviation between measured and expected/ predicted values for Hb. A sudden significant change (determined by statistical testing) can be either from sudden change of total water content or change of hemoglobin mass change or both.

Ad5. Non-invasive monitoring of Heart failure (HF) for flair ups and avoidance of admissions or readmission to the hospital has been the core element of cost reduction programs [43]. Frequently used strategy to reduce readmission rate includes behavior related recommendations: 1) Take medications as prescribed, 2) Monitor daily weights, 3) Stay active every day, 4) Follow low salt, fluid restricted diet, and 5) Recognize symptoms of heart failure and how to respond early. Our proposition regarding this issue is that the recommendations 2–5 could be helped with an ICPS Medical Software with appropriate sensor device. The bioimpedance measurement of ECW and ICW comes handy because of convenience and safety. As mentioned in Section 1. Introduction ODI has created BC-HS-A and gathered significant experience with this technology and improved the modeling and measurement technique by individualization of the measurement models [7–10]. The personalization can make bioelectric measurements extremely useful not just under physiological but also under pathophysiological conditions. For measuring cardiac function, we want to use Impedance Cardiography (ICG). Regarding accuracy of ICG it is stated in [44] that when ICG is used for intra-subject measurements with same device for continuous monitoring of cardiac stroke output the performance and accuracy is better and surpasses those of inter-subject measurements. The usage of ICG has been verified in clinical studies [45]. ICG can provide calculated SV's such as Cardiac Output, Cardiac Index, and other hemodynamic parameters. Our self-adapting process model of HF (SAM-HF) will capture metrics of HF in terms of cardiac output, weight, ECW, ICW, $VO_2$max, heart rate variability, Hb, oxygen delivery, and other hemodynamic indices by ICG. All these metrics can be integrated to an individualized HF score improving interpretation and facilitating clinical use.

### 3.2 Data flow

The flow of data in and out of ICPS as a Medical Software is like that one of ICPS ORI FIT-MET™. The sensor system consists of the following parts: 1. The heart rate and physical activity energy expenditure related data come from a wearable wristwatch-type fitness tracker or ODI's Sensor Belt (SB). 2. The body composition and hydration status related data come from our specialized Body Composition and Hydration Status Analyzer (BC-HS-A) and stand up scale [7–10]. 3. For noninvasive hemoglobin concentration measurement, one could use a smart phone app [41] or measuring device with lap top connection [42]. 4. Regarding Impedance Cardiography (ICG), development kits are available [46]. ODI has the vision to develop its own hemoglobin concentration measuring sensor device and ICG device and integrate all these sensors via Bluetooth wireless communication to BC-HS-A which serves also as a base unit communicating directly to ICPS Medical Software. The incoming data from the sensor system (SS) is processed by the ICPS Medical Software.

ODI wants to use the SV's and metrics of change from baseline and determine the physiological reserve of the variables on a continuum for preventive purposes before reaching significant disease, decompensation, or death. This concept is visualized in **Table 1**. entitled, "ICPS Medical Software".

The increasing risk of major morbidity/ mortality is represented by a thickening red stripe as the physiological reserve capacity diminishes. The tapering arrow in blue symbolizes diminishing reserve capacity and represents the target

| **Domains of health and MC models** | **Pathophysiological range metrics and possible interventions** | | **Major morbidity with crisis** |
|---|---|---|---|
| Morbidity mortality | | | |
| Physiological reserve | | | Organ failure and crisis |
| Cardio-Metabolic Health, CMFM & Metabolic Syndrome | W, L, F, WCF, R-, Rw-ratio, Fox/Cox, 24hRQ, DNL, Metrics & Risk Scoring | Behavior modification/ Lifestyle Change/ Dynamic behavioral modification with ICPS | Metabolic catastrophe with need for urgent intervention |
| Cardio-vascular Health CVFM & ASCD | $VO_2$max, Exercise Capacity, heart rate reserve Metrics & Risk Scoring | Cardiopulmonary exercise/ Dynamic exercises planning with ICPS | Cardiorespiratory failure with need for urgent intervention |
| Cardio-vegetative Stress CVSM & AD | HR, SDNN, LFr, HFr, Metrics & Risk Scoring | Care by cardiologist/ Dynamic planned interactions supported with metrics from ICPS | Nerve exhaustion/ pending sudden cardiac death needing urgent intervention |
| Chronic Anemia due to CKD & SAM-AC | Hb concentration Hb mass Metrics & Risk Scoring | Care by provider and supplementation of needed factor(s), Automatic alert by ICPS | Symptomatic anemia with need for urgent intervention |
| Heart Function& SAM-HF | Cardiac Output Cardiac Index Metrics & Risk Scoring | Care by provider and following guidelines Automatic alert by ICPS | Symptomatic Heart Failure with need for urgent intervention |

**Table 1.**
*ICPS medical software.*

for improvement. The diagram shows also major tools for how vanishing physiological reserve in each health category could be improved and potentially help restore health. ODI's leap ahead innovation is *to use ICPS to collect highly impactful data, compress them into MC models, and determine and predict the model parameters which become the target for optimization of physiological functioning to reduce risk for morbidity/mortality.*

**Table 1** also shows the MC models and the respective SV's which are used to calculate metrics of change and Risk Scores (see second column from the left in **Table 1**). The possible intervention types for each MC models are listed as well (see third column from the left in **Table 1**). Handling recognized major morbidities and crisis is shown in the rightmost column of **Table 1**.

### 3.3 Analysis and interpretation

MC modeling can provide special insight into physiological or pathophysiological processes alike, giving the expected direction of change of a data point in the future i.e. connecting the dots or putting them on a model trajectory and explaining the changes. The benefit is that instead of comparing the user's data against a group average, the individualized modeling and data trajectory creation allows for individualized interventions and support goals of person-centered, outcome-driven treatment as outlined by [14]. The MC models with trajectories and predictions allow for quantifying progress and for providing metrics for dynamic behavioral interventions supported by smart portable devices. The self-explaining context of SV's (metrics) have the potential to raise self-awareness and draw attention to risk reduction and individual responsibility in the fight against modifiable noncommunicative disease processes. The derived metrics provided by the MC models of ICPS have the potential to give the opportunity for education and learning about risks for health, development of new skills to fight risks, building motivation, as well as measuring self-efficacy in the fight against modifiable risks. The same ICPS metrics can be used by primary provider for teaching and guiding needed changes of lifestyle or behavior. A specialized sensor system such the Sensor Belt might provide important information to help manage also emerging emergency situations.

It is ODI's vision to develop its point-based risk-scoring system to summarize the relationship between SV's and the risk of the occurrence of a major morbidity event and have a Risk Score related to the five domains of functioning (in leftmost column of **Table 1**). The Risk Score calculation systems are popular among physicians and can facilitate evidence based clinical decision making [47]. The proposed Risk Score may permit effective risk stratification and assessing patient prognosis when the focus is on non-fatal outcomes because of specific causes [47].

Use of ICPS allows for machine learning to optimize the MC models to fit the best to the available data and enhance the accuracy and predictive value of the derived metrics and help maximize the control over results. **Table 2**. Entitled, "The Pathways to Maximize Control" gives a conceptual summary of how the collected data can be analyzed by ICPS and how the derived metrics can facilitate interventions across lifespan. In the future, an ICPS as a Medical Software could allow for Cyber-therapy i.e. to become a medical device allowing for diagnosis and therapy. Under such a scenario, an automated self-adaptive model will assess SV's at baseline and throughout pathophysiological changes. It is foreseen that autonomous computer-generated optimal control could be enabled to maximize improvements and realize individualized "precision" medicine with strict supervision by a health professional [10]. When the disease processes(es) enter crisis stage in a

| Intervention type | Physiological range methods of choice | Pathophysiological range possible interventions | Major morbidity with crisis |
|---|---|---|---|
| Self Care | Self-education, learning, following guidelines for healthy lifestyle | Self-healing with behavior modification and using ICPS | Optimized learned behaviors to secure survival until rescue |
| Managed Care/ therapy using information from ICPS medical device | Teaching/ learning how to improve health with use of ICPS | Interventions by health care provider/ team to guide therapy also using information from ICPS | Lifesaving interventions by rescue team using data also from ICPS |
| Cyber-therapy (ICPS medical device allowing for diagnosis and therapy) | Machine Learning of healthy baseline functioning | Autonomous computer-generated optimal control to maximize results and realize individualized "precision" medicine with strict supervision by health professional | Autonomous machine directed therapies which can be overruled by physician |

**Table 2.**
*The pathways to maximize control.*

home environment one can foresee the possibility of remote autonomous machine directed therapies which can be overruled by a physician.

## 4. Discussion

From person-centered, outcomes-driven treatment point of view of type 2 diabetes the innovation of the Integrated Cyber-Physical System Medical Software is that it can capture metrics in 5 intertwined domains of physiological or pathophysiological functioning in the user's natural environment non-invasively. Data can be obtained in the metabolic, cardiovascular, cardio-vegetative, hematological (circulating hemoglobin mass), and cardiac functioning health domains.

The ICPS non-Medical Software (ORI FIT-MET™) realizes already now the observation of metrics in the metabolic, cardiovascular, and cardio-vegetative health domains with preventative purpose. Input data regarding heart rate and physical activity energy expenditure come from a watch-type fitness tracker such as Garmin smart watch and from serially measured body composition and hydration data such as the Garmin Index scale. ICPS allows a quasi-real time monitoring of metrics of functioning for the user and personal trainer/primary provider and allowing for self-healing and directed lifestyle interventions. Analysis, prediction, and planning for change can be performed either at home or optionally in the personal trainer/primary provider's office through a web app and display of results on the user's smartphone. Unique to our effort is that our suggested state variables are connected to risks of morbidity and mortality and allow risk assessment continuously over a lifespan, raising self-awareness, enhancing motivation, and underscoring self-responsibility to reduce modifiable risks as much as possible. Metabolic health goals, like improved metabolic flexibility, improved insulin resistance along with greater lean mass and optimized fat versus carbohydrate burning can be approached with the help of ICPS ORI FIT-MET™ through feedback of information from a personalized self-adaptive mathematical model of the energy metabolism. ICPS can also help optimize cardiorespiratory fitness level by providing feedback of indirectly estimated maximum oxygen uptake from heart rate and measuring maximal activity energy expenditure. Knowing the fitness level by $VO_2$max can help set the optimal training loads for endurance training leading to improved resilience, fat oxidation and insulin sensitivity [31]. Cardio-vegetative stress level is estimated by time domain and frequency domain analysis providing metrics for the overall activation of the sympathetic system which is a non-specific marker of vegetative state and should not be interpreted without appropriate clinical context, but it has significant prognostic value for overall health status and change of it.

This chapter outlined the scope of an ICPS Medical Software which still must be built. The significance of this outlined plan is to show that with already existing technology, goals of [14] can be supported. The exciting perspective is that ICPS Medical Software or a similar device will undoubtedly allow for big data collection and data mining and thereby provide the foundation for truly individualized "precision" medicine. ICPS in its fully developed form could provide information about primary interlinked pathological processes of whole-body oxidative stress, inflammation, and insulin resistance. Multiple observational studies have demonstrated already that these primary pathological processes are intricately linked to metabolic syndrome, atherosclerotic disease, sympathetic nerve activation, anemia of chronic kidney disease, and heart failure. ICPS with its state variables and derived metrics & Risk Scoring can potentially give the opportunity to calculate risks of non-fatal major morbidity outcomes in the 5 studied domains and define clear targets for specific individualized interventions. Even treatments of complications of heart failure could be feasible at home, potentially avoiding frequent readmissions to the hospital.

Before making ICPS non-Medical Software (ORI FIT-MET™) available to the public several important problems need to be addressed. The technical hurdle is to create a scalable versatile mobile and cloud computing platform for ICPS which can potentially be used with a variety of mobile health products on the market. While ODI wants to make ICPS potentially usable with various mobile health products, this effort may be stifled because of a lack of interoperability of various fitness devices and because data are stored in "data silos," preventing users and health professionals from getting an integrated view of health and fitness data [48]. The current practice is for third-party developers to retrieve the data via an open API with permission of the owner of the API and the user. The key risk and challenge are to make users' data accessible for cloud computing systems like ICPS. A short list of other problems to be overcome is as follows: data privacy and security, to create a marketable product which is only a fitness device at this stage of development and remains a non-medical device category, creating tools for easy calorie intake counting, creating tools for visceral fat mass measurement, and educating future users and also physicians about the complex science behind ICPS.

To create an ICPS Medical Software would pose even more challenges. The needed sensor hardware components must be developed and interfaced with ICPS. The main reason for ODI developing its own hardware for ICPS Medical Software is to avoid the 3rd party API issues and to guarantee top security for data flow with the latest and possibly most up to date technology. The other reason to have self-developed hardware is to have information regarding errors of measurements. ODI uses intensively the Kalman filter technology which works best if the standard deviation of the error of the measuring instrument is known. This allows "tuning" the Kalman filter to have the best performance. The seemingly daunting proposition for ODI to build its own hardware is mitigated by the fact that major electronic device companies offer their sensors with fully developed reference designs for hardware and software. This should help to build the needed sensors such as the watch-type fitness tracker, the Sensor Belt for ECG and waist circumference monitoring, the body composition and hydration status measuring standup scale [9], the hemoglobin concentration measuring finger sensor, and the Impedance Cardiography which could be also designed as a wearable sensor belt for continuous use or it could be integrated into the afore mentioned stand up scale for one point in time use. Phase I clinical study is needed to verify accuracy and certify analytical performance and safety. Phase II study is desirable to demonstrate utility and create user guide for patients and physicians. Reimbursement for the use of ICPS is also an issue as insurance companies may want to have proof that ICPS is able to save cost and improve clinical outcome.

After proper consenting, secondary analysis of metabolic data could help not only clinical research and pursuing goals of Global Health [11], but also insurance companies to calculate costs and potentially reimburse the treatment/self-treatment and improvement of risk factors for prevention, treating type 2 diabetes and complications. A value-based health delivery system holds potential to incentivize participants to improve their lifestyle, especially if insurance companies would honor participants with a discount on the premiums for those who were successful in lowering their cardiometabolic, cardiovascular, and cardio-vegetative risk.

## 5. Conclusion

In conclusion, ICPS can serve as an appropriate quasi real-time tool to monitor and optimally adjust modifiable risk factors. The trends/trajectories of metabolic values calculated by the mathematical models can serve as tools, allowing for planning and executing dynamic changes of behavior for optimization and control of these values. All-encompassing Risk Scores calculated by the mathematical models can serve as outcome measures to be tracked by the user and personal trainer/primary provider to prevent and fight burdens of type 2 diabetes and optimize lifestyle quasi real-time.

## Acknowledgements

We would like to express our gratitude for the valuable related discussions with Professor Dr. John Buse, UNC-Chapel Hill. Further, we would like to thank Ilona Ori, JD, Ori Diagnostic Instruments, LLC, for editorial help.

## Conflict of interest

The author declares that there is no conflict of interest regarding the publication of this paper. No specific funding was provided for this research. This research was performed as part of the author's employment with Ori Diagnostic Instruments, LLC. The author is the inventor on patents [8, 9] and the patents are owned by Ori Diagnostic Instruments, LLC.

## Abbreviations

*System Variables:*

| | |
|---|---|
| aEEmax | maximal activity energy expenditure |
| AT | adaptive thermogenesis/thermal loss |
| DNL | de novo lipogenesis |
| ECW | extracellular water |
| F | fat weight |
| Fox/Cox | fat vs. carbohydrate oxidation |
| HFr | high frequency spectral power of heart rate variability |
| Hb | hemoglobin concentration |
| ICW | intracellular water |
| $K_k$ | Kalman gain provided by the Kalman filter |
| L | lean mass |
| LFr | low frequency spectral power of heart rate variability |
| PV | plasma volume |
| R | R-ratio |
| Rw | Rw-ratio |
| tHbmas | Total Hemoglobin Mass |
| 24hrRQ | 24 hr. respiratory quotient |
| SDNN | standard deviation of R-R intervals |
| $u_k$ | zero mean white noise sequence |
| $VO_2max$ | maximum oxygen uptake |
| $v_k$ | zero mean white noise sequence |
| W | weight |
| $w_k$ | zero mean white noise sequence |
| AD | Autonomic Dysfunction |

| | |
|---|---|
| ASCD | Atherosclerotic Cardiovascular Disease |
| BC-HC-A | Body Composition and Hydration Status Analyzer |
| CKD | Chronic Kidney Disease |
| CMD | Cardiometabolic Functioning and Disease |
| CMFM | Cardiometabolic Function Model |
| CVD | Cardiovascular Functioning and Disease |
| CVFM | Cardiovascular Fitness Model |
| CVS | Cardio-vegetative Functioning and Stress |
| CVSM | Cardio-vegetative Stress Model |
| CPS | Cyber-physical System |
| DM2 | type 2 diabetes |
| HF | Heart Failure |
| ICG | Impedance Cardiography |
| ICPS | Integrated Cyber-Physical System |
| MC | Medical Cybernetics |
| MHM | Metabolic Health Monitoring |
| MS | Metabolic Syndrome |
| MST | Metabolic Manager Software Tool |
| ODI | Ori Diagnostic Instruments, LLC |
| SAM-AC | Self-adaptive Model of Anemia of CKD |
| SAM-HF | Self-adaptive Model for Heart Failure |
| SAM-HEM | Self-adaptive models of the human energy metabolism |
| SB | Sensor Belt |
| SV | State Variable |
| WFE | Weight, Fat weight, Energy Balance calculation model |
| WFE-DNL-AT | WFE extended version |

## Author details

Zsolt P. Ori
Ori Diagnostic Instruments, LLC, Durham, NC, USA

*Address all correspondence to: ori.zsolt@oridiagnosticinstruments.com

## References

[1] Öri Z, Öri I. (2015). Self-directed weight management by feedback from a self-adaptive metabolic health monitoring system. Self-Adaptive and Self-Organizing Systems (SASO), 2015 IEEE 9th International Conference on. doi: 10.1109/SASO.2015.28

[2] Őri Z. (2017). Parametric recursive system identification and self-adaptive modeling of the human energy metabolism for adaptive control of fat weight. Medical and Biological Engineering and Computing. 2017 May 1; Volume 55, Issue 5: 759-767. DOI: 10.1007/s11517-016-1552-3

[3] Ori Z, Ori I. (2016). Canonical representation of the human energy metabolism of lean mass, fat mass, and insulin resistance. 2016 IEEE 7th Annual Ubiquitous Computing, Electronics & Mobile Communication Conference (UEMCON); 2016 Oct 20-22; New York, NY. IEEE; 2016 Dec 12. p. 1-8; DOI: 10.1109/UEMCON.2016.7777862. https://ieeexplore.ieee.org/Xplore/home.jsp4

[4] Ori Z, Ori I. (2016). Fighting weight problems and insulin resistance with the metabolic health monitor app for patients in the setting of limited access to health care in rural America. 2016 IEEE Global Humanitarian Technology Conference (GHTC); 2016 Oct 13-16; Seattle, WA. IEEE ISBN: 1-5090-2433-6, 978-1-5090-2433-9; 2017 Feb 16. p. 547-554. DOI: 10.1109/GHTC.2016.7857334. IEEE Xplore Digital Library https://ieeexplore.ieee.org/Xplore/home.jsp

[5] Ori, Z. (2018). Cyber-Physical System for Management and Self-Management of Cardio-metabolic Health. Published on-line and accepted for publication in "Type 2 Diabetes" by IntechOpen, DOI: http://dx.doi.org/10.5772/intechopen.84262

[6] Ori, Z. (2019). Metabolic Health Analysis and Forecasting with Mobile Computing. Published on-line in "Mobile Computing" by IntechOpen, https://www.intechopen.com/online-first/metabolic-health-analysis-and-forecasting-with-mobile-computing DOI: 10.5772/intechopen.88872

[7] Öri, Z. (2009). Portable Metabolic and Trauma Monitoring System. Leonard Wood Institute Research. Project Final Report [Unpublished final report]. "Phase 0" fund from the Leonard Wood Institute (197 Replacement Avenue, Fort Leonard Wood, Missouri 65473) subaward number: LWI-000-006, as part of a Prime Award of the Army Research Laboratory No.: W911NF-07-2-0062U

[8] Öri Z. (2018). "An Apparatus and Method for the Analysis of the Change of Body Composition and Hydration Status and for Dynamic Indirect Individualized Measurement of Components of the Human Energy Metabolism," U.S. Patent No.: 9,949,663 B1 Date: 4/24/2018, U.S. Patent No.: 10,716,491 B2 Date: 7/21/2020

[9] Ori Z. (2020). "Systems and methods for high frequency impedance spectroscopy detection of daily changes of dielectric properties of the human body to measure body composition and hydration status." U.S. Patent No.: US 10,653,333 B2. Date of Patent: May 19, 2020.

[10] Ori Z. (2020) Principles of Continuous Risk Monitoring of Insulin Resistance, Oxidative Stress and Nutrition for Cardiovascular Disease and Cancer Prevention in Primary Care [Forthcoming].

[11] Ori Z. (2020). Reaching for Cardio-Metabolic Fitness and Resilience through Self-Healing and Guided Individualized Cyber-Therapy – an

Opportunity to Reenergize Primary Care, Healthy Aging Research, Accepted for Publication, August 26, 2020. OPEN ACCESS Freely available online.

[12] Öri Z et al. (1992). Heart rate variability: Frequency Domain Analysis. Cardiology Clinics 1992. vol. 10, No 3, pp 499-537.

[13] Singer DH, Öri Z. (1995). Changes in heart rate variability associated with sudden cardiac death. In:nMalik M, Camm AJ, editors. Heart Rate Variability. Armonk, NY: Futura Publishing Company, Inc.; 1995. pp. 429-448.

[14] 100. Harris SB, Cheng AYY, Davies MJ, Gerstein HC, Green JB, Skolnik N. Person-Centered, Outcomes-Driven Treatment: A New Paradigm for Type 2 Diabetes in Primary Care. Arlington, Va., American Diabetes Association, 2020 (https://doi.org/10.2337/db2020-02)

[15] Ceriello A, Motz E: Is Oxidative Stress the Pathogenic Mechanism Underlying Insulin Resistance, Diabetes, and Cardiovascular Disease? The Common Soil Hypothesis Revisited. Arterioscler Thromb Vasc Biol. 2004; 24:816-823. DOI: 10.1161/01.ATV.0000122852.22604.78

[16] David E. Kelley: Skeletal muscle fat oxidation: timing and flexibility are everything. J. Clin. Invest. 115:1699-1702 (2005). doi:10.1172/JCI25758.

[17] Jose E. Galgani, Cedric Moro, and Eric Ravussin: Metabolic flexibility and insulin resistance. Am J Physiol Endocrinol Metab 295: E1009–E1017, 2008. First published September 2, 2008; doi:10.1152/ajpendo.90558.2008.

[18] Mary Madeline Rogge: The Role of Impaired Mitochondrial Lipid Oxidation in Obesity. Biological Research for Nursing, Volume 10 Number 4, April 2009 356-373 (2009). doi.org/10.1177/1099800408329408.

[19] Shook RP, Hand GA, Paluch AE, et al.: High respiratory quotient is associated with increases in body weight and fat mass in young adults. European Journal of Clinical Nutrition, 24 Nov 2015, 70(10):1197-1202. DOI: 10.1038/ejcn.2015.198

[20] Park K, Gross M. et al.: Oxidative Stress and Insulin Resistance. Diabetes Care 2009 Jul; 32(7): 1302-1307.https://doi.org/10.2337/dc09-0259

[21] Li Chen, Rui Chen, HuaWang, and Fengxia Liang: Mechanisms Linking Inflammation to Insulin Resistance. Hindawi Publishing Corporation. International Journal of Endocrinology, Volume 2015, Article ID 508409, 9 pages http://dx.doi.org/10.1155/2015/508409

[22] Shah AD, Langenberg C, Rapsomaniki E, et al. Type 2 diabetes and incidence of cardiovascular diseases: a cohort study in 1.9 million people. Lancet Diabetes Endocrinol 2015; 3:105-113; doi: 10.1016/S2213-8587(14)70219-0

[23] Bonora E, Kiechl S, Willeit J, et al. Insulin resistance as estimated by homeostasis model assessment predicts incident symptomatic cardiovascular disease in caucasian subjects from the general population: the Bruneck study. Diabetes Care. 2007; 30(2):318-324. doi:10.2337/dc06-0919

[24] Wei M, Kampert JB, Barlow CE et al: Relationship Between Low Cardiorespiratory Fitness and Mortality in Normal-Weight, Overweight, and Obese Men. JAMA. 1999;282(16):1547-1553. doi:10.1001/jama.282.16.1547

[25] Cerhan JR, Moore SC, Jacobs EJ, et al. A pooled analysis of waist circumference and mortality in 650,000 adults. Mayo Clin Proc.

2014;89(3):335-345. doi: 10.1016/j.mayocp.2013.11.011

[26] Carnethon MR, De Chavez PJ, Biggs ML, et al. Association of weight status with mortality in adults with incident diabetes [published correction appears in JAMA. 2012 Nov 28;308(20):2085]. JAMA. 2012;308(6):581-590. doi:10.1001/jama.2012.9282

[27] Khan SS, Ning H, Wilkins JT, et al. Association of Body Mass Index With Lifetime Risk of Cardiovascular Disease and Compression of Morbidity. *JAMA Cardiol.* 2018;3(4):280-287. doi:10.1001/jamacardio.2018.0022

[28] Fang SC, Wu YL, Tsai PS: Heart Rate Variability and Risk of All-Cause Death and Cardiovascular Events in Patients With Cardiovascular Disease: A Meta-Analysis of Cohort Studies. Biol Res Nurs. 2020 Jan; 22(1):45-56. doi: 10.1177/1099800419877442.

[29] Kwon SB, Ahn JW, Lee SM, et al. Estimating Maximal Oxygen Uptake From Daily Activity Data Measured by a Watch-Type Fitness Tracker: Cross-Sectional Study. JMIR Mhealth Uhealth. 2019;7(6):e13327. Published 2019 Jun 13. doi:10.2196/13327

[30] Clarke DC and Skiba PF: Rationale and resources for teaching the mathematical modeling of athletic training and performance. Adv Physiol Educ 37: 134-152, 2013; doi:10.1152/advan.00078.2011.

[31] Venables MC, Jeukendrup AE: Endurance Training and Obesity: Effect on Substrate Metabolism and Insulin Sensitivity. Medicine & Science in Sports & Exercise: March 2008 - Volume 40 - Issue 3 - p 495-502, doi: 10.1249/MSS.0b013e31815f256f

[32] McLellan SA and Walsh TS: Oxygen delivery and haemoglobin. Continuing Education in Anaesthesia, Critical Care & Pain | Volume 4 Number 4 2004. DOI 10.1093/bjaceaccp/mkh033

[33] Fidan-Yaylali G, Yaylali YT: The Association between Central Adiposity and Autonomic Dysfunction in Obesity. Med Princ Pract 2016; 25:442-448, DOI: 10.1159/000446915

[34] Tentolouris N, Liatis S: Sympathetic System Activity in Obesity and Metabolic Syndrome. Ann. N.Y. Acad. Sci. 1083: 129-152 (2006). New York Academy of Sciences. doi:10.1196/annals.1367.010

[35] Skinner JE, Pratt CM, Vybiral T. A reduction in the correlation dimension of heartbeat intervals precedes imminent ventricular fibrillation in human subjects. Am Heart J. 1993;125(3):731-743. doi:10.1016/0002-8703(93)90165-6

[36] Pereira AA, Sarnak MJ. Anemia as a risk factor for cardiovascular disease. Kidney Int Suppl. 2003;(87):S32-S39. doi:10.1046/j.1523-1755.64.s87.6.x

[37] Rehman, K., Akash, M.S.H. Mechanisms of inflammatory responses and development of insulin resistance: how are they interlinked? J Biomed Sci 23, 87 (2016). https://doi.org/10.1186/s12929-016-0303-y

[38] Christy AL, Manjrekar PA et al: Influence of Iron Deficiency Anemia on Hemoglobin A1C Levels in Diabetic Individuals with Controlled Plasma Glucose Levels. Iran Biomed J. 2014 Apr; 18(2): 88-93. doi: 10.6091/ibj.1257.2014

[39] Otto JM, Montgomery HE, Richards T. Haemoglobin concentration and mass as determinants of exercise performance and of surgical outcome. Extrem Physiol Med. 2013;2(1):33. Published 2013 Nov 26. doi:10.1186/2046-7648-2-33

[40] Cattadori G, Agostoni P, Corrà U, et al. Heart failure and anemia: Effects

on prognostic variables. Eur J Intern Med. 2017; 37:56-63. doi:10.1016/j.ejim.2016.09.011

[41] Wang EJ, Li W et al: HemaApp: HemaApp: Noninvasive Blood Screening of Hemoglobin Using Smartphone Cameras. UBICOMP '16, September 12-16, 2016, Heidelberg, Germany. DOI: http://dx.doi.org/10.1145/2971648.2971653

[42] Timm U, McGrath D et al: Sensor System for Non-Invasive Optical Hemoglobin Determination. SENSORS, 2009 IEEE, 25-28 Oct. 2009, IEEE Xplore: 22 January 2010, DOI: 10.1109/ICSENS.2009.5398321

[43] Ziaeian B, Fonarow GC. The Prevention of Hospital Readmissions in Heart Failure. Prog Cardiovasc Dis. 2016;58(4):379-385. doi: 10.1016/j.pcad.2015.09.004

[44] Miller JC, Horvath SM: Impedance Cardiography. Psychophysiology. Volume15, Issue1, January 1978. Pages 80-91, https://doi.org/10.1111/j.1469-8986.1978.tb01340.x

[45] Yancy C, Abraham WT. Noninvasive hemodynamic monitoring in heart failure: utilization of impedance cardiography [published correction appears in Congest Heart Fail. 2004 May-Jun;10(3):139]. *Congest Heart Fail*. 2003;9(5):241-250. doi:10.1111/j.1751-7133.2003.tb00021.x

[46] Hafid A, Benouar S, Kedir-Talha M, Abtahi F, Attari M, Seoane F. Full Impedance Cardiography measurement device using Raspberry PI3 and System-on-Chip biomedical Instrumentation Solutions. IEEE J Biomed Health Inform. 2018;22(6):1883-1894. doi:10.1109/JBHI.2017.2783949

[47] Austin PC, Lee DS, D'Agostino RB, Fine JP. Developing points-based risk-scoring systems in the presence of competing risks [published correction appears in Stat Med. 2018 Apr 15;37(8):1405]. *Stat Med*. 2016;35(22):4056-4072. doi:10.1002/sim.6994

[48] Gay V and Leijdekkers P: Bringing Health and Fitness Data Together for Connected Health Care: Mobile Apps as Enablers of Interoperability. J Med Internet Res. 2015 Nov; 17(11): e260. Published online 2015 Nov 18. doi: 10.2196/jmir.5094